SHOULDER AND ELBOW TRAUMA

SHOULDER AND ELBOW TRAUMA

William N. Levine, MD
Vice Chairman and Professor of Orthopaedic Surgery
Center for Shoulder, Elbow and Sports Medicine
Department of Orthpaedic Surgery
New York Presbyterian/Columbia University Medical Center
New York, NY
USA

Edwin R. Cadet, MD
Assistant Professor of Clinical Orthopaedic Surgery
Assistant Attending Orthopaedic Surgeon
Center for Shoulder, Elbow and Sports Medicine
Columbia University
New York Presbyterian/Columbia University Medical Center
New York, NY
USA

Christopher S. Ahmad, MD
Associate Professor of Orthopaedic Surgery
Center for Shoulder, Elbow and Sports Medicine
Department of Orthopaedic Surgery
New York Presbyterian/Columbia University Medical Center
New York, NY
USA

JP medical publishers

London • St Louis • Panama City • New Delhi

Published by JP Medical Ltd, 83 Victoria Street, London, SW1H 0HW, UK
Tel: +44 (0)20 3170 8910 Fax: +44 (0)20 3008 6180
Email: info@jpmedpub.com Web: www.jpmedpub.com

ISBN: 978-1-907816-09-3

British Library Cataloguing in Publication Data
A catalogue record for this book is available from the British Library

Library of Congress Cataloging in Publication Data
A catalog record for this book is available from the Library of Congress

JP Medical Ltd is a subsidiary of Jaypee Brothers Medical Publishers (P) Ltd, New Delhi, India (www.jaypeebrothers.com).

Publisher:	Geoff Greenwood
Development Editor:	Gavin Smith
Design:	Designer's Collective Ltd

Indexed, typeset, printed and bound in India.

Preface

Trauma of the shoulder and elbow continues to challenge orthopaedic surgeons given the complex anatomy, often osteoporotic bone, and limited bone available for fixation when internal fixation surgery is required. *Shoulder and Elbow Trauma* has been created, therefore, with the practicing orthopaedic surgeon in mind. Our goal was very simple. We did not want to create another 'textbook' of shoulder and elbow trauma, but instead the 'go to' practical resource for busy practitioners who need to quickly read up on how to manage the case but also avoid pitfalls along the way. We have recruited leaders in shoulder, elbow and trauma surgery who are not only thought of as experts in their field, but also experienced clinical practitioners ideally placed to share their pearls of wisdom and help demystify these challenging injuries.

The first part of the book begins with the shoulder and starts with the classification of proximal humeral fractures. We have organized the chapters into highly focused areas to make it easy for the reader to look up the exact fracture and the treatment required to manage it (e.g. Chapter 4: *Open reduction and internal fixation of greater and lesser tuberosity fractures*). Part one therefore contains chapters on the management of every possible injury from acute proximal humeral fractures to clavicle fractures, scapular fractures, and the management of proximal humeral malunions and non-unions.

The second part of the book covers elbow trauma and again, we have recruited recognized leaders in the field to share their personal approaches to some of the most challenging fractures that orthopaedic surgeons must treat. It begins with an excellent chapter on the anatomy and surgical approaches, setting the stage for the following chapters. Focused chapters again allow the reader to easily find the topic of their choice, for example coronoid fractures, capitellum fractures, terrible triad, malunion, non-union, or even total elbow replacement for complex distal humeral fractures.

We are indebted to the authors of these chapters for helping us to create a book which we feel will serve as a definitive, stand-alone reference for all orthopaedic surgeons who manage shoulder and elbow trauma.

William N. Levine, MD
Edwin R. Cadet, MD
Christopher S. Ahmad, MD

Contents

Contributors

Christopher S. Ahmad, MD
Associate Professor of Orthopaedic Surgery
Center for Shoulder, Elbow and Sports Medicine
Department of Orthopaedic Surgery
New York Presbyterian/Columbia University Medical Center
New York, NY
USA

Shahryar Ahmadi, MD
Assistant Professor of Orthopaedics
Director, Shoulder and Elbow Surgery
Department of Orthopaedics
University of Arkansas for Medical Sciences
Little Rock, AR
USA

George S. Athwal, MD, FRCSC
Associate Professor
Hand and Upper Limb Centre
University of Western Ontario
London, Ontario
Canada

Jeffrey M. Bair, MD
Orthopaedic Trauma Surgeon
ProMedica Toledo Hospital
Toledo, OH
USA

Knut Beitzel, MA, MD
Research Fellow Orthopedic Sports Medicine
Department of Orthopaedic Surgery
University of Connecticut Health Center
Farmington, CT
USA

John-Erik Bell, MD, MS
Assistant Professor of Orthopaedic Surgery
Department of Orthopaedic Surgery
Shoulder and Elbow Surgery
Dartmouth-Hitchcock Medical Center
Lebanon, NH
USA

Louis U. Bigliani, MD
Chairman and Professor of Orthopaedic Surgery
Center for Shoulder, Elbow and Sports Medicine
Department of Orthopaedic Surgery
New York Presbyterian/Columbia University Medical Center
New York, NY
USA

Robert E. Boykin, MD
Fellow, Sports Medicine
The Steadman Clinic
Steadman Philippon Research Institute
Vail, CO
USA

Jeffrey M. Bradley, MD
Orthopaedic Surgery Resident
Grand Rapids Medical Education Partners - Michigan State University College of Human Medicine
Grand Rapids, MI
USA

Edwin R. Cadet, MD
Assistant Professor of Clinical Orthopaedic Surgery
Assistant Attending Orthopaedic Surgeon
Center for Shoulder, Elbow and Sports Medicine
Columbia University
New York Presbyterian/Columbia University Medical Center
New York, NY
USA

Andrew Kai-Hong Chan, BSc
Medical Student
Center for Shoulder, Elbow and Sports Medicine
Department of Orthopaedic Surgery
Columbia University
New York, NY
USA

Peter A. Cole, MD
Chief of Orthopaedic Surgery, Regions Hospital
Professor, University of Minnesota
Department of Orthopaedic Surgery
Regions Hospital
University of Minnesota
St Paul, MN
USA

Patrick M. Connor, MD
The Shoulder and Elbow Center
The Sports Medicine Center
OrthoCarolina
Charlotte, NC
USA

Jason D. Doppelt, MD
Fellow
Department of Orthopaedic Surgery
The Cleveland Clinic
Cleveland, OH
USA

Thomas J. S. Durant, MPT
Physical Therapist
The University of Connecticut Health Center/New England Musculoskeletal institute
Farmington, CT
USA

Sara L. Edwards, MD
Assistant Professor of Orthopaedic Surgery
Department of Orthopaedic Surgery
Northwestern University Feinberg School of Medicine
Chicago, IL
USA

T. Bradley Edwards, MD
Attending Shoulder Surgeon
Fondren Orthopedic Group, L. L. P.
Texas Orthopedic Hospital, Houston, TX
USA

Peter J. Evans, MD, PhD
Staff
Department of Orthopaedic Surgery
The Cleveland Clinic, Cleveland, OH
USA

Michael S. Ferrell, MD
The Shoulder and Elbow Center
The Sports Medicine Center
OrthoCarolina
Charlotte, NC
USA

Leesa M. Galatz, MD
Associate Professor of Orthopedic Surgery
Shoulder and Elbow Service
Washington University Orthopedics
Barnes-Jewish Hospital
St. Louis, MO
USA

Michael J. Gardner, MD
Assistant Professor, Orthopaedic Surgery
Department of Orthopaedic Surgery
Washington University School of Medicine
St. Louis, MI
USA

Trevor R. Gaskill. MD
Assistant Professor of Surgery
Bone and Joint Sports Medicine Institute
Naval Medical Center Portsmouth
Portsmouth, VA
USA

Michael R. Hausman, MD
Robert K. Lippmann Professor of Orthopedic Surgery
Department of Orthopedic Surgery
Mount Sinai Medical Center
New York, NY
USA

Stephanie H. Hsu, MD
Fellow, Orthopedic Surgery
Center for Shoulder, Elbow and Sports Medicine
Columbia University
New York, NY
USA

Joseph P. Iannotti, MD, PhD
Maynard Madden Professor and Chair
Orthopaedic and Rheumatologic Institute
Department of Orthopaedic Surgery
Cleveland Clinic
Cleveland, OH
USA

Aaron R. Jacobson, DC
Trauma Researcher
Orthopaedic Surgery
Regions Hospital
University of Minnesota
St Paul, MN
USA

Peter S. Johnston, MD
Southern Maryland Orthopaedics and Sports Medicine
Leonardtown, MD
USA

Clifford B. Jones, MD, FACS
Orthopaedic Associates of Michigan
Clinical Professor, Michigan State University/CHM
Adjunct Professor, Van Andel Research Institute
Research Director, Spectrum Orthopaedic Surgery Department
Grand Rapids, MI
USA

Graham J. W. King, MD, MSc, FRCSC
Professor of Orthopaedic Surgery
Hand and Upper Limb Centre
University of Western Ontario
London, Ontario
Canada

G. Yves Laflamme, MD, FRSCS
Associate Professor
Department of Surgery
University of Montreal
Montreal , Quebec
Canada

Jared T. Lee, MD
Resident in Orthopedic Surgery
Harvard Combined Orthopedic Residency Program
Harvard School of Medicine
Boston, MA
USA

William N. Levine, MD
Vice Chairman and Professor of Orthopaedic Surgery
Center for Shoulder, Elbow and Sports Medicine
Department of Orthpaedic Surgery
New York Presbyterian/Columbia University
Medical Center
New York, NY
USA

Guido Marra, MD
Associate Professor of Orthopaedic Surgery
Loyola University Medical Center
Maywood, IL
USA

Augustus D. Mazzocca, MS, MD
Associate Professor of Orthopaedic Surgery,
University of Connecticut
Orthopaedic Team Physician, University of
Connecticut Athletics
Director of the Human Soft Tissue
Research Laboratory
Director of Orthopaedic Resident Education,
Shoulder and Elbow Surgery
Department of Orthopaedic Surgery
University of Connecticut Health Center
Farmington, CT
USA

Bradley R. Merk, MD
Associate Professor of Orthopaedic Surgery
Department of Orthopaedic Surgery
Northwestern University Feinberg School of Medicine
Chicago, IL
USA

Peter J. Millett, MD, MSc
Director of Shoulder Surgery
Shoulder, Knee, and Sports Medicine
Orthopaedic Surgery
The Steadman Clinic
Steadman Philippon Research Institute
Vail, CO
USA

Ash K. Moaveni, BHB, MBChB, FRACS, FAOrthA
Orthopaedic Surgeon
Department of Orthopaedic Surgery
Alfred Hospital
Monash University
Melbourne, Victoria
Australia

Todd C. Moen, MD
Orthopaedic Surgeon
The Carrell Clinic
Dallas, TX
USA

Bernard F. Morrey, MD
Professor of Orthopedic Surgery, Mayo Clinic
Rochester, MN
Professor of Orthopedic Surgery, University of Texas
Health Science Center
San Antonio, TX
USA

Anand M. Murthi, MD
Attending Orthopaedic Surgeon
Director, Shoulder and Elbow Service
Department of Orthopaedic Surgery
Medstar Union Memorial Hospital
Baltimore, MD
USA

Andrew S. Neviaser
Assistant Professor of Orthopaedic Surgery
Mount Sinai School of Medicine
New York, NY
USA

Thomas S. Obermeyer, MD
Resident, Orthopaedic Surgery
Department of Orthopaedic Surgery
Loyola University Medical Center
Maywood, IL
USA

Reza Omid, MD
Assistant Professor of Orthopaedic Surgery
Shoulder and Elbow Reconstruction, Sports Medicine
University of Southern California
Keck School of Medicine
Department of Orthopaedic Surgery
Los Angeles, CA
USA

Surbhi Panchal, MD
Orthopaedic Surgery Resident
Department of Orthopaedic Surgery
Medstar Union Memorial Hospital
Baltimore, MD
USA

Bradford O. Parsons, MD
Assistant Professor of Orthopaedic Surgery
Mount Sinai School of Medicine
New York, NY
USA

Matthew L. Ramsey, MD
Professor of Orthopaedic Surgery
Rothman Institute
Shoulder and Elbow Service
Thomas Jefferson University
Philadelphia, PA
USA

Lauren H. Redler, MD
Resident
Center for Shoulder, Elbow and Sports Medicine
Columbia University
New York, NY
USA

Eric T. Ricchetti, MD
Associate Staff
Department of Orthopaedic Surgery
The Cleveland Clinic
Cleveland, OH
USA

Clayton Riley, MD
Orthopedic Surgeon
Martin Knee and Sports Medicine Center, P. A.
Arkansas Surgical Hospital
Little Rock, AR
USA

Arnaldo I. Rodríguez-Santiago, MD
Shoulder and Elbow Surgeon
Department of Orthopaedic Surgery
HIMA San Pablo Caguas
Puerto Rico
USA

Joaquin Sanchez-Sotelo, MD, PhD
Consultant and Associate Professor
Shoulder and Elbow Fellowship Director
Mayo Clinic and Mayo Graduate Medical School
Rochester, MN
USA

Felix H. Savoie III, MD
Lee C. Schlesinger Professor of Orthopaedics
Tulane University School of Medicine
Department of Orthopaedic Surgery
Tulane Institute of Sports Medicine
New Orleans, LA
USA

Daniel G. Schwartz, MD
Department of Orthopaedic Surgery
Northwestern University Feinberg School of Medicine
Chicago, IL
USA

Scott P. Steinmann, MD
Professor of Orthopedic Surgery
Department of Orthopedic Surgery
Mayo Clinic
Rochester, MN
USA

Douglass E. Stull, MD
OrthoKansas
Lawrence, KS
USA

Olivier A. J. van der Meijden, MD
Resident in Orthopedic Surgery
Steadman Philippon Research Institute
Vail, CO
USA

Marco Vennettilli, MD, FRCSC
Clinical Fellow
Hand and Upper Limb Centre
London, Ontario
Canada

Ilya Voloshin, MD
Bob Yin, MD
Associate Professor of Orthopaedics
Post-Doctoral Residency Fellow
Shoulder and Elbow Division
Department of Orthopedic Surgery
University of Rochester
Columbia University Medical Center
Rochester, NY
New York
USA

Gerald R. Williams, Jr, MD
Professor of Orthopaedic Surgery
Chief, Shoulder and Elbow Division
Department of Orthopaedic Surgery
The Rothman Institute
Jefferson Medical College
Philadelphia, PA
USA

Acknowledgements

The editors would like to acknowledge the tireless efforts of their Administrative Coordinator, Mrs Michele Roberts-Ravelo.

Chapter 1 Fractures of the proximal humerus: anatomy, classification, and surgical approaches

John-Erik Bell

ANATOMY

Detailed knowledge of pertinent anatomy is required in order to understand, classify, and perform surgical procedures for fractures of the proximal humerus. In 1934, Codman described the epiphyseal lines of the proximal humerus, which demarcate the proximal humerus into the articular segment, the greater tuberosity, the lesser tuberosity, and the humeral shaft (Codman 1934). (This description formulated the basis for Neer's classic paper on the classification of fractures of the proximal humerus, described below.) These four 'parts' of the proximal humerus displace after fracture in predictable ways, based on the tendinous attachments. The greater tuberosity tends to displace superiorly and posteriorly, due to the pull of the supraspinatus and infraspinatus, respectively. The lesser tuberosity tends to displace anteriorly and medially, due to the pull of the subscapularis. The humeral shaft displaces proximally and medially with anterior angulation, due to the pull of the pectoralis major and deltoid.

An understanding of the vascular supply of the proximal humerus is also critical. The AO classification system described below is primarily based on degrees of vascular compromise of the articular segment. The risk of osteonecrosis is higher in some fracture patterns than in others, and this risk is an important prognostic factor; it is also taken into account when determining indications for surgery. Laing (1956) described the vascular supply of the proximal humerus. The arcuate artery, a branch of the anterior circumflex humeral artery, was described as the primary vascular supply of the humeral head. The anterolateral branch of the anterior circumflex humeral artery ascends along the lateral aspect of the long head of the biceps tendon and penetrates the head at the junction of the intertubercular groove and the greater tuberosity proximally. It then becomes the arcuate artery as it assumes an intraosseous course. More recently, the important role of the posterior humeral circumflex artery has also been described (Brooks et al. 1993, Hettrich et al. 2010). While Laing (1956) and Brooks et al. (1993) agree that the anterior blood supply via the arcuate artery predominates, Hettrich et al. (2010) found that the posterior humeral circumflex contributes 64% of the articular segment blood supply, which may explain why osteonecrosis does not develop after some fractures with complete disruption of the anterior blood supply via the arcuate artery.

Rates of osteonecrosis in the humeral head tend to increase with increasing complexity of the fracture (Lee and Hansen 1981). Hertel et al. (2004) described radiographic predictors of vascular compromise. The best were length of the metaphyseal head extension (less than 8 mm), the fracture type, and the integrity of the medial hinge. Fracture types that were predictive of osteonecrosis included anatomic neck fractures, four-part displaced fractures, and all three-part fractures except those in which there was no fracture between the tuberosities. The overall degree of displacement was not as important as these factors. They theorized that increasing length of the metaphyseal extension correlated with preservation of the posteromedial blood supply via the posterior humeral circumflex artery.

A good understanding of the neurologic anatomy is similarly critical to the safe treatment of fractures of the proximal humerus. The incidence of neurologic injury associated with these fractures is generally underestimated. Visser et al. (2001) found that the rate of axillary nerve abnormality, as document by electromyography (EMG), was 58%, and suprascapular nerve abnormality was as high as 48%.

CLASSIFICATION

Classification systems are helpful for several reasons. They provide a common terminology for colleagues to discuss fractures in both clinical and research contexts. They also help surgeons devise appropriate treatment strategies and advise patients on prognosis. This chapter focuses on the two most widely used classification systems for fractures of the proximal humerus, that proposed by Neer, and that of the Arbeitsgemeinschaft für Osteosynthesefragen (AO). It is important to note, however, that neither is ideal, and so the advantages and shortcomings of each are discussed. The ideal classification system is one that is easy to use, reproducible, comprehensive, able to guide treatment, and that offers reliable prognostic information to patients and physicians. Shortcomings of classification systems include poor reliability, inability to include all variations, and inability to account for important variables, such as bone quality, patient age, and comorbidities.

The Neer classification system

The most widely used classification (**Fig. 1.1**) is that of CS Neer, originally described in his classic 1970 paper on the radiographic and intraoperative anatomic findings from 300 displaced fractures of the proximal humerus and fracture dislocations (Neer 1970). Neer's work was actually based on previous work by EA Codman, who in 1934 introduced the critical concept that fractures of the proximal humerus typically separate one, two, three, or four major segments from the rest (Codman 1934). These segments are the head, shaft, greater tuberosity, and lesser tuberosity. Neer then defined a 'part' as a segment that is displaced from another segment by at least 1 cm or 45°. Precise anatomic or radiographic points at which to measure these amounts of displacement were not specified by Neer. Any other fracture lines

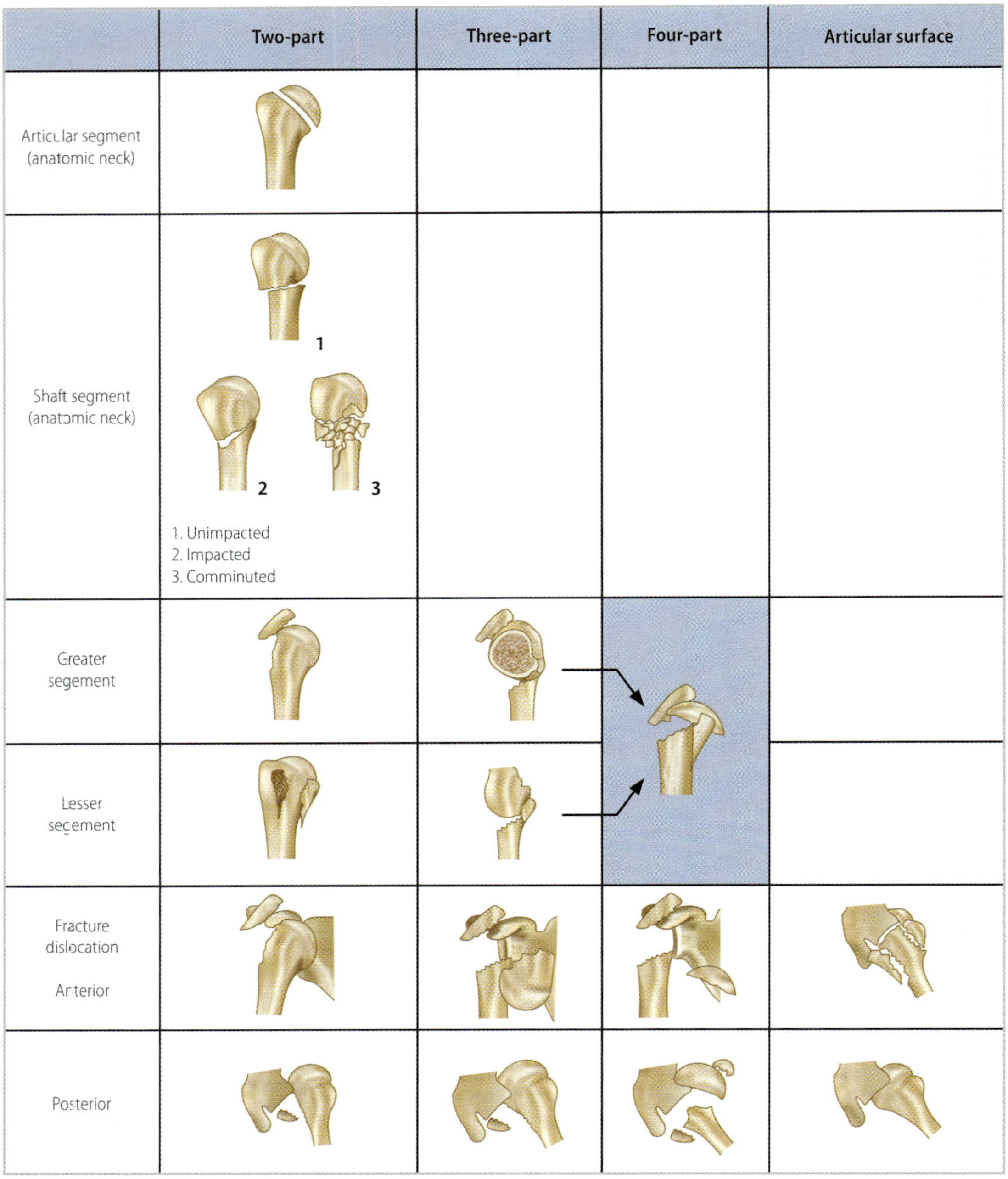

Figure 1.1 The Neer classification system. From Neer CS. Four-segment classification of proximal humerus fractures: purpose and reliable use. J Shoulder Elbow Surg 2002;11:391. Adapted by Robinson BC, Athwal GS, Sanchez-Sotelo J, Rispoli DM. Classification and imaging of proximal humerus fractures. Orthop Clin North Am 2008;39:393–403.

that did not meet these criteria were classified as non-displaced. Neer admitted that these criteria for displacement were arbitrarily set, based on an editorial suggestion (Neer 2002). He also listed modifiers of his classification method, including associated dislocation and articular injury, which was termed 'head-split' injury.

Neer's classification, in contrast to the traditional systems, which had been based on the mechanism of injury or fracture level, allowed surgeons to focus on more pertinent anatomic characteristics of the fracture, such as soft-tissue attachments and deforming forces, fragment vascularity, and involvement of the articular surface. In 2002, Neer, in a statement on the purpose of his classification system, wrote that it was a '"concept" or mental picture of the actual pathomechanics and pathoanatomy of displaced proximal humerus fractures and the terminology to identify each category' (Neer 2002).

The interobserver and intraobserver reliabilities of Neer's classification system have been called into question. Sidor et al. (1993) reported interobserver reliability of 0.43–0.58 and intraobserver reliability of 0.50–0.83, while Siebenrock and Gerber (1993) reported values of 0.40 and 0.60, respectively.

The valgus impacted fracture of the proximal humerus is also important to understand. It did not feature in the original Neer classification but was included in the revised version (Neer 2002). It is typically a three- or four-part fracture in which the head is displaced into valgus angulation and impacted on the shaft fragment. In this type of fracture, the greater tuberosity is typically superiorly displaced (**Fig. 1.2**). Rates of osteonecrosis are typically lower in valgus impacted four-part fractures than in displaced four-part fractures and fracture dislocations (DeFranco et al. 2006). This is

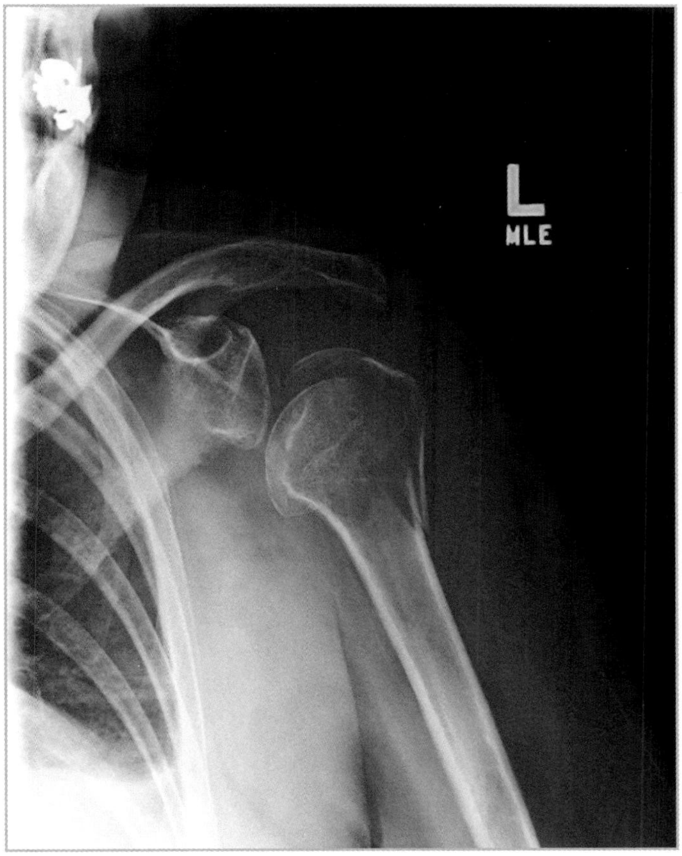

Figure 1.2 Anteroposterior radiograph demonstrating a typical four-part valgus impacted fracture of the proximal humerus. The head is displaced by more than 45° of valgus angulation and the greater tuberosity is displaced superiorly.

because the articular segment is not laterally displaced, but simply angulated, with preservation of the posteromedial blood supply (Jakob et al. 1991). In a recent multicenter study of 509 fractures of the proximal humerus, the valgus impacted pattern was found in 17 (3.3%) (Tamai et al. 2009).

The AO classification system

The AO classification system is predominantly used in Europe. It is based on fracture complexity and vascular supply of the humeral head (**Fig. 1.3**). Type A fractures are extracapsular with an intact vascular supply, and involve two of the four segments. Type B fractures are partially intracapsular with possible vascular compromise, and involve three of the four segments. Type C fractures are intracapsular, have a high probability of vascular compromise, and involve all four of the segments. Each type is subdivided into groups and subgroups, according to severity (location, displacement, dislocation, angulation, and impaction). This system was initially adopted by the Orthopaedic Trauma Association (OTA) in 1996, but was modified in 2007 by Marsh et al. (2007). Strengths of the AO system include its comprehensiveness, and ability to correlate with outcomes and avascular necrosis. Its weaknesses are, as with the Neer system, its inter- and intraobserver reliabilities (indeed, they are actually worse in most studies), and it, too, fails to account for the valgus impacted fracture pattern. Further, it lacks criteria to define displacement, and is complex.

Impaction fractures and fractures through the articular surface

Impaction fractures are frequently seen following anterior and posterior dislocations. In an anterior dislocation, the posterolateral impaction fracture is often referred to as a 'Hill–Sachs' lesion. In a posterior dislocation, the impaction fracture is typically anterior and is called a 'reverse Hill–Sachs' lesion. When small, these are often inconsequential, but larger lesions may require surgical management. Before closed reduction or surgical treatment is planned, care should be taken ensure that such fractures are not accompanied by a non-displaced fracture line through the surgical neck (**Fig. 1.4**).

Fractures of the proximal humerus may also involve the articular surface of the humeral head. These can be difficult to treat, and can be overlooked in the setting of significant extra-articular comminution. These 'head-splitting' fractures carry a worse prognosis in general than fractures that spare the articular surface.

TECHNIQUE

The workhorse for fractures of the proximal humerus is the deltopectoral approach. This can be used for open reduction and internal fixation, as well as arthroplasty. It is extensile and is associated with minimal morbidity. Furthermore, through the same skin incision an anterolateral approach can be made in combination, as described below (Bell et al. 2007).

Deltopectoral approach

This standard approach for fractures of the proximal humerus exploits the internervous plane between the axillary (deltoid) and medial/lateral pectoral nerves (pectoralis major). The incision typically begins at the lateral border of the coracoid process and extends down the arm in an oblique fashion, directed toward the antecubital fossa. Full-thickness flaps are made medially and laterally using needle-tip electrocautery. The superficial dissection extends superiorly to the clavicle, and inferiorly to the insertion of the pectoralis major. The deltopectoral interval is then identified, heralded by a stripe of fat overlying the cephalic vein. The cephalic vein is preserved, and retracted either medially or laterally, depending on the surgeon's preference. If vigorous lateral retraction is needed, as is sometimes required when locked plating is used to treat the fracture, trauma to the vein may be minimized by retracting the vein medially. However, for arthroplasty procedures, the vein is typically retracted laterally with the deltoid because there are fewer venous tributaries from the pectoralis than from the deltoid.

The subdeltoid bursal space is then identified and developed, beginning in the subacromial space, and sweeping laterally and distally. A Richardson retractor is placed beneath the deltoid, and a second retractor is placed deep to the pectoralis muscle, revealing the clavipectoral fascia. This fascia is then incised just lateral to the conjoint tendon, and a medium Richardson retractor is placed to retract the conjoint tendon medially. The musculocutaneous nerve and axillary nerve can be palpated at this point, to ensure that the retractor is not putting pressure on them. With the conjoint tendon retracted medially, the coracoacromial ligament is identified and should be preserved because it is an important part of the coracoacromial arch. A Darrach retractor is then placed beneath the deltoid and used to gently lever the humeral head anteriorly. The anterior bursa is completely removed, affording clear visualization of the proximal humerus and subscapularis.

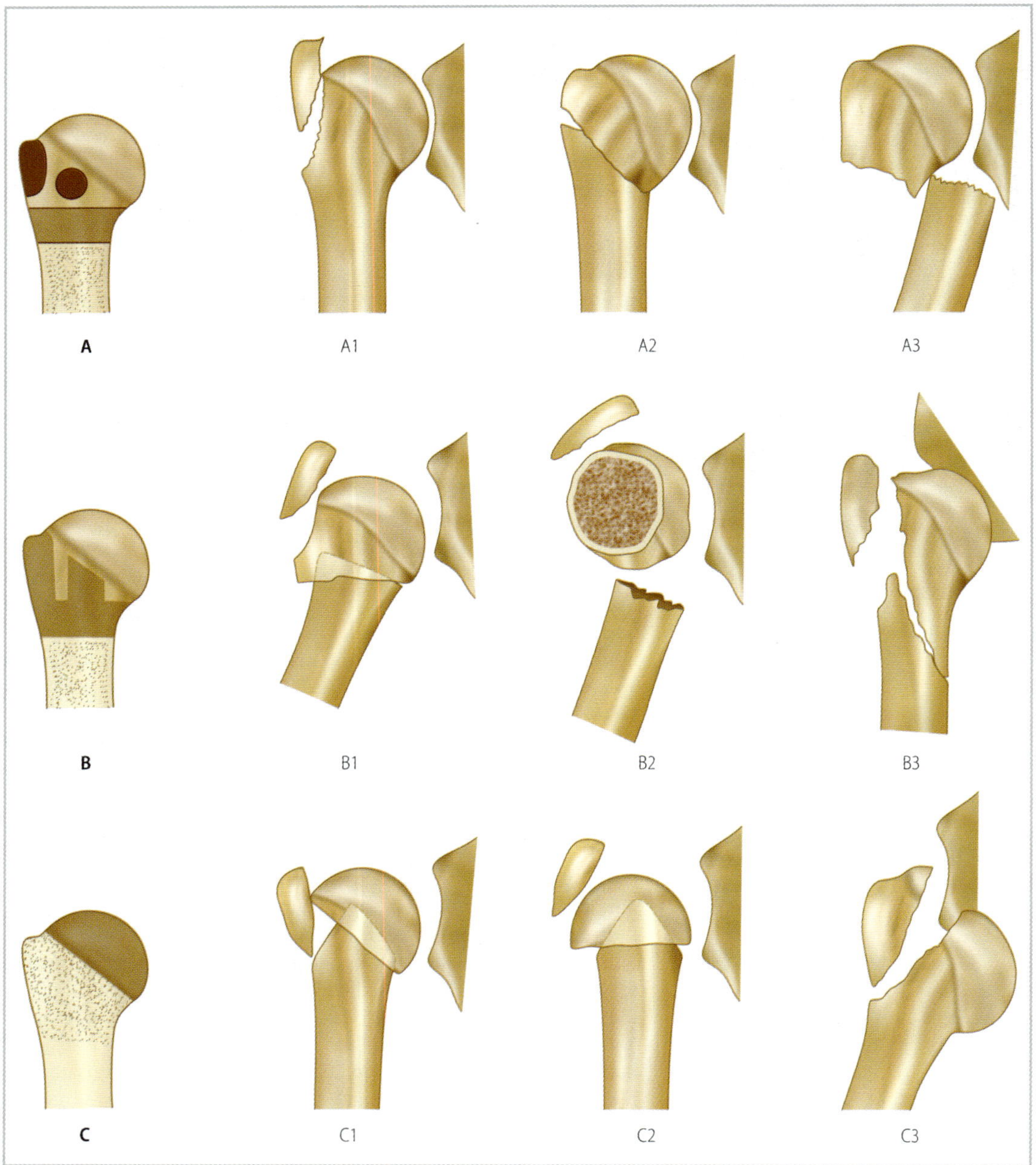

Figure 1.3 The AO classification system. Type A, B, and C fractures. From Muller ME. Appendix A: The comprehensive classification of fractures of long bones. In: Muller ME, Allgower M, Schneider R, Willenegger H, eds. Manual of Internal Fixation: Techniques Recommended by the AO-ASIF Group. Berlin: Springer-Verlag, 1991: 118–125. Adapted by Nho SJ, Brophy RH, Barker JU, et al. Innovations in the management of displaced proximal humerus fractures. J Am Acad Orthop Surg 2007;15:12–26.

In four-part fracture dislocations, the articular head segment can be displaced significantly. The head is sometimes found adjacent to the axillary artery and nerves of the brachial plexus. Extreme caution should be observed if this is the case, since the axillary artery can be lacerated by the sharp fracture edges of the head while it being removed. If it is not felt that removal can be done safely, it should be done with a vascular surgeon readily available.

In surgery for fractures of the proximal humerus, the subscapularis typically does not need to be divided. The best way to define the anatomy of the fracture is to identify the long head of the biceps, which runs between the fragments of the greater and lesser tuberosities. Access to the glenohumeral joint is obtained by following the long head of the biceps to the rotator interval. The rotator interval consists of the coracohumeral and superior glenohumeral ligaments, in addition to the transverse ligament, and lies between the superior rolled edge of the subscapularis and the anterior border of the supraspinatus. Opening this tissue does not result in damage to the rotator cuff, and is a safe means of accessing and inspecting the humeral articular segment. With surgery in the anterior aspect of the shoulder, care must be taken to protect the axillary nerve and posterior circumflex humeral artery, which run under the muscular portion of the subscapularis, towards the quadrangular space.

Extensile deltopectoral approach

For complex fractures extending into the diaphyseal humerus, the deltopectoral approach may need to be extended distally. This is done by extending the incision along the lateral border of the biceps. The interval between biceps and brachialis is identified, the biceps is retracted medially, and the brachialis is split in its midline, taking advantage of the dual innervation of the brachialis (radial nerve on

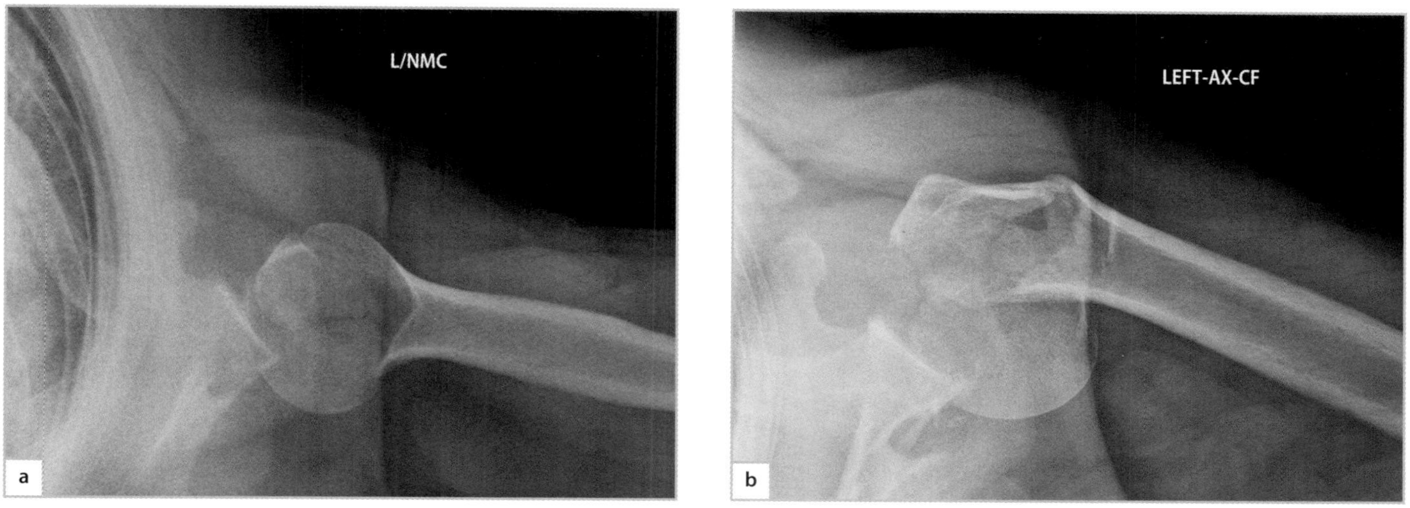

Figure 1.4 Importance of identifying non-displaced fracture lines prior to reduction maneuvers. (a) Axillary radiograph demonstrating a locked posterior fracture dislocation. Note the non-displaced crack through the head to the surgical neck. (b) After attempted closed reduction, the fracture has displaced.

the lateral aspect, and musculocutaneous nerve on the medial aspect). Subperiosteal dissection allows safe exposure of the humeral shaft. The radial nerve pierces the intermuscular septum 10 cm proximal to the lateral epicondyle of the humerus.

Anterosuperior approach

This approach can be utilized for locked plating of fractures of the surgical neck, and for fractures of the greater tuberosity. The skin incision extends from the anterior lip of the acromion 8 cm distally, in line with the deltoid fibers. The subcutaneous tissue is divided with needle-tip electrocautery, and full-thickness flaps are raised anteriorly and posteriorly until the superficial deltoid fascia is exposed. The avascular raphe separating the anterior and middle thirds of the deltoid is incised from its acromial attachment distally to a point approximately 4 cm from the acromion. If dissection needs to be carried more distally than this, as is typically the case for locked plating, the axillary nerve must be identified as it crosses the field, and protected. If exposure is needed only for open reduction and internal fixation of the greater tuberosity, an antipropagation stitch can be placed in the deltoid, approximately 4 cm from the acromion, to avoid damaging the axillary nerve from retraction of the deltoid division. Richardson retractors are placed to retract the anterior deltoid anteriorly, and the middle deltoid posteriorly. This allows exposure of the bursa and proximal humerus. Detachment of the deltoid origin from the lateral acromion is considered a last resort for increased exposure, because of the postoperative complication of deltoid dehiscence, which may not be salvageable. If some fibers of deltoid origin are detached, detachment should be done strictly subperiosteally, so that a cuff of stout tissue remains for repair.

Combined approach

In certain situations, the advantages of both the deltopectoral and anterosuperior approaches can be exploited. The problem with the deltopectoral approach for surgery to fractures of the proximal humerus is that exposure of a fragment of the greater tuberosity may be poor and access to the correct angle for screw placement in the locked plating may be difficult, especially in large or muscular patients. By using a combined approach, this access to the posterior structures can be improved. If the combined approach is planned preoperatively, the deltopectoral skin incision is made slightly more laterally; however, the combined approach can be done through a standard deltopectoral incision (see above). The standard deltopectoral procedure is then followed but with the addition of a second interval created between the anterior and middle deltoid, as described for the anterosuperior approach (see above). Both fascial intervals are entered through the same skin incision.

CONCLUSION

Knowledge of anatomy is critical to understanding classification systems and surgical approaches for fractures of the proximal humerus. An understanding of the epiphyseal lines, the vascularity of the proximal humerus, and the typical fracture patterns is important for making thoughtful decisions regarding the role of surgery and the best surgical plan.

REFERENCES

Bell J-E, Edwards SL, Blaine SA. Surgical exposures of the shoulder. In: D Berry, S Steinman, eds. Adult Reconstruction. Philadelphia, PA: Lippincott, Williams and Wilkins, 2007: 213–219.

Brooks CH, Revell WJ, Healtey FW. Vascularity of the humeral head after proximal humeral fractures. An anatomical cadaver study. J Bone Joint Surg Br 1993;75:132–136.

Codman E. The Shoulder: Rupture of the Supraspinatus Tendon and Other Lesions In or About the Subacromial Bursa. New York: Miller, 1934.

DeFranco MJ, Brems JJ, Williams GR Jr, Iannoitti JP. Evaluation and management of valgus impacted four-part proximal humerus fractures. Clin Orthop Relat Res 2006;442:109–114.

Hertel R, Hempfing A, Stiehler M, Leunig M. Predictors of humeral head ischemia after intracapsular fracture of the proximal humerus. J Shoulder Elbow Surg 2004;13:427–433.
Hettrich CM, Boraiah S, Dyke JP, et al. Quantitative assessment of the vascularity of the proximal part of the humerus. J Bone Joint Surg Am 2010;92:943–948.
Jakob RP, Miniaci A, Anson PS, et al. Four-part valgus impacted fractures of the proximal humerus. J Bone Joint Surg Br 1991;73:295–298.
Laing PG. The arterial supply of the adult humerus. J Bone Joint Surg Am 1956;38:1105–1116.
Lee CK, Hansen HR. Post-traumatic avascular necrosis of the humeral head in displaced proximal humeral fractures. J Trauma 1981;21:788–791.
Marsh JL, Slongo TF, Agel J, et al. Fracture and dislocation classification compendium – 2007: Orthopaedic Trauma Association classification, database and outcomes committee. J Orthop Trauma 2007;21(10 suppl):S1–133.
Neer CS 2nd. Displaced proximal humeral fractures. I. Classification and evaluation. J Bone Joint Surg Am 1970;52:1077–1089.
Neer CS. Four-segment classification of proximal humeral fractures: purpose and reliable use. J Shoulder Elbow Surg 2002;11:389–400.
Sidor ML, Zuckerman JD, Lyon T, et al. The Neer classification system for proximal humeral fractures. An assessment of interobserver reliability and intraobserver reproducibility. J Bone Joint Surg Am 1993;75:1745–1750.
Siebenrock KA, Gerber C. The reproducibility of classification of fractures of the proximal end of the humerus. J Bone Joint Surg Am 1993;75:1751–1755.
Tamai K, Ishige N, Kuroda S, et al. Four-segment classification of proximal humeral fractures revisited: a multicenter study on 509 cases. J Shoulder Elbow Surg 2009;18:845–850.
Visser CP, Coene LN, Brand R, Tavy DL. Nerve lesions in proximal humeral fractures. J Shoulder Elbow Surg 2001;10:421–427.

Chapter 2 Percutaneous treatment of proximal humerus fractures

Bob Yin, Christopher S. Ahmad

INDICATIONS

For patients with displaced fractures of the proximal humerus, anatomic reduction and stable fixation are generally essential for a satisfactory functional outcome (Neer 1970, Leyshon 1984). While open reduction and internal fixation afford direct visualization and manipulation of fracture fragments, both the open exposure and the use of plate fixation are associated with well described complications that may adversely affect final clinical outcome or lead to reoperation. Open approaches have greater potential for scarring, which clinically manifests as postoperative stiffness; they also carry a greater risk of infection.

Compared with open reduction and internal fixation, minimally invasive percutaneous techniques are associated with less operative time and shorter hospitalization. Furthermore, the open approach may increase the risk of avascular necrosis (AVN) of the humeral head (Jakob et al. 1991, Hertel et al. 2004). AVN is a devastating complication in younger, more active patients, who are not ideal candidates for humeral head replacement. The main vascular supply to the humeral head is the ascending branch of the anterior humeral circumflex artery, along with its interosseous continuation, called the arcuate artery (Brooks et al. 1993). These small vessels are often disrupted during the injury, and then further compromised as part of the approach and dissection for open reduction. Closed reduction and percutaneous fixation, when performed on the appropriate patient, may reduce the risk of humeral head AVN, since it requires less soft-tissue dissection and therefore results in less disruption of vascularity.

Open approaches typically employ rigid fixation with conventional or locked plates. Plate fixation is prone to complications caused by technical errors in initial fracture reduction, plate positioning, and screw length. Screw cut-out and joint penetration are common complications of locked plating, occurring in over 10% of cases in the series reported by Agudelo et al. (2007), Owsley and Gorczyca (2008), and Clavert et al. (2010). The same series reported rates of mal-reduction between 13.7% and 25% when utilizing locking plates and screws. Although plate fixation may provide greater rigidity than percutaneous implants, the high rigidity of the construct predisposes it to pseudoarthrosis and plate breakage, the latter occurring most commonly across metaphyseal or disphyseal screw holes that are left empty in a locked-plate construct. These complications are strongly correlated with the need for reoperation and with poor clinical results. For appropriately selected injuries, percutaneous treatment can avoid many of the complications associated with plate fixation. A number of case series have reported good or excellent outcomes in the majority of patients undergoing percutaneous treatment for fractures of the proximal humerus (Jaberg et al. 1992, Resch et al. 1997, Chen et al. 1998, Fenichel et al. 2006, Calvo et al. 2007, Keener et al. 2007, Kayalar et al. 2009, Brunner et al. 2010).

Adequate strength of fixation is a greater concern with percutaneous pinning than with open reduction and internal fixation. Kavol et al. performed biomechanical shear loading on simulated two-part fractures in cadaveric humeri, and concluded that internal fixation with a T-plate and screws was significantly stronger than with a construct utilizing four Schanz pins (Koval et al. 1996). Subsequent biomechanical studies were performed to determine the best percutaneous pin configuration for maximum fixation strength. One study employed pins 2.5 mm long, in four different configurations, and determined that the addition of bicortical tuberosity pins to two laterally inserted pins resulted in significantly greater torsional and rotational rigidity (Naidu et al. 1997). More recently, Jiang et al. (2007) demonstrated that parallel pins placed 1 cm apart provided greater strength against torsional loads than did converging ('fan-shaped') pins. These studies support the use of terminally threaded Schanz pins in a parallel configuration across the fracture site, with bicortical fixation whenever possible.

The indications for percutaneous pinning require consideration of patient factors and fracture characteristics. In general, younger patients who have better bone quality are more appropriate for percutaneous treatment, since this technique relies on obtaining fixation with threaded pins or cancellous screws. Bone quality must be sufficient to provide firm purchase for the percutaneous implants in order to avoid loss of fixation and pin migration. Patients who are candidates for percutaneous treatment need to be compliant and reliable because they will require frequent postoperative follow-up. Weekly visits are needed to verify fracture reduction, and for pin surveillance and removal.

Fractures selected for percutaneous treatment must be reducible with closed techniques. These include two- and three-part fractures involving the surgical neck, with little or no metaphyseal comminution. An intact medial calcar provides critical mechanical support to aid the reduction, and a vascular envelope that lowers the risk of AVN (Brooks et al. 1993, Hertel et al. 2004). In addition, medial support is necessary to avoid loss of fixation for percutaneous implants.

Although most four-part fractures carry a high risk of AVN and are treated with hemiarthroplasty in the older patient, the valgus impacted four-part fracture is usually amenable to percutaneous fixation because it is associated with a lower risk of AVN (Jakob et al. 1991), and can be well reduced and fixed with percutaneous techniques. The articular fragment is centered over the shaft, resulting in a more intact soft-tissue envelop, and less damage to the critical blood vessels in the posteromedial calcar.

Valgus impacted four-part fractures do not have significant displacement of the lateral humeral head, and are associated with less disruption of soft tissues and blood supply to the humeral head (see Fig. 2.8, below). Jakob et al. (1991) reported 74% satisfactory or excellent outcomes in a series of patients with valgus impacted four-part fractures treated with closed reduction or limited open reduction, and suggested that these fractures do not require humeral head arthroplasty because they exhibit a relatively low rate of AVN. Internal fixation is the preferred surgical treatment, since humeral head arthroplasty can always be performed in the future, should AVN develop. Primary replacement of the humeral head should be avoided in younger patients with this injury, since they are more likely to outlive the implant, resulting in obligatory revision surgery. A preoperative computerized tomography scan is helpful in assessing the fracture pattern and to confirm that the fracture is indeed valgus impacted and amenable to internal fixation.

In summary, the relative indications for percutaneous fixation include:

- patient characteristics –
  - adequate bone quality to provide sufficient pin fixation;
  - ability to comply with postoperative follow-up and rehabilitation;
  - ability to attend follow-up visit for pin removal;
- fracture characteristics –
  - feasible reduction with closed and percutaneous techniques;
  - two- and three-part fractures with no medial metaphyseal comminution (surgical neck plus greater tuberosity);
  - intact medial calcar;
  - valgus impacted four-part fractures.

CONTRAINDICATIONS

The main contraindications to percutaneous treatment include diffuse osteopenia that prohibits adequate fixation, and extensive metaphyseal comminution that prevents anatomic reduction and stability. Generally, severely displaced three- and four-part fractures are not amenable to closed reduction, especially if the humeral head is dislocated. Fractures that contain a split in the humeral head or that extend across the anatomic neck are better treated with open reduction and internal fixation. Finally, injuries over three weeks old are difficult to reduce percutaneously due to scarring and early callous formation, and may require open reduction and internal fixation.

In summary, relative contraindications include:

- osteopenia/osteoporosis;
- extensive metaphyseal comminution;
- severely displaced three- and four-part fractures and fracture dislocations;
- head-splitting fractures;
- fractures of the anatomic neck;
- injuries that are over three weeks old or that show early callous formation.

TECHNIQUE

Preoperative evaluation and planning

The features of the fracture are evaluated with a standard trauma series of the injured shoulder (anteroposterior, scapular-Y lateral, and axillary views). Almost all patients being considered for surgery undergo computerized tomography with three-dimensional reconstruction to further characterize the fracture. As discussed above, special attention is paid to characterizing the fracture type, measuring the degree of displacement and angulation of fragments, and assessing comminution and medial calcar status. The patient is counseled on the operative technique and the use of pins that need to be monitored and removed. Where the indications for pinning are in doubt, the procedure may still be attempted, but with the option to convert to plating or hemiarthroplasty during surgery, although this should be discussed with the patient preoperatively.

Instruments and equipment

An elevator such as a small Cobb and pointed hook retractors are needed to perform the reduction percutaneously. For fixation of the shaft to the head fragment, we prefer to use 2.8 mm terminally threaded Schanz pins. For fixation of the tuberosities, we use 4.0 mm or 4.5 mm cannulated screws, because they do not require hardware removal, and they permit patients to have greater range of motion postoperatively.

A large image intensifier (large C-arm) is needed throughout the procedure (**Fig. 2.1**). A second, smaller image intensifier (mini C-arm) can be placed in an orthogonal position to the large C-arm, to obtain simultaneous orthogonal views (**Fig. 2.2**).

Implants and equipment for open reduction and internal fixation, and for hemiarthroplasty, must be available in the event that adequate reduction and fixation cannot be obtained with percutaneous techniques.

Patient positioning

Regional interscalene block supplemented with sedation for surgical anesthesia is used. The patient is placed in a modified beach-chair position, with the head of the bed at approximately 45° and the patient's head gently attached to a headrest; care is needed to keep the neck in neutral flexion/extension (**Fig. 2.1**). The patient must be moved laterally to the edge, such that a true anteroposterior (AP) fluoroscopy view of the shoulder can be obtained without obstruction. The large C-arm is brought in from a cephalad direction parallel

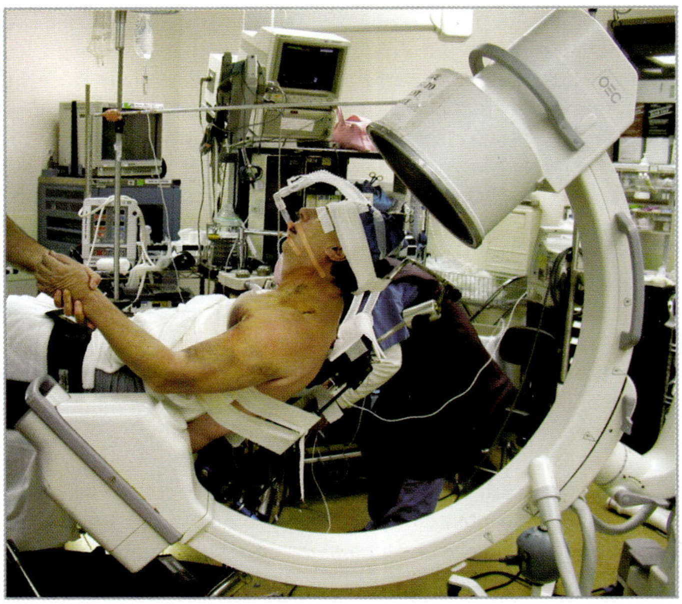

Figure 2.1 Modified beach-chair position. The head of the bed is raised to approximately 45°, and the patient is lateralized to the edge of the table so that the shoulder is fully accessible to reduction maneuvers and intraoperative imaging. The large C-arm is brought in from a cephalad direction. Adequate orthogonal images of the entire proximal humerus and glenohumeral joint should be obtained prior to prepping and draping, to verify appropriate patient and C-arm positioning.

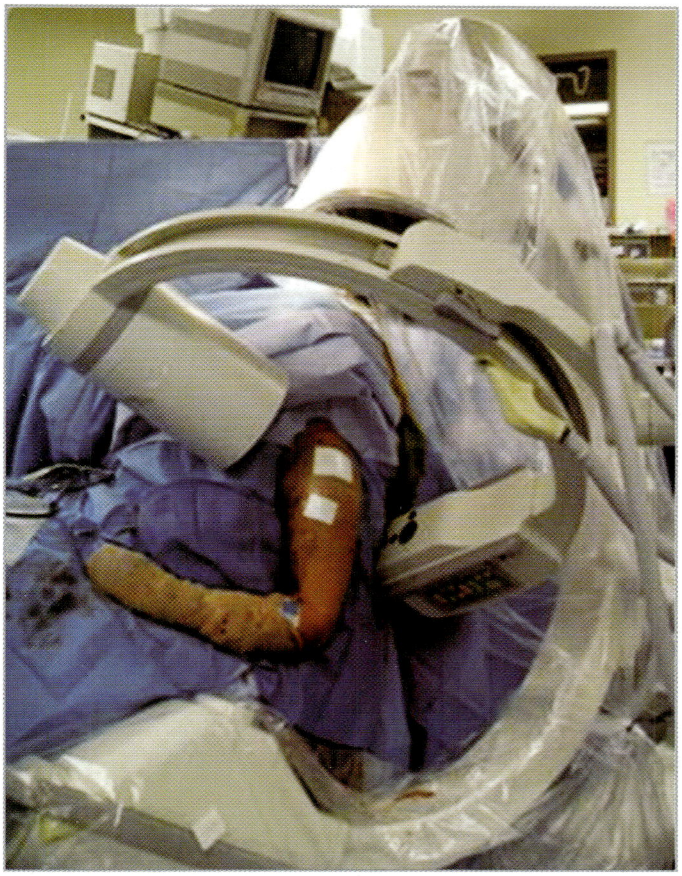

Figure 2.2 Dual C-arm configuration. A second C-arm is brought in to take simultaneous orthogonal images during the procedure.

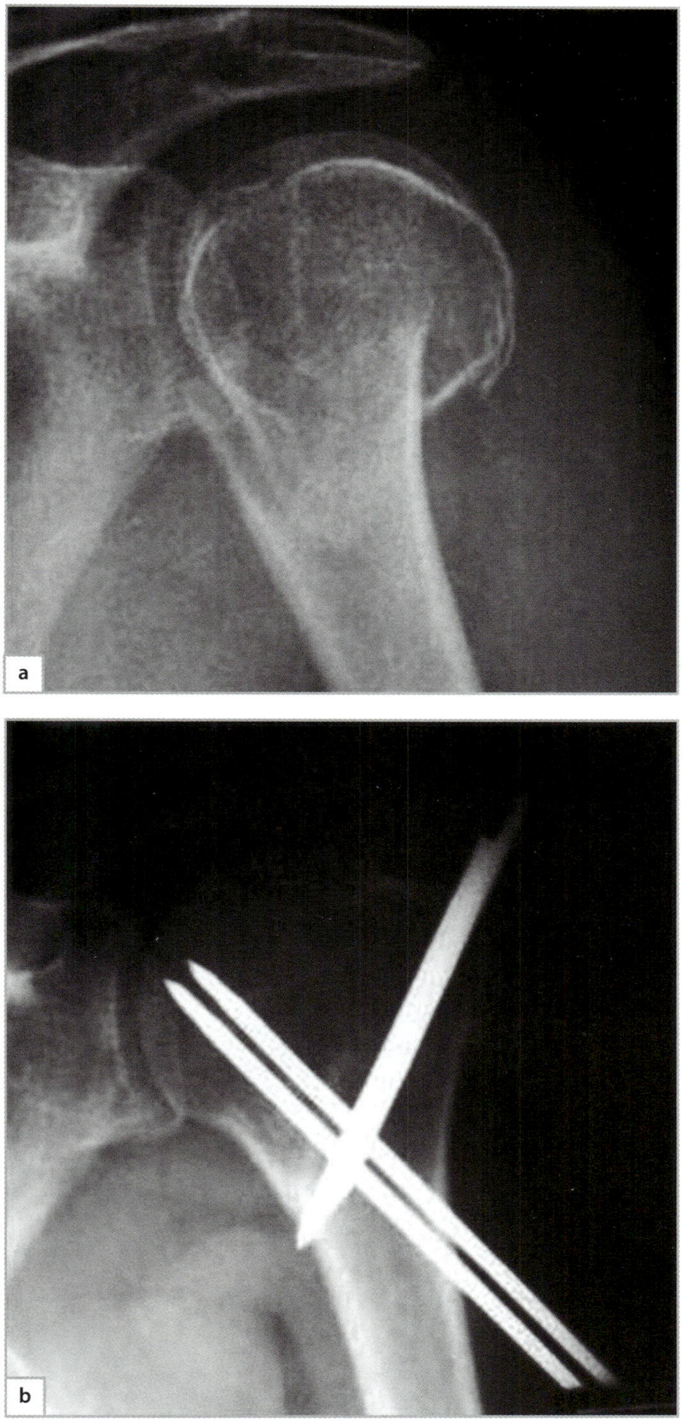

Figure 2.3 Two-part fracture of the surgical neck in the dominant arm of a healthy, active, 67-year-old woman. (a) Anteroposterior view demonstrates the typical medial displacement of the shaft caused by the pull of the pectoralis as well as internal rotation of both the head and shaft. (b) Postoperative anteroposterior radiograph showing anatomic reduction with fixation provided by two retrograde lateral pins ending in subchondral bone, and two antegrade superior pins ending in the dense bone of the medial humeral cortex.

to the operating table (**Fig. 2.1**). The mini C-arm may be brought in orthogonally to the large C-arm, to allow instant assessment of the fracture in two planes (**Fig. 2.2**). Prior to prepping and draping the patient, ability to obtain AP and axillary views is verified.

Two-part fractures of the surgical neck

For a fracture of the surgical neck, the humeral head is usually pulled into slight varus by the unopposed force of the supraspinatus. The pectoralis major displaces the shaft anteriorly and medially (**Fig. 2.3a**). A closed reduction maneuver is performed by applying a posteriorly directed force to the humerus (**Fig. 2.4**). To reduce the head to the shaft, the shoulder is brought into adduction, internal rotation, and flexion. The head may be gently pushed into the shaft when the shoulder is in this position. A skin hook may be percutaneously introduced through an incision 2 cm lateral to the anterior acromion, and used to hook the supraspinatus and pull the head out of varus. Once the head is reduced to the shaft, the arm is brought into neutral rotation and a variable amount of abduction, depending on the degree of varus of the humeral head.

Retrograde lateral pins are inserted first. The starting point is on the lateral humeral shaft, just proximal to the deltoid insertion. This location represents a safe zone between the axillary nerve, whose average location is 5 cm from the inferior edge of the acromion (Burkhead et al. 1992), and the radial nerve, which courses through the spiral groove distally. Fluoroscopic imaging with a pin overlying the arm is used to localize the desired starting point (**Fig. 2.5a**). Following a small skin incision, a fine clamp is used to bluntly dissect down to bone, and a drill guide is inserted to act as a soft-tissue protector during pin insertion (**Fig. 2.5b**). The lateral pin is directed posteromedially to account for

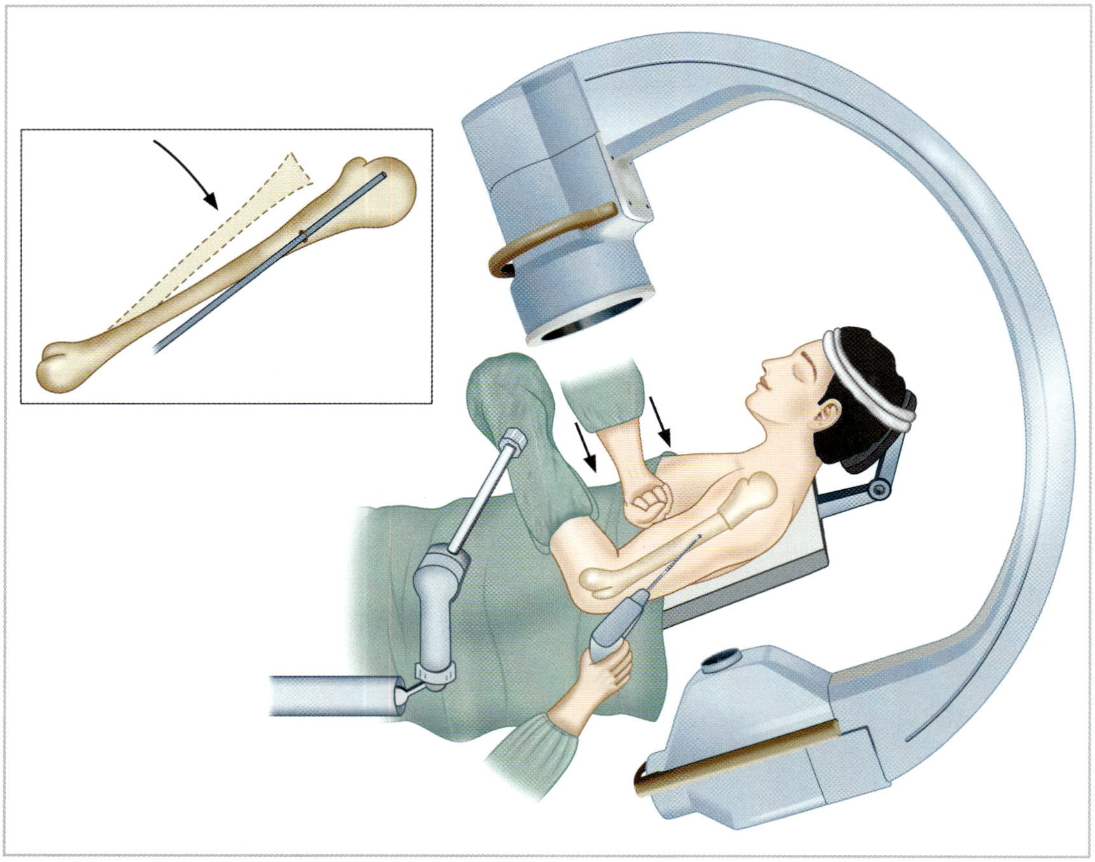

Figure 2.4 Shaft reduction and fixation. A posteriorly directed external force (arrows) will correct the anterior displacement and apex anterior angulation of the shaft piece (inset) caused by the pull of the pectoralis muscles. Once this deformity is corrected and anatomic reduction has been confirmed on imaging, the lateral pin may be advanced into the humeral head to fix the reduction in place.

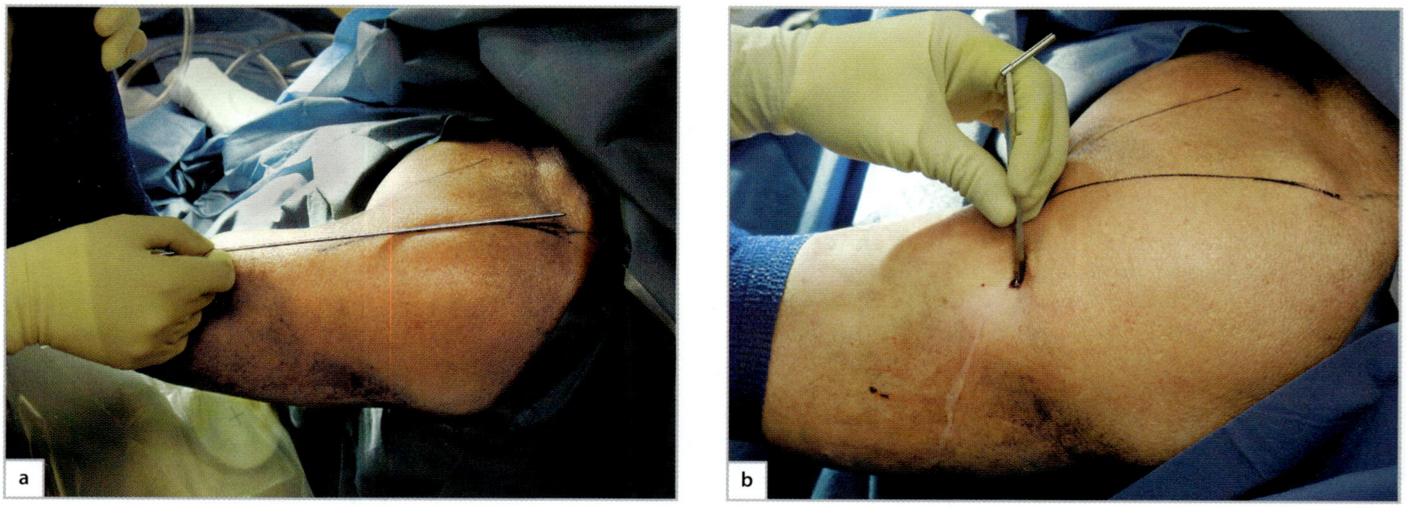

Figure 2.5 Determining pin orientation and starting point. (a) Images taken with the pin against the skin can localize the skin incision needed to reach the ideal starting point on bone, which should be just proximal to the deltoid insertion on the lateral edge of the humerus. (b) A drill guide is used as a soft-tissue protector during pin insertion.

humeral retroversion, and is advanced just short of the fracture site, at which time the final reduction is performed, as described above. Once the anatomic reduction has been verified with imaging, the lateral pin, which has been 'waiting' near the fracture site, is advanced past the fracture, stopping in the dense subchondral bone of the medial humeral head. A second lateral pin is inserted parallel to the first to provide additional fixation and rotational stability (**Fig. 2.3b**). Stability is improved if the pins do not converge near the fracture site.

If the fracture is particularly unstable, several pin configurations can augment fixation. A third retrograde pin can be inserted from the anterior humeral cortex, at the same level as the lateral pins, and advanced into the humeral head. Another option, shown in **Fig. 2.3b**, is antegrade insertion of superior pins through the greater tuberosity. The pin is inserted just lateral to the acromion, and directed medially across the fracture into the thick medial humeral calcar, which is especially well suited for pin fixation. Care must be taken to insert these antegrade pins with enough inclination so that they end below the interior margin of the articular surface, to prevent joint penetration.

Once all the pins have been inserted, the shoulder is taken through a gentle range of motion, with repeated imaging to confirm the stability of the fracture and that the pins are contained in the humeral head. The pins are cut just beneath the level of the skin, and the skin closed.

Two-part fractures of the greater tuberosity

Assessment of this fracture must ensure that a concomitant fracture of the surgical neck does not exist. If a non-displaced fracture exists, percutaneous pins to fix the head to the shaft may be selected at the start of the procedure, as their use will avoid displacing the fracture of the surgical neck. The greater tuberosity must be large enough and of adequate bone quality to be fixed with screws. If it is too small, or if the bone quality is poor, or if comminution is appreciable, the fracture should be fixed or supplemented with a suture fixation technique. In these situations, open or arthroscopic treatment techniques must be employed, and are discussed elsewhere in this (Chapters 3–9).

The greater tuberosity displaces superiorly and posteriorly, due to the pull of the rotator cuff attachments. Fractures with more than 5 mm of displacement or significant angulation generally require operative treatment. To reduce the fracture percutaneously, an incision is made 2–3 cm distal to the anterolateral edge of the acromion, and a skin hook is inserted to manipulate the tuberosity (**Fig. 2.6a**). External rotation of the shoulder can aid in the reduction by bringing the fracture site on the humeral head posteriorly to meet the displaced fragment of tuberosity. It can be difficult to assess the quality of a reduction of the greater tuberosity on AP imaging. Two signs that suggest an adequate reduction are that the bone density does not abruptly change between the head and the tuberosity fragment, and that the contour of the humeral head assumes an anatomic appearance.

Once reduced, two guide wires from a cannulated screw system are inserted to provisionally stabilize the fracture. The wires are placed just lateral to the edge of the acromion, and directed into the medial humeral cortex when possible or into the subchondral bone of the medial humeral head (**Fig. 2.6b**). The starting point should be just lateral to the greater tuberosity's most superior aspect, to avoid postoperative impingement of the screw. Imaging with multiple orthogonal views is performed to confirm that the guide wires have not penetrated the joint, and that the tuberosity is no longer displaced posteriorly. Small skin incisions are made at the wire sites to allow for insertion of the measuring device. Once screw lengths have been determined, drilling proceeds over a soft-tissue protector. The appropriate 4.0 mm cannulated screws are inserted over the guide wires for final fixation. Washers are used if the bone quality is less than average. Final imaging is obtained to rule out joint penetration, and to assess the stability of the reduction when the shoulder is brought through a gentle range of motion.

Three-part fractures of the surgical neck and greater tuberosity

Three-part fractures involving the surgical neck and greater tuberosity are usually associated with superior and posterior displacement of the fragment of the greater tuberosity, along with internal rotation of the humeral head due to the unopposed force of the subscapularis (**Fig. 2.7a**). The humeral shaft may demonstrate the typical anterior and medial displacement, as well as apex anterior angulation, owing to the strong pull of the pectoral muscles.

First, the shaft and head must be reduced, and lateral pins placed, using the same technique described above for two-part fractures of the surgical neck. Following reduction and fixation of the shaft and head, the fragment of the tuberosity is percutaneously reduced using the techniques discussed for isolated fractures of the greater tuberosity. A skin hook is introduced 2–3 cm lateral to the acromion (**Fig. 2.7c,d**). If the greater tuberosity is not easily reducible to its anatomic position, the quality of the shaft–head reduction must be reassessed. A poor reduction there will lead to an inadequate reduction of the fragment of the greater tuberosity. If necessary, the percutaneous incision may be extended to directly visualize and palpate the fragment, to obtain an anatomic reduction. Once reduced, the piece of greater tuberosity is fixed with cannulated screws, with fixation to the medial humeral shaft when possible (**Fig. 2.7e,f**). Frequent fluoroscopic imaging is performed throughout the procedure and at its conclusion, to verify appropriate implant position without joint penetration or loss of reduction.

Valgus impacted four-part fractures

Valgus impacted four-part fractures have a fracture pattern where the head is displaced into valgus, and the greater and lesser tuberosities are minimally displaced in relation to the shaft. Therefore, once the head is reduced relative to the shaft, the tuberosities are also reduced, typically without any manipulation.

Percutaneous reduction begins with the introduction of a small bone elevator under the impacted head fragment, to raise the head and restore the height of the articular surface (**Fig. 2.8c,d**). The shaft is reduced to the head with a combination of internal rotation, adduction, and flexion, while a posterior force is directed onto the shaft to counteract the pull of the pectoralis. Judicious imaging during this process will help ensure the proper height of the humeral head is attained relative to the shaft. Once a satisfactory reduction has been obtained, the retrograde lateral pins are advanced past the fracture, coming to a stop in the subchondral bone of the medial humeral head. Imaging is used again to confirm the reduction; it is important to assess the height of the humeral articular surface, and to ensure that the pins are not penetrating the joint (**Fig. 2.8e**).

The lesser tuberosity is not significantly displaced in these fractures, due to the integrity of the medial humeral calcar, so this piece generally does not need to be fixed with separate implants. Attention is turned to the greater tuberosity, which is reduced percutaneously with a skin hook and fixed with one or two cannulated screws. Final fluoroscopic images are taken to confirm maintenance of satisfactory reduction during gentle shoulder range of motion, and proper implant depth outside of the joint space.

Pearls and pitfalls

Indication

- The surgeon should be prepared to switch to an alternative, open approach and fixation technique, or arthroplasty, for fractures with compromised stability – for example because of osteoporosis or medial calcar comminution.

Technique

- Patient positioning should allow for perfect fluoroscopic imaging of the shoulder.

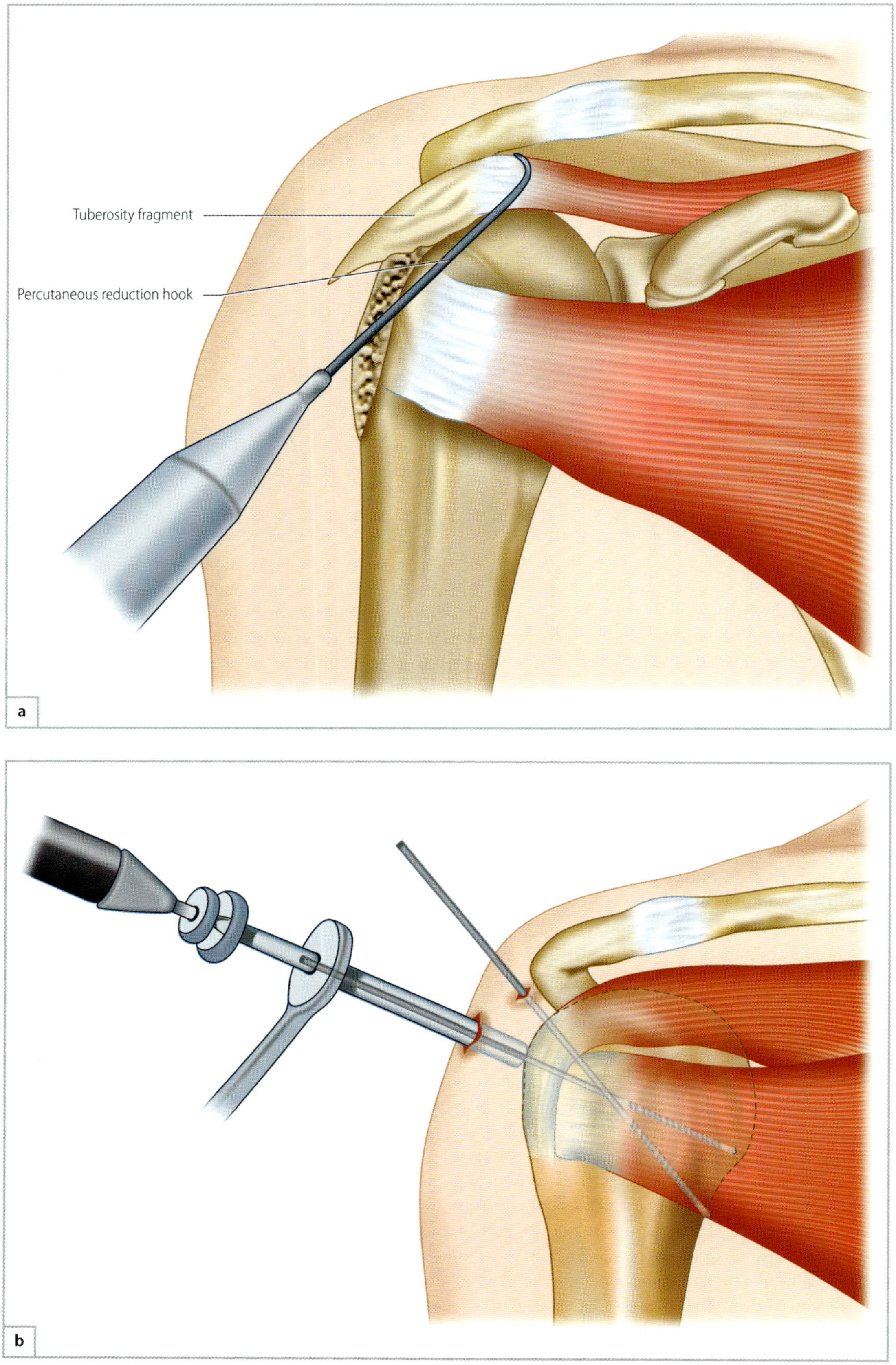

Figure 2.6 Two-part fracture of the greater tuberosity. (a) A percutaneous reduction hook is used to bring the fragment of the tuberosity down from its superoposterior position. Reduction can be aided by externally rotating the humerus. (b) Kirschner wires are inserted through the tuberosity over a soft-tissue protector, with the ideal starting point just lateral to the anterolateral edge of the acromion. The wires are advanced to subchondral bone or medial cortex, and screw lengths are measured. Reduction should be verified by imaging before drilling and screw insertion.

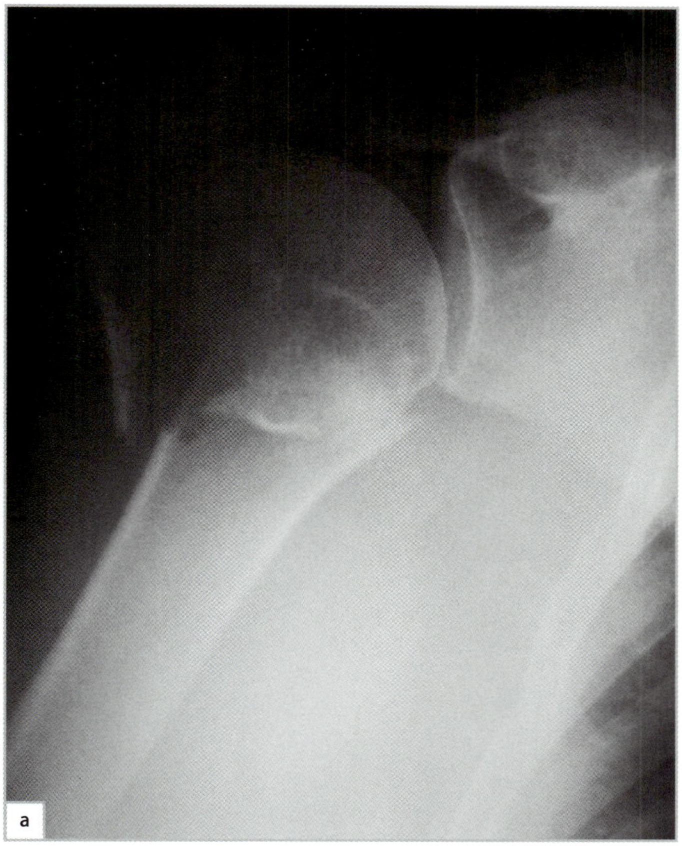

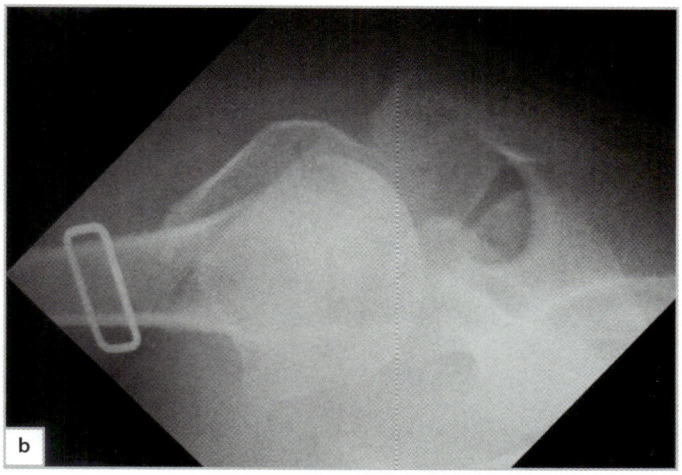

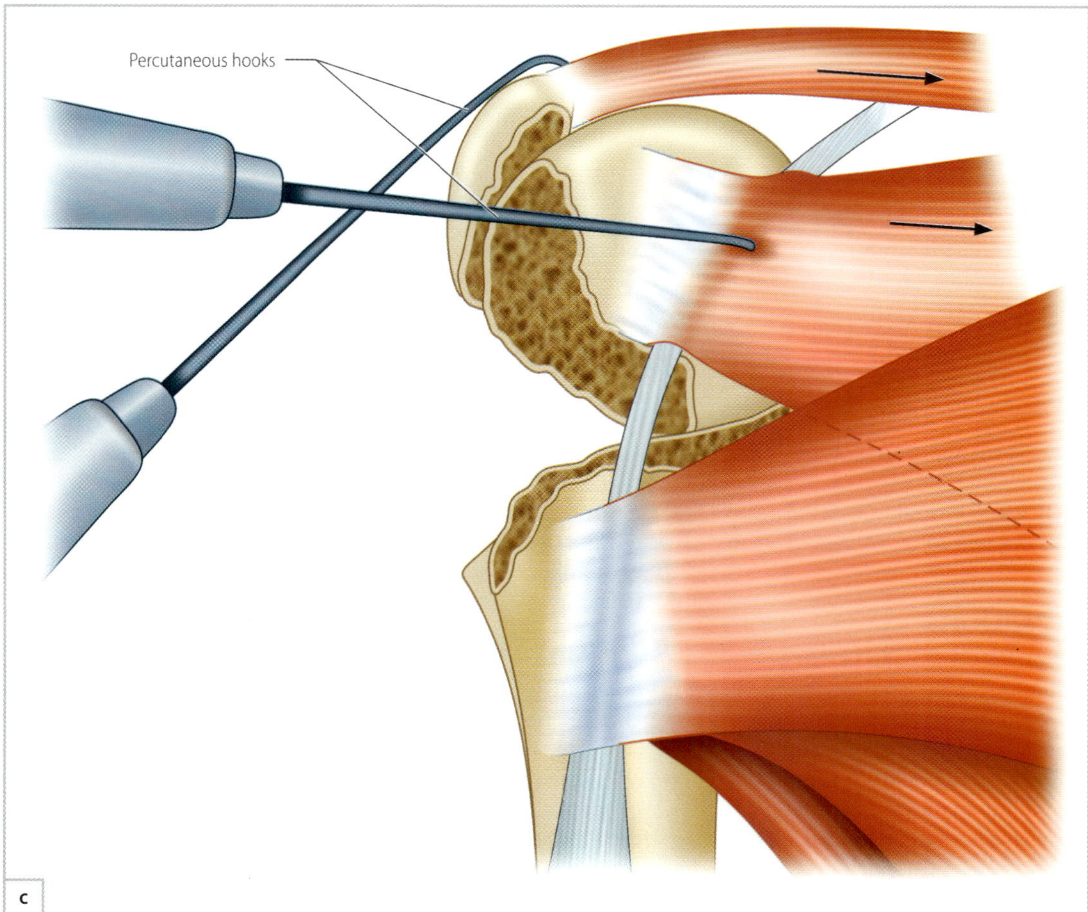

Figure 2.7 Three-part fracture of the greater tuberosity and surgical neck, in the dominant arm of a 52-year-old male who is an active fly fisherman. *Contd...*

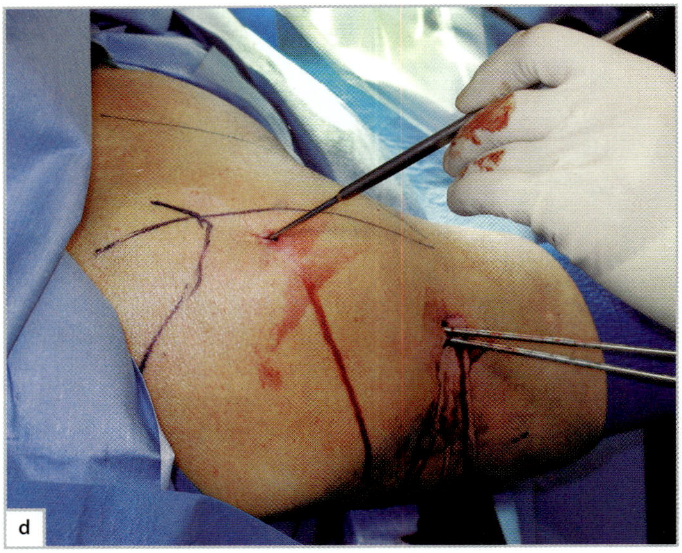

d

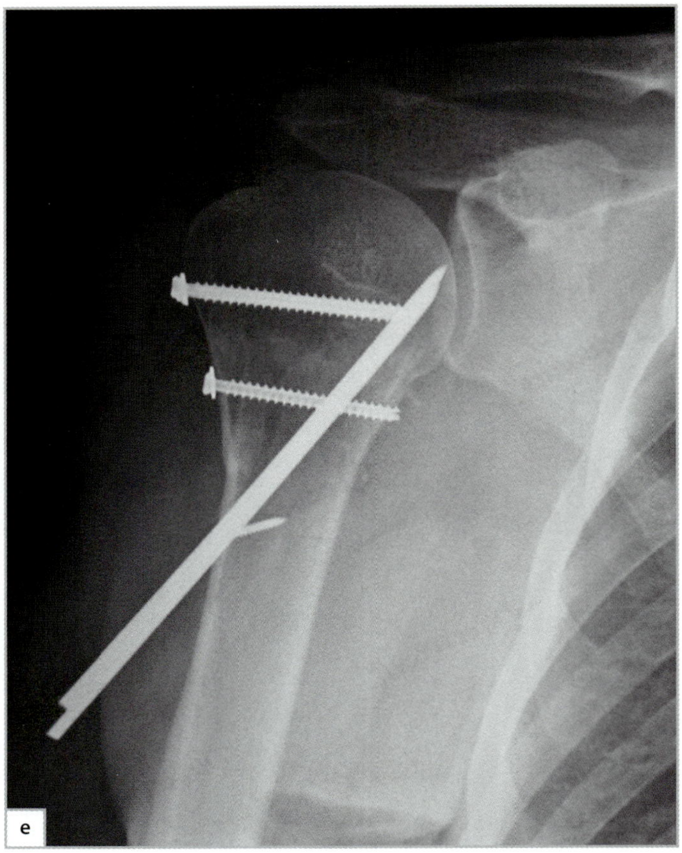

e

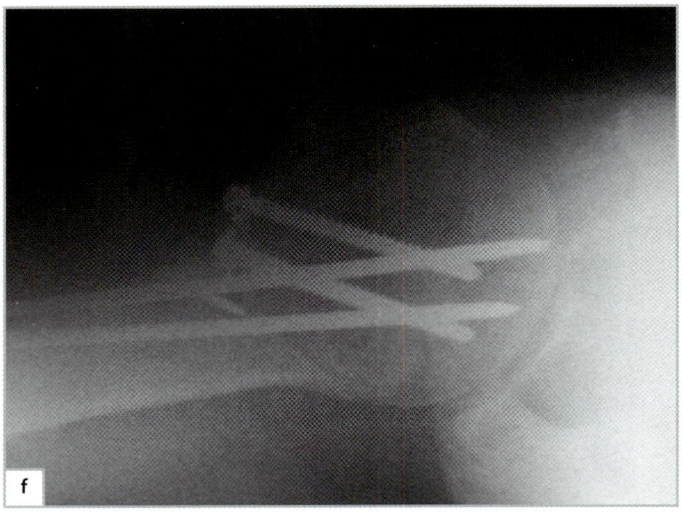

f

Figure 2.7 Three-part fracture of the greater tuberosity and surgical neck, in the dominant arm of a 52-year-old male who is an active fly fisherman. (a) Preoperative anteroposterior radiograph and (b) axillary radiograph demonstrating the typical deformity. (c) Schematic demonstrating the use of a percutaneous hook to bring the greater tuberosity inferiorly to its footprint, and a second hook to bring the fragment of the humeral head out of internal rotation. (d) Reduction of the tuberosity fragment is best achieved after stable fixation of the shaft to the head with lateral pins. (e) Postoperative anteroposterior radiograph after anatomic reduction and fixation with two lateral pins across the surgical neck, and two 4.0 mm cannulated screws across the greater tuberosity. (f) Postoperative axillary radiograph showing anatomic restoration of the proximal humeral relationships.

- Fluoroscopy with dual C-arms can save time, and allow for easier reduction and fixation.
- Surgeons who have a good knowledge of the radial and axial nerve anatomy, and who place pins in the safe zone, are less likely to injure a nerve.

Pin placement considerations

- A common error is to place the pins too medially so that only a small portion of the head is captured.
- Other common errors include using too few pins, placement of pins too close together, and having two pins converge at the fracture site.
- The entry point for the lateral retrograde pin should be just proximal to the deltoid insertion, to avoid injury to the radial nerve in the spiral groove distally, or to the transverse branches of the axillary nerve proximally.
- Retrograde lateral pins should be provisionally placed in the humeral shaft distal to the fracture, so that they are 'waiting' for the reduction and therefore can be readily advanced across the fracture once anatomic reduction is obtained. This minimizes the risk of inadvertently losing the reduction during pin placement.

Adequate fixation

- Adequate fixation must be achieved because it provides the best chance of restoring anatomy. Fixation strength should be maximized to facilitate accelerated rehabilitation.
- Adequate fixation is achieved not only with the use of more pins or screws, but with the proper placement of the implants into dense subchondral or cortical bone that is well suited for implant fixation.

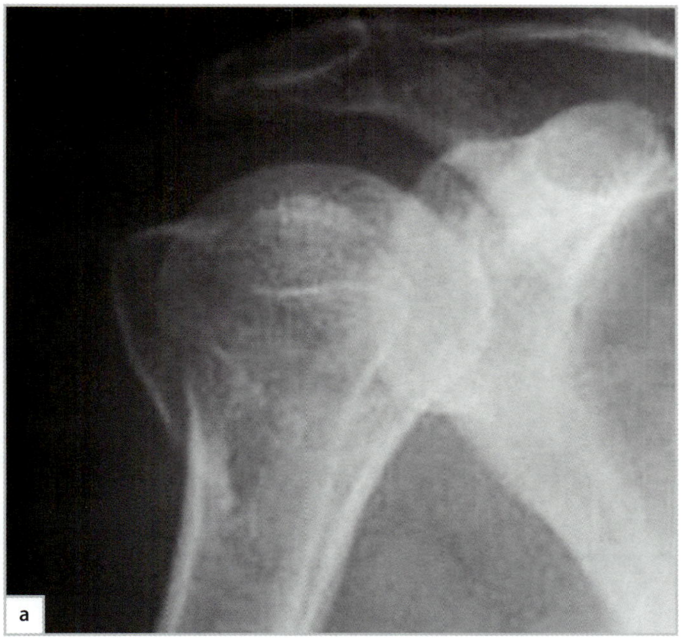

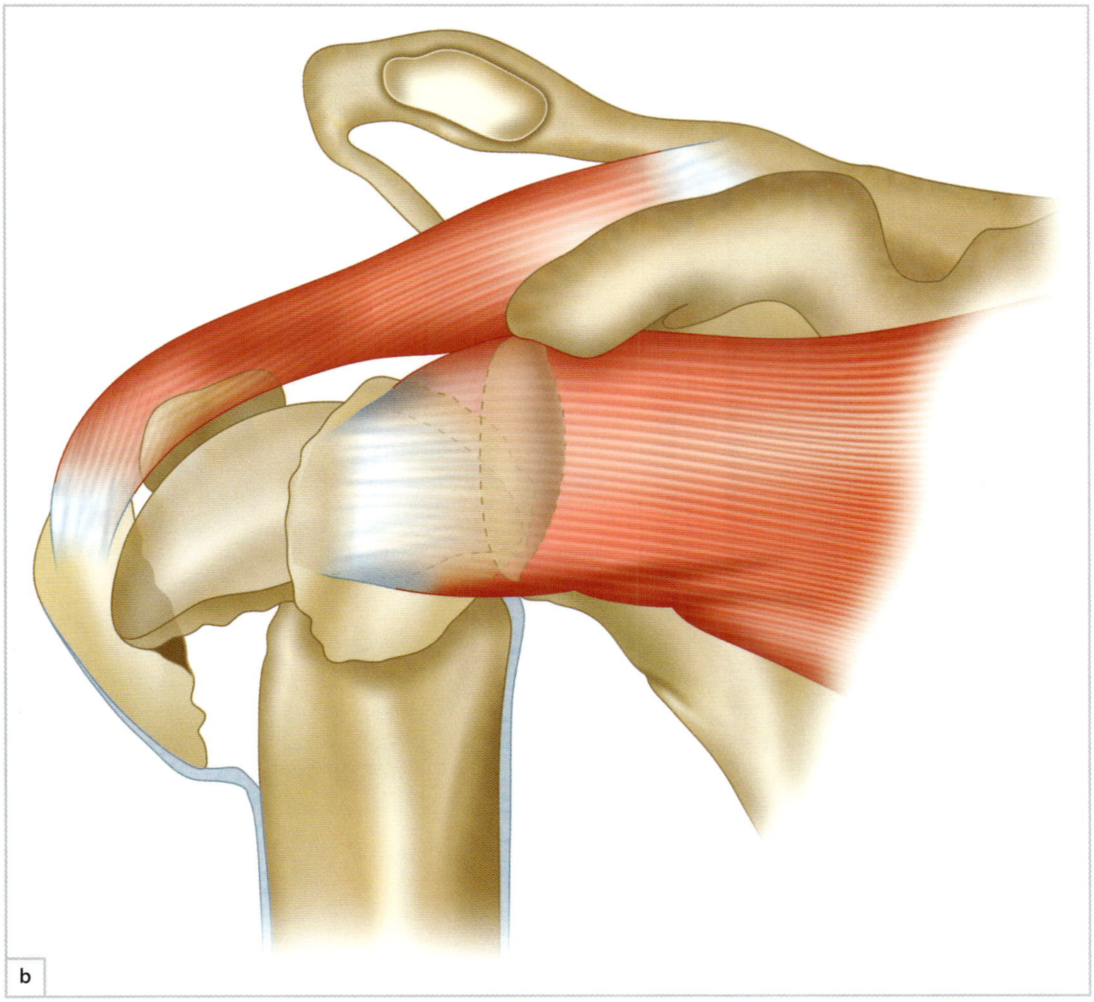

Figure 2.8 Four-part valgus impacted fracture in the dominant arm of a 53-year-old female office assistant. *Contd...*

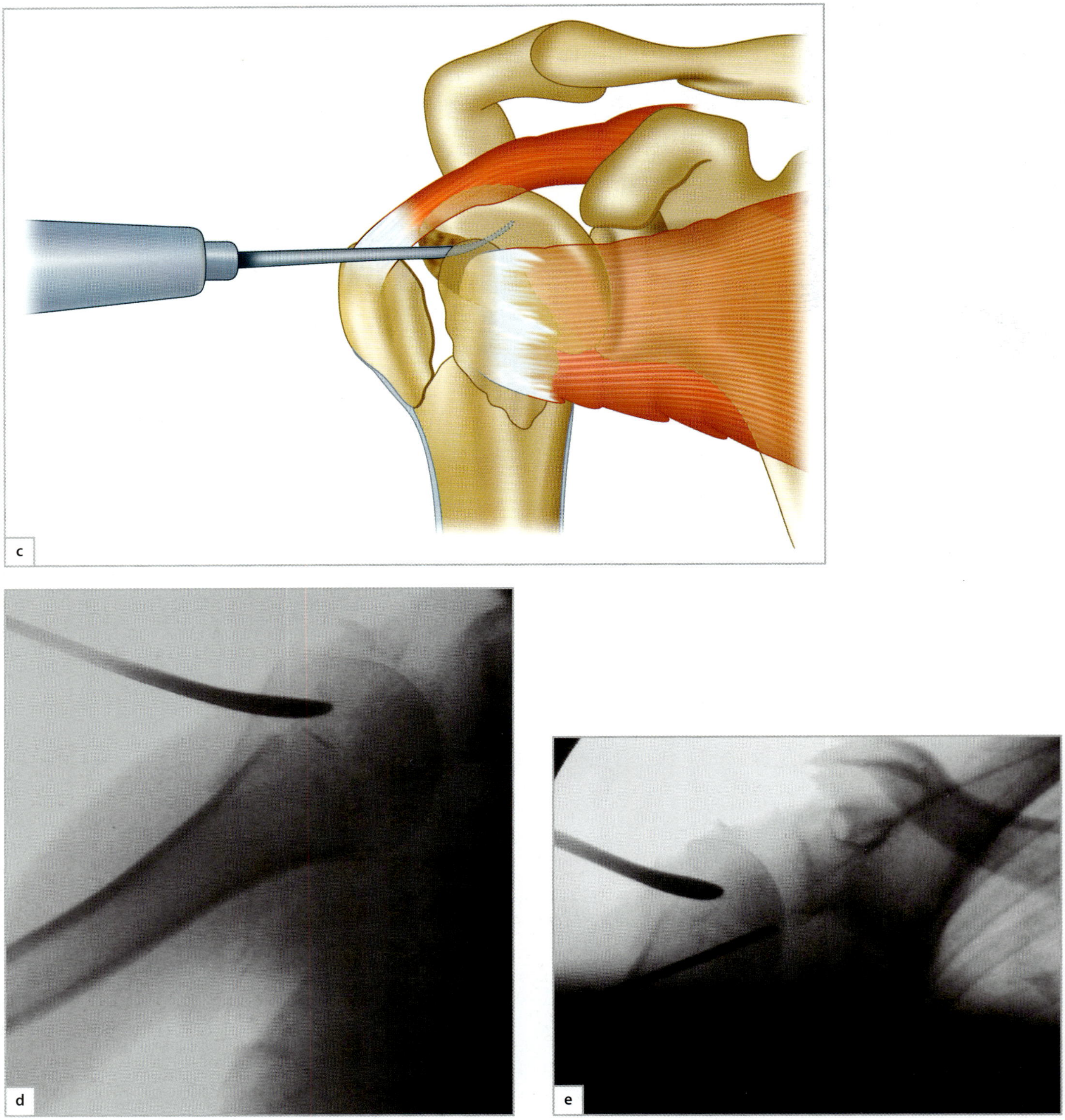

Figure 2.8 Four-part valgus impacted fracture in the dominant arm of a 53-year-old female office assistant. *Contd...*

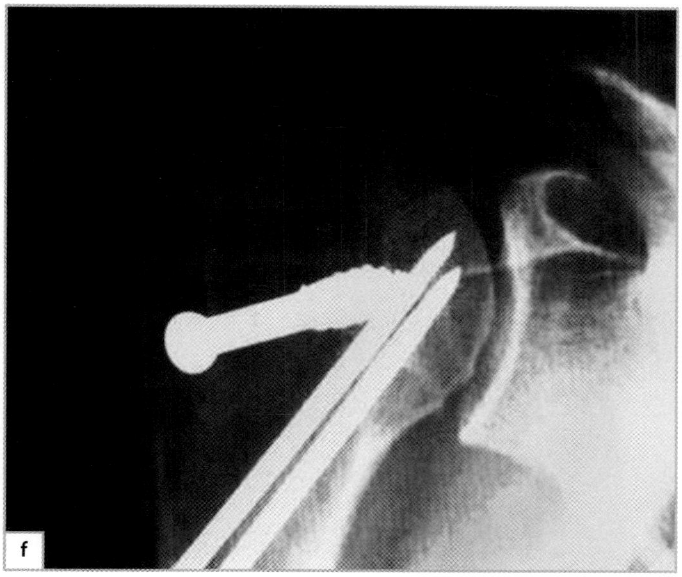

Figure 2.8 Four-part valgus impacted fracture in the dominant arm of a 53-year-old female office assistant. (a) Anteroposterior radiograph and (b) schematic showing valgus impaction of the articular fragment, resulting in loss of articular height without significant lateral displacement of the humeral head relative to the shaft, resulting in a preserved medial calcar and soft tissues. (c) Schematic and (d) intraoperative fluoroscopic image showing a bone elevator inserted percutaneously into the fracture between the greater and lesser tuberosities to raise the articular fragment. (e) Once the height of the humeral head has been restored, the shaft is reduced to the head, and a lateral pin is inserted across the surgical neck, ending in medial subchondral bone. (f) The final anteroposterior radiograph shows anatomic reduction and fixation of the greater tuberosity with a cannulated screw.

- Insufficient fixation is associated with loss of reduction, pin migration, and the need to limit postoperative motion, leading to stiffness.

Postoperative care

- It is important to obtain weekly radiographs to assess pin position and fracture reduction.
- Early range of motion should be encouraged as long as the surgeon has maximized fixation strength.

REHABILITATION

Patients return for weekly radiographs to check pin position and verify fracture reduction. Pendulum exercises are initiated immediately after surgery if fixation is adequate. During postoperative weeks 2–4, gentle passive external rotation is initiated. Patients with superior pins through the greater tuberosity will have these removed at postoperative week 3 or 4, at which time passive forward elevation exercises are initiated. At postoperative week 6 all remaining pins are removed, and the patient begins full active and passive range-of-motion exercises without restrictions.

Pin removal is routinely performed in the office under local anesthesia with lidocaine if pins are easily palpable and the patient is comfortable. Alternatively, the pins are removed in the operating room with sedation and local anesthesia. A scalpel is used to make a small incision over the palpable pin site to aid in visualization, and pliers or a T-handle chuck are used to grasp and unscrew the pins. The incision is closed with nylon sutures.

REFERENCES

Agudelo J, , Schürmann M, Stahel P, et al. Analysis of efficacy and failure in proximal humerus fractures treated with locking plates. J Orthop Trauma 2007;21:676–681.

Brooks CH, Revell WJ, Healtey FW. Vascularity of the humeral head after proximal humeral fractures. An anatomical cadaver study. J Bone Joint Surg Br 1993;75:132–136.

Brunner A, Weller K, Thormann S, et al. Closed reduction and minimally invasive percutaneous fixation of proximal humerus fractures using the Humerusblock. J Orthop Trauma 2010;24(7): 407–413.

Burkhead WZ Jr, Scheinberg RR, Box G. Surgical anatomy of the axillary nerve. J Shoulder Elbow Surg 1992;1:31–36.

Calvo E, de Miguel I, de la Cruz JJ, López-Martín N. Percutaneous fixation of displaced proximal humeral fractures: indications based on the correlation between clinical and radiographic results. J Shoulder Elbow Surg 2007;16(6):774–781.

Chen CY, Chao EK, Tu YK, et al. Closed management and percutaneous fixation of unstable proximal humerus fractures. J Trauma 1998;45:1039–1045.

Clavert P, Adam P, Bevort A, et al. Pitfalls and complications with locking plate for proximal humerus fracture. J Shoulder Elbow Surg 2010;19(4):489–494.

Fenichel I, Oran A, Burstein G, Perry Pritsch M. Percutaneous pinning using threaded pins as a treatment option for unstable two- and three-part fractures of the proximal humerus: a retrospective study. Int Orthop 2006;30:153–157.

Hertel R, Hempfing A, Stiehler M, Leunig M. Predictors of humeral head ischemia after intracapsular fracture of the proximal humerus. J Shoulder Elbow Surg 2004;13:427–433.

Jaberg H, Warner JJ, Jakob RP. Percutaneous stabilization of unstable fractures of the humerus. J Bone Joint Surg Am 1992;74:508–515.

Jakob RP, Miniaci A, Anson PS, et al. Four-part valgus impacted fractures of the proximal humerus. J Bone Joint Surg Br 1991;73:295–298.

Jiang C, Zhu Y, Wang M, Rong G. Biomechanical comparison of different pin configurations during percutaneous pinning for the treatment of proximal humeral fractures. J Shoulder Elbow Surg 2007;16:235–239.

Kayalar M, Toros T, Bal E, et al. [The importance of patient selection for the treatment of proximal humerus fractures with percutaneous technique]. [Article in Turkish.] Acta Orthop Traumatol Turc 2009;43:35–41.

Keener JD, Parsons BO, Flatow EL, et al. Outcomes after percutaneous reduction and fixation of proximal humeral fractures. J Shoulder Elbow Surg 2007;16:330–338.

Koval KJ, Blair B, Takei R, et al. Surgical neck fractures of the proximal humerus: a laboratory evaluation of ten fixation techniques. J Trauma 1996;40:778–783.

Leyshon RL. Closed treatment of fractures of the proximal humerus. Acta Orthop Scand 1984;55:48–51.

Naidu SH, Bixler B, Capo JT, et al. Percutaneous pinning of proximal humerus fractures: a biomechanical study. Orthopedics 1997;20:1073–1076.

Neer CS 2nd. Displaced proximal humeral fractures. II. Treatment of three-part and four-part displacement. J Bone Joint Surg Am 1970;52:1090–1103.

Owsley KC, Gorczyca JT. Fracture displacement and screw cutout after open reduction and locked plate fixation of proximal humeral fractures [corrected]. J Bone Joint Surg Am (2008);90:233–240.

Resch H, Povacz P, Fröhlich R, Wambacher M. Percutaneous fixation of three- and four-part fractures of the proximal humerus. J Bone Joint Surg Br 1997;79:295–300.

Chapter 3 Arthroscopically assisted open reduction and internal fixation of fractures of the proximal humerus, glenoid and acromion

Felix H. Savoie III

INDICATIONS

Although almost any articular fracture may be considered for arthroscopic management, there are certain fracture patterns of the humerus and glenoid that are best managed by arthroscopically assisted techniques. In the proximal humerus, fractures of the greater tuberosity, avulsion injuries of the lesser tuberosity, and head-splitting fractures without detachment from the humeral shaft are all injuries that benefit from arthroscopic techniques.

There are also several fractures on the scapular side that benefit from arthroscopic techniques. In the glenoid, anterior or posterior avulsion injuries, coracoid base fractures that extend into the glenoid, and vertical split injuries are amenable to arthroscopic management. Acromial apophyseal separation injuries may also be managed via arthroscopic techniques.

CONTRAINDICATIONS

Arthroscopy is quite useful in many articular fractures. In the case of the shoulder, fractures that separate the shaft from the rest of the proximal humerus represent a contraindication to arthroscopic management. While it may be useful to 'take a quick peek' into the joint using arthroscopy, the severity of the damage and the displacement of the shaft toward the neurovascular structures make arthroscopic management less than ideal. Most three- and four-part fractures are not amenable to management solely using arthroscopic techniques, but management may be helped by dry visualization of the articular surface during open surgery. Dry visualization, while indeed also useful in many two-part fractures that require open or percutaneous fixation, is difficult in most operating theatres.

TECHNIQUE

General principles

Preoperative planning is essential for successful arthroscopic surgery. Patient positioning, fluoroscopic access and visualization, and hypotensive anesthesia are key. We prefer to place the patient in the lateral decubitus position for most fractures. Suspension of the arm using a traction tower often assists in reduction of the fracture by bringing the distal fragment (arm) to the proximal fragment. The anesthesiologist is positioned near the waist, away from the beam of the x-ray device. The fluoroscopy unit is brought in from the patient's head, which allows a true posteroanterior (PA) view of the shoulder, and also oblique and lateral views with rotation of the arm.

With the patient in the beach-chair position, the fluoroscopy unit is brought in from the side rather than over the head. It is important that the unit can rotate and cant into positions that allow axillary views of the humerus (**Fig. 3.1**).

A 'game plan' for fixation of the fracture should be in place before surgery. The images may be copied on paper, and a sketch of the proposed fixation written on the page. Listing the sequence of the procedure, and sharing this information with the crew of the operating room, are key to a successful procedure.

Once the team and the fluoroscopy unit are ready, the procedure may commence. It is often helpful to 'spear' the movable fragments with a Kirschner wire (K-wire) under fluoroscopic guidance prior to commencing the arthroscopy, in order to minimize swelling and also to make the reduction more efficient.

Fractures of the greater tuberosity

The arthroscope is introduced into the joint via a standard posterior portal. An anterior portal is established from outside in, via direct visualization, to evacuate the hematoma, and to allow complete diagnostic arthroscopy from both the posterior and the anterior portals. In young patients with a high-velocity injury, one will often find an anterior labral tear, damage to the biceps, and damage to the intrinsic supraspinatus or infraspinatus tendon, in addition to the fracture. If there is significant damage to the biceps, a tenotomy should be performed. A labral tear should be repaired quickly and efficiently. In the more common lower-energy fractures, these injuries will not be present.

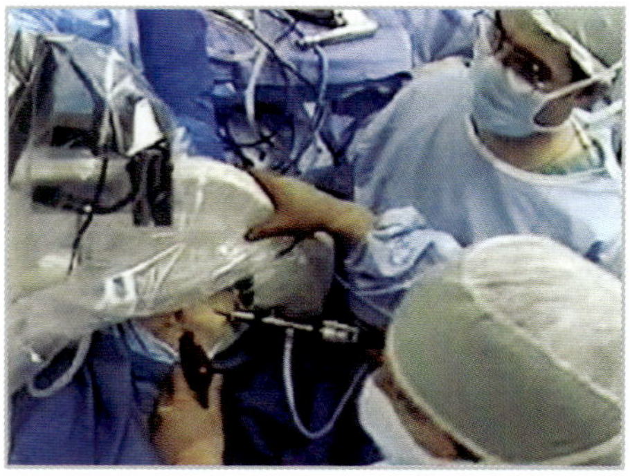

Figure 3.1 A patient being prepped for arthroscopically assisted fixation of a fracture of the proximal humerus. The most efficient position of the patient, anesthesiologist, fluoroscopy unit, and arthroscopy tower are shown.

The arthroscope is then moved to the subacromial space. An anterior lateral portal is established, and the fracture bed debrided of hematomas and adhesions (**Fig. 3.2**).

We feel a careful release of the subdeltoid bursa allows better visualization, but this must be carefully performed with the shaver facing away from the axillary nerve on the undersurface of the deltoid muscle, to prevent injury.

The arthroscope is then moved to the anterior lateral portal to visualize the fracture. A grasper, placed through the anterior portal or via a posterior lateral portal (or both), can be used to pull the fracture back toward the avulsion bed (**Fig. 3.3**). Lateral visualization allows the fragment to be placed anatomically into the site. Provisional fixation may be accomplished with a K-wire. The reduction is then evaluated via fluoroscopy (**Fig. 3.4**).

Two additional wires for cannulated screws are then placed, under fluoroscopic control, through the fragment and into the medial cortex. These are overdrilled through the fragment and into the humeral shaft, and 6.5 mm cannulated screws with washers are placed over the wires, through the fragment, and into the medial cortex (**Fig. 3.5**).

Using a switching stick (via the posterior lateral portal) as a retractor to keep the deltoid away from the humerus and a probe to guide the washer through the retracted deltoid will prevent accidental incorporation of the muscle into the fracture fixation, and preserve visualization of the fracture. Where the bone is inadequate to hold the screw, suture anchors may be inserted into the bed and the sutures retrieved through the soft, osteoporotic bone, and the fracture pulled into the bed as the sutures are tied.

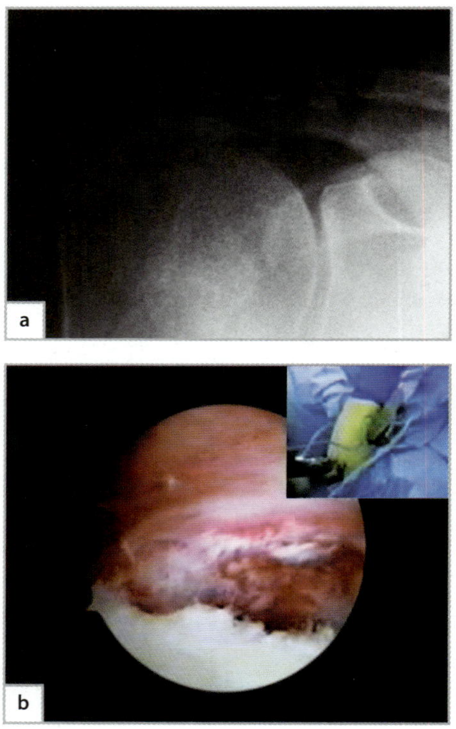

Figure 3.2 Fracture bed from an avulsion injury of the greater tuberosity. (a) Lateral view. (b) Associated hemorrhage and adhesions.

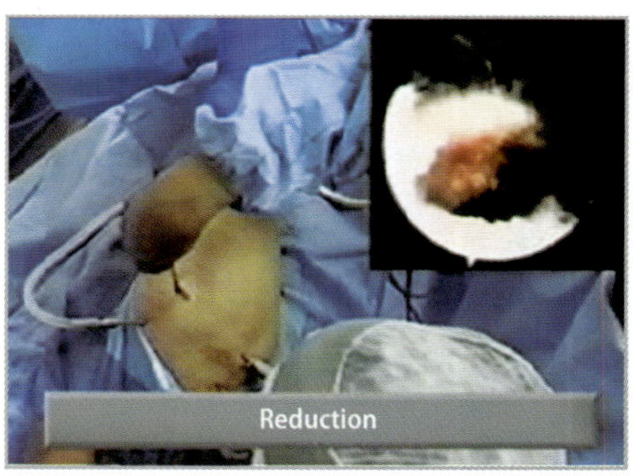

Figure 3.3 Fragment of the greater tuberosity being positioned anatomically. In this view from the lateral portal (inset), the fragment is being positioned via a joystick technique, in preparation for fracture reduction and fixation.

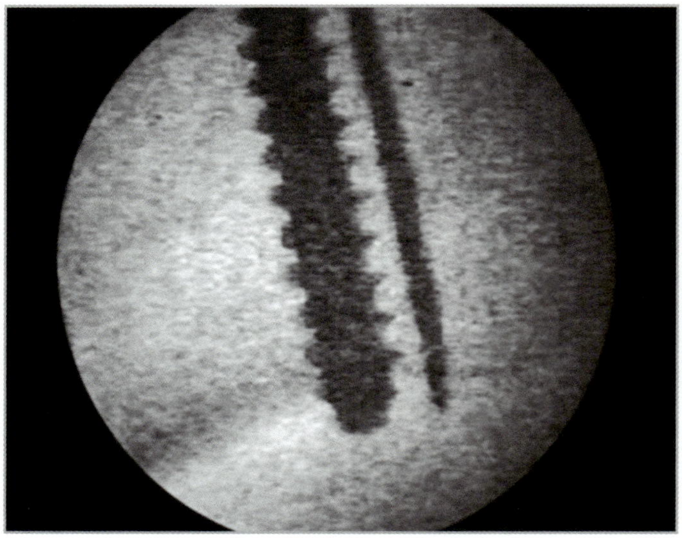

Figure 3.4 Fluoroscopic view of a cannulated screw and washer being inserted into the fragment of the greater tuberosity for fixation of the fracture.

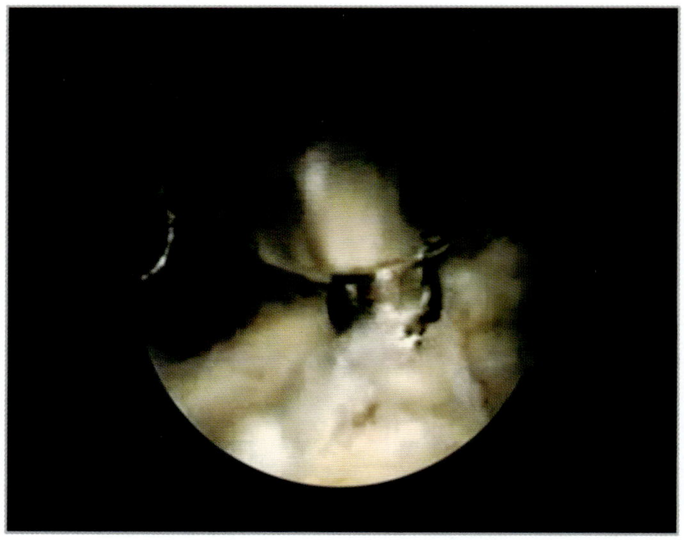

Figure 3.5 Arthroscopic view of a screw fixation for a fracture of the lesser tuberosity. Avulsions of the lesser tuberosity are an excellent indication for arthroscopically assisted fixation.

Fractures of the lesser tuberosity

The basic setup and principles are the same as for fractures of the greater tuberosity. In glenohumeral arthroscopy, careful attention must be paid to the location of the biceps tendon, as it is often caught within the fracture in these injuries. In some cases these may be managed with a 70° scope from within the joint. A good understanding of three-dimensional anatomy is extremely important when doing this technique, to prevent damage to the conjoined tendon or even to the brachial plexus. In this technique, the fracture is manipulated with a K-wire from directly anterior into the fracture bed. In the 'inside view' technique, we use a large, 8 mm cannula in the anterior portal, and insert the wire and the 3.5 or 4.0 mm cannulated screw through the cannula.

In the 'outside view' technique, the arthroscopy visualization portal is anterior lateral. The viewing portal is located 3 cm distal and 1 cm anterior to the anterior lateral corner of the acromion. Anterior, straight lateral, and anterior superior portals allow access for graspers to manipulate the fragment. As with the 'inside view' technique, an 8 or 8.5 mm cannula is used in the anterior inferior portal to protect the deltoid and the conjoined tendon during screw insertion. The fragment is held in place by a percutaneous K-wire. The first cannulated screw wire is then placed through the cannula, through the fragment, and into the humeral head. It is usually necessary to obtain a full-length wire of the same size, as the one from the cannulated screw set is often too short to pass through the cannula. A wire of similar length is used for measurement of screw length.

Head-splitting fractures

The arthroscope provides excellent visualization of head-splitting fractures without destroying the rotator cuff. We have found three-dimensional computerized tomography to be extremely useful in planning surgery, as it is otherwise not always clear which part of the head will be mobile and allow for reduction. In these cases the use of K-wire joysticks is invaluable. The fracture is visualized via glenohumeral arthroscopy (**Fig. 3.6**). The wires are then used to reduce the fracture under arthroscopic visualization. Screws are usually placed from posterior to anterior for fixation.

Fractures of the glenoid

Arthroscopy may be useful in managing fractures of the glenoid (**Fig. 3.7a**). Anterior or posterior rim fractures can be easily visualized and repaired using standard suture anchor techniques (**Fig. 3.7b**). If the fragment is of sufficient size, screw fixation with or without a washer may be of benefit.

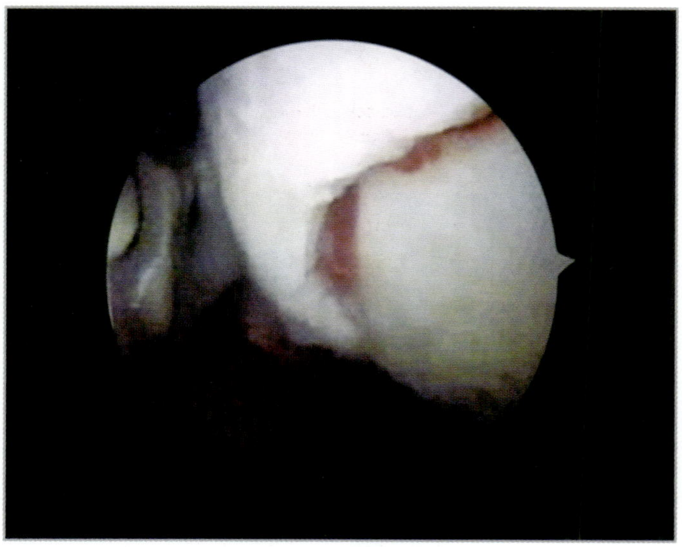

Figure 3.6 Arthroscopic view of a head-splitting fracture prior to reduction.

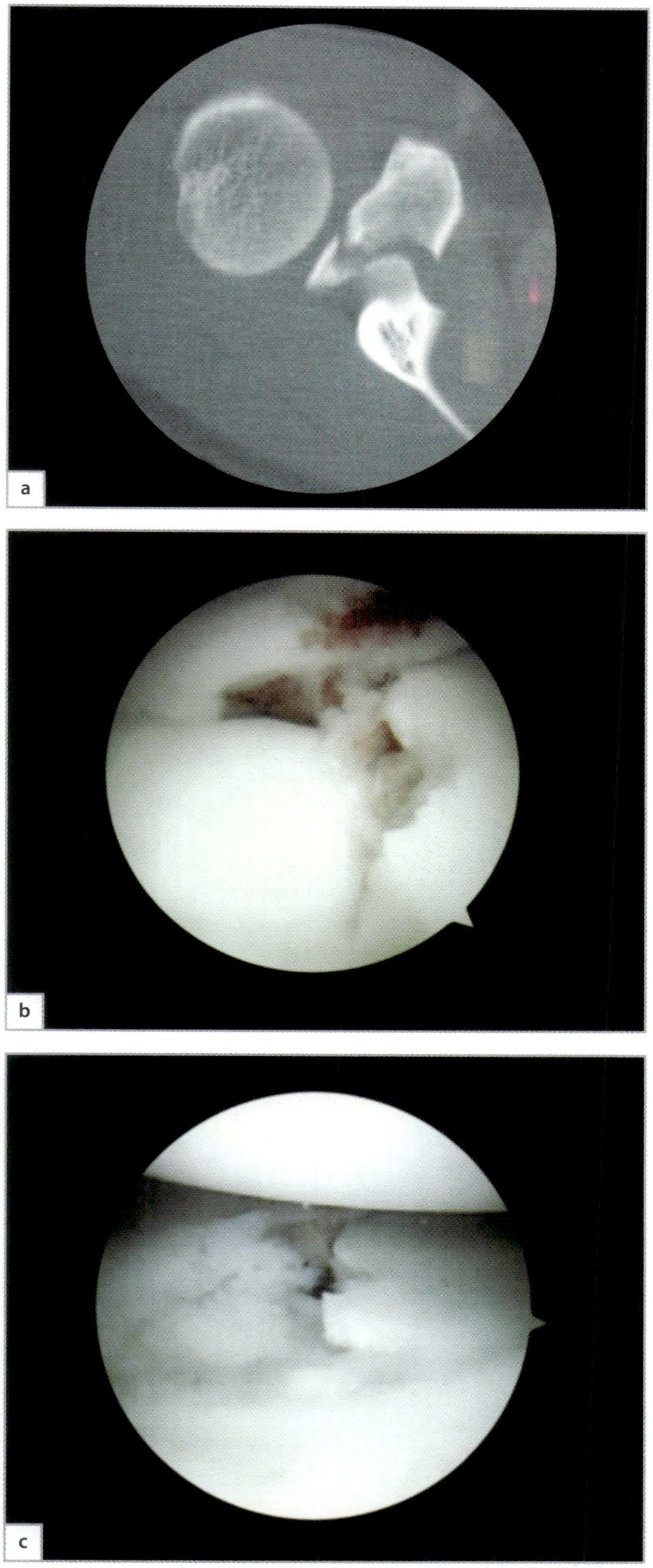

Figure 3.7 Arthroscopic treatment of a glenoid fracture. (a) Computerized tomography scan. (b) Arthroscopic view of the fracture. (c) Arthroscopic view of the fracture after fixation.

Metal screws used for glenoid fixation should be removed relatively early, to prevent worsening of potential arthritis. In this technique the arthroscope is best placed into a superior portal, as a panoramic view of the joint allows a probe to be placed through the posterior portal. The tip can be placed over the anterior rim of the fragment, and used to reduce and hold the fragment while a K-wire is placed percutaneously for provisional stabilization. Then 3.5 or 4.0 mm cannulated screws are inserted via the anterior inferior cannula by the usual technique. **Fig. 3.8** shows the sequence of steps.

For posterior rim fractures, the arthroscope remains in the same portal but the instrument portals are reversed.

In central-split glenoid fractures, it is important to make sure the articular surface is not detached completely from the glenoid neck. These fractures are managed similarly to the rim fractures, but the screws may be placed more medially, from either anterior or posterior, eliminating the need for early removal (**Fig. 3.9**).

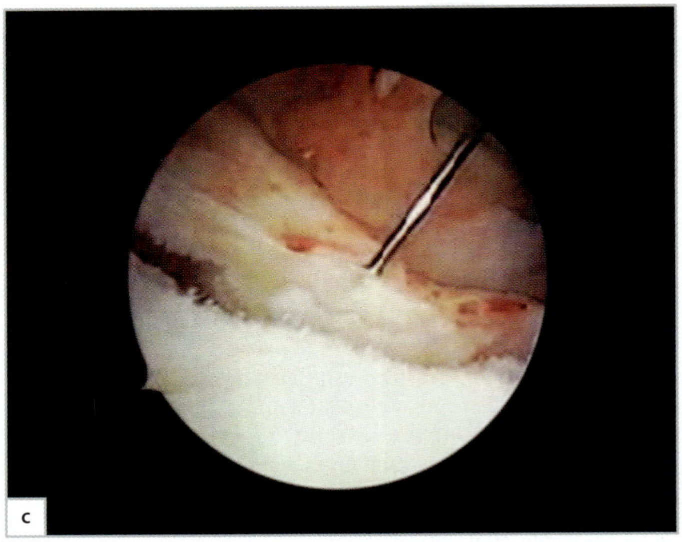

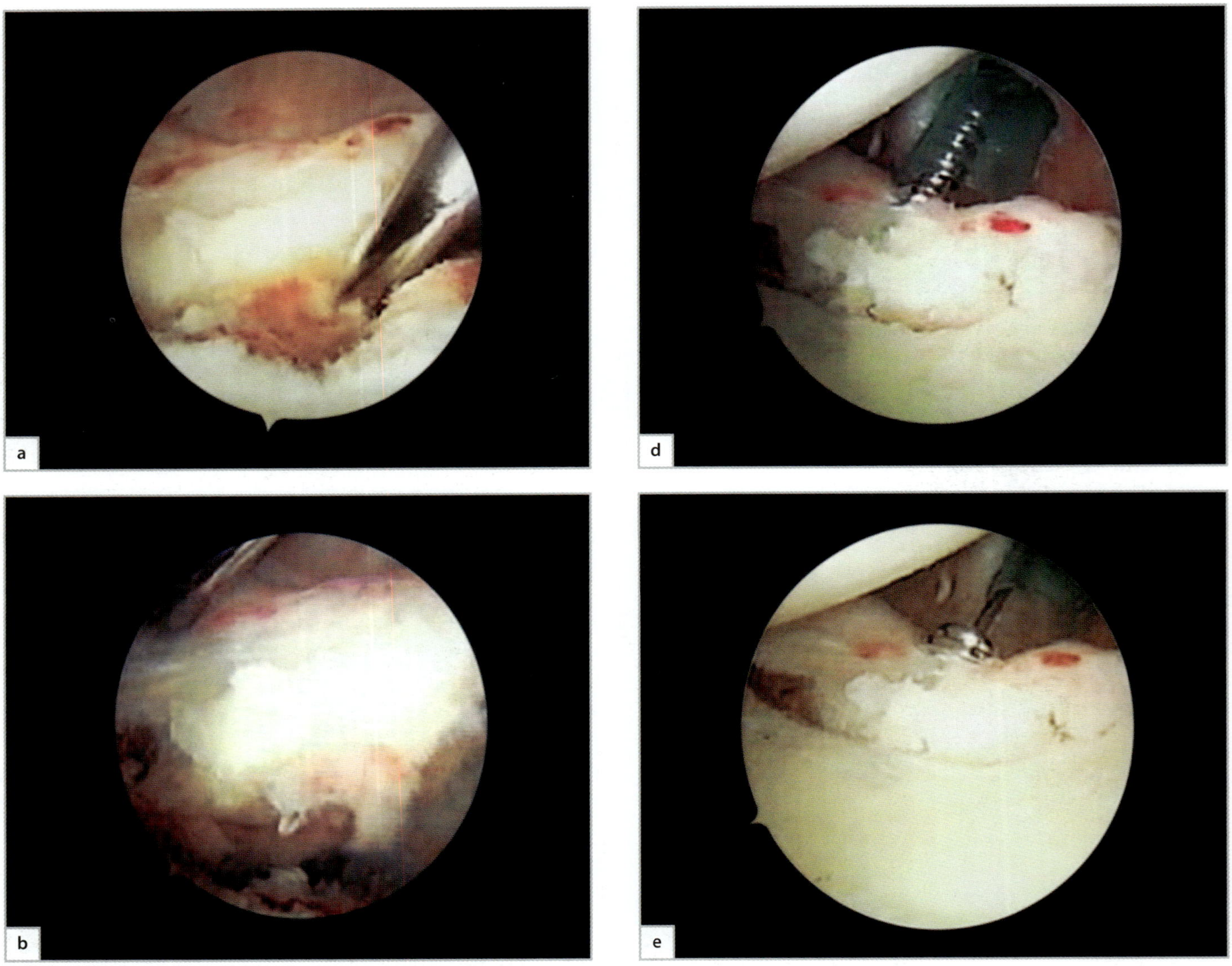

Figure 3.8 Repair of an anterior glenoid fracture. (a) The tip can be placed over the anterior rim of the fragment, and used to reduce and hold the fragment (b) while a Kirschner wire is placed percutaneously for provisional stabilization (c). Then 3.5 mm or 4.0 mm cannulated screws are inserted via the anterior inferior cannula by the usual technique (d,e).

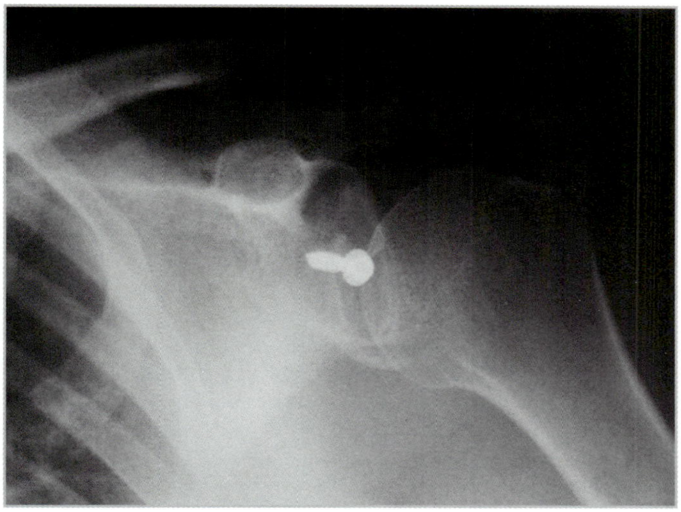

Figure 3.9 Central-split glenoid fracture. These fractures are managed similarly to rim fractures, but the screws may be placed more medially, from either anterior or posterior.

Fractures of the acromion

Fractures of the acromion that require fixation almost always involve an unfused os acromionale that was injured and has become unstable. In many cases, simple excision of a small fragment is the best form of treatment. However, when 50% or more of the acromion is involved, fixation (**Fig. 3.10**) may be indicated, especially in young, active individuals.

The area of separation may be readily identified in acute injuries by hemorrhage. In more chronic cases, cautery may be necessary to expose the site of injury.

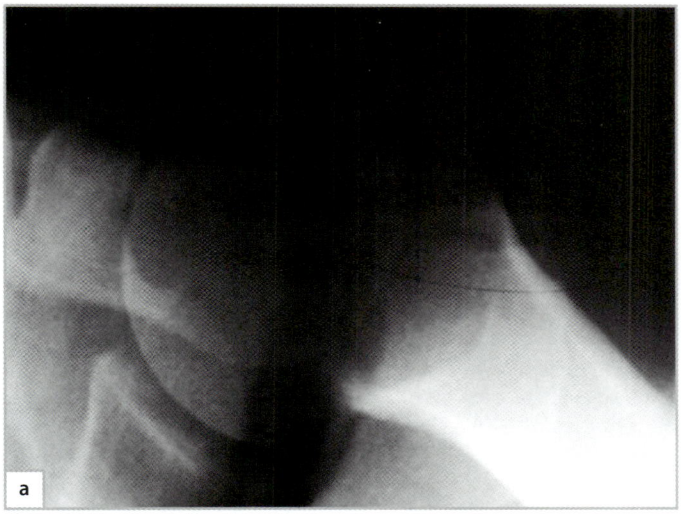

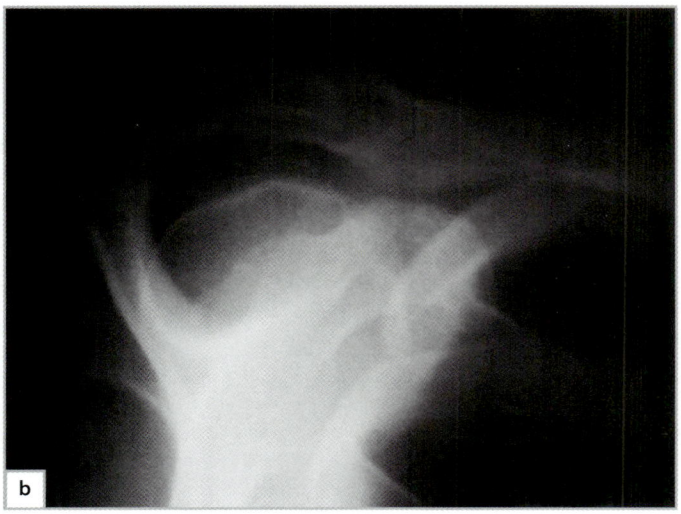

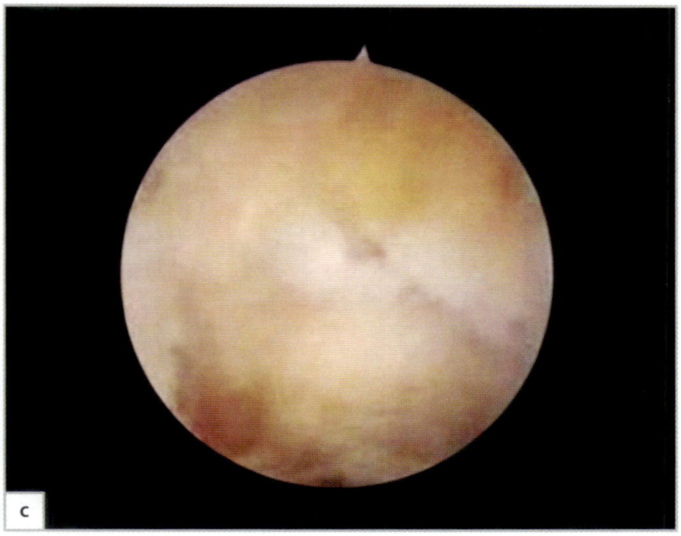

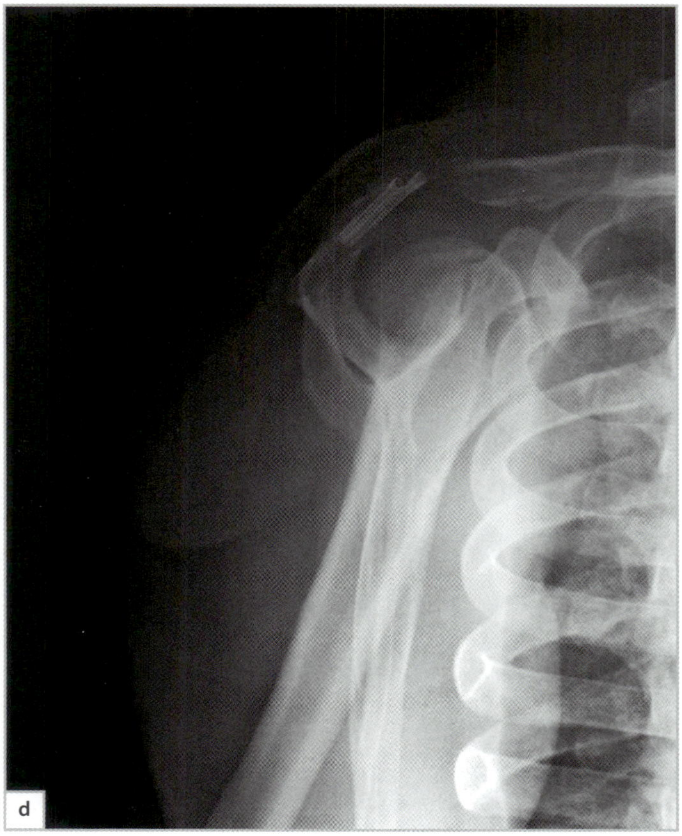

Figure 3.10 Fixation of a fracture of the acromion. *Contd.*

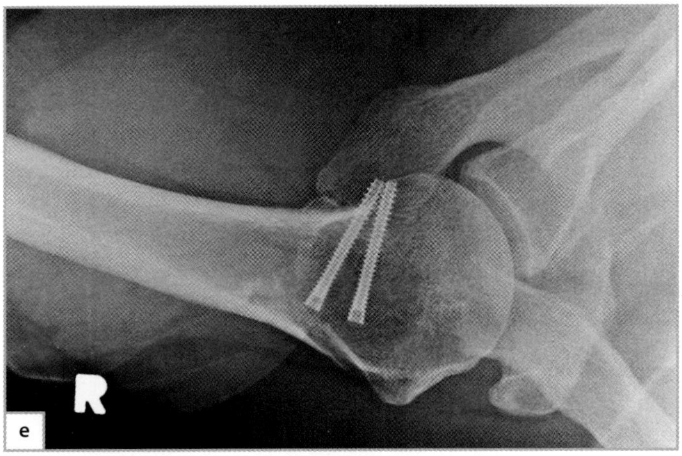

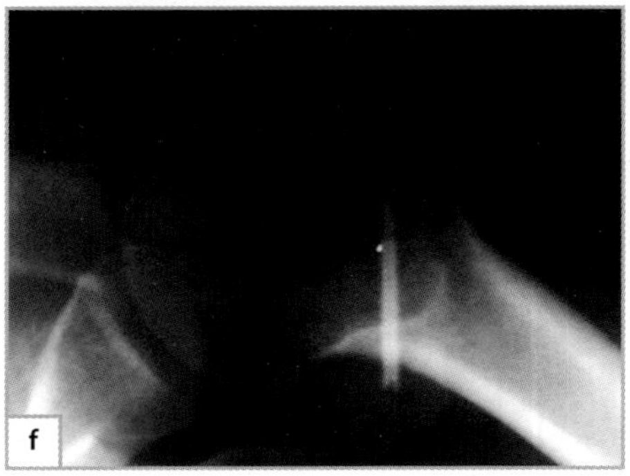

Figure 3.10 Fixation of a fracture of the acromion. (a) Unfused os acromionale that was injured and became unstable. (b) The area of separation on the axillary view. (c) Arthroscopic view subacromially from a lateral portal of fixation (helpful in debriding of the cartilage surfaces, and in monitoring the insertion and fixation). (d–f) Three views of the completed repair.

Arthroscopically assisted fixation is accomplished while viewing subacromially from a lateral portal (**Fig. 3.10c**). The shaver may be introduced from superiorly, directly through the separation, in order to prepare each side for fixation. A large tenaculum clamp is then placed with the hook tips on the front and back edges of the acromion, to reduce and compress the two fragments of the os once the wires have been passed. Two cannulated screw guide wires are inserted from anterior to posterior across the os under arthroscopic control. The fracture is reduced with a tenaculum once the wires have been properly positioned. Cannulated compression screws are then inserted over the wires, with the tenaculum in place to prevent inadvertent downward tilting of the anterior fragment during fixation (**Fig. 3.10d–f**).

Pearls and pitfalls

Pearls

- Preoperative planning of fixation is essential.
- A wide variety of fixation tools should be available.
- The patient is best positioned to allow both arthroscopy and fluoroscopy before beginning the surgery.
- The surgeon should identify and spear the movable fragment with a K-wire under fluoroscopic control before beginning the arthroscopy, to minimize associated edema.
- Visualization of the fracture is essential. The surgeon should find the best portal for visualization of the injury.
- Damage should be repaired in order of significance: spending an hour repairing a small labral tear in a patient with a displaced fracture of the greater tuberosity is inappropriate use of surgical time - the main problem should be fixed first.

Pitfalls

- Swelling. (Arthroscopic management of fractures is a race between swelling and fixation. It is very easy to spend too much time 'cleaning up' for visualization. Planning and efficiency are essential.)
- Accepting less than adequate fixation due to swelling and time.
- Failure to gain control of the movable fragment before starting the arthroscopy.
- Failure to open when the arthroscopy becomes ineffective: if there is too much swelling or blood, the surgeon should stop and finish open. It is better to add a scar than to do an inadequate job.

REHABILITATION

Rehabilitation is no different from that after open surgery, other than being easier for the patient and the therapist. Most fractures managed by arthroscopically assisted fixation heal much more rapidly than those managed using open procedures, so we tend to follow these patients at more frequent early intervals, in order to advance as rapidly as the fracture allows.

We usually get patients to start scapular retraction exercises the day after surgery, although they keep wearing an abduction sling. Passive range of movement without rotation (in order to avoid torsion stress to the fracture fixation) is started at week 1, and rotation is usually added between weeks 3 and 6, depending on bone and fixation quality, and the rapidity of healing.

Active rehabilitation starts between weeks 4 and 6, and progresses until full functional restoration is achieved. Adding aquatic therapy early helps the patient to regain range of motion without increasing pain.

FURTHER READING

Carrera EF, Matsumoto MH, Netto NA, Faloppa F. Fixation of greater tuberosity fractures. Arthroscopy 2004;20:e109–e111.

Carro LP, Nunez MP, Llata JL. Arthroscopic-assisted reduction and percutaneous external fixation of a displaced intra-articular glenoid fracture. Arthroscopy 1999;15:211–214.

Dawson FA. Four-part fracture dislocation of the proximal humerus: an arthroscopic approach. Arthroscopy 2003;19:662–666.

Jones CK, Savoie FH III. Arthroscopically assisted open reduction and internal fixation of proximal humerus fractures. In: WH Levine et al., eds. Fractures of the Shoulder Girdle. New York: Marcel Dekker, 2003: 146–154.

Kato S, Kobayashi T, Gonoji Y, Amaya S. Arthroscopy-assisted reduction of impression fracture of the humeral head: a case report. J Shoulder Elbow Surg 2008;17:e11–e14.

Keener JD, Parsons BO, Flatow EL, et al. Outcomes after percutaneous reduction and fixation of proximal humeral fractures. J Shoulder Elbow Surg 2007;16:330–338.

Song HS, Williams GR Jr. Arthroscopic reduction and fixation with suture-bridge technique for displaced or comminuted greater tuberosity fractures. Arthroscopy 2008;24:956–960.

Weber SC. The ten millimeter rule revisited: nonoperative treatment of the displaced greater tuberosity fractures. Paper presented at the 14th Open Meeting of the American Shoulder and Elbow Surgeons, 15 February 1997, San Francisco.

Chapter 4 Open reduction and internal fixation of fractures of the greater and lesser tuberosities

Jeffrey M. Bair, Ilya Voloshin

FRACTURES OF THE GREATER TUBEROSITY

Diagnosis and assessment

Isolated fractures of the greater tuberosity (GT) account for approximately 15–20% of all fractures of the proximal humerus (Bahrs et al. 2006) but few (roughly 5%) require surgical treatment (Bahrs et al. 2006, Gruson et al. 2008). Diagnosis of isolated GT fractures can be difficult radiographically; small fragment size, superimposition of fracture fragments over the intact humeral head, or calcium deposits within the rotator cuff tendon may contribute to misdiagnosis or under-appreciation of the severity of injury (Green and Izzi 2003, Bahrs et al. 2006, Gruson et al. 2008). A study by Ogawa et al. (2003) found that as many as 59% of isolated GT fractures were missed upon initial presentation, and often misdiagnosed as contusions, rotator cuff tears or tendinitis. While a large portion of the missed fractures were Neer one-part fractures, over 25% of Neer two-part GT fractures were misdiagnosed (see Chapter 1 for the Neer classification). The authors found that smaller fragments limited to the supraspinatus facet were at greatest risk of misdiagnosis. In contrast, fractures extending posteriorly to involve the infraspinatus and teres minor facets were less commonly missed.

Accurate diagnosis of isolated GT fractures can be aided by a physical examination (with a finding of severe localized tenderness to palpation at the lateral wall of the GT) and adequate radiographs (Ogawa et al. 2003). Radiographs in three planes are important for the identification and characterization of isolated GT fragments: a true anteroposterior (AP) view in the plane of the scapula, a lateral (scapular Y) view of the scapula, and an axillary lateral view. If it is not possible to position the patient for the axillary view, Velpeau views may be substituted. AP radiographs obtained with 30° humeral external rotation provide the best profile view of the GT, and allow accurate assessment of displacement in the frontal plane, although an axillary lateral view may be beneficial in an assessment of posterior retraction (Flatow et al. 1991, George 2007). Where only limited, inadequate radiographs are available, computerized tomography (CT) may help to characterize and quantify fracture displacement (Green and Izzi 2003, Gruson et al. 2008).

Proposed mechanisms for GT fractures include shear, impaction, and avulsion. Shear forces may occur as a result of a fall onto an outstretched arm or a direct blow to the lateral arm in which the GT is driven into the acromion or glenoid surface. Impaction against the anterior glenoid and avulsion by the rotator cuff muscles may occur with anterior dislocations (George 2007). A recent study found that 57% of isolated GT fractures occurred in combination with anterior glenohumeral dislocations (**Fig. 4.1**). Additionally, the displacement patterns in that study suggested shearing against the glenoid rim as the mechanism, rather than avulsion by the rotator cuff (Bahrs et al. 2006).

Longitudinal tears within the rotator interval are present in more than half of patients with GT fractures. Complete avulsions involving supraspinatus or infraspinatus were also seen, although less frequently (Dimakopoulos et al. 2009).

Indications

Indications for the surgical management of isolated GT fractures include: open fractures, injuries associated with vascular compromise necessitating surgical intervention, and displacement of the GT fragment. Non-displaced GT fractures can be reliably treated non-operatively, generally with a short period of immobilization (1–3 weeks), with the initiation of pendulum and passive range-of-motion exercises in the days after injury, followed by the initiation of active motion and strengthening over 6–12 weeks, depending on radiographic signs of healing. Platzer et al. (2008) found that 97% of isolated GT fractures with <5 mm displacement had a good or excellent outcome when treated non-operatively. However, associated intra-articular pathology such as labral tears and partial tears of the rotator cuff may contribute to lingering pain and disability, even after minimally displaced fractures have healed. Patients presenting with persistent symptoms after fracture healing should be evaluated with a careful physical examination and a magnetic resonance scan to rule out these associated injuries (Green and Izzi 2003).

Neer's classic criteria of 1 cm or 45° to define fragment displacement has proven useful with respect to fractures of the proximal humerus; however, an increasing number of studies, both cadaveric and clinical, have suggested that the definition of displacement for GT fractures should be more stringent. Anatomically, the humeral articular surface rises approximately 8 mm above the top of the GT, suggesting that even smaller amounts of GT displacement may lead to impingement within the subacromial space (Iannotti et al. 1992). Dynamic cadaveric studies demonstrate mechanical blocks to abduction and external rotation with 1 cm of GT displacement superiorly or posteriorly, respectively. Furthermore, a nearly 30% increase in deltoid force was required to achieve humeral abduction with 1 cm of GT displacement (Bono et al. 2001).

Few clinical studies have compared the outcomes of isolated, displaced GT fractures when treated operatively or non-operatively. One such study demonstrated unsatisfactory outcomes in 33% of patients with fractures displaced more than 5 mm treated non-operatively (Platzer et al. 2008). Current accepted definitions for displacement of GT fractures is >5 mm, or >3 mm in athletes or patients who perform frequent overhead activities (Platzer et al. 2005).

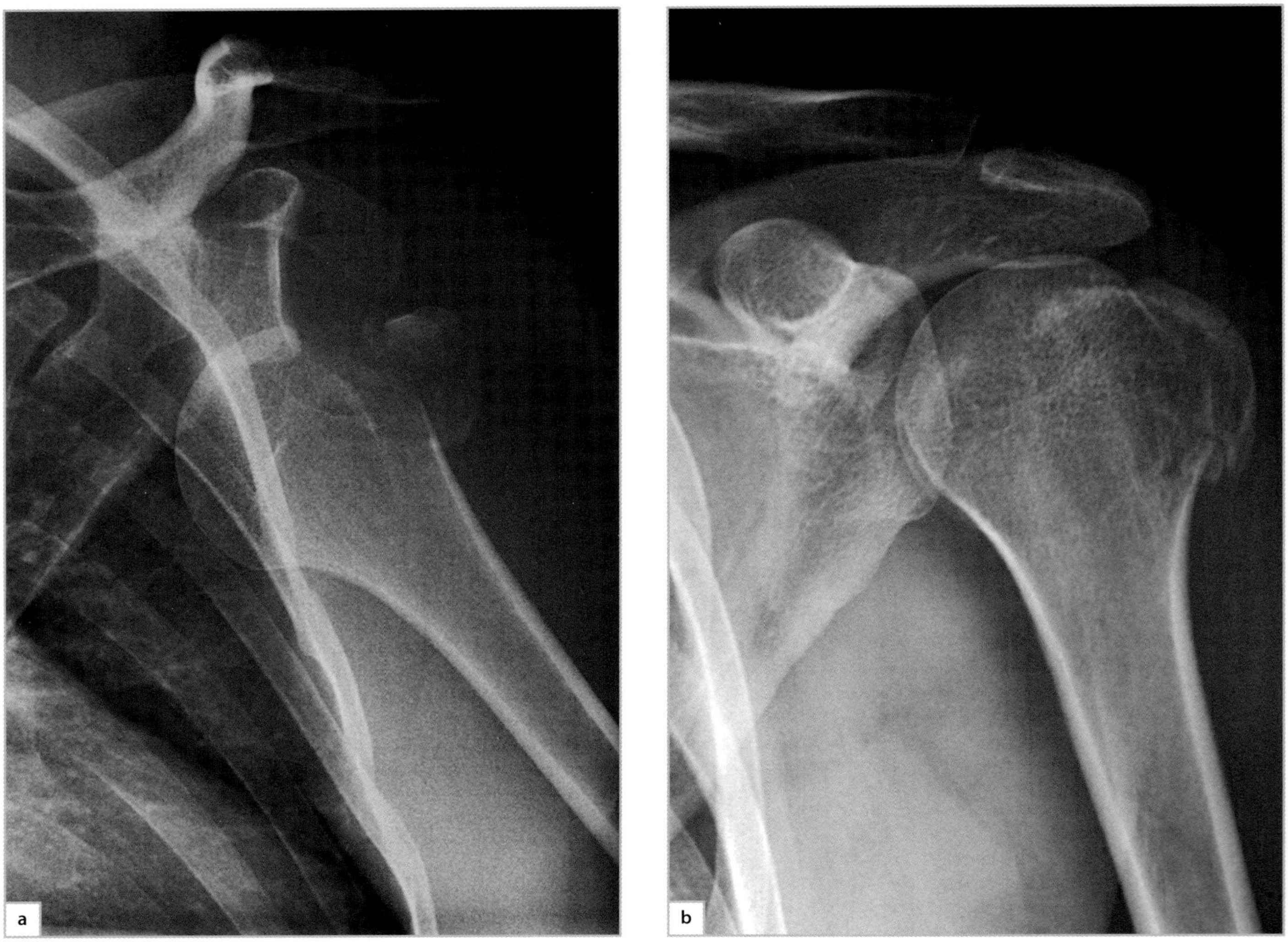

Figure 4.1 Isolated fracture of the greater tuberosity with anterior glenohumeral dislocation. (a) Pre-reduction view; (b) after reduction. Reduction of the dislocation often improves the position of the fragment of the greater tuberosity. Care should be taken to evaluate the injury radiographically for non-displaced fractures of the surgical neck, to prevent displacement with attempts at reduction.

Indications for surgical management relate to patient characteristics, fracture qualities, and surgeon experience. Patient-specific considerations include age, associated comorbidities, activity level, functional demands, hand dominance, and bone quality. Characteristics of the fracture to consider include degree of displacement, anatomic location, presence of comminution, and deforming forces (Gruson et al. 2008).

Contraindications

Patient-specific factors that may lead to decisions to treat fractures non-surgically include medical comorbidities that contribute to risk profiles in the perioperative period that outweigh the potential benefits of surgery. Additionally, patients who lack the mental capacity to comply with postoperative management protocols should be considered for non-operative management.

Non-displaced fractures are unlikely to benefit from surgical stabilization, as they are often stable and amenable to early, progressive mobilization.

Technique

Open reduction and internal fixation techniques remain the gold standard for the management of displaced, isolated GT fractures, with closed reduction and percutaneous fixation providing an alternative for large GT fragments. Also, several studies describe arthroscopic techniques for the management of displaced GT fractures (see Chapter 3); these are associated with less soft-tissue disruption, although they are technically demanding, due to constraints within the subacromial space.

Patients are placed in the beach-chair position for open surgical management. The patient's head should be positioned at the top of the bed, with the operative limb positioned with the shoulder off the edge of the operating table, to facilitate exposure and to achieve adequate intraoperative imaging. The free arm should be supported intraoperatively with a padded Mayo stand or a hydraulic, articulated arm-holder. A fluoroscope should be positioned prior to draping the patient, to ensure adequate imaging. A large fluoroscopy C-arm unit positioned parallel with the operating table, entering from a cephalad position, will give AP and axillary lateral views (**Fig. 4.2**). Exposure of the fracture site can be achieved using either of two well described surgical techniques: an anterosuperior deltoid-splitting approach, or a standard anterior deltopectoral approach.

The authors' preferred approach utilizes an anterosuperior ('bra-strap' or 'saber') skin incision (**Fig. 4.3**) at the lateral margin of the acromion, along Langer's lines, followed by splitting of the deltoid muscle fibers, which provides direct access to the fractured GT, including exposure of the posterior portion and rotator cuff for possible repair. Distal extension of the deltoid split is limited by the axillary nerve located 4–5 cm distal to the acromion; a stay suture should be placed at the distal extent of the deltoid fascial split to limit inadvertent propagation and iatrogenic injury to the axillary nerve. The anterosuperior incision gives direct exposure of the fracture site, with the ability to address posterior displacement and concomitant rotator cuff pathology. Disadvantages of this approach are the risk of axillary nerve injury, possible detachment of the deltoid origin, and limited distal exposure, which makes management of fractures with extension to the surgical neck more difficult. However, an extended exposure, to the lateral aspect of the proximal humerus, has been described that facilitates identification and protection of the axillary nerve, while utilizing a deltoid-splitting anterolateral approach to gain access distal to the surgical neck of the humerus (Gardner et al. 2008).

Alternatively, a standard deltopectoral approach (**Fig. 4.4**) allows anterior exposure of the proximal humerus, including the surgical neck, which may be advantageous for large GT fragments. The skin incision is made anteriorly, starting superior and lateral to the coracoid process, and extending along the deltopectoral interval towards the deltoid muscle insertion. Care should be taken to identify and protect the cephalic vein within the interval; retraction of the vein laterally with the deltoid may minimize the number of venous perforations requiring ligation. The clavipectoral fascia is incised, permitting exposure of the subscapularis, access to the subacromial space, and exposure of the fracture.

With adequate exposure of the fracture site from either surgical approach, the fracture bed is debrided of hematoma, and the fragment is mobilized and debrided of overlying bursal tissue. Many fixation techniques have been described, including cancellous screws, tension-band wiring, and transosseous suture methods. With large fragments in younger patients with optimal bone quality, cancellous screws placed through the GT fragment extending into the subchondral bone of the humeral head can be used. Washers are often used to distribute compression forces over a larger surface area (**Fig. 4.5**).

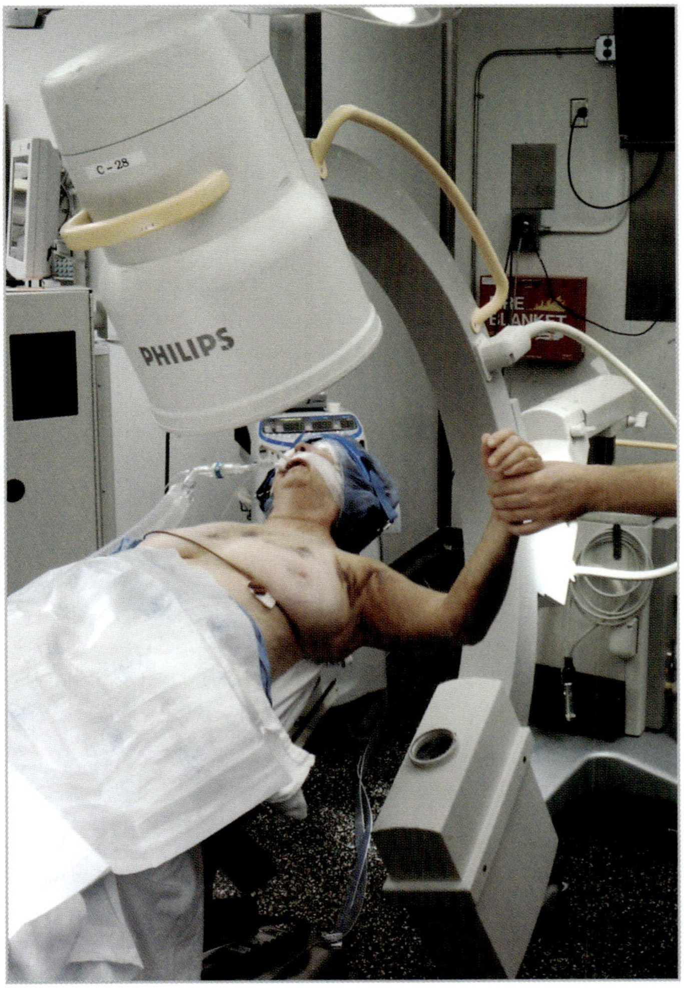

Figure 4.2 Preoperative setup demonstrating a supine, beach-chair position. A large fluoroscopy C-arm is positioned to enter from a cephalad position. Anteroposterior and axillary lateral images may be obtained by rotating the C-arm over the top or under the limb.

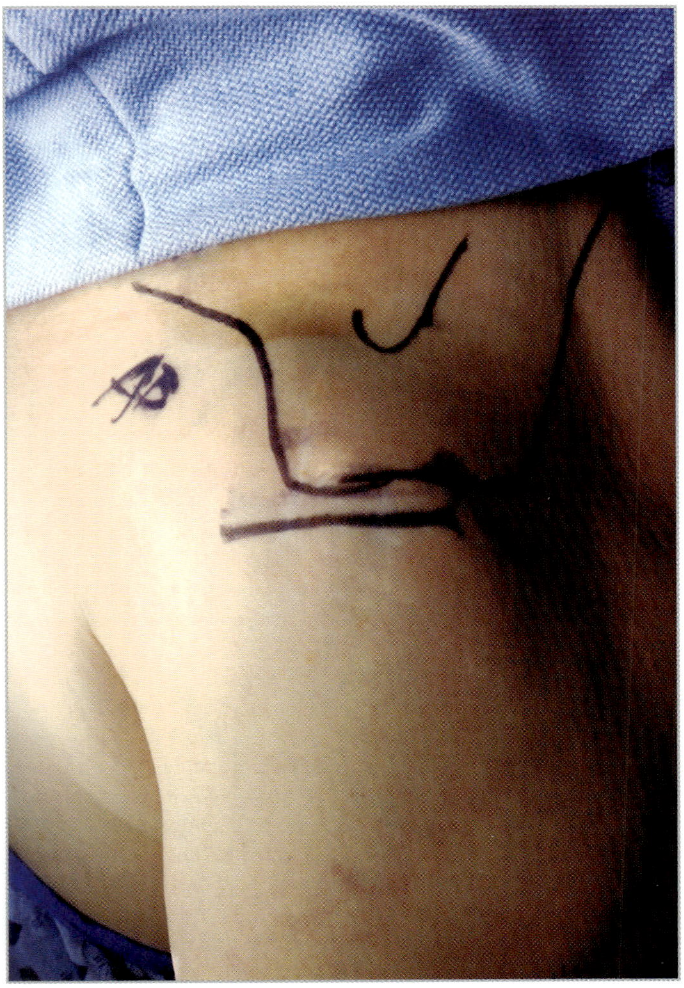

Figure 4.3 Anterosuperior (saber) incision. Landmarks are drawn to define the bony outlines of the acromion, clavicle, and coracoid process. The skin incision is placed at the lateral margin of the acromion.

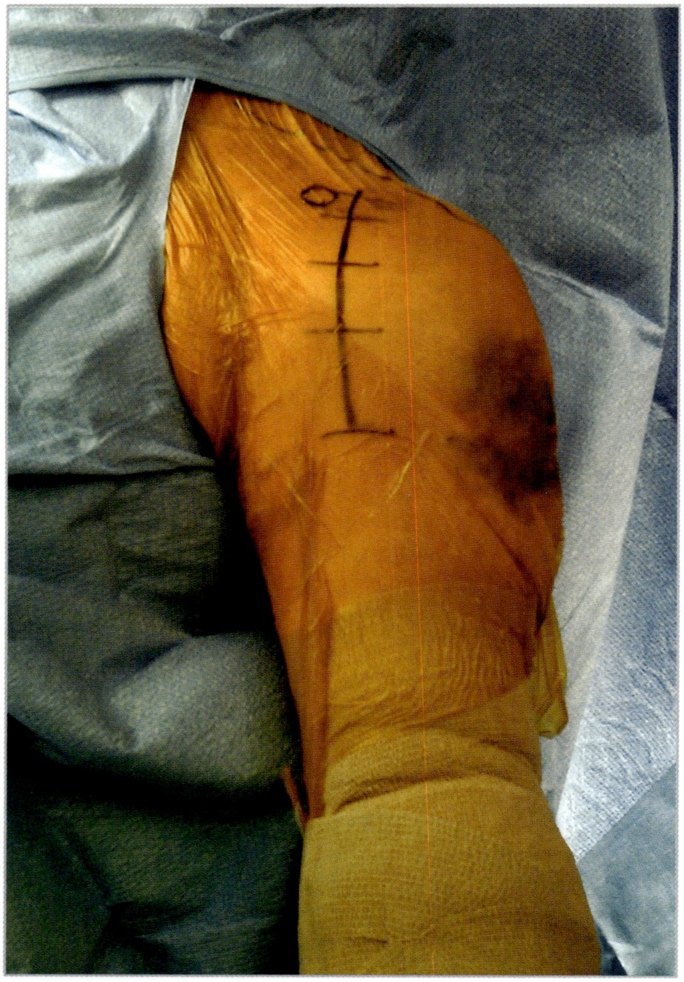

Figure 4.4 Deltopectoral approach. Bony landmarks are outlined, including the acromion, clavicle, and coracoid process. The skin incision is placed superolateral to the coracoids, and extends distally toward the deltoid insertion on the humerus.

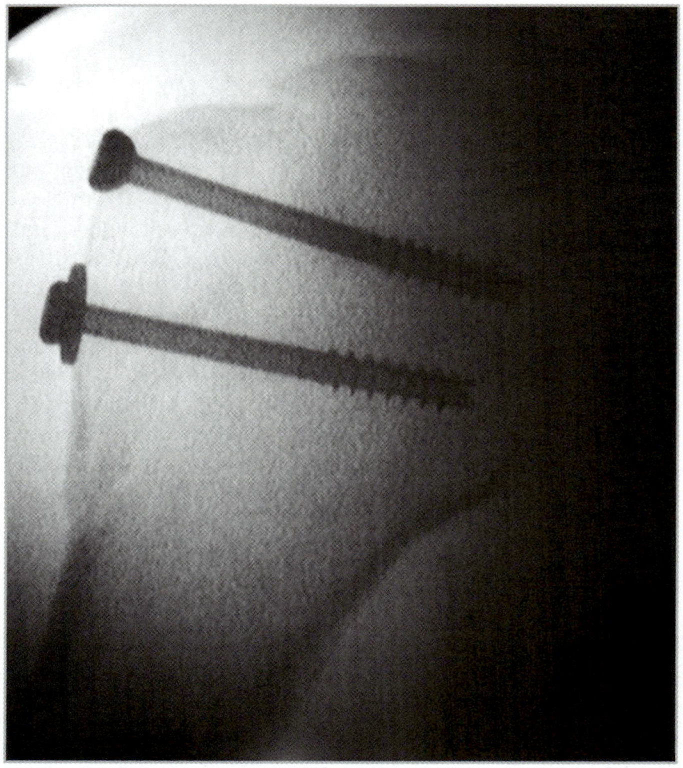

Figure 4.5 Fixation with screws for a fracture of the greater tuberosity. Large, isolated fragments of the greater tuberosity may be stabilized using 4.0 mm cancellous screws. The use of washers may facilitate distribution of compressive forces over a larger surface area. Courtesy of Columbia Center for Shoulder, Elbow and Sports Medicine.

However, the GT fragment is often comminuted, is of poor bone quality, or is too small to facilitate screw fixation, and compromises fixation if screws are used. Tension-band wiring utilizes 18 G wire passed proximally at the bone–tendon interface of the fragment, through drill holes, or around a screw placed distal to the fracture bed. Fragment reduction is facilitated as the wire is tensioned over the fragment (**Fig. 4.6**).

Suture methods utilize heavy non-absorbable suture passed through the fragment at the bone–tendon interface, and passed transosseously through drill holes. They may be accomplished using open or arthroscopic techniques. Commercially available suture anchors provide an alternative to transosseous suturing techniques and allow for double-row suture fixation. (Flatow et al. 1991). In one method the suture is passed through the GT fragment, entering the cancellous fracture bed, and exiting through cortical drill holes (**Fig. 4.7**). Sutures are strategically placed at the superior and inferior margins of the fragment, and passed through tunnels that provide a spread of fixation points along the fracture bed. In total, five separate sutures are used to secure the superior, midportion, and inferior aspects of the fragment (Dimakopoulos et al. 2009). Other suture techniques pass the suture in a 'figure of eight' through the fracture site in an effort to prevent overcompression (Green and Izzi 2003).

Suture anchors have also been demonstrated to be helpful for suture fixation of isolated GT fractures, eliminating the need for transosseous drill holes for fixation, or direct passage through a comminuted GT fragment. One double-row technique places two or three suture anchors within the proximal portion of the fracture bed, passing the suture strands through the supraspinatus tendon approximately 5 mm proximal to the insertion site. These sutures are tied in horizontal 'mattress' fashion, providing a medial row of fixation. Double-row fixation is achieved by placing an additional suture anchor or two in the cortical bone at the distal margin of the fracture site. The fracture is then secured by tying the proximal row of suture strands to the distal row of sutures, or by passing one limb of the distal row of sutures through the bone–tendon junction and tying (as with simple sutures) (Bhatia et al. 2006).

Our preferred technique utilizes suture anchors placed at the medial border of the fracture bed, and suture-locking anchors placed distal to the fracture bed, to achieve transosseous equivalent fixation. Suture-locking anchors are commercially available products, designed to capture the free limb(s) of a previously placed suture within the anchor, and provide fixation to bone by inserting the anchor into a hole drilled into the bone, thus achieving friction-based fixation of the free suture limb(s) to the bone surface. These types of anchor allow fixation methods that achieve compression over a larger area of tendon footprint, and in effect are equivalent to a transosseous repair technique. The proximal row of sutures is passed through the bone–tendon interface and tied as horizontal mattress stitches, with the free limbs tensioned over the fragment, and secured distally using suture-locking anchors placed within the lateral cortex distal to the fracture bed (**Fig. 4.8**).

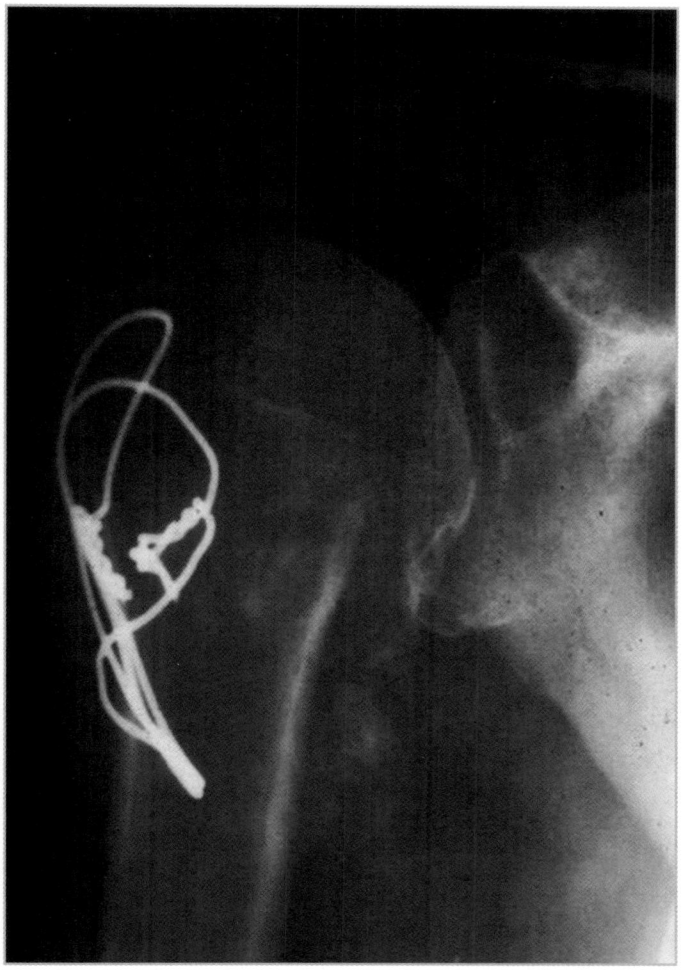

Figure 4.6 **Tension-band wiring technique.** Isolated fragments of the greater tuberosity may be repaired using 18 G wire to provide compressive forces over the fracture fragment. Courtesy of Columbia Center for Shoulder, Elbow and Sports Medicine.

Suture-anchor techniques may be performed arthroscopically with encouraging results, despite being technically challenging due to the limited amount of room within the subacromial space. The author's preference is to place the patient in the beach-chair position, although the lateral decubitus position is an alternative (George 2007). Intra-articular examination is performed through a posterior viewing portal; an anterior working portal is used for debridement and examination of the articular surface of the rotator cuff and fracture fragment debridement. The extent of the fracture and rotator cuff tear is marked by passing sutures from the glenohumeral joint into the subacromial space for later identification. Sutures anchors may be placed into the fracture bed through the anterior portal (or percutaneously via a transtendinous insertion), and suture strands passed through the rotator cuff into the subacromial space to establish medial row fixation. The arthroscope is then placed into the subacromial space and a standard lateral working portal is created. After subacromial bursectomy/debridement to facilitate visualization, the fracture bed and fragment are debrided of hematoma. A lateral row of suture anchors is placed at the distal extent of the fracture bed at the anterior and posterior aspects, with the suture strands passed through the rotator cuff bone–tendon junction and between the previously passed (untied) medial row of sutures and the bone fragment. The medial row of sutures are tied in horizontal mattress fashion to establish first reduction of the medial footprint of the rotator cuff, followed by reduction of the fragment, under direct arthroscopic visualization. Arthroscopic graspers or a blunt trocar may be used to maintain fracture reduction. Kirschner wires (K-wires) may be utilized for provisional fixation (Carrera et al. 2004). Intraoperative fluoroscopy should be used to confirm fracture reduction before the lateral row of sutures is tied. Stability is achieved after tying the medial and lateral rows of sutures. The arthroscope may be returned to the glenohumeral joint for intra-articular confirmation of fracture reduction (Ji et al. 2007). A similar arthroscopic suture fixation technique utilizes suture-locking anchors in lieu of a laterally placed, second row of suture anchors (Kim et al. 2008).

Careful repair of the longitudinally torn rotator interval using side-to-side sutures should be performed after fracture stabilization, for both open and arthroscopic fixation techniques (George 2007, Ji et al. 2007, Kim et al. 2008).

Pearls and pitfalls

- Preoperative preparation should include adequate images to define the fracture size, location, and pattern.
- Both the patient and a large fluoroscopy C-arm unit should be positioned to ensure optimal intraoperative fluoroscopic images in the AP and axillary planes, prior to prepping and draping the patient.
- Exposure and visualization of the fracture are key, and are a priority when using either the open or the arthroscopic approach.
- Adequate stability will facilitate early mobilization (through a postoperative rehabilitation program) to prevent stiffness.
- Excision of bone fragments should be avoided, as bone-to-bone healing is more reliable than tendon-to-bone healing.
- Over-reduction of the fracture fragment into the fracture bed or distal malreduction should be avoided, as this can lead to over-tensioning of the rotator cuff.
- Excessive retraction may injure the axillary nerve, leading to motor and sensory deficits postoperatively.

Rehabilitation

Postoperatively, patients should be managed with sling immobilization; an abduction immobilizer with an abduction pillow will minimize the tension across the repair site that occurs with adduction of the arm. Rehabilitation protocols closely mimic those of rotator cuff repairs. Sling immobilization usually lasts for six weeks, during which time it is removed only for therapy exercises. Pendulum exercises are initiated within the immediate postoperative period (1–3 days), with progression to supine passive forward elevation and external rotation as tolerated. Restriction of humeral adduction and internal rotation is necessary to avoid stress across the repair site. Active and active assisted motion with further stretching is initiated 6–8 weeks after surgery. Strengthening of the shoulder girdle and specific strengthening of the rotator cuff muscles begins 8–12 weeks after surgery. Patients should be advised preoperatively that recovery may take up to a year (Green and Izzi 2003, Gruson et al. 2008).

FRACTURES OF THE LESSER TUBEROSITY

Diagnosis and assessment

Fractures of the lesser tuberosity (LT) are rarely isolated (i.e. Neer two-part fractures) as they tend to occur in combination (Neer three- and four-part fractures). The estimated annual incidence in adults is 0.46

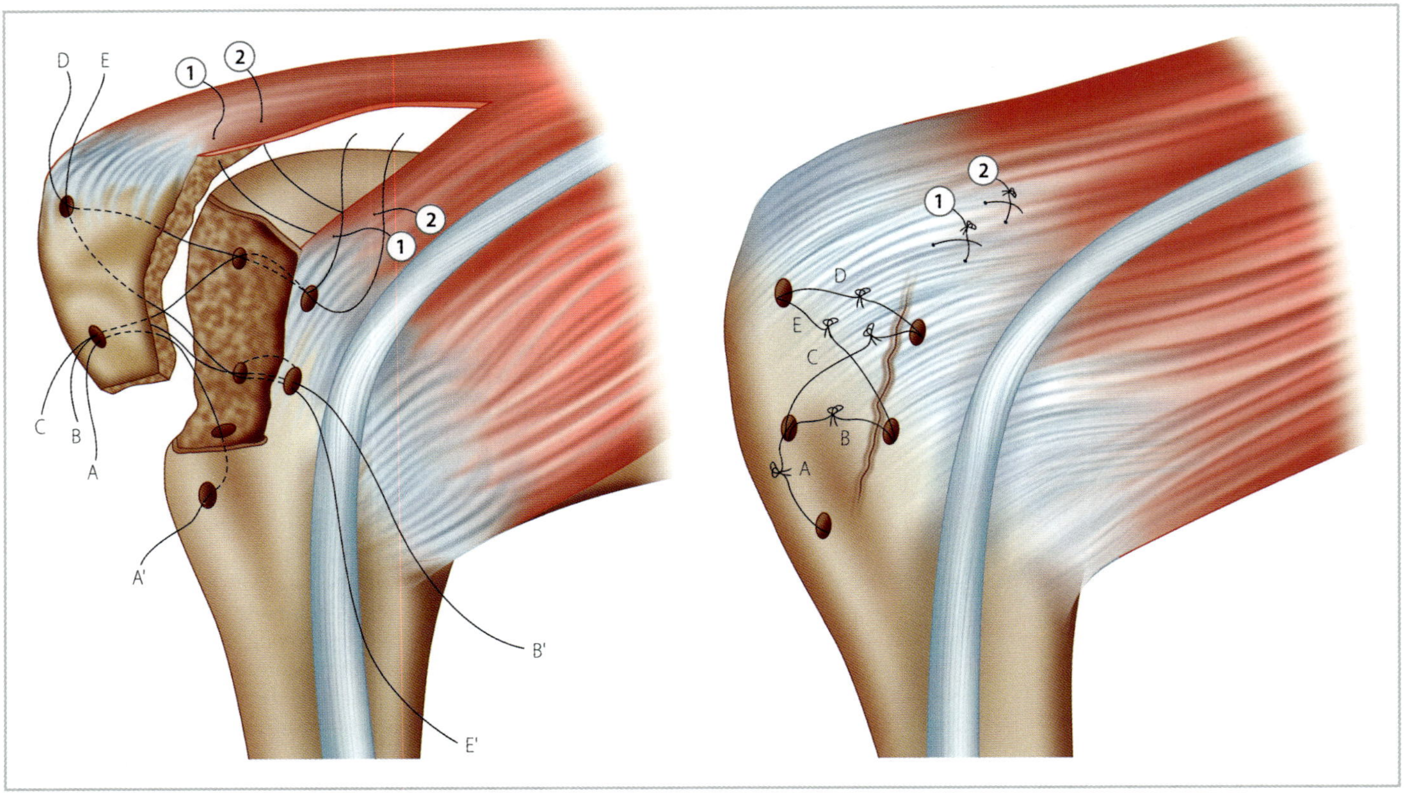

Figure 4.7 Illustration of the suture technique for larger fractures of the greater tuberosity. Heavy non-absorbable suture is passed directly through the fracture fragment and into the fracture bed, exiting through drill holes at the periphery of the fracture. The five sutures (A–E) pass through two entry points in the fragment of the greater tuberosity, and exit through three points around the periphery of the fracture bed. Sutures 1 and 2 represent figure-of-eight techniques to repair a longitudinal tear in the supraspinatus or rotator interval.

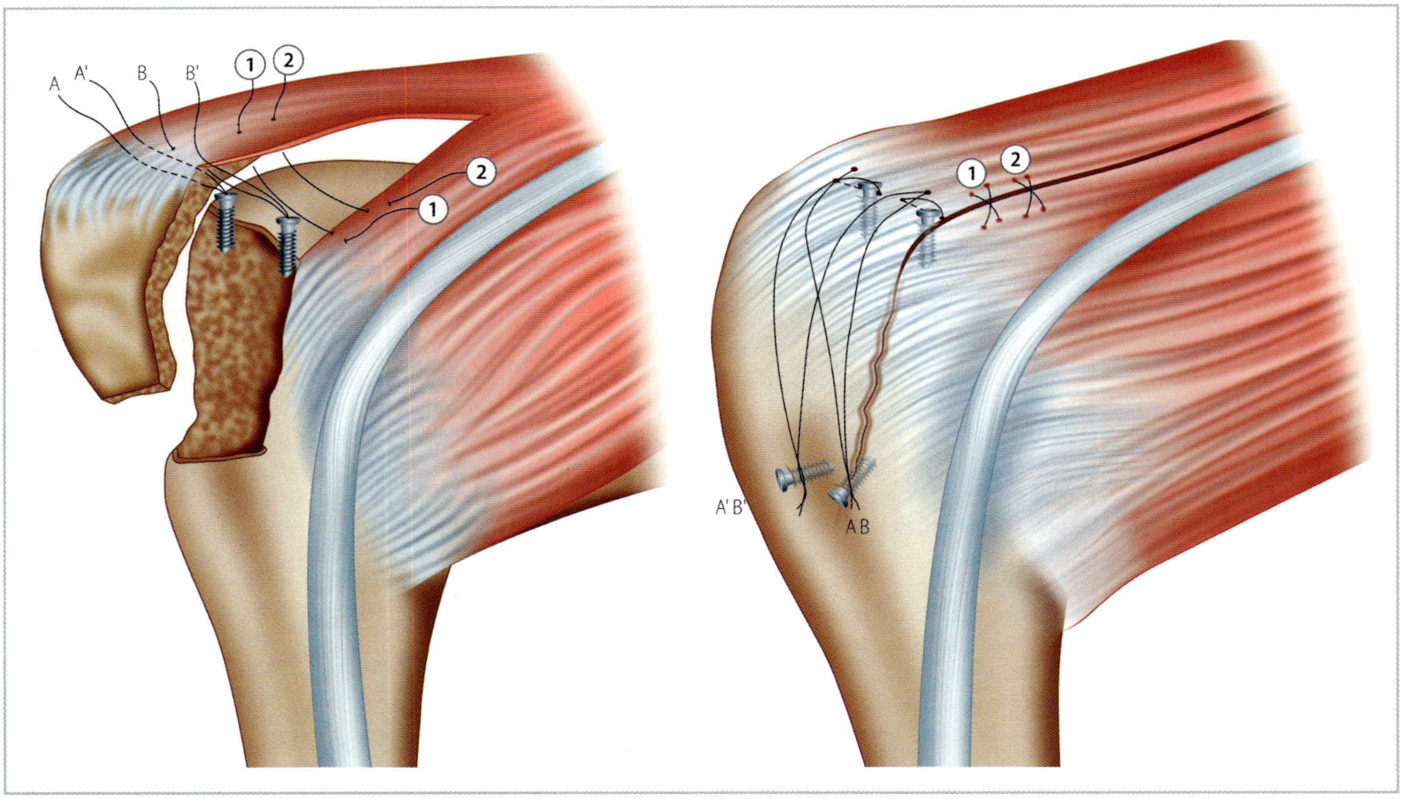

Figure 4.8 Illustration of double-row suture anchor fixation. A row of suture anchors is placed medial to the fracture bed. Suture limbs are passed through supraspinatus at the bone–tendon junction. The sutures are then tied, creating a horizontal mattress stitch establishing the medial row. Limbs of the sutures are then passed over the fragment using suture-locking anchors that allow tensioning, to establish double-row fixation at the distal margin of the fracture bed and compression of the tendon's footprint.

per 100,000 (Robinson et al. 2009). Most current literature is limited to case reports or small case series; there are no reports of controlled studies comparing operative with non-operative management, and no studies have directly compared stabilization techniques. Reported mechanisms of injury include LT avulsion due to forced abduction and external rotation of the arm, forceful contraction of the subscapularis, and shearing of the LT against the anterior glenoid rim; fractures can also occur with a posterior shoulder dislocation, with a large associated reverse Hill-Sachs lesion (Robinson et al. 2009).

Most reported injuries are the result of falls from moderate heights (e.g. from ladders or off bicycles or motorcycles or horses, or down a couple of steps) but assault-related causes are also common (Ogawa and Takahashi 1997, Robinson et al. 2009). Diagnosis may be difficult in the trauma setting, because the history the patient gives is often non-specific regarding the mechanism of injury, and physical examination is frequently limited by pain with palpation and attempted range of motion. Axillary lateral radiographs are the diagnostic key to identify isolated LT fractures and to gauge the degree of displacement. It is recommended that an axillary lateral view should be included for all shoulder traumas. Additional details of the fracture size and morphology and involvement of the articular surface or bicipital groove may be obtained with computerized tomography of the shoulder (van Laarhoven et al. 1995, Robinson et al. 2009).

Associated injuries of the shoulder include posterior dislocation (which often goes unrecognized), proximal biceps tendon pathology, including rupture or instability due to disruption of the medial wall of the bicipital groove, and tear of the rotator interval (Ogawa and Takahashi 1997, Gruson et al. 2008, Robinson et al. 2009).

Indications

Traditional criteria of >1 cm or angulation >45° should be considered as operative indications for isolated LT fractures (Robinson et al. 2009). However, recent reports suggest that any amount of radiographically visible displacement of the LT should be considered for operative stabilization, given the limited results of delayed reconstruction and the potential for progressive displacement by the unopposed pull of the subscapularis, as well as the potential development of subcoracoid impingement (van Laarhoven et al. 1995, Ogawa and Takahashi 1997, Kowalsky et al. 2007, Robinson et al. 2009). Motor weakness or blocks to motion - signs of a displaced fracture - are indications for surgical management (Gruson et al. 2008).

Contraindications

Surgical stabilization of isolated LT fractures should be avoided in medically complex patients with non-modifiable surgical risk factors that outweigh the benefits of operative management. Additionally, operative treatment should be avoided in patients who are unwilling or unable to comply with the postoperative rehabilitation protocols and activity restrictions that apply.

Technique

Displaced, isolated fractures of the LT are most easily approached through the deltopectoral interval to the anterior shoulder. Fractures associated with posterior dislocations may be irreducible using closed methods thus requiring open reduction. In such cases, an extended deltoid-splitting technique may be used to reduce the head (Robinson et al. 2009) but we prefer a deltopectoral approach with a Wissinger rod introduced through a posterior stab incision (standard posterior arthroscopy portal) to facilitate reduction of the humeral head.

Patients are positioned supine in beach-chair fashion, with a padded Mayo stand or a hydraulic, articulating arm-holder used to support the limb. A standard deltopectoral approach is performed, as described above. The clavipectoral fascia is incised to facilitate exposure of the proximal humerus. The LT fragment and fracture bed should be readily identifiable in acute cases. The fracture fragments are gently debrided of hematoma to facilitate anatomic reduction. A traction suture placed at the bone–tendon junction of the subscapularis may be advantageous for reduction maneuvers. Provisional stabilization is obtained using large, pointed reduction forceps or K-wires, but may be difficult where there are multiple smaller fragments. In cases with larger fragments (>2 cm), the use of 3.5 mm cancellous screws (with or without washers) will provide adequate stabilization for early motion. Multiple screws may be placed, depending upon fracture size and orientation. Screw trajectory is anterior to posterior with 45° shoulder external rotation, to prevent overtensioning of the subscapularis. Emphasis should be placed on achieving bicortical fixation when available, while avoiding penetration of the articular surface; this often requires screws 40–50 mm in length (Robinson et al. 2009).

Fragments of the LT that preclude screw fixation because of their small size or comminution may be stabilized using suture techniques, similar to those described above for GT fractures (Flatow et al. 1991). Heavy, non-absorbable suture is passed through the bone–tendon junction of the subscapularis (which provides optimal tissue), through drill holes placed at the lateral and inferior margins of the fracture bed (**Fig. 4.9**). Similar to stabilization with screws, a transosseous suture repair should be performed with the shoulder at 45° of external rotation to prevent overtightening of the subscapularis (Robinson et al. 2009). An arthroscopic technique has also been described which utilizes suture anchors placed into the fracture bed, with mattress sutures passed through the bone–tendon

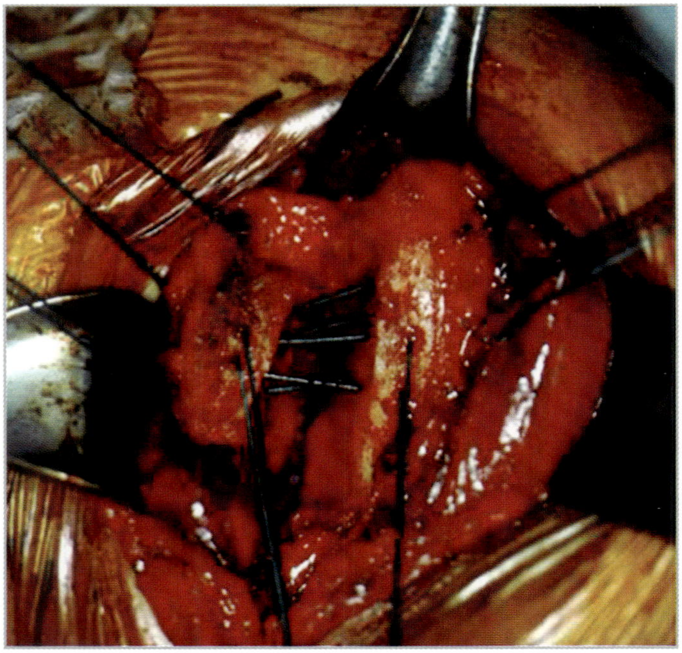

Figure 4.9 Suture repair techniques for fractures of the lesser tuberosity. Sutures are passed through the bone–tendon junction and through the fracture bed, exiting through 2.7 mm drill holes. Courtesy of Columbia Center for Shoulder, Elbow and Sports Medicine.

junction of the subscapularis for stabilization of the osseous fragment (Scheibel et al. 2005).

Intraoperatively, attention should be given to restoration of the congruity of the articular surface, and to the integrity of the bicipital groove, as these two structures are commonly involved (Robinson et al. 2009). Large LT fragments may include an anteromedial portion of the articular surface; if so, it should be anatomically reduced and stabilized under direct visualization, to minimize the risks of late post-traumatic arthrosis.

One particular consideration when performing this arthroscopic technique is the recognition of an intact 'pulley' to maintain reduction of the biceps tendon within the intertubercular groove. Injuries involving the superior aspect of the LT and the medial wall of the bicipital groove may disrupt the 'pulley', permitting medial displacement of the biceps tendon. Reduction and stabilization (via arthroscopic or open techniques) of the LT may restore tendon stability within the groove, although tenodesis or tenotomy may be required if persistent instability is noted. In these cases, the authors' preference is for subpectoral biceps tenodesis, to avoid the risk of anterior shoulder pain, which may occur with scarring or incarceration of the biceps tendon within the bicipital groove.

Fractures resulting from posterior dislocations should be assessed for shoulder stability intraoperatively, as patients with large, engaging reverse Hill-Sachs lesions may require additional procedures for restoration of glenohumeral stability.

Pearls and pitfalls

- Radiographic imaging is required for diagnosis and evaluation. An axillary lateral view should be included for the evaluation of shoulder trauma. Computerized tomography should be used for further evaluation of the morphology and extent of isolated LT fractures.
- Adequate exposure, achieved by open or arthroscopic techniques, is necessary for anatomic reduction of the fracture.
- To prevent stiffness, sufficient stability is necessary to allow early mobilization postoperatively with passive pendulum exercises.
- Biceps tendon pathology should be identified - including ruptures and instability - and treated accordingly, to minimize the risk of persistent anterior shoulder pain.

Rehabilitation

Postoperatively, patients should be managed in an immobilizer in neutral positions for abduction, rotation, and shoulder flexion. The immobilizer should be used for six weeks. Passive pendulum exercises should be initiated immediately postoperatively (1-3 days), with progression to active assisted exercises after two weeks. External rotation and abduction of the shoulder should be avoided to minimize tension across the fracture repair site. These limitations may be determined with an intraoperative examination to assess repair site tension during external rotation and abduction. Further isometric strengthening and active range-of-motion rehabilitation of the shoulder girdle and rotator cuff muscles should continue over the next four to six months, similar to rehabilitation after surgery to repair an isolated rotator cuff.

REFERENCES

Bahrs C, Lingenfelter E, Fischer F, et al. Mechanism of injury and morphology of the greater tuberosity fracture. J Shoulder Elbow Surg 2006;15:140–147.

Bhatia DN, van Rooyen KS, du Toit DF, de Beer JF. Surgical treatment of comminuted, displaced fractures of the greater tuberosity of the proximal humerus: a new technique of double-row suture-anchor fixation and long-term results. Injury 2006;37:946–952.

Bono CM, Renard R, Levine RG, Levy AS. Effect of displacement of fractures of the greater tuberosity on the mechanics of the shoulder. J Bone Joint Surg Br 2001;83:1056–1062.

Carrera EF, Matsumoto MH, Netto NA, Faloppa F. Fixation of greater tuberosity fractures. Arthroscopy 2004;20:e109–e111.

Dimakopoulos P, Panagopoulos A, Kasimatis G. Transosseous suture fixation of proximal humeral fractures. Surgical technique. J Bone Joint Surg Am 2009;91 Suppl 2:8–21.

Flatow EL, Cuomo F, Maday MG, et al. Open reduction and internal fixation of two-part displaced fractures of the greater tuberosity of the proximal part of the humerus. J Bone Joint Surg Am 1991;73:1213–1218.

Gardner MJ, Boraiah S, Helfet DL, Lorich DG. The anterolateral acromial approach for fractures of the proximal humerus. J Orthop Trauma 2008;22:132–137.

George MS. Fractures of the greater tuberosity of the humerus. J Am Acad Orthop Surg 2007;15:607–613.

Green A, Izzi J Jr. Isolated fractures of the greater tuberosity of the proximal humerus. J Shoulder Elbow Surg 2003;12:641–649.

Gruson KI, Ruchelsman DE, Tejwani NC. Isolated tuberosity fractures of the proximal humeral: current concepts. Injury 2008;39:284–298.

Iannotti JP, Gabriel JP, Schneck SL, et al. The normal glenohumeral relationships. An anatomical study of one hundred and forty shoulders. J Bone Joint Surg Am 1992;74:491–500.

Ji JH, Kim WY, Ra KH. Arthroscopic double-row suture anchor fixation of minimally displaced greater tuberosity fractures. Arthroscopy 2007;23:1133.e1–4.

Kim KC, Rhee KJ, Shin HD, Kim YM. Arthroscopic fixation for displaced greater tuberosity fracture using the suture-bridge technique. Arthroscopy 2008;24:120.e1–3.

Kowalsky MS, Bell JE, Ahmad CS. Arthroscopic treatment of subcoracoid impingement caused by lesser tuberosity malunion: a case report and review of the literature. J Shoulder Elbow Surg 2007;16:e10–14.

Ogawa K, Takahashi M. Long-term outcome of isolated lesser tuberosity fractures of the humerus. J Trauma 1997;42:955–959.

Ogawa K, Yoshida A, Ikegami H. Isolated fractures of the greater tuberosity of the humerus: solutions to recognizing a frequently overlooked fracture. J Trauma 2003;54:713–717.

Platzer P, Kutscha-Lissberg F, Lehr S, et al. The influence of displacement on shoulder function in patients with minimally displaced fractures of the greater tuberosity. Injury 2005;36:1185–1189.

Platzer P, Thalhammer G, Oberleitner G, et al. Displaced fractures of the greater tuberosity: a comparison of operative and nonoperative treatment. J Trauma 2008;65:843–848.

Robinson CM, Teoh KH, Baker A, Bell L. Fractures of the lesser tuberosity of the humerus. J Bone Joint Surg Am 2009;91:512–520.

Scheibel M, Martinek V, Imhoff AB. Arthroscopic reconstruction of an isolated avulsion fracture of the lesser tuberosity. Arthroscopy 2005;21:487–494.

van Laarhoven HA, te Slaa RL, van Laarhoven EW. Isolated avulsion fracture of the lesser tuberosity of the humerus. J Trauma 1995;39:997–999.

Chapter 5 Open reduction and internal fixation of fractures of the surgical neck

Andrew Kai-Hong Chan, Edwin R. Cadet

INTRODUCTION

The surgical neck is involved in the majority of fractures of the proximal humerus seen clinically. It has been estimated that 65% of fractures of the proximal humerus involve the surgical neck alone. These fractures can occur following high-energy trauma (e.g. a motor vehicle accident) in younger individuals, or low-energy trauma in elderly individuals (as the sequela of underlying osteopenia or osteoporosis). Fractures involving displacement of the surgical neck occur secondary to deforming forces exerted on fracture 'parts' by the surrounding musculature. In fractures of the surgical neck, the rotator cuff remains attached to the tuberosities, thus maintaining the humeral head in neutral rotation. The insertion site of the pectoralis major lies just lateral to the bicipital groove and, as a result, medializes and internally rotates the humeral shaft. The humeral head abducts as a result of shaft displacement. Translation of the shaft from the pull of the pectoralis major causes the characteristic deformity seen in fractures of the surgical neck (**Fig. 5.1**). In high-energy cases, there may be significant varus deformity, with the shaft translating laterally, and impacted against the abducted humeral head (**Fig. 5.2**).

Open reduction and internal fixation of these fractures can often be challenging, as there is potential for malreduction, with iatrogenic surgical error causing complications, necessitating further surgery. The indications for surgery, operative technique, 'tricks of the trade', and rehabilitation protocols are presented in this chapter.

INDICATIONS

Isolated fractures of the surgical neck, in the absence of significant displacement, are usually managed non-operatively, with a short course of immobilization and the early initiation of passive range-of-motion exercises (Bigliani 1990, Chun 1994, Koval et al. 1997). According to Neer (1970a), 'significant' displacement of proximal humerus fractures has been defined as fracture fragments displaced more than 1 cm and angulated more than 45°. It has been estimated that approximately 85% of fractures of the surgical neck fall into this category (Bigliani 1990, Chun 1994, Koval et al. 1997). Larger degrees of displacement are well tolerated in elderly, lower-demand patients (Neer 1970b, Keene 1983), and in pediatric and adolescent patients with open physes. In the pediatric and adolescent populations, conservative treatment is generally accepted with angulation measuring: less than 70° in children aged under 5 years; 40–70° in children between 5 and 12 years old; and more than 45° in children over 12 years old (Van Heest 2005).

Operative management for these fractures is indicated for fracture patterns exhibiting significant displacement (i.e. greater than 1 cm and 45° angulation), polytrauma, comorbid ipsilateral arm injuries (e.g. floating shoulder), vascular compromise, open fractures, metastatic fractures (**Fig. 5.3**), and fractures that have failed non-operative management.

With the exception of metastatic fractures, our current preference is to treat displaced fractures of the surgical neck via osteosynthesis with a fixed-angle construct. Proximal humerus locking plates provide a good option to ensure rigid fracture stabilization, particularly in the setting of osteopenic bone and early mobilization. Fixed-angled locking plates neutralize forces exerted on fracture fragments from the pull of the rotator cuff and surrounding musculature, to provide rigid fixation, so that mobilization can begin in the early postoperative period. Proper surgical technique is essential, as complication rates as high as 40% have been cited using locked-plate techniques for fractures of the proximal humerus (Sudkamp et al. 2009).

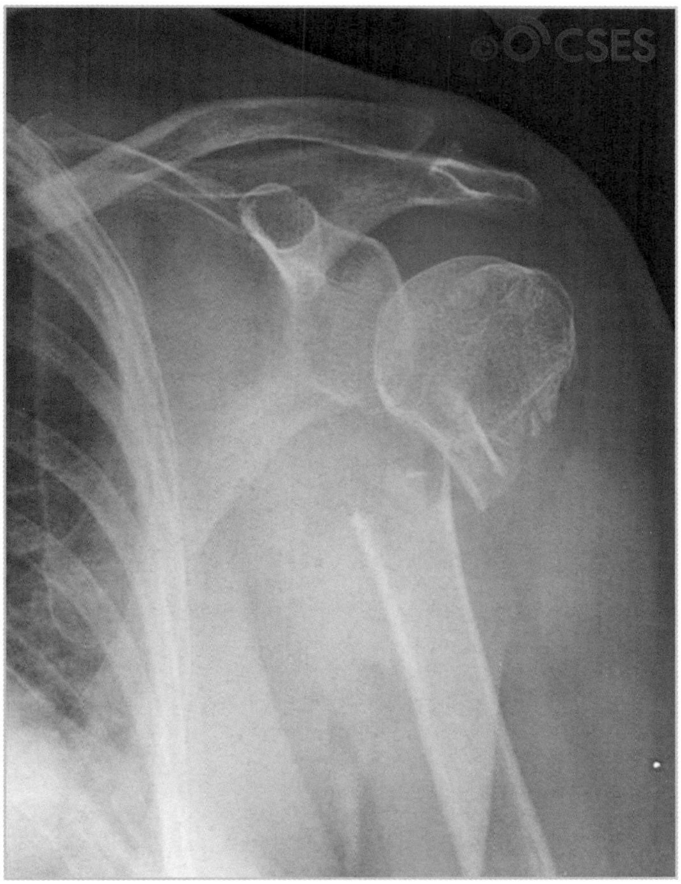

Figure 5.1 Medial shaft displacement. Anteroposterior radiograph of the left humerus demonstrating medial shaft displacement with the humeral head in neutral rotation. Courtesy of the Center for Shoulder, Elbow and Sports Medicine.

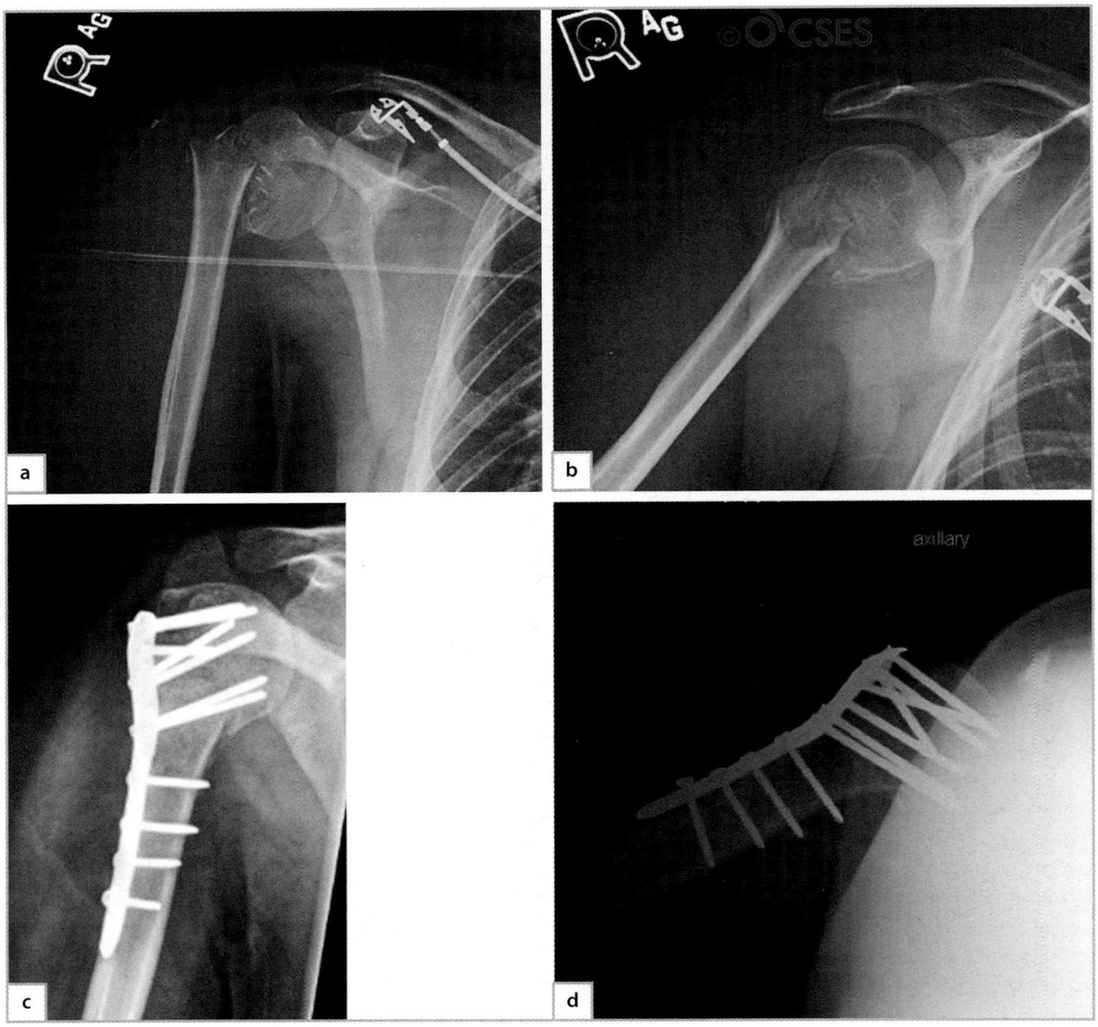

Figure 5.2 Varus deformity with the humerus shaft impacted against the head of the humerus. Anteroposterior view (a) and axillary view (b) of the right shoulder of a 17-year-old male pedestrian who was struck by a motor vehicle. (c,d) Three-month postoperative radiographs following open reduction and internal fixation, demonstrating callus at the medial metaphyseal region and satisfactory placement of locking screws. Courtesy of the Center for Shoulder, Elbow and Sports Medicine.

CONTRAINDICATIONS

The main contraindications for osteosynthesis of fractures of the surgical neck with locking plates are the following scenarios:

- inability to achieve an acceptable reduction intraoperatively, secondary to severe medial calcar comminution, despite structural endosteal strut support or optimal screw position;
- pre-existing poor bone quality that will not support adequate screw fixation;
- metastatic fractures;
- grossly contaminated open fractures that would benefit from preliminary external fixation;
- patients who are unable to comply with postoperative rehabilitation protocols.

Medial calcar support via proper screw placement, or with anatomic reduction, and metaphyseal calcar segment integrity, are necessary for successful outcomes following osteosynthesis with locked plates for fractures of the proximal humerus (Gardner et al. 2007, Gardner et al. 2008, Solberg et al. 2009a, Solberg et al. 2009b). When medial calcar support is not achieved, failure rates are significantly greater (Gardner et al. 2007). Strategies for re-establishing medial calcar support in the setting of comminution are discussed below. Furthermore, in some cases, severely osteopenic bone will not support screw fixation. When the extent of osteoporosis compromises screw fixation, open reduction with suture fixation using strong, non-absorbable sutures yields acceptable results (Park et al. 2003).

TECHNIQUE

Proper patient positioning is the first of many critical steps to achieve a successful result for open reduction and internal fixation with locked plating. Osteosynthesis of fractures of the surgical neck using a fixed-angle locking plate can be accomplished with the patient in either a supine or a modified beach-chair position. The supine position is particularly advantageous when performing concomitant surgery for upper- and lower-extremity trauma. When performing open reduction and internal fixation of fractures of the surgical neck with the patient in the supine position, a radiolucent table is necessary, as it gives the ability easily to obtain proper fluoroscopic imaging throughout. Our preference is for the Jackson table with a radiolucent extremity extension. With the patient supine, a large fluoroscopic unit (C-arm) is best positioned opposite to the operated arm. An additional small C-arm can be positioned on the ipsilateral side to obtain a valid axillary view. Regional or general anesthesia is administered. Regional anesthesia offers the benefits of postoperative pain management. General anesthesia can provide greater muscle relaxation, which aids reduction in cases of significant displacement and deformity, and allows for an accurate immediate neurologic postoperative examination.

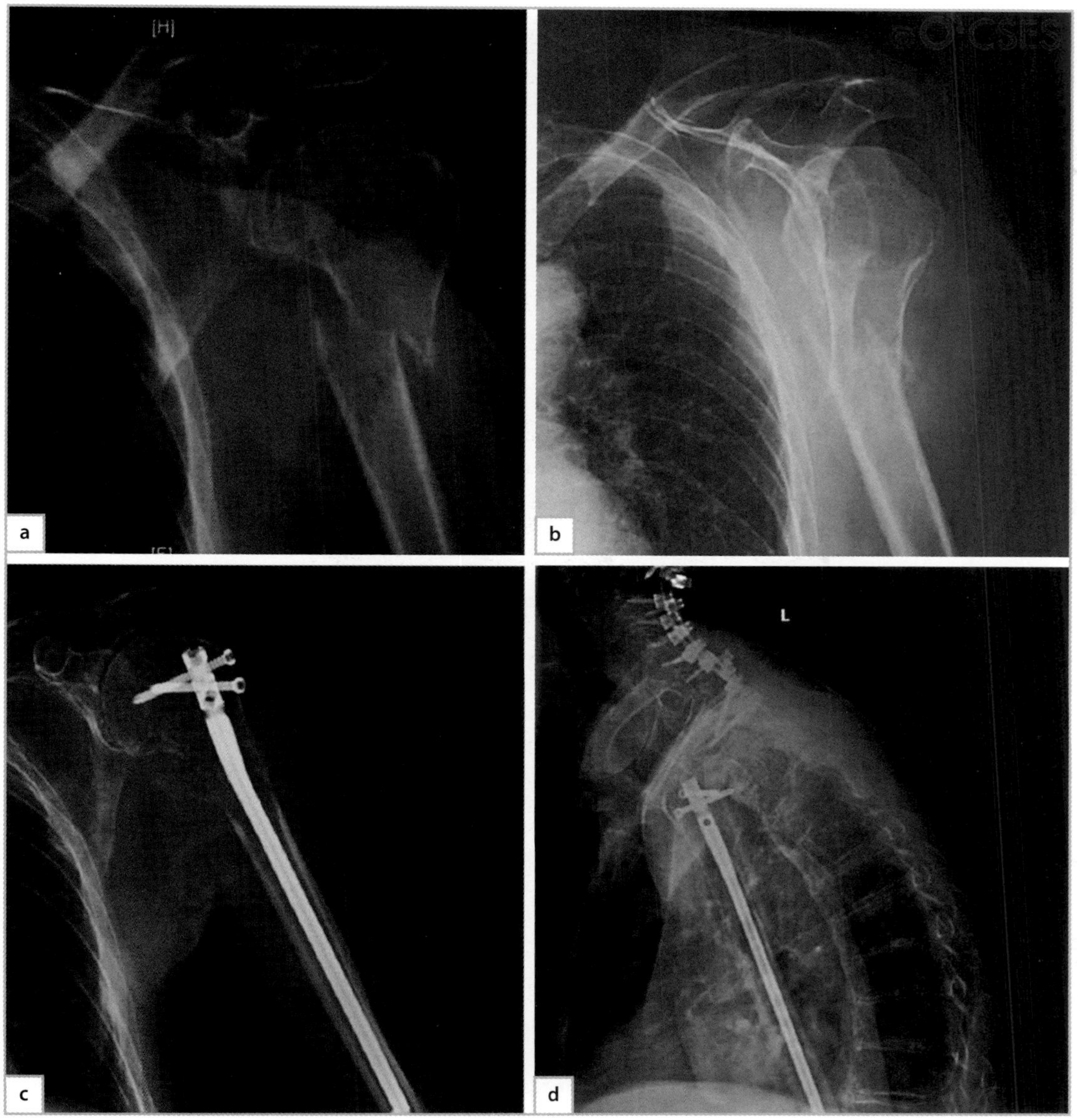

Figure 5.3 Metastatic fracture of the surgical neck. (a) Anteroposterior and (b) outlet views. (c,d) Stabilization was achieved using an intramedullary nail. Courtesy of the Center for Shoulder, Elbow and Sports Medicine.

In the setting of an isolated surgical neck fracture in the absence of concomitant lower-extremity trauma stabilization surgery, our preference is to use the modified beach-chair position, with the trunk flexed and the back of the table raised to approximately 45°. An advantage of the beach-chair position over the supine position is that venous return is less, thus potentially lowering intraoperative blood loss. We use an inflatable bean bag to help maintain custom patient positioning, regardless of body habitus, during the entire procedure; this can also facilitate unobstructed fluoroscopic views of the operated shoulder, by bringing the bean bag as far lateral as possible to avoid capturing radio-opaque components of the operating table in the fluoroscopic field of view. A large C-arm is positioned on the ipsilateral side of the operated shoulder and can be positioned either at the head of the table and aimed in the caudal direction, or at the foot of the table and aimed in the cephalad direction (**Fig. 5.4**). Our preference is to position the C-arm at the head of the table, so that the surgeon and assistants can work in concert with fluoroscopic imaging. Adequate anteroposterior (AP) and axillary fluoroscopic images are usually easily obtained with this setup, but the ability to do so should be confirmed prior to sterile draping of the patient. We routinely use a pneumatic arm-holder (Spider, Smith and Nephew) to aid arm positioning during surgery.

Our preference is to use a standard deltopectoral approach to the proximal humerus when addressing fractures of the surgical neck. The osseous anatomical landmarks (clavicle, acromion, and coracoid) are palpated and marked. A longitudinal incision is made starting at the anteroinferior border of the clavicle and extending distally and laterally toward the deltoid tuberosity. If the fracture is found to extend to the humeral shaft, distal exposure can be accomplished by supplementing the deltopectoral incision with an anterior approach to the humerus. The cephalic vein is identified and can be retracted either medially or laterally. In many cases, the upper third of the pectoralis major tendon is released, leaving a cuff of tendon to the humeral shaft for later reattachment. Releasing the proximal third of the pectoralis major tendon both improves fracture exposure and decreases some of the deforming forces on the humeral shaft, which in turn will aid in fracture reduction.

The clavipectoral fascia is often hemorrhagic; once it has been removed, fracture fragments become easily visualized. The long head of the biceps tendon is also identified and mobilized from the bicipital sheath, located in the intertubercular groove. The tendon of the long head of the biceps often serves as an impediment to reduction, and can be a source of pain following osteosynthesis. Thus, we routinely

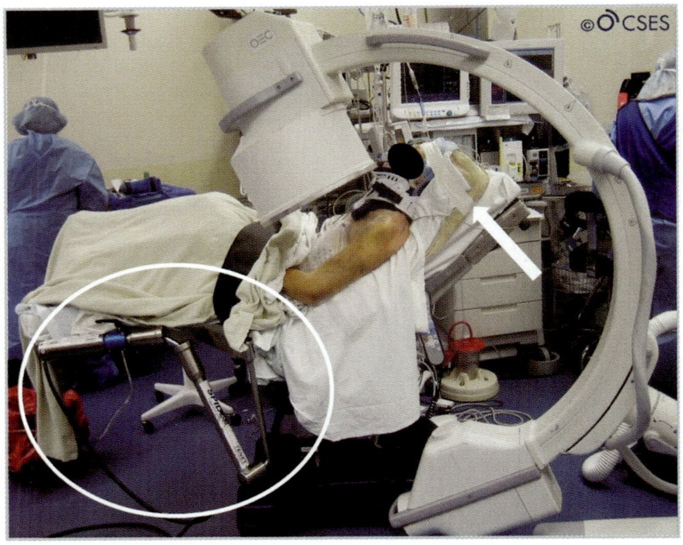

Figure 5.4 Patient position for open reduction and internal fixation of the surgical neck. Note the presence of an inflatable bean bag (white arrow) contoured to the shape of the patient, with stabilization of the head, a pneumatic arm-holder located at the foot of the bed (white circle), and the C-arm positioned on the ipsilateral side at the head of the surgical table. Courtesy of the Center for Shoulder, Elbow and Sports Medicine.

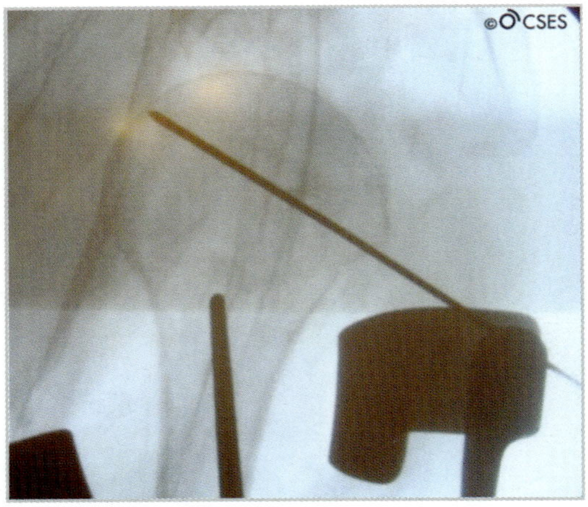

Figure 5.5 Use of a bone hook at the shaft and the position of a Kirschner wire to achieve reduction. Intraoperative fluoroscopic image. Courtesy of the Center for Shoulder, Elbow and Sports Medicine.

perform a biceps tenodesis at the end of surgery. Our recent preference has been to tenodese the long head of the biceps to the conjoint tendon (Verma et al. 2005, Drakos et al. 2008). This affords soft-tissue-to-soft-tissue healing (rather than soft-tissue-to-bone healing), and secure fixation without having to protect motion. The vector of pull for the long head of the biceps tendon is similar to that of the conjoint tendon.

The humeral shaft is generally displaced in one of two positions: superior and impacted at the lateral edge of the abducted humeral head; or medial and impacted against the medial metaphyseal flare of the proximal fragment. Reduction of the humeral shaft to the head can be accomplished with gentle downward traction of the arm. Occasionally, the use of a small bone hook with accompanying gentle traction can aid disimpaction of fracture fragments (**Fig. 5.5**). Extreme care must be taken when using the bone hook, as comminution and poor bone quality often coexist in these fractures. When the shaft is medialized, manual lateral translation of the humeral shaft with distraction will often manipulate the fracture fragments into the proper alignment. A 2 mm Kirschner wire (K-wire) placed centrally in the humeral head can also facilitate manipulation of the fragment of the proximal humeral head, with abduction, adduction, or rotation (**Fig. 5.5**). The end of the K-wire should be placed either at the lesser tuberosity or at the bicipital groove, and the wire is then aimed toward a center–center position within the humeral head. This position will ensure rigid K-wire fixation, which will allow manipulation of the head and, furthermore, will not interfere with subsequent lateral plate placement.

Preliminary fixation of the shaft to the head is necessary to stabilize the desired reduction prior to lateral plate placement and screw fixation. Preliminary fixation is performed using several 2.0 mm smooth K-wires. The starting point for these K-wires should be on the anterior shaft of the humerus, several centimeters distal to the shaft fracture line. The K-wires are aimed from caudad to cephalad, toward the center of the humeral head, on the subchondral line, just shy of the articular surface. The wires should diverge, to maximize fixation strength between these two points (**Fig. 5.6**). Additional K-wire fixation can be provided to increase the rigidity of the reduction. The starting point for additional K-wire fixation should be at the most superior and medial edge of the greater tuberosity, aiming toward a point several centimeters distal to the fracture line (**Fig. 5.7**).

Once preliminary K-wire fixation has been accomplished, the cortex of the lateral humeral shaft must be prepared for placement of the locking plate. The deltoid insertion can sometimes impair direct lateral placement of the plate via a deltopectoral approach. Occasionally, a limited release (2–3 mm) of the most anterior edge of the deltoid insertion from the lateral cortex along Sharpey's fibers can be performed to avoid anterior plate placement, which is a common pitfall when using a deltopectoral approach. However, a more aggressive release (>3 mm) can create iatrogenic deltoid insufficiency. If extensive plate coverage of the lateral shaft is necessary, a direct lateral approach to the shaft may be more appropriate.

Our preferred fixation device is a proximal humerus locking plate. Contoured plates are commercially available that closely mimic the geometry of the proximal humerus to allow proper screw placement in the humeral head. The screws in the plate are positioned at fixed angles. Plate location on the shaft is critical to ensure adequate screw fixation in the humeral head, and to avoid impingement of the proximal extent of the plate in the subacromial space. The locking plate should be placed so that its proximal edge does not impinge on the undersurface of the acromion with maximum abduction, and so that the inferior screws are parallel to the inferior calcar. The plate can also be positioned inferior, so that its proximal edge lies parallel to a line drawn through the center of the proximal humerus, to ensure multiple fixed-angle screws can be placed in the central and inferior quadrants of the humeral head (**Fig. 5.8b**). When performing this technique, we frequently augment locked-screw fixation with 4.0 mm, fully threaded cancellous screws directed along the medial metaphyseal cortex, and from the lateral shaft toward the center–center position in the humeral head (**Fig. 5.8c**).

An anatomic reduction and fracture fragment compression *must* be achieved prior to screw and plate placement when using a locked-plating technique. Malreduction is a frequent complication following locked-plate osteosynthesis. Using cortical shaft screws to translate the 'shaft to the plate' will frequently cause losses in reduction. Anatomic reduction prior to plate placement best assures that the reduction obtained will be maintained during screw placement, and will allow the surgeon more freedom over where to locate the plate for optimal screw placement (see below).

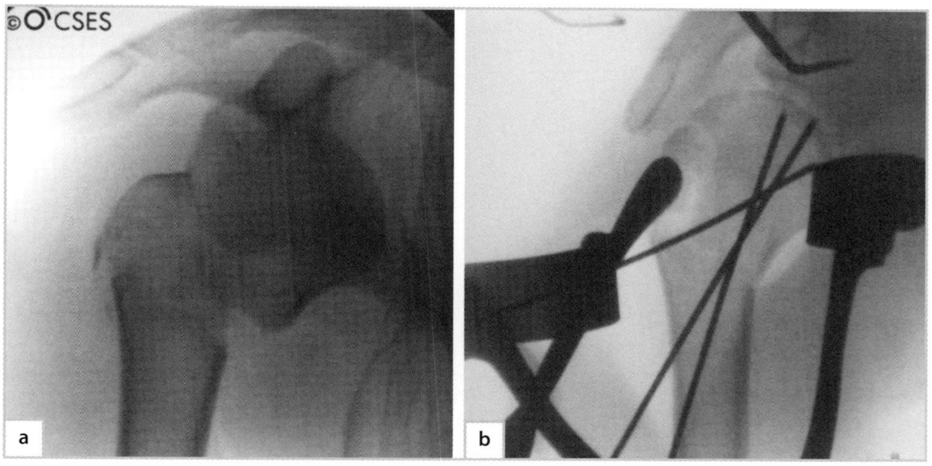

Figure 5.6 Fracture dislocation involving the surgical neck with a large Hill–Sachs lesion. Fluoroscopic images from a 33-year-old female. (a) Preoperative view. (b) Preliminary fixation of the fracture with two anteriorly placed Kirschner wires aimed toward the center of the head with disimpaction of the Hill–Sachs lesion.

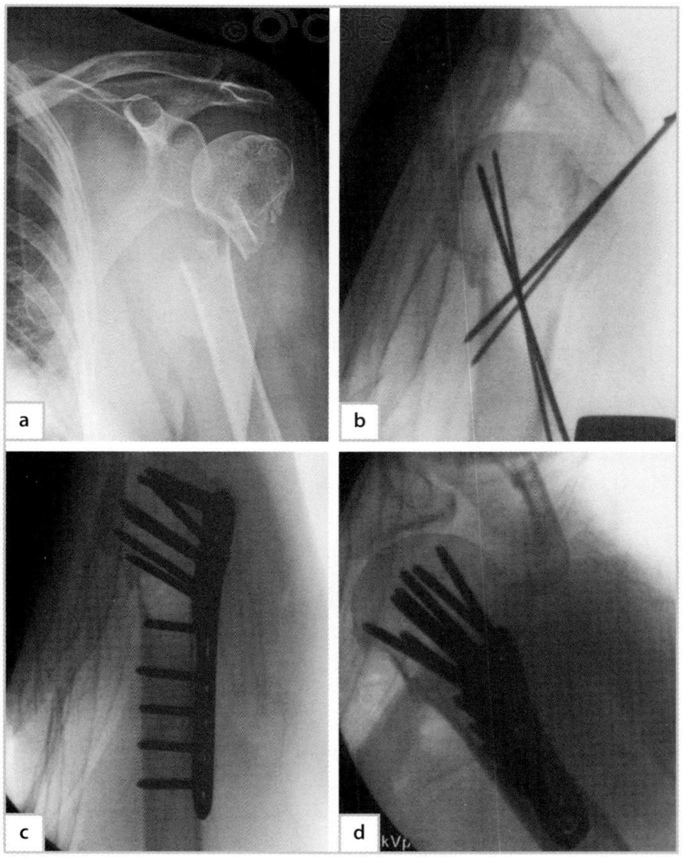

Figure 5.7 Fracture of the surgical neck with a minimally displaced greater tuberosity. Fluoroscopic images from a 68-year-old female. (a) Preoperative view. (b) Note the position of the Kirschner wires (anteroinferior to central, and superolateral to inferomedial) to obtain preliminary fixation. (c,d) Final construct. Courtesy of the Center for Shoulder, Elbow and Sports Medicine.

The length of the plate will be determined by fracture extension toward the humeral shaft. For fractures without significant extension, four or five optimally placed locking screws in the humeral head with a minimum of six cortices at the humeral shaft should be sufficient. Patients with significant osteoporosis may require additional locking or fully threaded cancellous screws in the head and shaft. As stated above, *screw position* in the humeral head is critical when determining the success of locked plating for fractures of the surgical neck. The highest bone density is located in the central quadrant of the proximal humerus, and the poorest bone quality in the anterosuperior quadrant (Tingart et al. 2006). Tingart et al. (2006) demonstrated increased cancellous screw pullout strength in regions with higher bone mineral density; thus, the least number of screws should be placed in the region with the poorest bone quality (i.e. the anterosuperior quadrant) (**Figs 5.8**, **5.9**).

The success of osteosynthesis for surgical neck fractures is dependent on establishing medial support (Gardner et al. 2007). This extremely important step is accomplished by achieving an anatomic reduction of the medial metaphyseal calcar, inferomedial calcar screw placement or endosteal support using a structural cortical allograft (in the setting of significant inferomedial comminution) (Gardner et al. 2007, Gardner et al. 2008, Mathison et al. 2010). Re-establishing medial support has been shown to be a strong factor in preventing complications following locked plating for fractures of the proximal humerus (Gardner et al. 2007). We have occasionally used an intramedullary fibular strut allograft to provide additional medial support in patients with significant osteoporosis and/or comminution. In addition, the allograft serves as a good tool for indirect reductions of the fracture without disrupting the medial soft tissues. This technique has been shown to improve the biomechanical properties of the construct, with good clinical results (Gardner et al. 2008, Mathison et al. 2010). The allograft can be positioned and manipulated into the intramedullary canal using forceps, bone reduction clamps, or a broad K-wire. A cortical or locking screw is placed at the inferior margin of the allograft to prevent migration of the graft down the intramedullary canal. An additional locking screw is used to move the allograft toward the inferomedial calcar. Screw placement can then ensue, with or without drilling through the allograft (**Fig. 5.10**).

A thorough fluoroscopic examination of the final repair construct must follow final screw placement. Intra-articular or extra-articular screw penetration is the most common complication following osteosynthesis for fractures of the proximal humerus, given the unique, 'global' anatomy of the humeral head. Live fluoroscopy with the joint placed at the extremes of rotation is essential to detect any evidence of screw perforation. It is also crucial to obtain satisfactory orthogonal views, including true anteroposterior and axillary views, in the operating room, to confirm proper screw length and position. In general, screw perforation is present if the screw appears to be 'out', even if on only one view.

We routinely use a drain for less than 24 hours. The deltopectoral interval is closed with non-absorbable number 2 suture. The subcutaneous layer is closed with a braided 2-0 suture and 3-0 monofilament absorbable suture, respectively. The arm is immobilized in a sling with an abduction pillow to neutralize the pull of the rotator cuff. Overnight admission is generally recommended for pain management, the administration of postoperative antibiotics, and exercise education by a trained physiotherapist and/or occupational therapist.

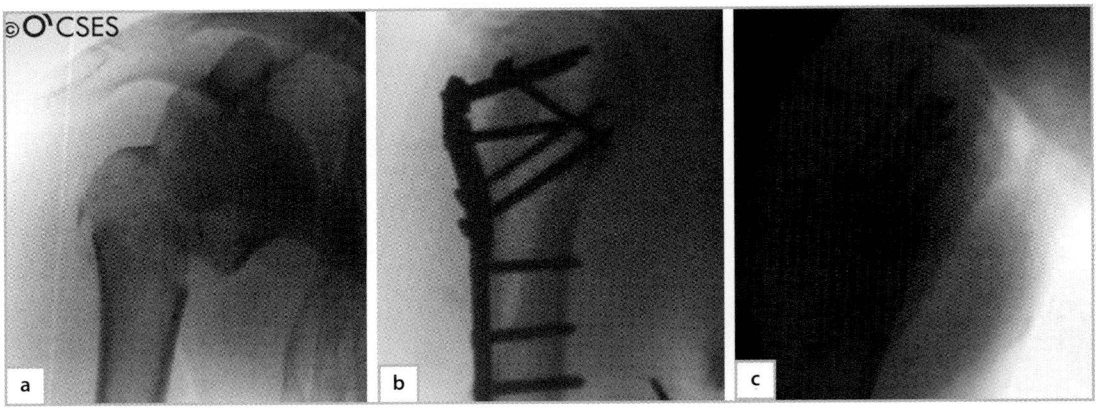

Figure 5.8 Open reduction and internal fixation of the proximal humerus using fibular cortical strut, intramedullary allograft. Fluoroscopic images from an 82-year-old female. (a) Preoperative view. (b,c) Note the slight inferior position of the plate to allow clustering of screws in the central and inferior medial calcar region. Courtesy of the Center for Shoulder, Elbow and Sports Medicine.

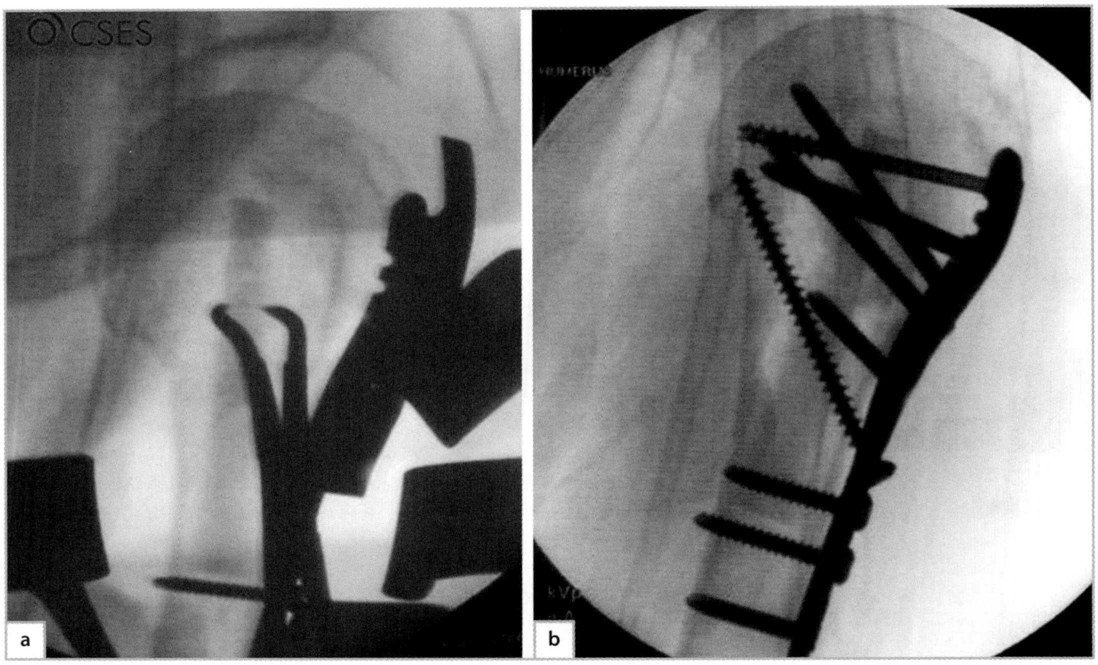

Figure 5.9 Open reduction and internal fixation of a fracture dislocation of the proximal humerus, involving the surgical neck. (a,b) Fluoroscopic films following the procedure. Note that only one screw is placed in the anterosuperior quadrant of the humeral head. Courtesy of the Center for Shoulder, Elbow and Sports Medicine.

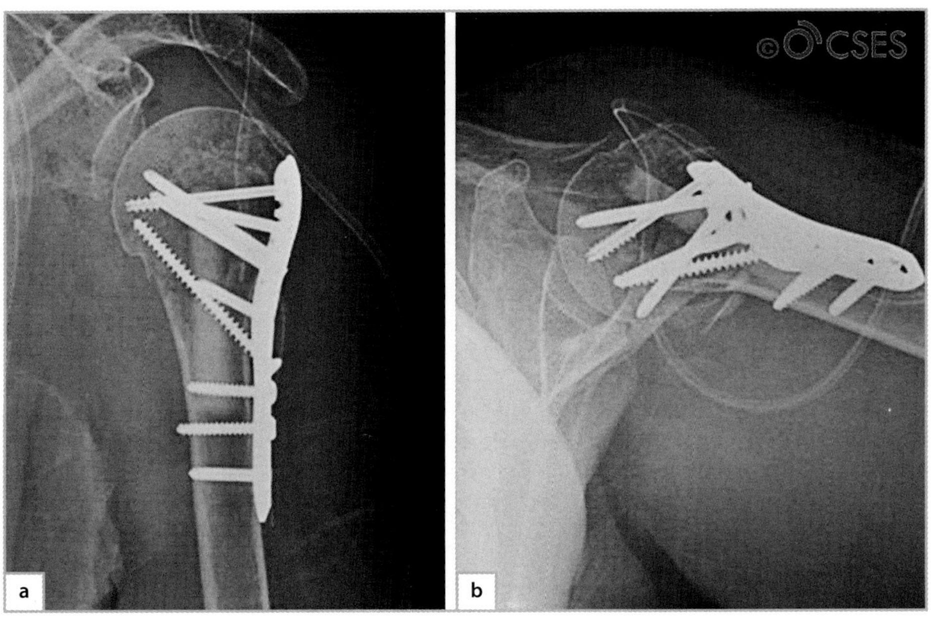

Figure 5.10 Use of a fibular cortical strut, intramedullary allograft to enhance medial support. Fluoroscopic images. (a) Placement and manipulation of allograft in the intramedullary canal. (b) Final fluoroscopic image. Courtesy of the Center for Shoulder, Elbow and Sports Medicine.

Pearls and pitfalls

Pearls

- Use of a bean bag in the beach-chair position can facilitate adequate orthogonal fluoroscopic views, especially the axillary view, in the operating room.
- A skilled assistant is critical for maintaining fracture reduction and screw placement.
- Identifying the long head of the biceps tendon and releasing it from the intertubercular groove is helpful when placing K-wires on the anterior humeral shaft for preliminary fixation.
- Manipulation of the arm without a pneumatic arm positioner may aid fracture reduction.
- The anterior K-wires can serve as a guide to prevent anterior plate positioning.
- The use of an intramedullary, structural cortical allograft can help support the medial calcar in the setting of significant comminution.
- An anatomic reduction and fracture compression must be achieved prior to plate fixation and screw placement, to prevent malreduction and non-union.
- The ideal *inferior* screw placement (along the medial calcar) should be identified first, to confirm the proper height of the plate.
- A 4.0 mm fully threaded cancellous screw can be used with greater flexibility in humeral placement when striving to achieve optimal screw positioning in the humeral head.

Pitfalls

- Fractures with significant osteopenia/osteoporosis may not benefit from locked-plate fixation, and may be best managed with suture fixation or non-operative management.
- Inadequate fluoroscopy secondary to poor patient positioning can increase the risk of failure to recognize penetration of a humeral head screw.
- Improper and inadequate screw placement and/or lack of medial calcar support can lead to iatrogenic causes of failure.
- Inadequate soft-tissue release may increase the risk of an anterior plate position using the deltopectoral approach.
- Potential complications include humeral head screw penetration (most common), infection, plate impingement, adhesive capsulitis, implant failure, malreduction, and varus subsidence (Sudkamp et al. 2009, Solberg et al. 2009a, Solberg et al. 2009b, Sproul et al. 2011, Yang et al. 2011).

REHABILITATION

Pendulum exercises are permitted immediately following surgery. Active and passive elbow, wrist and finger motion is encouraged to prevent stiffness. The affected arm is kept non-weight-bearing for six weeks. It has been our experience that cryotherapy significantly decreases the need for pain medication. Gentle passive range of motion is initiated two weeks after surgery. We generally restrict motion to 0–120° of forward elevation in the plane of the scapula, and 30° of external rotation with the arm adducted for the first two weeks; this can advance to 140° of forward elevation in the first month, depending fixation strength and bone quality. At six weeks, passive range of motion can advance, with the goal of achieving the full range of motion between 8 and 12 weeks. Improvements in range of motion can be seen as late as three months to a year later (Sudkamp et al. 2009). Active range of motion and isometric strengthening can begin after six weeks, following radiographic confirmation of preservation of proper fracture alignment. Abundant callus will not be observed secondary to the rigid, locked construct. Scapulothoracic strengthening can also commence. Resisted rotator cuff strengthening should not start until 10–12 weeks postoperatively.

REFERENCES

Bigliani L. Shoulder trauma. In: Orthopedic Knowledge Update 2. Park Ridge, IL: American Academy of Orthopedic Surgeons, 1987: 195–206.

Bigliani L. Fractures of the proximal humerus. In: Rockwood CA, Matsen FA, eds. The Shoulder, 2nd edn, vol 2. Philadelphia, PA: WB Saunders, 1990: 278–334.

Chun J. Two-part fractures of the proximal humerus. J Shoulder Elbow Surg 1994;3:273–287.

Cofield RH. Comminuted fractures of the proximal humerus. Clin Orthop Relat Res 1988;(230):49–57.

Drakos MC, Verma NN, Gulotta LV, et al. Arthroscopic transfer of the long head of the biceps tendon: functional outcome and clinical results. Arthroscopy 2008;24:217–223.

Gardner MJ, Weil Y, Barker JU, et al. The importance of medial support in locked plating of proximal humerus fractures. J Orthop Trauma 2007;21:185–191.

Gardner MJ, Boraiah S, Helfet DL, Lorich DG. Indirect medial reduction and strut support of proximal humerus fractures using an endosteal implant. J Orthop Trauma 2008;22:195–200.

Keene J. Proximal humeral fractures. A correlation of residual deformity with long-term function. Orthopaedics 1983;6:173–178.

Koval KJ, Gallagher MA, Marsicano JG, et al. Functional outcome after minimally displaced fractures of the proximal part of the humerus. J Bone Joint Surg Am 1997;79:203–207.

Mathison C, Chaudhary R, Beaupre L, et al. Biomechanical analysis of proximal humeral fixation using locking plate fixation with an intramedullary fibular allograft. Clin Biomech (Bristol, Avon) 2010;25:642–646.

Mills HJ, Horne G. Fractures of the proximal humerus in adults. J Trauma 1985;25:801–805.

Neer CS 2nd. Displaced proximal humeral fractures. I. Classification and evaluation. J Bone Joint Surg Am 1970a;52:1077–1089.

Neer CS. Displaced proximal humeral fractures. II. Treatment of three-part and four-part displacement. J Bone Joint Surg Am 1970b;52:1090–1003.

Park MC, Murthi AM, Roth NS, et al. Two-part and three-part fractures of the proximal humerus treated with suture fixation. J Orthop Trauma 2003;17:319–325.

Razemon J. Les fractures et les fractures-luxations de l'extremite superieure de l'humerus. Rev Chir Orthop 1969;5:387–496.

Solberg BD, Moon CN, Franco DP, Paiement GD. Surgical treatment of three- and four-part proximal humeral fractures. J Bone Joint Surg Am 2009a;91:1689–1697.

Solberg BD, Moon CN, Franco DP, Paiement GD. Locked plating of 3- and 4-part proximal humerus fractures in older patients: the effect of initial fracture pattern on outcome. J Orthop Trauma 2009b;23:113–119.

Sproul RC, Iyengar JJ, Devcic Z, Feeley BT. A systematic review of locking plate fixation of proximal humerus fractures. Injury 2011;42:408–413.

Sudkamp N, Bayer J, Hepp P, et al. Open reduction and internal fixation of proximal humeral fractures with use of the locking proximal humerus plate. Results of a prospective, multicenter, observational study. J Bone Joint Surg Am 2009;91:1320–1328.

Tingart MJ, Lehtinen J, Zurakowski D, et al. Proximal humeral fractures: regional differences in bone mineral density of the humeral head affect the fixation strength of cancellous screws. J Shoulder Elbow Surg 2006;15:620–624.

Van Heest A. Shoulder and humerus: pediatrics. In: Orthopedic Knowledge Update 8. Rosemont, IL: American Academy of Orthopedic Surgeons, 2005: 697–703.

Verma NN, Drakos M, O'Brien SJ. Arthroscopic transfer of the long head biceps to the conjoint tendon. Arthroscopy 2005;21:764.

Yang H, Li Z, Zhou F, et al. A prospective clinical study of proximal humerus fractures treated with a locking proximal humerus plate. J Orthop Trauma 2011;25:11–17.

Chapter 6 Open reduction and internal fixation of three- and four-part fractures of the proximal humerus

Eric T. Ricchetti, Gerald R. Williams, Jr

INTRODUCTION

Fractures of the proximal humerus are the second most common fracture of the upper extremity, following fractures of the distal radius, and the third most common fracture overall in patients over 65 years of age, trailing only fractures of the hip and distal radius (Ricchetti et al. 2009, Ricchetti et al. 2010). The frequency of these fractures is expected to rise as the elderly population increases. More than 80% of fractures of the proximal humerus are minimally or non-displaced and can be treated non-operatively; however, displaced fractures typically require some form of surgical intervention (Ricchetti et al. 2009). Closed reduction and non-operative management of significantly comminuted or displaced fractures can be difficult and produce poor functional results (**Fig. 6.1**) (Ricchetti et al. 2009). Numerous surgical options have been described to treat displaced fractures, and no single technique has proven to be the optimal choice; moreover, the quality of the evidence supporting any particular treatment is generally low (Lanting et al. 2008, Handoll and Ollivere 2010).

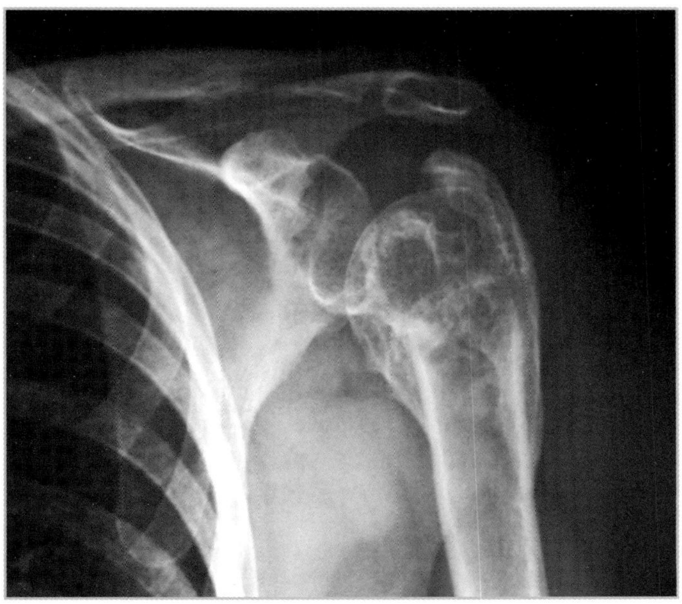

Figure 6.1 Anteroposterior radiograph showing the malunion of the proximal humerus. Here, the greater tuberosity has healed in a superiorly migrated position. (From Ricchetti ET, Warrender WJ, Abboud JA. Use of locking plates in the treatment of proximal humerus fractures. J Shoulder Elbow Surg 2010;19S:66–75. © Elsevier 2010.)

Open reduction and internal fixation using locking plates has demonstrated promise in the treatment of three- and four-part fractures of the proximal humerus, with several potential advantages over more traditional open techniques (Ricchetti et al. 2009, Thanasas et al. 2009, Ricchetti et al. 2010, Sproul et al. 2011). Its benefits can include improved fracture stability (due to the fixed-angle construct), a shorter period of immobilization (with the opportunity for earlier rehabilitation), lower risk of damage to the rotator cuff, lower risk of a later need for implant removal, and the potential avoidance of hemiarthroplasty in more complex fractures (Ricchetti et al. 2009, Ricchetti et al. 2010). Despite such benefits, however, complications have been reported with this technique, including varus malunion, avascular necrosis (AVN) of the humeral head, screw penetration into the glenohumeral joint, subacromial plate impingement, infection, non-union, and implant failure (Ricchetti et al. 2009, Thanasas et al. 2009, Ricchetti et al. 2010, Sproul et al. 2011). The frequency of complications reported in the literature has varied, depending in part on the definitions and inclusion criteria utilized in a given study (Ricchetti et al. 2009, Thanasas et al. 2009, Ricchetti et al. 2010, Sproul et al. 2011).

With the use of locking plates becoming more common in the treatment of these fractures, precise knowledge of and experience with the surgical technique is required to maximize clinical outcomes. The purpose of this chapter is to describe the use of locking plates in the treatment of three- and four-part fractures of the proximal humerus, including indications, contraindications, pearls and pitfalls, and postoperative rehabilitation.

INDICATIONS AND CONTRAINDICATIONS

Indications for the use of proximal humerus locking plates in the treatment of three- and four-part fractures include almost all displaced fractures or fracture dislocations that meet the criteria as defined by Neer (1970) (see Chapter 1), particularly those fractures with significant metaphyseal comminution or insufficient osseous contact and/or a disrupted medial hinge, in which other fixation techniques may be inadequate. Relative contraindications for their use include fractures in which arthroplasty may be a more appropriate surgical option because of concern about AVN or non-union. Certain fracture dislocations, such as a dislocated fracture of the humeral head through the anatomic neck (**Fig. 6.2**), comminuted head-splitting fractures, and impression fractures that involve over 40% of the articular surface typically fall into this arthroplasty category (Ricchetti et al. 2009).

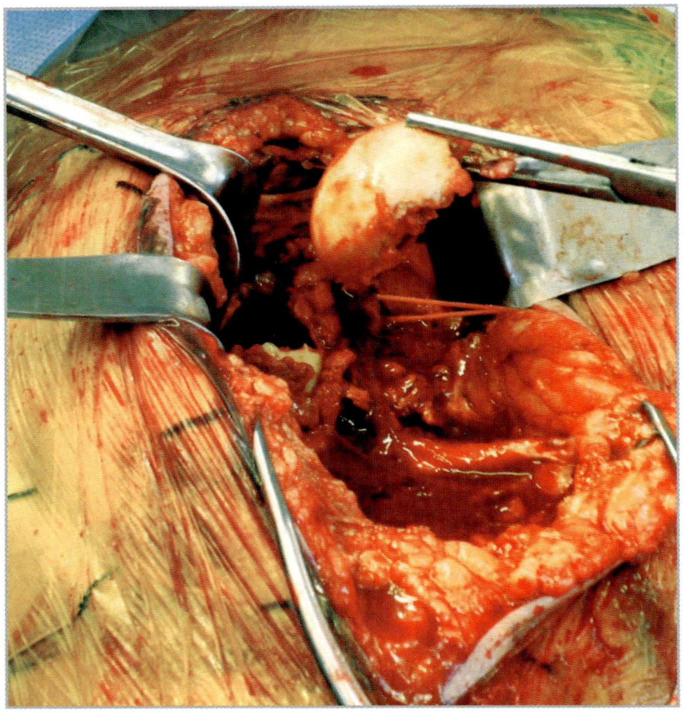

Figure 6.2 Intraoperative view of a fracture of the proximal humerus with complete detachment of a large fragment of the humeral head. Fractures with significant disruption of the fragment(s) of the humeral head, including comminuted head-splitting fractures and impression fractures that involve over 40% of the articular surface, are a relative contraindication to open reduction and internal fixation because of the risk of avascular necrosis. (From Ricchetti ET, Warrender WJ, Abboud JA. Use of locking plates in the treatment of proximal humerus fractures. J Shoulder Elbow Surg 2010;19S:66–75. © Elsevier 2010.)

Extremely osteoporotic bone may also be a contraindication to locking plates (for any three- or four-part fracture, with or without fracture comminution) if the poor bone quality does not permit stable fracture fixation with the implant. In such instances, the humeral head can essentially behave as a hollow shell that does not allow adequate fixation points for the proximal locking screws.

Other relative contraindications include young age, severe debilitation, and multiple medical comorbidities. Some patients will have little scope to benefit from surgery because of neurologic or other functional impairment, and others will be at high risk of local complications because of infected or deficient soft tissues (Ricchetti et al. 2009).

While reported rates of AVN following three- and four-part fractures of the proximal humerus have ranged from 0% to 34% (Hettrich et al. 2010), many of these fractures can be managed with open reduction and internal fixation. Hertel et al. (2004) attempted to determine predictors of humeral head ischemia following a displaced fracture of the proximal humerus by evaluating the intraoperative perfusion of 100 acute fractures that underwent open reduction and internal fixation. The most relevant predictors of ischemia were found to be the length of the posteromedial metaphyseal extension of the humeral head component (<8 mm), loss of integrity of the medial hinge (defined by greater than 2 mm of shaft displacement in any direction), and fractures involving the anatomic neck of the humerus. When all three of these criteria were present, the positive predictive value for humeral head ischemia was 97% (Hertel et al. 2004). In a follow-up study, however, the authors found that the presence of ischemia initially following fracture was not predictive of future humeral head collapse from AVN (Bastian and Hertel 2008). Forty of the fractures from the original study were followed for a mean of five years; 30 were considered perfused and 10 considered ischemic at the time of surgery. Radiographic evidence of collapse was seen in four of the 30 perfused fractures, and in two of the 10 ischemic fractures. Radiographic changes without collapse were seen in the other eight ischemic fractures, suggesting that revascularization had occurred. The authors concluded that open reduction and internal fixation of proximal humerus fractures initially thought to be ischemic can be a viable treatment option, and that revascularization of these fractures can occur with adequate reduction and stable fixation (Bastian and Hertel 2008).

TECHNIQUE

Preoperative evaluation

A thorough preoperative evaluation should be performed in every patient; it should include history and physical examination, radiographic evaluation, and surgical planning. Important components of the history are mechanism of injury, patient age, handedness, preinjury shoulder function, functional demands, and medical comorbidities. The physical examination should evaluate: whether the fracture is open or closed and whether there is an associated dislocation; areas of swelling, ecchymosis, or tenderness; neurovascular status of the arm; and other injuries in the same arm or other body part. Preoperative radiographs should include standard anteroposterior (AP), axillary, and scapular Y views to determine the fracture pattern and presence of a dislocation, as well as to evaluate bone quality. Fine-cut computerized tomography (CT) of the shoulder with coronal and sagittal reconstructions should be performed if intra-articular involvement is suspected, if the glenoid is fractured, or if the fracture pattern and tuberosity displacement are difficult to appreciate on plain radiographs (**Fig. 6.3**). A CT scan may also be needed to confirm the presence of a dislocation if plain radiographs are equivocal. The information obtained from these imaging studies is essential in determining a preoperative surgical plan, including the appropriate reduction maneuvers and fixation techniques.

Implants and equipment

Regardless of manufacturer, the current proximal humerus locking plates are precontoured to fit the proximal humeral anatomy. They consist of a proximal end, with locking holes designed to create a locked construct in the humeral head, and a distal shaft end, with multiple holes that may be locking or non-locking (**Fig. 6.4**). Although these plates are anatomically precontoured, a patient's proximal humeral anatomy may not always precisely fit the plate, due to normal anatomical variations. In these instances, plates can be further contoured using plate benders.

Differing diverging or converging screw patterns in the humeral head can be created, depending on the particular plate design, as well as the choice of locking holes utilized in the proximal end of the plate. Certain plates offer variable-angle locking-screw options, which allow the surgeon to dictate the screw pattern; however, their added clinical value has not yet been demonstrated. Diverging patterns are typically preferred, as they increase the spread of screws into the humeral head (Ricchetti et al. 2009). Smaller, peripheral holes around the proximal end of the plate are also present to allow placement of Kirschner wires for temporary intraoperative fixation,

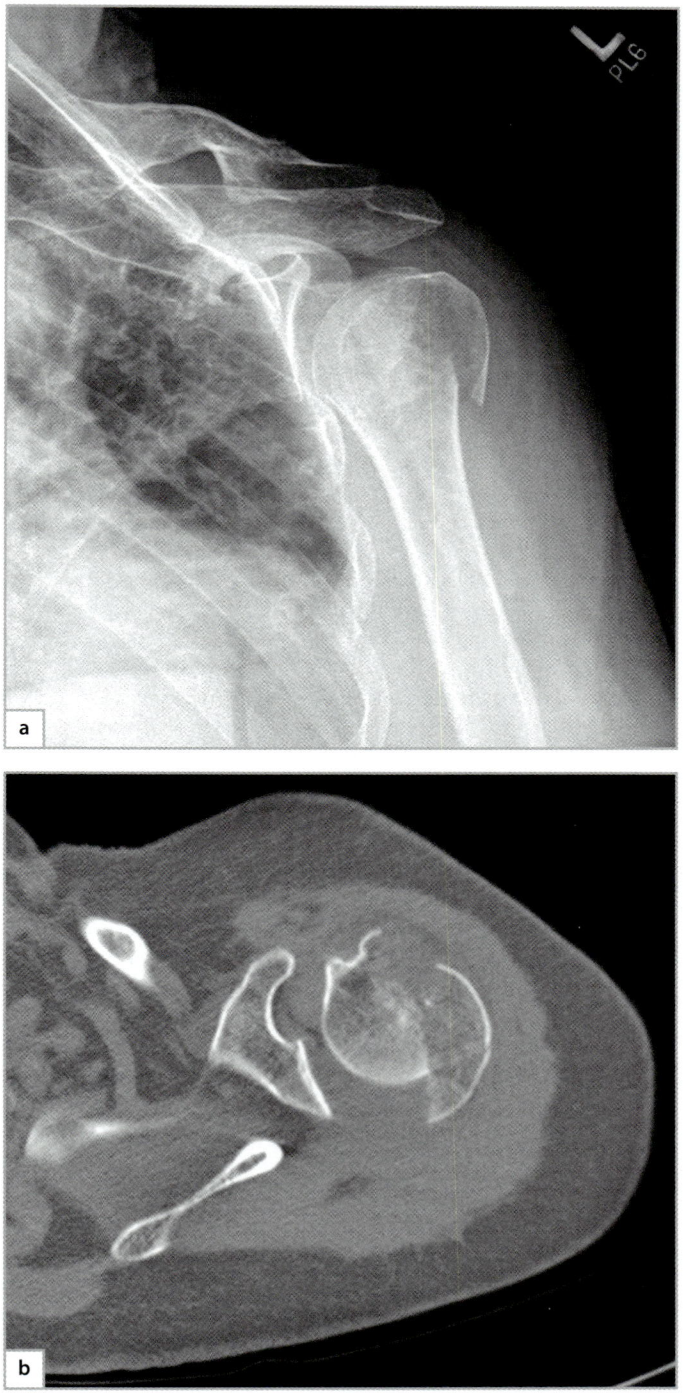

Figure 6.3 A displaced, valgus impacted, three-part fracture of the proximal humerus through the surgical neck and greater tuberosity. (a) An anteroposterior radiograph suggested that open reduction and internal fixation was a treatment option. (b) A computerized tomography scan, however, showed that the fracture line on the greater tuberosity extended into the articular surface of the humeral head. This head-splitting fracture was therefore treated with hemiarthroplasty.

or for passage of suture for additional fixation. To increase fracture stability, the locking-plate construct can be augmented with sutures passed through the rotator cuff and proximal plate. These sutures are recommended for additional tuberosity fixation in three- and four-part fractures. Heavy, non-absorbable suture is preferred, such

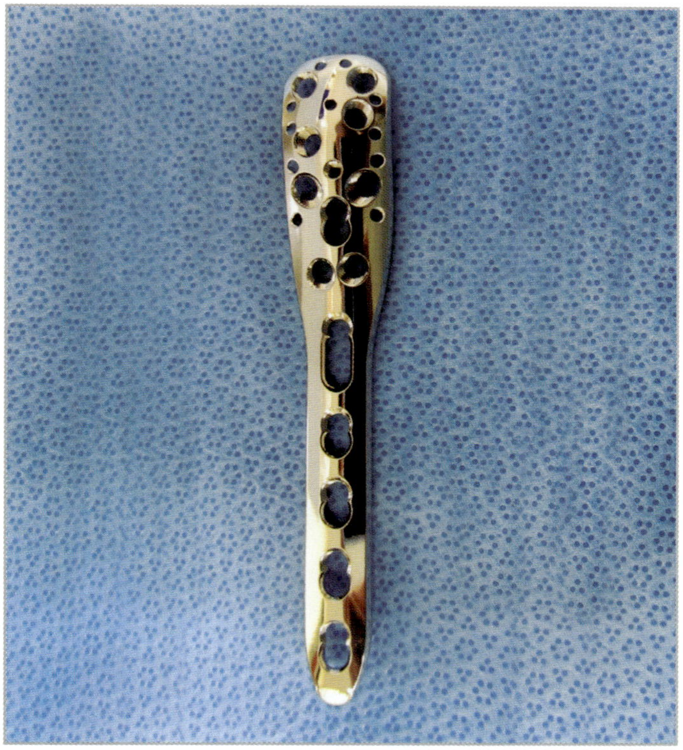

Figure 6.4 Precontoured proximal humerus locking plate. The proximal end of the plate has locking holes that enable the creation of a locked construct in the humeral head, while the distal shaft end has holes that may be used for locking or non-locking screws.

as 1 mm Cottony II Dacron (Deknatel, Mansfield, MA) or number 2 FiberWire (Arthrex, Naples, FL). Bone graft or bone graft substitutes – such as demineralized bone matrix, Norian SRS (Synthes, West Chester, PA) – can also be placed at the fracture site to further increase fracture stability and stimulate healing.

Patient positioning and setup

Patients are typically placed under general anesthesia for the procedure, with or without the use of a regional interscalene nerve block in the affected extremity for postoperative pain control. Surgeons may prefer to avoid the use of regional anesthesia, to allow evaluation of the postoperative neurological status of the extremity. This may be particularly true if a neurologic deficit existed in the extremity preoperatively. The patient is then placed in the beach-chair position, with the head of the bed elevated approximately 35–45° relative to the horizontal, and the shoulder off the edge of the table to allow full range of motion (ROM) of the extremity during the operation. Use of a mechanical arm-holding device allows the arm to be held in almost any position that is needed during surgery.

Once the patient has been positioned, the fluoroscopy machine should be brought in prior to sterile draping to confirm that adequate fluoroscopic images, including AP and axillary views, can be obtained during the procedure. The unit can be positioned at the head of the bed and rotated over the shoulder to allow for intraoperative use without being blocked by the bed or the patient's body, and to avoid the risk of contamination (**Fig. 6.5**). Alternatively, the machine can be placed on the opposite side of the bed and brought across the patient's body to obtain images.

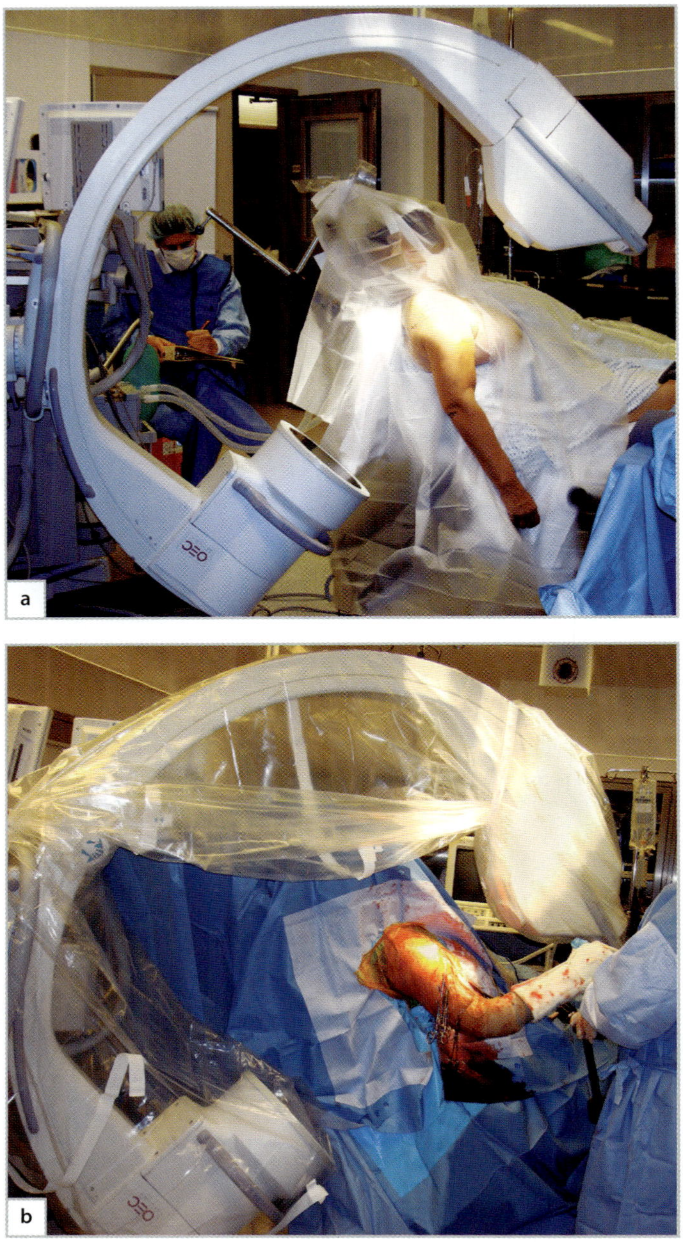

Figure 6.5 Arrangement of the fluoroscope. (a) The unit can be positioned at the head of the bed and rotated over the shoulder to allow for intraoperative use. (b) It must be sterilely draped to eliminate the risk of contamination. (From Ricchetti ET, DeMola PM, Roman D, Abboud JA. The use of precontoured humeral locking plates in the management of displaced proximal humerus fracture. J Am Acad Orthop Surg 2009;17:582–590. © 2009 American Academy of Orthopaedic Surgeons.)

Surgical approach

Several surgical approaches have been described for open reduction and internal fixation of fractures of the proximal humerus with locking plates, including deltopectoral, anterolateral deltoid-splitting, and two-incision techniques (Gallo et al. 2005, Gardner et al. 2008a, Hepp et al. 2008, Laflamme et al. 2008, Sudkamp et al. 2009). The anterolateral and two-incision approaches were developed with the goal of minimizing soft-tissue dissection and muscle retraction, and thereby to decrease the risk of AVN, as well as to provide better visualization laterally for plate placement and reduction of the greater tuberosity (Gallo et al. 2005, Gardner et al. 2008a, Laflamme et al. 2008). Two-incision techniques have been described that include an anterolateral deltoid-splitting incision with a more distal shaft incision (Laflamme et al. 2008), or a deltopectoral incision with a straight lateral deltoid-splitting incision (Gallo et al. 2005). Identification and protection of the axillary nerve are required, particularly in deltoid-splitting approaches, if dissection is carried more than 4–5 cm distal to the acromion (Gallo et al. 2005, Gardner et al. 2008a, Laflamme et al. 2008). Percutaneous two-incision techniques may, however, fail to facilitate filling of all plate holes because of the course of the axillary nerve. Therefore, such minimally invasive approaches may not be appropriate in certain three- and four-part fractures where use of these screw holes is required for fixation (Laflamme et al. 2008). While an increased rate of injury to the axillary nerve has not been observed with deltoid-splitting techniques (Gallo et al. 2005, Gardner et al. 2008a, Laflamme et al. 2008), improved outcomes, including lower rates of AVN, have also not been clearly demonstrated with these approaches in comparison with the deltopectoral approach (Hepp et al. 2008, Sudkamp et al. 2009).

The deltopectoral approach is the most commonly used for fracture exposure. The skin incision is approximately 10–15 cm long and starts at the tip of the coracoid process proximally and extends distally to the deltoid tuberosity. Once the skin and the subcutaneous tissues have been incised, the cephalic vein, deltoid, and pectoralis major are identified. As a major draining vein of the upper extremity, the cephalic vein should be preserved. It is typically retracted laterally to protect its many deltoid branches that come in on this side. The internervous plane between the deltoid (axillary nerve) and the pectoralis major (medial and lateral pectoral nerves) is developed to expose the proximal humerus (**Fig. 6.6**). If the fracture has not disrupted the clavipectoral fascia, this layer can be opened up and the conjoint tendon retracted medially to further expose the fracture site. Typically, no deltoid or pectoralis major detachment is needed during the approach. An extensive fracture hematoma is usually encountered. This blood should be evacuated, and important neurovascular structures, particularly the axillary and musculocutaneous nerves and circumflex vessels, should be identified and protected throughout the procedure. Digital palpation can verify the integrity of the axillary nerve deep to the conjoint tendon, as the nerve courses from anteromedial to posterolateral before passing under the lower border of the subscapularis tendon. The musculocutaneous nerve enters the conjoint tendon approximately 5–8 cm distal to the tip of the coracoid process. As its proximity to the coracoid can be highly variable, the nerve can sometimes be palpated along the undersurface of the conjoint tendon, but it is often too distal to be located within the surgical field.

Fracture exposure, mobilization, and reduction

Several techniques can be utilized for sufficient exposure of the fracture site and fracture reduction. Adequate muscle paralysis by anesthesia is helpful, for both soft-tissue retraction and fracture reduction. A self-retaining retractor should be used to retract the deltoid laterally, and the pectoralis major and conjoint tendon medially. Care should be taken when retracting the conjoined tendon to avoid excessive traction on the musculocutaneous nerve, particularly if the nerve has been identified close to the tip of the coracoid. An additional deltoid retractor is often necessary for adequate proximal exposure of the humeral head. Slight abduction of the arm will also relax the deltoid muscle, and improve access to the humeral head.

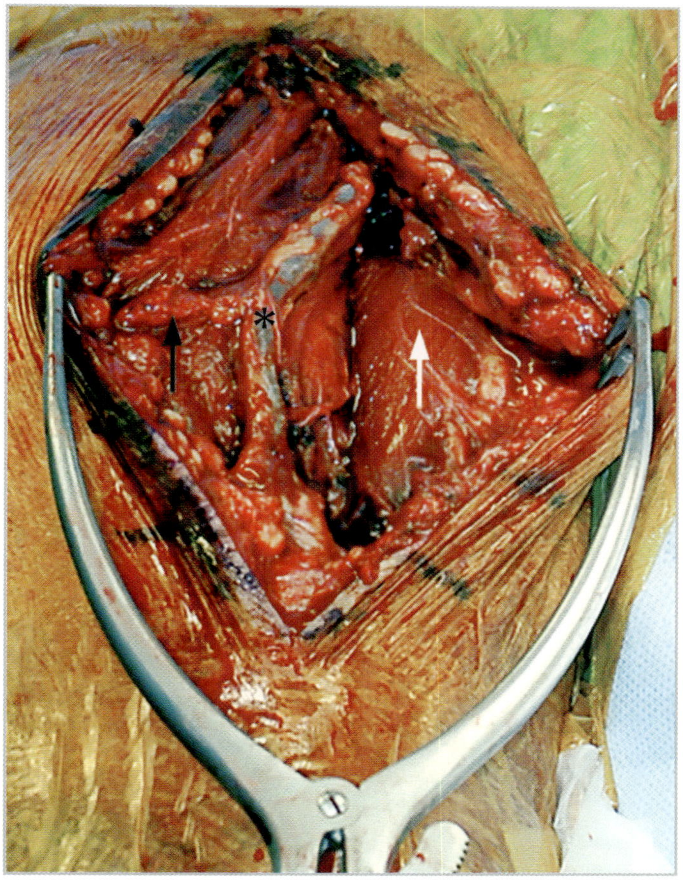

Figure 6.6 Exposure of the deltopectoral interval in a patient with a fracture of the proximal humerus. The deltoid (black arrow) appears laterally and the pectoralis major appears (white arrow) medially. The cephalic vein (asterisk) is shown overlying the deltoid, lateral to the interval (From Ricchetti ET, DeMola PM, Roman D, Abboud JA. The use of precontoured humeral locking plates in the management of displaced proximal humerus fracture. J Am Acad Orthop Surg 2009;17:582–590. © 2009 American Academy of Orthopaedic Surgeons.)

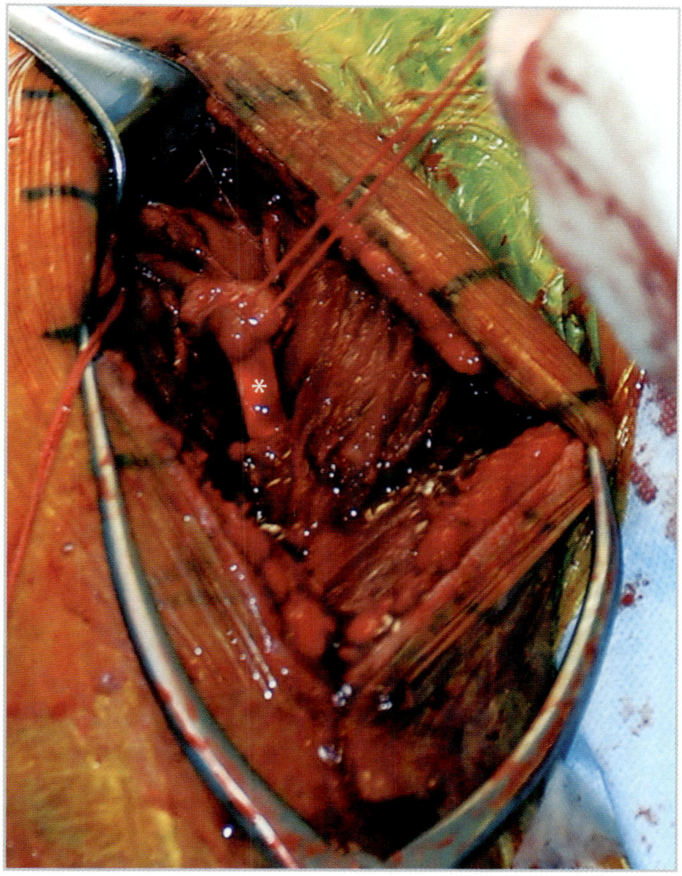

Figure 6.7 The long head of the biceps tendon identified and tagged with suture. The tendon (flagged here with the asterisk) is important in orienting the anatomy of the proximal humerus following three- and four-part fractures, particularly the location of the greater and lesser tuberosities. The tendon is most easily identified deep to the upper border of the pectoralis major tendon insertion on the humerus, and can then be followed proximally. (From Ricchetti ET, DeMola PM, Roman D, Abboud JA. The use of precontoured humeral locking plates in the management of displaced proximal humerus fracture. J Am Acad Orthop Surg 2009;17:582–590. © 2009 American Academy of Orthopaedic Surgeons.)

Identification of the long head of the biceps tendon is essential in orienting the anatomy of the proximal humerus, as it defines the location of the bicipital groove and, therefore, the relationship between the greater and lesser tuberosities (**Fig. 6.7**). The tendon is particularly useful as a landmark in highly comminuted three- and four-part fractures, where bony anatomy can be significantly distorted. In these fractures, one fracture line usually runs close to the bicipital groove, and separates the fracture fragments of the greater and lesser tuberosities. The long head of the biceps tendon is most easily located deep to the upper border of the pectoralis major tendon insertion on the humerus, and can then be followed proximally. The tendon is typically mobilized up to its origin on the superior glenoid by unroofing the tendon and performing a rotator interval release. This rotator interval release can further assist with fracture reduction, by allowing digital palpation within the glenohumeral joint to confirm appropriate orientation of the humeral head, and to confirm that intra-articular screw penetration has not occurred when locking screws are placed into the humeral head. Release of the rotator interval is also beneficial for shoulder ROM in the postoperative period. The long head of the biceps is tenotomized from its origin on the superior glenoid following rotator interval release, and tagged for tenodesis at the end of the case.

Next, the rotator cuff is generously tagged with heavy, non-absorbable sutures anteriorly, posteriorly, and superiorly, to assist with reduction of fracture fragments, and, ultimately, to reinforce fixation of the fracture to the plate (**Fig. 6.8**). Typically, at least one suture is passed through each of the rotator cuff tendons at the tendon-bone junction, so that there is a minimum of one suture through the lesser tuberosity (subscapularis), and three sutures through the greater tuberosity (supraspinatus, infraspinatus, teres minor). These traction sutures allow for improved control of the humeral head and fracture fragments of the tuberosity, and for improved reduction of the fragments to the humeral shaft and to each other (Ricchetti et al. 2009, Ricchetti et al. 2010). Once the fracture fragments have been tagged with rotator cuff sutures, the fractures lines must still be adequately mobilized to allow for appropriate reduction. The fracture of the surgical neck is first freed up, so that the humeral head can be brought back into an anatomic position on the humeral shaft. A combination of electrocautery, elevator instruments, curettes, and rongeurs can be used to mobilize the fracture of the surgical neck, with care not to disrupt the posteromedial soft-tissue sleeve, as it has been shown to be an important blood supply to the humeral head (Hettrich et al. 2010). The same instruments can also be utilized to free up the tuberosity fractures, as needed.

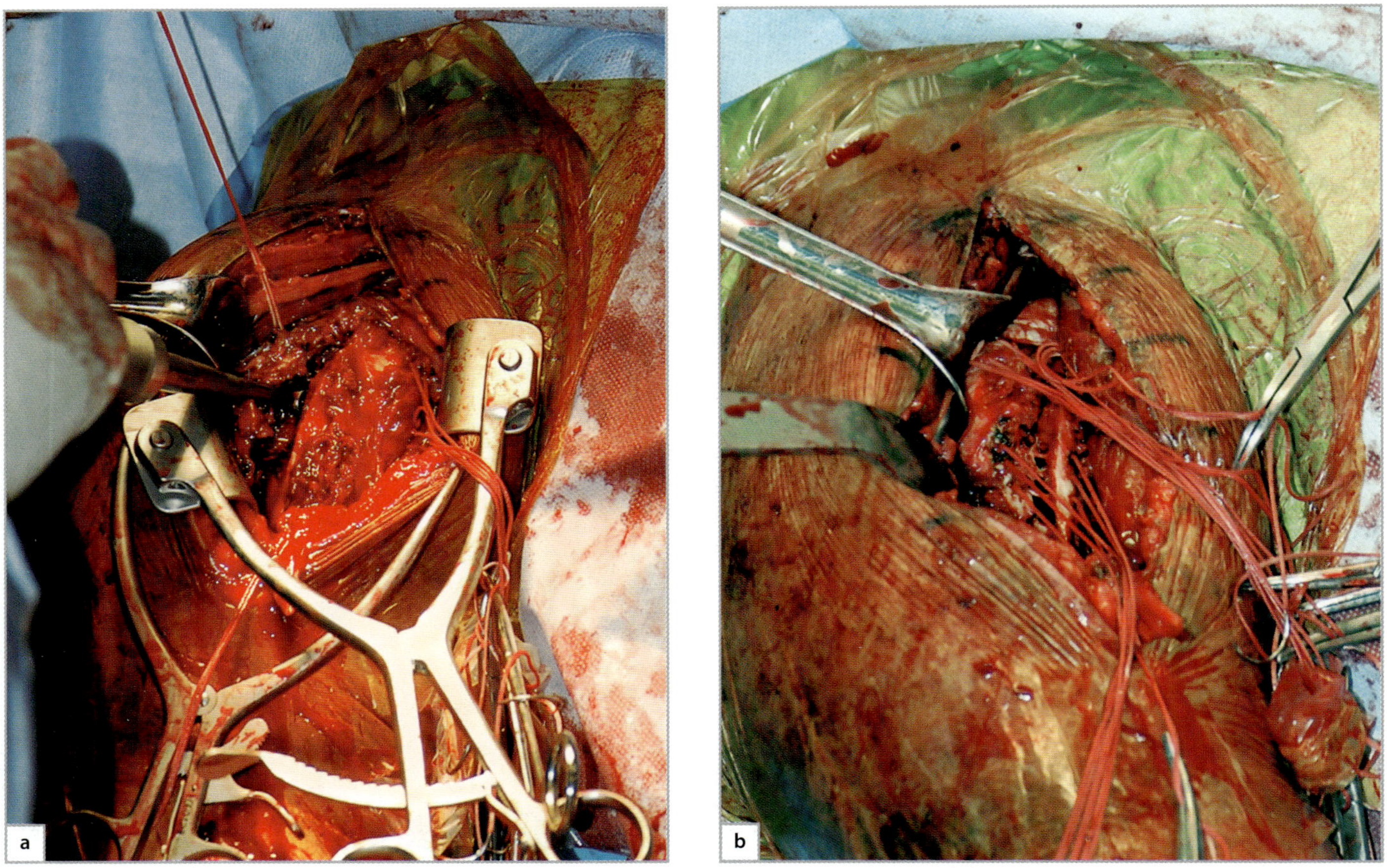

Figure 6.8 Tagging of the rotator cuff with non-absorbable sutures prior to attempted reduction of a fracture of the proximal humerus. (a,b) Intraoperative views. Each of the four rotator cuff tendons is tagged to assist with reduction of fracture fragments, and to reinforce fixation of the fracture to the locking plate. (From Ricchetti ET, DeMola PM, Roman D, Abboud JA. The use of precontoured humeral locking plates in the management of displaced proximal humerus fracture. J Am Acad Orthop Surg 2009;17:582–590. © 2009 American Academy of Orthopaedic Surgeons.)

Once all fracture fragments have been adequately mobilized, reduction maneuvers can be performed. If an impacted fragment of the humeral head is present, it can be gently disimpacted with an elevator instrument, such as a Cobb, placed into the fracture gap in the surgical neck. A combination of levering with this instrument and simultaneous traction on the sutures in the rotator cuff will typically bring the humeral head out of its impacted position (usually varus and retroversion) and into anatomical alignment. Further reduction maneuvers can be performed to align the tuberosity fragments and to fine-tune fracture alignment; these maneuvers include longitudinal traction of the extremity, shoulder abduction–adduction, and/or external–internal rotation, and lateral translation of the humeral shaft. Simultaneous digital manipulation and/or traction on the sutures in the rotator cuff can assist with any of these reduction maneuvers. Lateral translation of the humeral shaft is typically necessary in fractures involving the surgical neck, as pull of the pectoralis major often displaces the shaft medially. Correction of the varus tilt of a fragment of the humeral head, or superior displacement of a fragment of the greater tuberosity, can be assisted by traction on superiorly placed sutures in the rotator cuff (supraspinatus, infraspinatus), while correction of the rotational alignment of the fragments of the humeral head and/or tuberosity can be assisted with traction on anteriorly and posteriorly placed sutures in the rotator cuff (subscapularis, teres minor, infraspinatus).

Tuberosity reduction is essential to good functional outcomes following fixation (Gerber et al. 1998, Ricchetti et al. 2010). Once appropriate fracture alignment is achieved with reduction maneuvers, the adequacy of the reduction must be confirmed by fluoroscopic imaging prior to placing any hardware. AP fluoroscopic views should be used to confirm an appropriate neck–shaft angle, while axillary images are necessary to confirm appropriate version of the humeral head, and adequate alignment between the head and shaft. If necessary, temporary fixation of Kirschner wires can be utilized to hold the reduction in place before plate placement. Wires should be placed to avoid interference with plate positioning.

Placement of the locking plate

After adequate fracture alignment is confirmed by fluoroscopy, a precontoured locking plate is positioned approximately 5–10 mm lateral to the bicipital groove and 15–20 mm distal to the tip of the greater tuberosity. Placement with respect to the tip of the greater tuberosity will depend on the particular plate utilized and the angle of the proximal locking screws. The sutures in the rotator cuff can be passed through the smaller peripheral holes around the proximal end of the plate at this point, but will not typically be tied down until all screws have been placed. If necessary, the plate can also be further contoured with the use of large plate benders to better match the patient's anatomic-neck–shaft angle. The deltoid insertion may need to be partially released in order to position the plate in a sufficiently lateral position. Proper plate placement is important: placing the plate too high increases the risk of subacromial impingement or violation of the rotator cuff, while placing it too low can lead to inadequate screw purchase and fixation in the humeral head.

Plate position should be assessed with fluoroscopic imaging prior to placing any screws through the plate, including AP views to confirm correct proximal–distal plate position, and axillary views to confirm centering of the plate on the humeral shaft in the anterior–posterior direction (**Fig. 6.9**). Kirschner wires can be temporarily placed through the small periphery holes at the proximal end of the plate to hold the plate in position during imaging and subsequent screw placement.

Typically, the shaft screw hole on the plate just distal to the surgical neck fracture line is filled first, prior to placing any locking screws proximally. This screw hole is typically oblong, and at the level of the proximal shaft. A 3.5 mm non-locking, cortical screw placed in this hole will reduce the humeral shaft to the plate, and will correct any residual medial translation of the shaft relative to the proximal humerus. Tightening of the 3.5 mm cortical screw in this hole may occasionally lead to a slight upward migration of the plate on the greater tubercle. The oblong hole allows any upward migration to be corrected by loosening the screw slightly and repositioning the plate, avoiding the need to remove the screw completely. Adequate plate position and fracture reduction should be reconfirmed with fluoroscopic imaging if plate repositioning is necessary.

Proximal and distal screw holes in the plate are next sequentially drilled and filled. Typically, the proximal locking screws into the humeral head are placed first. It is essential that all fracture fragments are reduced and the plate correctly aligned prior to placement of locking screws, as these screws will prevent any further reduction of the fracture, or reduction of the plate to bone. Most implant systems have an insertion guide to facilitate placement of the proximal locking screws (**Fig. 6.10**). Differing diverging or converging screw patterns in the humeral head can be created, depending on the particular plate design and locking holes utilized; however, divergent patterns of five

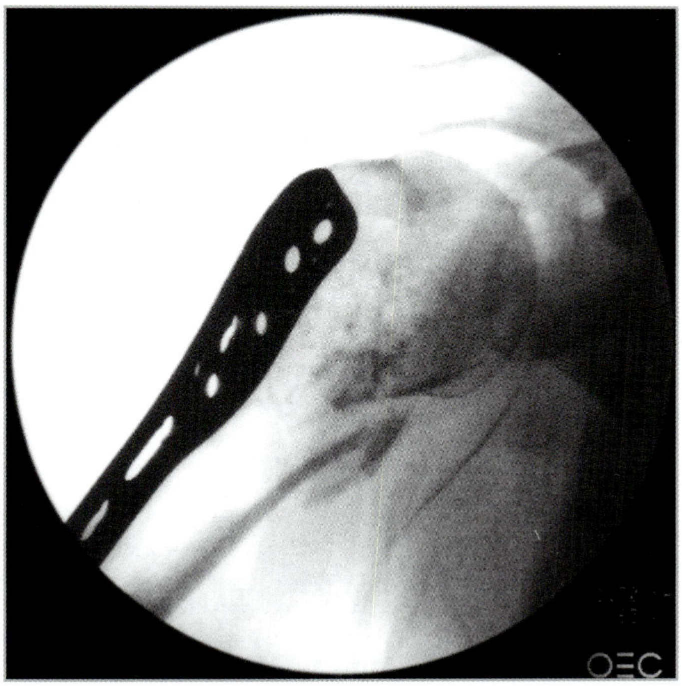

Figure 6.9 Intraoperative fluoroscopic image of a fracture of the proximal humerus with provisional placement of the locking plate. Adequate fracture reduction and plate positioning should be confirmed on fluoroscopy before any screws are placed through the plate. (From Ricchetti ET, DeMola PM, Roman D, Abboud JA. The use of precontoured humeral locking plates in the management of displaced proximal humerus fracture. J Am Acad Orthop Surg 2009;17:582–590. © 2009 American Academy of Orthopaedic Surgeons.)

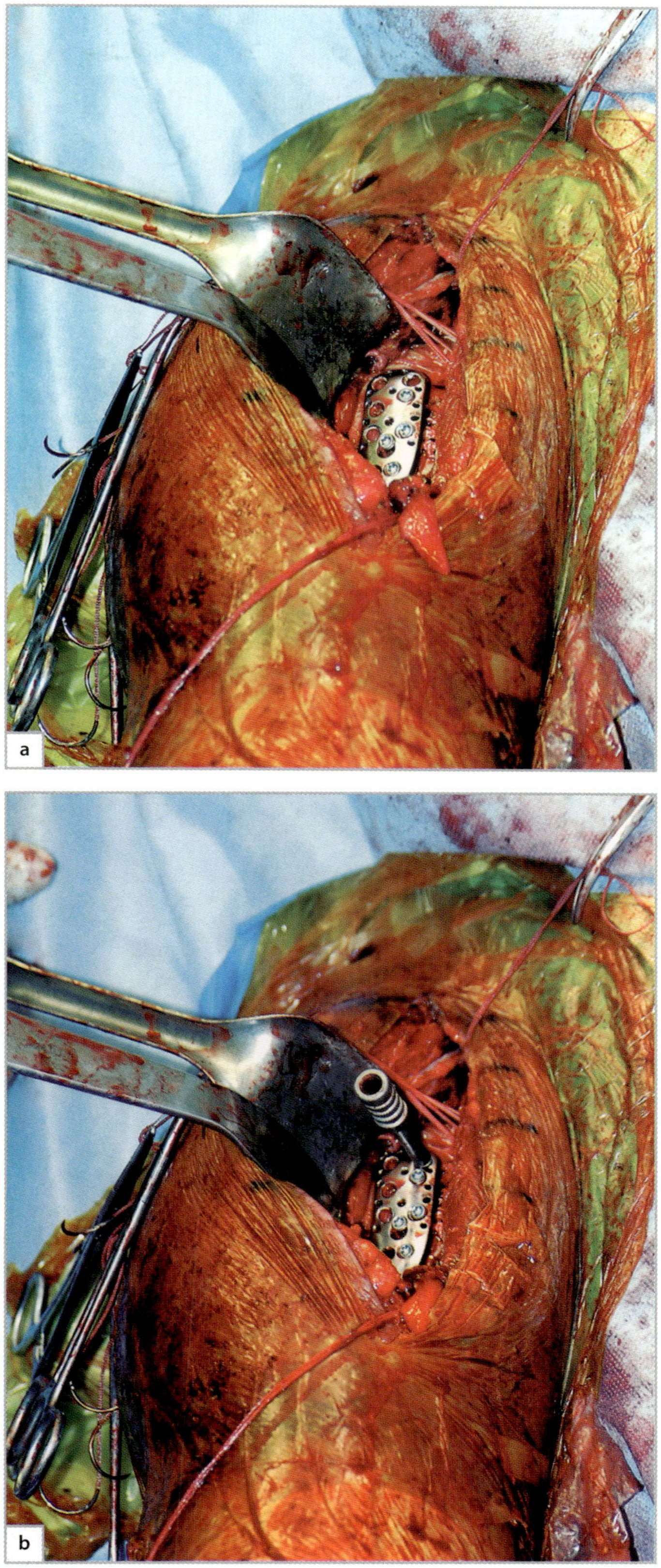

Figure 6.10 Plate fixation for a fracture of the proximal humerus. (a) Intraoperative view of locking screws in the proximal end of the plate. (b) A guide sleeve can be inserted into the locking screw holes to ensure proper placement of the locking screws into the screw holes. (From Ricchetti ET, DeMola PM, Roman D, Abboud JA. The use of precontoured humeral locking plates in the management of displaced proximal humerus fracture. J Am Acad Orthop Surg 2009;17:582–590. © 2009 American Academy of Orthopaedic Surgeons.)

to seven locking screws are typically recommended to maximize construct stability. In drilling the proximal screw holes into the humeral head, stepwise advancement of the drill bit should be utilized until resistance from subchondral bone is felt. Screw length is determined with a depth gauge, and should be at least 5–10 mm short of subchondral bone, to avoid intra-articular penetration. Intraoperative fluoroscopy is used to confirm that intra-articular screw penetration has not occurred, and digital palpation of the articular surface of the humeral head through the rotator interval should be performed as a final confirmation that none of the proximal locking screws has penetrated into the glenohumeral joint. Screw penetration into the glenohumeral joint has been reported at a relatively high rate in several studies (Sudkamp et al. 2009, Thanasas et al. 2009, Ricchetti et al. 2010, Sproul et al. 2011), from either intraoperative error (primary penetration) or subsidence/collapse of the humeral head fragment postoperatively (secondary penetration) (**Fig. 6.11**). These techniques help to minimize this complication (Ricchetti et al. 2010).

The shaft end of the plate may be filled with locking or non-locking screws. A minimum of three bicortical screws should be used to prevent hardware failure. Insertion of locking screws into the shaft creates a fixed-angle construct for bridging of metaphyseal comminution, if present. Holes at the metaphyseal level should not be filled in these instances, in order to allow the plate to function as a bridging device. The segment of the plate not filled with screws allows for absorption of bending moments, thus preventing implant breakage due to excessive stress concentration at the bone–implant interface (Ricchetti et al. 2009, Ricchetti et al. 2010). A longer plate may be necessary in fractures with a significant zone of metaphyseal comminution.

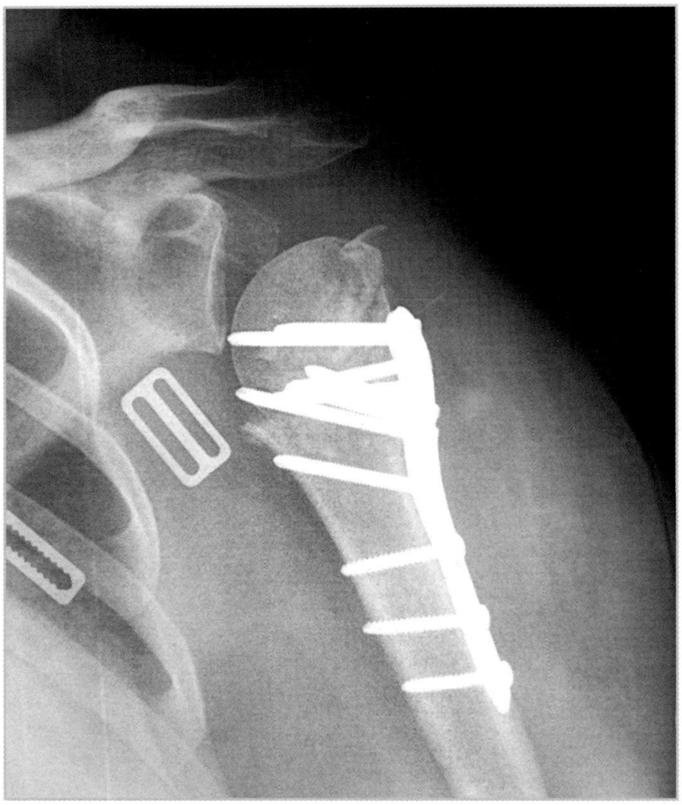

Figure 6.11 Anteroposterior radiograph of a fracture of the proximal humerus following unsatisfactory open reduction and internal fixation with a locking plate. The collapse of the humeral head fragment is due to avascular necrosis and subsequent screw penetration through the humeral head into the glenohumeral joint. (From Ricchetti ET, Warrender WJ, Abboud JA. Use of locking plates in the treatment of proximal humerus fractures. J Shoulder Elbow Surg 2010;19S:66–75. © Elsevier 2010.)

Augmentation techniques

When all screws have been placed in the locking plate, the sutures in the rotator cuff should be tied down for additional fracture fixation. Sutures can be tied down through the small peripheral holes in the proximal end of the plate or directly through fracture fragments. The natural deforming forces of the rotator cuff can be counteracted by tying these sutures through the plate, further increasing the stability of the construct. Indications for suture use and fixation in the rotator cuff should be generous, as the added stability allows for early postoperative exercises, and decreases the risk of loss of reduction or malunion (Ricchetti et al. 2009, Ricchetti et al. 2010).

The presence of significant comminution, bone loss, or osteoporotic bone in the humeral head or metaphysis, common in three- and four-part fractures of the proximal humerus, should lend consideration in certain instances to the use of other augmentation techniques to maximize stability of the locking-plate construct. Significant bone defects that are well contained, in either the humeral head or the metaphyseal region, can be filled with auto- or allograft cancellous bone or bone graft substitutes to further increase fracture stability and stimulate healing. Typically, the graft material can be placed through an anterior or lateral cortical window in the metaphyseal region that is present due to fracture comminution. Metaphyseal comminution can also lead to loss of the medial cortex in this region and, therefore, a lack of medial support, which can lead to loss of fracture reduction. Gardner et al. (2007) defined the presence of medial support as any one of three sets of conditions: (1) the medial cortex is anatomically reduced and no comminution is present; (2) the fragment of the head of the proximal humerus is impacted laterally into the distal humeral shaft fragment; or (3) an oblique locking screw is positioned inferomedially in the head fragment ('kickstand screw'). They found that a lack of medial support was a significant predictor of loss of reduction following open reduction and internal fixation with locking plates (Gardner et al. 2007). In a subsequent study, Gardner et al. (2008b) described the use of an intramedullary, structural fibular allograft as another method to obtain reduction and support of the medial cortex in cases of significant comminution. Other authors have also advocated this technique to support the humeral head, and to provide additional fixation for the distal shaft screws in cases of severe comminution and poor bone quality (Boileau et al. 2006, Badman et al. 2011).

Wound closure

When fixation is complete, the shoulder should be taken through a full, passive ROM to assess the stability of the locking-plate construct. Final fluoroscopic images should also be taken to confirm adequate fracture reduction, plate positioning, and length of the proximal locking screws (to ensure there is no penetration into the glenohumeral joint). The long head of the biceps is then tenodesed to the pectoralis major tendon. We prefer biceps tenodesis in most cases, as either the bicipital groove cannot be perfectly restored with fracture reduction and fixation, or the proximal tendon has been significantly damaged by the fracture. The wound is copiously irrigated, and a drain is placed deep to the deltopectoral interval to close down any dead space and prevent hematoma formation. The wound is then closed in layers and covered with sterile dressings, and the arm is placed in a sling for immobilization.

Pearls and pitfalls

Pearls

- Use of a mechanical arm-holding device facilitates surgery by providing support of the arm and shoulder girdle throughout the procedure.
- Knowledge of the precise location of neurovascular structures is critical. Failure to identify the axillary nerve, musculocutaneous nerve, and humeral circumflex vessels may lead to neurovascular injury, particularly if dissection strays too far medially.
- Adequate muscle paralysis throughout surgery is helpful in fracture exposure, mobilization, and reduction.
- Other keys to adequate fracture reduction include identifying the long head of the biceps tendon to help define proximal humeral anatomy, appropriately mobilizing fracture fragments, use of rotator cuff sutures, and intraoperative fluoroscopy.
- Inadequate reduction and stabilization of the fracture must be avoided. The fracture should not be plated prior to obtaining adequate reduction. The plate must be long enough for the fracture pattern, and an adequate number of screws must be used within the humeral head and shaft.
- Sutures should be placed in the rotator cuff not only for fracture reduction but also to increase construct stability. These sutures can be tied down through the peripheral holes in the locking plate to help neutralize the deforming forces of the rotator cuff.
- Bone graft or bone graft substitutes should be used when needed to fill cavitary defects in the humeral head or metaphysis, or for structural support (intramedullary fibular allograft).
- The risks and benefits to the patient must be considered when contemplating revision of fracture reduction and improved positioning of the implant.

Pitfalls

- Excessive exposure and soft-tissue stripping of the fracture fragments may interrupt the blood supply to the fragments, particularly if the posteromedial soft-tissue sleeve is disrupted.
- Inadequate reduction of a displaced humeral head fragment, particularly if left in varus malposition, can lead to poor functional results and possible loss of reduction.
- Displaced tuberosity fragments that have been insufficiently reduced or inadequately fixed to the plate may secondarily displace, and also lead to poor functional outcomes, including subacromial impingement.
- Subacromial plate impingement during arm elevation can result from a failure to place the locking plate in an appropriately distal position in relation to the top of the humeral head and greater tuberosity. Attempting to reduce a medially displaced fragment of the humeral shaft to the plate with a bicortical, non-locking screw can also cause proximal displacement of the plate as the screw is tightened.
- Incorrect threading of the locking screws in the screw holes can result in failure of the locking mechanism between plate and screws, cold welding, and/or screw loosening.
- Too few bicortical screws in the humeral shaft can lead to hardware failure and displacement of the plate from the shaft.
- Lack of medial support has been shown to be a significant predictor of loss of reduction following open reduction and internal fixation with a locking plate.
- Appropriate length of the screws in the humeral head should be confirmed with intraoperative fluoroscopy to avoid screw perforation into the glenohumeral joint and iatrogenic damage to the articular cartilage. Digital palpation of the articular surface of the humeral head through the rotator interval can be used as an additional measure to determine whether intra-articular screw penetration has occurred.

REHABILITATION

Postoperatively, the arm is initially placed in a sling to immobilize the shoulder. The drain is removed one to two days after surgery. Active shoulder use and lifting with the affected arm are prohibited for the first four to six weeks after surgery, but passive ROM exercises of the shoulder are begun early, with the exact timing dictated by fracture stability, bone quality, and patient compliance (Ricchetti et al. 2009, Ricchetti et al. 2010). Passive stretching is typically started within the first two weeks postoperatively to avoid shoulder stiffness, and initially consists of pendulum exercises, passive supine forward elevation, and passive supine external rotation at the side. Patients can usually be taught how to perform these simple exercises on their own at home, and one should be cautious of overaggressive formal physiotherapy during the early postoperative period, as this may lead to loss of fracture reduction or construct failure. Active ROM of the elbow, wrist, and hand can also be started in the early postoperative period, to avoid the development of stiffness.

Active shoulder ROM exercises begin at approximately four to six weeks postoperatively, after radiographic evidence of fracture healing is evident, and include stretching exercises in all planes (forward flexion and extension, external and internal rotation, abduction and adduction). Strengthening or resistive exercises are not initiated on the shoulder until approximately 10–12 weeks postoperatively, after significant bony consolidation has been confirmed on plain radiographs, and adequate coordination of the extremity has been achieved. Shoulder ROM should be maximal or near maximal at that point. Resistive exercises include rotator cuff, deltoid, and scapular strengthening, and are advanced as tolerated. Return to unrestricted activity with the arm occurs around five to six months postoperatively.

Standard AP, axillary, and scapular Y radiographic views of the shoulder are taken immediately after surgery and at routine outpatient follow-up visits, typically six weeks, three months, and six months postoperatively, in order to follow fracture healing (**Fig. 6.12**). After bony union is complete, plate removal is generally not necessary, unless subacromial plate impingement or adhesive capsulitis develops.

CONCLUSION

The primary goal of surgery for the treatment of fractures of the proximal humerus should be to create a construct stable enough to maintain fracture alignment and allow early ROM of the shoulder. Age, fracture pattern and displacement, bone quality, humeral head vascular status, pre-existing rotator cuff disease or degenerative changes, associated injuries, and patient function are important factors to consider in selecting the optimal surgical technique and implant to achieve this goal (Ricchetti et al. 2009). Locking plates may be ideal for three- and four-part fractures where adequate fixation to allow early rehabilitation is not possible with other techniques, non-operative or operative.

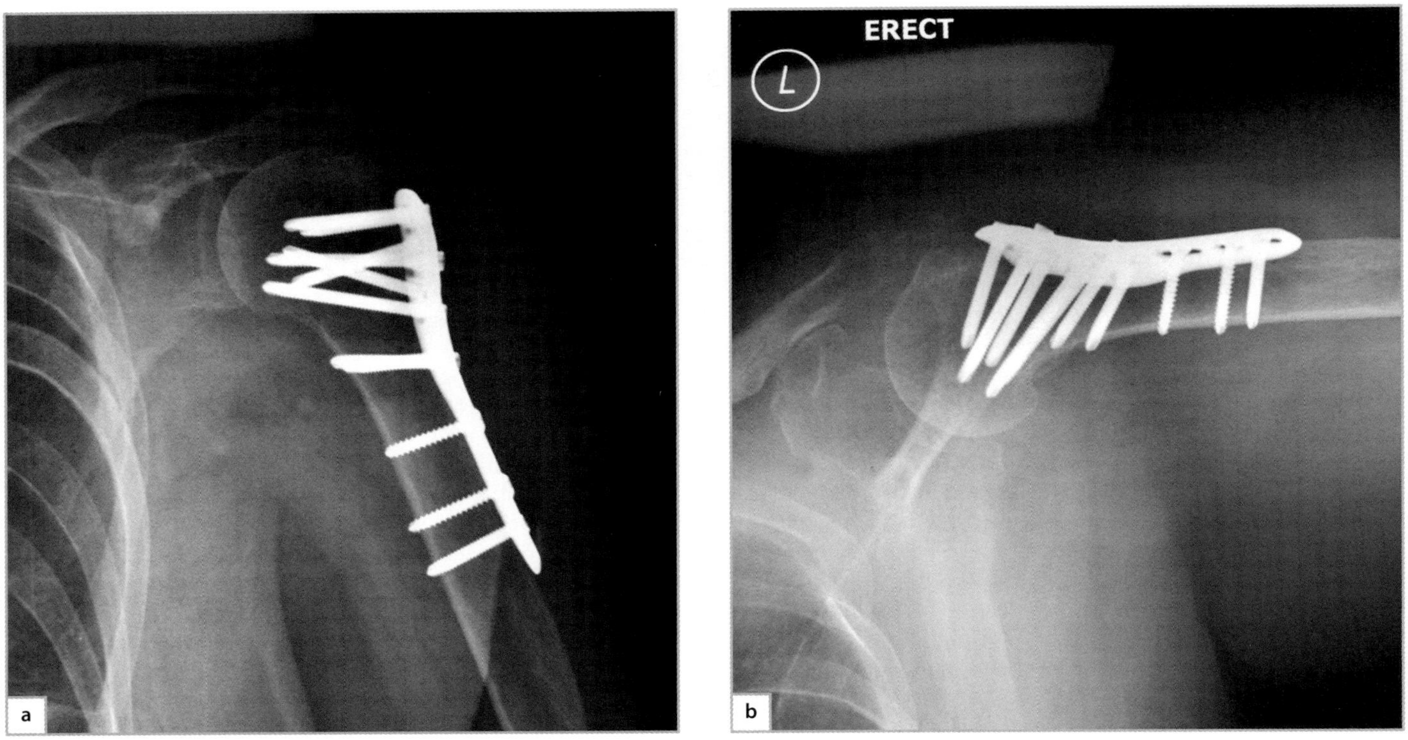

Figure 6.12 Radiographs of a healed fracture of the proximal humerus following fixation with a locking plate. (a) Anteroposterior view and (b) axillary view. The fracture and plate show good alignment, without evidence of screw penetration into the glenohumeral joint. (From Ricchetti ET, Warrender WJ, Abboud JA. Use of locking plates in the treatment of proximal humerus fractures. J Shoulder Elbow Surg 2010;19S:66–75. © Elsevier 2010.)

REFERENCES

Badman B, Frankle M, Keating C, et al. Results of proximal humeral locked plating with supplemental suture fixation of rotator cuff. J Shoulder Elbow Surg 2011;20:616–624.

Bastian JD, Hertel R. Initial post-fracture humeral head ischemia does not predict development of necrosis. J Shoulder Elbow Surg 2008;17:2–8.

Boileau P, Chuinard C, Le Huec JC, et al. Proximal humerus fracture sequelae: impact of a new radiographic classification on arthroplasty. Clin Orthop Relat Res 2006;442:121–130.

Gallo RA, Zeiders GJ, Altman GT. Two-incision technique for treatment of complex proximal humerus fractures. J Orthop Trauma 2005;19:734–740.

Gardner MJ, Weil Y, Barker JU, et al. The importance of medial support in locked plating of proximal humerus fractures. J Orthop Trauma 2007;21:185–191.

Gardner MJ, Boraiah S, Helfet DL, Lorich DG. The anterolateral acromial approach for fractures of the proximal humerus. J Orthop Trauma 2008a;22:132–137.

Gardner MJ, Boraiah S, Helfet DL, Lorich DG. Indirect medial reduction and strut support of proximal humerus fractures using an endosteal implant. J Orthop Trauma 2008b;22:195–200.

Gerber C, Hersche O, Berberat C. The clinical relevance of posttraumatic avascular necrosis of the humeral head. J Shoulder Elbow Surg 1998;7:586–590.

Handoll HH, Ollivere BJ. Interventions for treating proximal humeral fractures in adults. Cochrane Database Syst Rev 2010;12:CD000434.

Hepp P, Theopold J, Voigt C, et al. The surgical approach for locking plate osteosynthesis of displaced proximal humeral fractures influences the functional outcome. J Shoulder Elbow Surg 2008;17:21–28.

Hertel R, Hempfing A, Stiehler M, Leunig M. Predictors of humeral head ischemia after intracapsular fracture of the proximal humerus. J Shoulder Elbow Surg 2004;13:427–433.

Hettrich CM, Boraiah S, Dyke JP, et al. Quantitative assessment of the vascularity of the proximal part of the humerus. J Bone Joint Surg Am 2010;92:943–948.

Laflamme GY, Rouleau DM, Berry GK, et al. Percutaneous humeral plating of fractures of the proximal humerus: results of a prospective multicenter clinical trial. J Orthop Trauma 2008;22:153–158.

Lanting B, MacDermid J, Drosdowech D, Faber KJ. Proximal humeral fractures: a systematic review of treatment modalities. J Shoulder Elbow Surg 2008;17:42–54.

Neer CS 2nd. Displaced proximal humeral fractures. I. Classification and evaluation. J Bone Joint Surg Am 1970;52:1077–1089.

Ricchetti ET, DeMola PM, Roman D, Abboud JA. The use of precontoured humeral locking plates in the management of displaced proximal humerus fracture. J Am Acad Orthop Surg 2009;17:582–590.

Ricchetti ET, Warrender WJ, Abboud JA. Use of locking plates in the treatment of proximal humerus fractures. J Shoulder Elbow Surg 2010;19S:66–75.

Sproul RC, Iyengar JJ, Devcic Z, Feeley BT. A systematic review of locking plate fixation of proximal humerus fractures. Injury 2011;42:408–413.

Sudkamp N, Bayer J, Hepp P, et al. Open reduction and internal fixation of proximal humeral fractures with use of the locking proximal humerus plate. Results of a prospective, multicenter, observational study. J Bone Joint Surg Am 2009;91:1320–1328.

Thanasas C, Kontakis G, Angoules A, et al. Treatment of proximal humerus fractures with locking plates: a systematic review. J Shoulder Elbow Surg 2009;18:837–844.

Chapter 7

Open reduction and internal fixation of fractures of the proximal humerus: the anterolateral acromial approach

Michael J. Gardner

INTRODUCTION

Operative fixation of displaced and unstable fractures of the proximal humerus can be a challenge. Possibly more than in any other anatomic region in the body, the combination of small volume and poor quality bone in the humeral head often compromises stable fixation. Additionally, many fracture patterns contain displaced tuberosity fractures, for which reduction and fixation are critical for acceptable shoulder function.

Dozens of implants and techniques have been developed for fixation of fractures of the proximal humerus. Recently developed locking plates are ideally suited for maintaining fixation in short, osteoporotic end-segments by providing fixed-angle screws and multiple oblique potential fixation points in the humeral head. Despite the theoretical advantages of locking plates in these fractures, relatively high rates of both mechanical and biological complications persist (Egol et al. 2008, Owsley and Gorczyca 2008, Solberg et al. 2009). It has become clear that locking plates are not a panacea for these fractures, and that technical aspects of the operative procedure remain paramount (Gardner et al. 2007a). Specifically, accurate reduction of the fracture fragments is necessary to decrease stresses on the implant and at the bone–screw interfaces, and thereby to minimize the risk of implant failure.

INDICATIONS

The deltopectoral approach is the workhorse approach to the shoulder, and is familiar to most orthopaedic surgeons. It is extensile and is effective for many operative procedures around the shoulder. However, it is suboptimal for locked plating of fractures of the proximal humerus, for a variety of reasons. It involves anterior shoulder access, in which the anterior humeral circumflex arteries, which contribute to the critical humeral head vascularity (Gerber et al. 1990), are directly in the surgical dissection (Gardner et al. 2006). To access the lateral aspect of the proximal humerus, vigorous retraction to the large deltoid muscle mass is often necessary. The greater tuberosity most commonly retracts posteriorly, due to rotator cuff muscular forces, making it difficult to access from an anterior approach. This has prompted some authors to recommend an accessory incision to mobilize this fragment (Gallo et al. 2005). Additionally, fracture lines often require extraosseous reduction instruments, which can add to the biological insult.

To address some of these issues, the anterolateral acromial (ALA) approach was developed (Gardner et al. 2005, Gardner et al. 2008). By exploiting the interval between the anterior and middle heads of the deltoid, the intertuberosity fracture line is accessed directly. This facilitates mobilization of both the greater and lesser tuberosities. Additionally, access to the cancellous fracture surface of the fragments of the humeral head, through either the anatomic or the surgical neck fracture line, allows reduction maneuvers with minimal biological disturbance (Gardner et al. 2007b). The anterior circumflex vessels are not in the surgical field (Gardner et al. 2006). The ALA approach is directly in line with the plating zone and vector of the locking screws, allowing the plate to be used as an indirect reduction tool.

Indications for using the ALA approach include displaced two-, three-, and four-part fractures of the proximal humerus. Fractures of both the surgical and the anatomic neck are accessible through this approach. Metaphyseal non-unions are also fully accessible for debridement, fixation, and bone grafting after exposure of the axillary nerve. In our experience, glenohumeral fracture dislocations are also facilitated through the ALA approach. Because the surgical plane is lateral to the subscapularis insertion, the glenoid is easily visualized, providing a point for counterforce on the glenoid when reducing the humeral head into the shoulder joint.

CONTRAINDICATIONS

The main contraindication to the ALA approach is if an arthroplasty procedure is being planned or is highly likely. Hemiarthroplasty and reverse shoulder arthroplasty are both possible through this approach, but are generally more reproducible through a deltopectoral approach. Additionally, if the lesser tuberosity is displaced more than 1 cm medially, accessing the fragment or the subscapularis tendon deep to the anterior deltoid can be difficult through the ALA approach without undue tension on the axillary nerve.

TECHNIQUE

The preferred patient positioning is supine on a reversed cantilever-type operating table (**Fig. 7.1**). Beach-chair positioning is also possible, but we have found fluoroscopic imaging more cumbersome with that setup. General anesthesia with full muscle paralysis is used to minimize

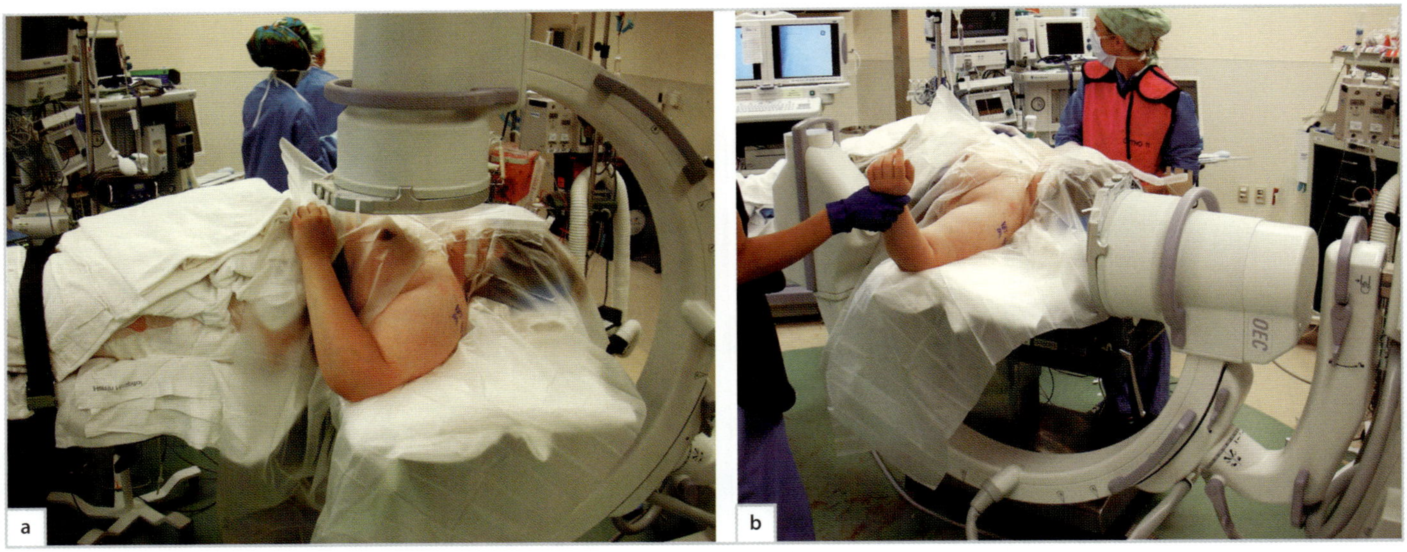

Figure 7.1 Patient positioning for the anterolateral acromial (ALA) approach. The supine position is preferred. The patient is brought to the edge of the bed on the operative side with the arm resting on a Plexiglas extension. Prior to prepping and draping, the anteroposterior (a) and axillary views (b) are checked to ensure fluoroscopic visualization is adequate.

deforming forces on the fracture fragments. The patient is brought to the edge of the table, with a Plexiglas or other radiolucent arm-board to support the operative upper extremity. Fluoroscopy views are checked prior to preparation and draping, to ensure visualization is adequate.

The incision is marked; it begins just proximal to the anterolateral corner of the acromion, and extends distally 12–15 cm toward the deltoid tuberosity, in line with the palpable humeral shaft. The approximate location at which the axillary nerve is crossed is marked on the skin 65 mm from the edge of the acromion (**Fig. 7.2**). The skin and subcutaneous tissue are incised. The avascular raphe between the anterior and middle heads of the deltoid is then identified (**Fig. 7.3**). This plane is developed bluntly to the level of the deep deltoid fascia. The interval is then opened proximally until the acromion is palpated, to ensure the skin marking was correct. Deep in the wound the bursa is identified (**Fig. 7.4**). The bursa must be incised to identify any fracture lines proximal to the surgical neck (e.g. in the tuberosities), as well as to appose the plate to the bone.

With the proximal window exposed, the deltoid raphe is carefully developed from superficial to deep, and from proximal to distal, to expose the axillary nerve. When the level of the nerve is reached, retraction on the anterior and middle deltoid heads should be minimized, as this can stretch the nerve. Distal to the nerve, the humeral shaft is identified and prepared for later plate and screw application (**Fig. 7.5**).

Attention is then turned back to the proximal window for reduction and fixation of the fracture. The bursa can be elevated anteriorly and posteriorly to fully expose the fracture lines, and can be partially excised if it is hypertrophic and redundant. In almost all patients and fracture patterns, placing several traction sutures in the rotator cuff tendons is beneficial. These allow for mobilization and control of the tuberosities, if present, or of the entire humeral head fragment if the tuberosities are intact. These sutures are tied to the plate after final fixation, to provide an additional tension band to offset the varus force of the rotator cuff. With traction on the rotator cuff, a wide elevator or the surgeon's finger is gently passed in the subacromial space to break up any adhesions. Fracture reduction then proceeds using a variety of instruments and maneuvers, depending on the fracture pattern.

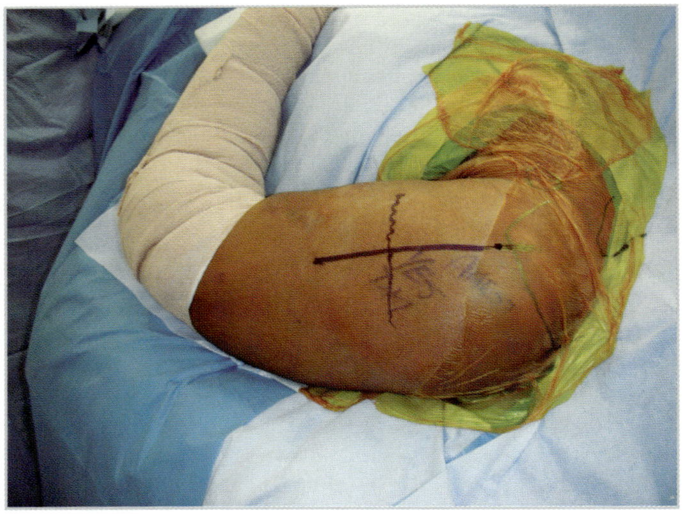

Figure 7.2 Marking of the skin incision. The incision extends distally from the anterolateral acromion to the deltoid tuberosity. The approximate position of the crossing axillary nerve is marked on the skin 65 mm from the acromial edge.

Valgus – surgical neck

The most straightforward fracture reduction maneuver is with displaced two-part fractures of the surgical neck. The typical displacement pattern is humeral head valgus, medial translation of the humeral shaft, and apex anterior. The ALA approach is ideally suited for this fracture pattern, as the plate can be used as in indirect reduction tool. With both windows exposed proximal and distal to the axillary nerve, the plate is applied in the appropriate position just posterior to the biceps tendon, and 5–10 mm distal to the apex of the greater tuberosity. The plate is secured proximally using 1.6 mm (0.062 in) Kirschner wires (K-wires) (this can additionally be done distally at this stage). The sagittal plane alignment is checked on the axillary view, and reduced if necessary. A cortical screw is then placed through the plate

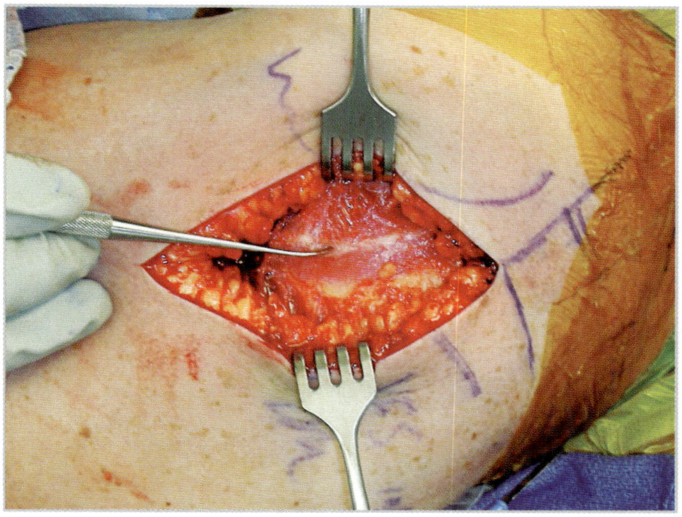

Figure 7.3 After the skin and subcutaneous tissue is incised, the raphe between the anterior and middle heads of the deltoid is identified.

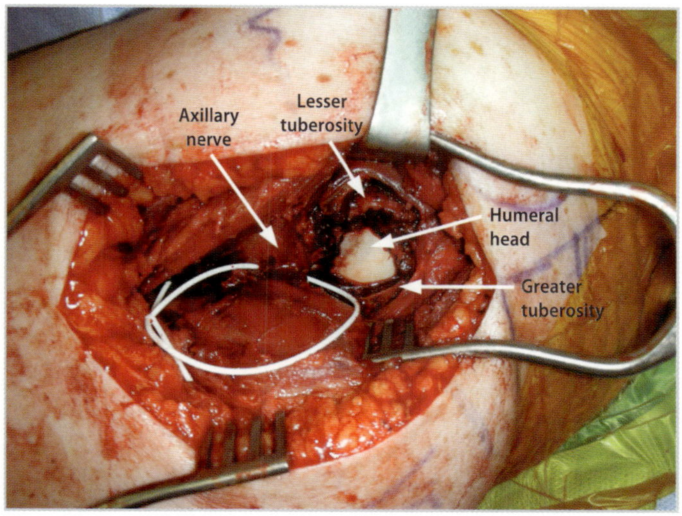

Figure 7.5 Distal to the axillary nerve, the humeral shaft is exposed for later plate and screw application.

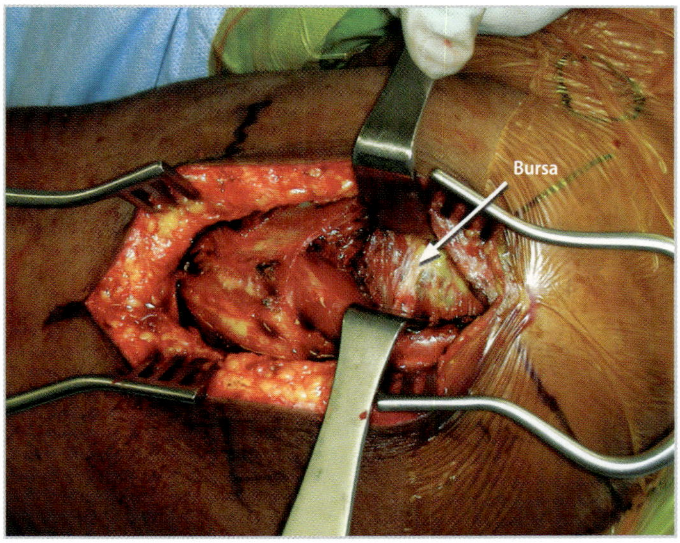

Figure 7.4 Proximally in the wound, the raphe is bluntly developed to expose the deep bursal tissue.

to draw the shaft to the plate, indirectly reducing the surgical neck (**Fig. 7.6**). Additional screws are then placed proximally and distally to complete the fixation.

Valgus – anatomic neck

Fractures that involve the anatomic neck are nearly always associated with fractures of the greater and/or lesser tuberosities. These patterns are typically easier to maintain reduced once anatomic reduction is obtained (Solberg et al. 2009). The key is restoring the 'ring' of the tuberosity fractures, which has been likened to an egg cup that provides a stable base on which to support the fragment of the humeral head (Hertel 2005). After incising the bursa, frequently the articular surface of the humeral head is directly in the wound (**Fig. 7.7**). Traction sutures are placed into the subscapularis and infraspinatus tendons to control the lesser and greater tuberosities, respectively. The head fragment is then disimpacted and reduced with an elevator (**Fig. 7.8**). During this step, care should be taken to restore the version of the humeral head relative to the humeral axis, which is frequently in excessive retroversion (**Fig. 7.9**). With the humeral head elevated, the tuberosities are brought together and reduced with the sutures (**Fig. 7.10**). These sutures can be tied to each other to maintain the tuberosities' reduced positions.

The plate is then applied in the correct position relative to the head fragment. At this point, the humeral head and tuberosities have been reconstructed and provisionally stabilized, leaving a two-part fracture at the surgical neck. A cortical reduction screw is used in the shaft, as described above, to reduce the shaft medialization, and locking screws are placed to complete the fixation (**Fig. 7.11**).

Varus

Varus fracture patterns require special attention to avoid varus malreductions. Due to the pull of the rotator cuff tendons, any residual varus deformity of the head segment predisposes to subsequent fixation failure. As a general principle, efforts are made to over-reduce the fracture into valgus, and indirect maneuvers are subsequently used to 'dial' out the valgus of the neck to achieve an anatomic-neck–shaft angle.

Through an ALA approach, the first step is to access the cancellous surface of the humeral head through the intertuberosity split. The head fragment is elevated out of varus using a broad flat elevator along the inferior region of the head. If the greater tuberosity is intact, rotator cuff sutures are useful for applying a valgus moment to the humeral head. Stout K-wires or threaded Steinmann pins (2.0 mm or greater) are also valuable as joysticks. If the greater tuberosity is fractured, it is reduced to the head fragment using dental picks and sutures, and K-wires are placed provisionally and strategically to avoid obstructing the plate position. The lesser tuberosity is reduced in a similar fashion. With the humeral head reconstructed, the arm is abducted to over-reduce the metaphysis into valgus, with medial shaft translation. A reduction screw is then inserted and slowly tightened to achieve a slow, controlled metaphyseal reduction. Locking screws are then placed into the shaft to maintain the reduction. The initial cortical reduction screw frequently needs to be changed to a shorter screw. Multiple locking screws are then placed into the humeral head, and the rotator cuff sutures are tied to the plate to augment fixation (**Fig. 7.12**).

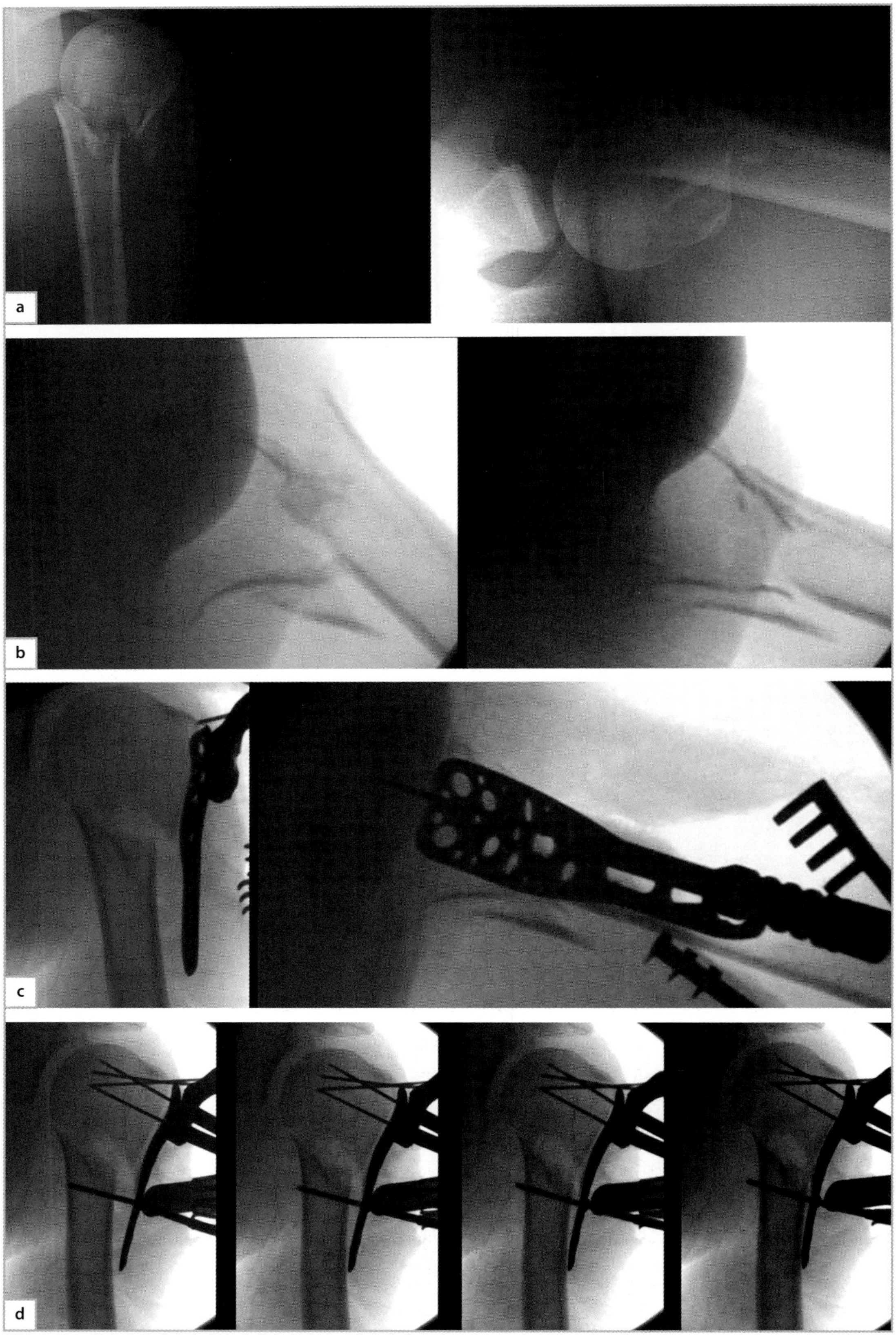

Figure 7.6 Displaced two-part fracture of the surgical neck of the humerus. A 42-year-old man was involved in a motor vehicle collision, resulting in the fracture (a). In such cases the axillary view should be checked early on in the reduction process; the sagittal alignment can be reduced indirectly using arm manipulation and towel bumps under the elbow (b). The plate is then positioned relative to the head on both views and stabilized provisionally (c). A cortical screw is placed through the shaft to indirectly reduce the shaft medialization at the surgical neck (d).

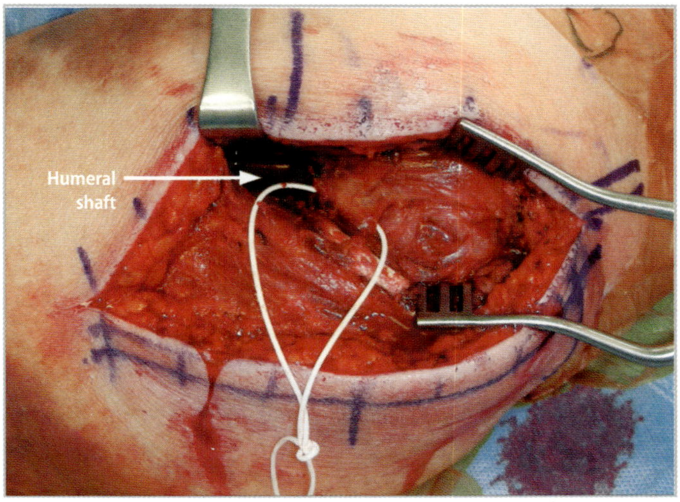

Figure 7.7 After incision of the bursal tissue in the proximal window, the intertuberosity fracture line, and often the articular fragment of the humeral head, are directly visualized.

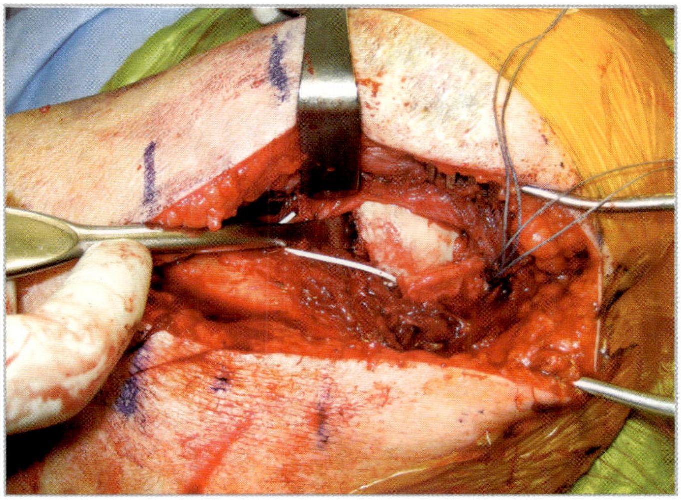

Figure 7.8 In valgus four-part fractures, the humeral head segment can be elevated and de-rotated for reduction using an elevator.

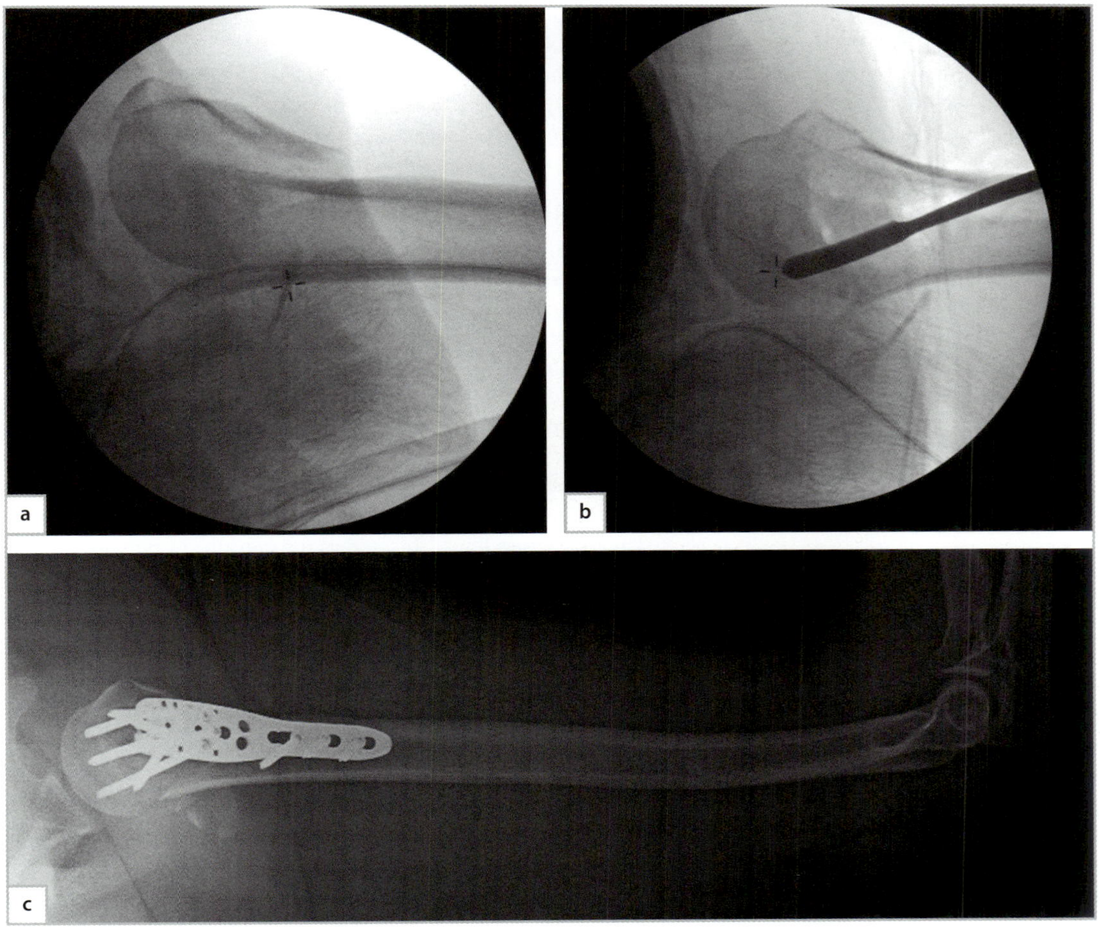

Figure 7.9 Excessive retroversion of the humeral head. This is a frequent deformity pattern (a). An elevator placed posteriorly on the cancellous surface can de-rotate the humeral head into an anatomic position, approximately 20° relative to the transepicondylar axis (b). Following open reduction and internal fixation, anatomic retroversion is restored (c).

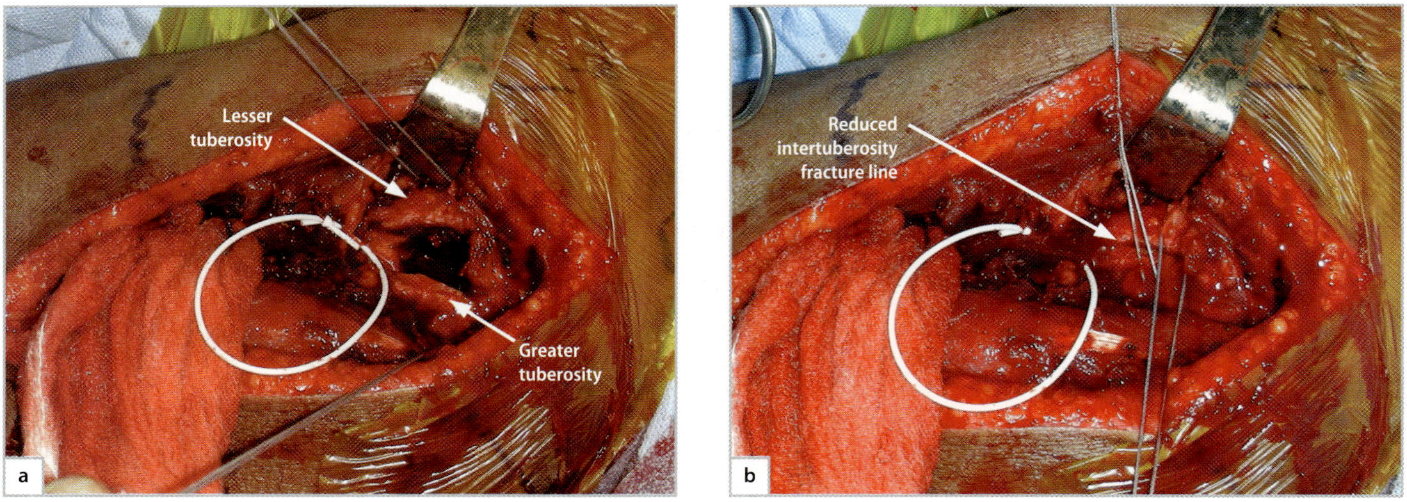

Figure 7.10 Mobilization, reduction, and stabilization of an intertuberosity fracture. (a) With the humeral head elevated, the greater and lesser tuberosities are mobilized using traction sutures in the respective rotator cuff tendon insertions. (b) The intertuberosity fracture line is reduced and stabilized using the sutures, and these are subsequently tied to each other for provisional stabilization.

Fracture dislocations

Upon incision of the bursa through the ALA approach, the glenoid is visible deep in the wound due to the displacement of the humeral head out of the joint space. Three or four threaded Steinmann pins are placed into the cancellous surface of the dislocated fragment of the humeral head, whether it is anterior or posterior to the glenoid. The wires are gathered together and inserted into a universal T-handled chuck to allow for manipulation of the humeral head. Because the dislocated head is frequently incarcerated anterior and inferior to the coracoid, lateral traction on the head tends to translate the entire scapula. To overcome this, a blunt instrument can be placed against the glenoid to allow for a counterforce. While the glenoid is pushed medially, the multiple Steinmann pins are pulled laterally to reduce the humeral head back into the glenoid (**Fig. 7.13**). Fracture reduction can then proceed based on the fracture pattern.

Pearls and pitfalls

Axillary nerve

- The nerve is adherent to the deep deltoid fascia, at a relatively constant position (around 65 mm from the acromion).
- Once the proximal window is opened proximal to the nerve, the surgeon's finger can be placed deep to the deltoid and swept from posterior to anterior, and the nerve can be palpated as a transverse band adherent to the undersurface of the deltoid.
- After the position of the nerve is identified by palpation and visualization, it does not need to be fully dissected. It is enveloped in a sleeve of alveolar tissue and is adjacent to the posterior humeral circumflex artery, which should be preserved when possible.
- A vessel loop should be placed around the nerve to maintain the surgical team's awareness of its position. Care must then be taken not to use the vessel loop for excessive traction.
- In most plating systems, the nerve overlies several screw holes in the plate. These are often screws that are directed along the calcar. The nerve should be gently retracted when the locking guides are inserted and these important screws placed.
- Some plates feature 'block' guides that are bulky and often impinge on the nerve when used with the ALA approach. These guides should be avoided in favor of attaching the threaded locking guides free-hand.
- The humeral shaft distal to the axillary nerve should be identified early in the procedure, during the surgical approach, so when the time comes to place the plate, this region will already be exposed.

Reduction maneuvers

- Sutures are invaluable for reducing and stabilizing the tuberosities. To reduce the tuberosities to each other, sutures in the rotator cuff tendons can be used and tied to each other. Additional rotator cuff sutures should be tied to the plate.
- When using K-wires as joysticks in the humeral head, these should be placed proximal to the anticipated position of the plate, so the reduction can be held while fixation is applied into the humeral head.
- If a cancellous elevator is used to reduce the humeral head out of valgus or varus, it should be placed along the anterior aspect of the lateral fracture lines. This allows the elevator to remain in place anterior to the plate for maintenance of reduction while screws are inserted though the plate.
- A varus fracture should be over-reduced into valgus, using instruments, K-wires, traction sutures in the rotator cuff, and arm abduction. The alignment can then be reduced back to anatomic in a controlled fashion, with frequent fluoroscopic views. This minimizes the risk of leaving a fracture in varus intraoperatively.

Implant placement

- Placing the plate too proximally will result in impingement on the acromion. Too distal plate placement may preclude the preferred positioning of the inferomedial calcar screws.
- When using a cortical screw as a reduction screw, the screw tip will often 'grow' as the diaphysis translates laterally into a reduced position. This screw should then be swapped for a screw of appropriate length at the completion of the procedure.

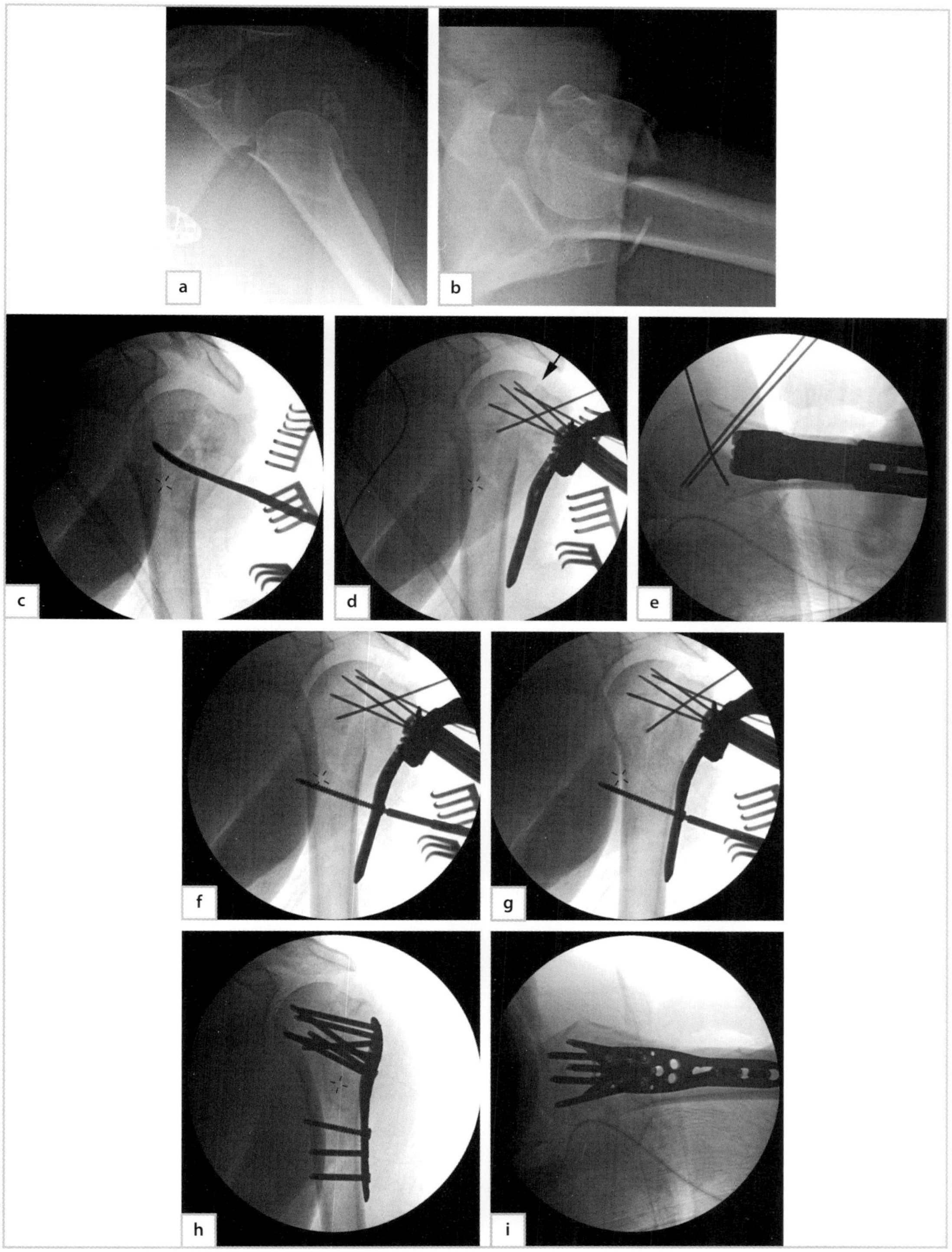

Figure 7.11 Treatment of a displaced four-part valgus impacted fracture of the proximal humerus. A 28-year-old female was involved in a motor vehicle accident, and sustained this fracture (a,b). Through an anterolateral acromial approach, the intertuberosity fracture was identified, and the humeral head fragment was elevated with an elevator (c). The tuberosities were manipulated using sutures in the rotator cuff and K-wire joysticks, until reduced to each other and to the humeral head fragment (arrow, d). Next, the plate was applied in the appropriate position relative to the reconstructed proximal fragment (d). At this point, it is crucial to check the axillary view to assess sagittal plane reduction and plate position (e). Next, a cortical reduction screw was placed through the plate into the humeral shaft (f) and was tightened until a metaphyseal reduction was achieved (g). Final fluoroscopic views demonstrate accurate reductions and implant positions (h,i).

- When locking screws are placed into the humeral head, the drill bit is typically used with tactile feedback to reach the subchondral bone. However, in osteoporotic bone, tactile sensation is minimal, and it is easy to perforate the humeral head and obtain an inaccurate measurement for the screw. To avoid this, a blunt K-wire can be placed as a 'sound', and the screw length measured indirectly.
- The sutures in the rotator cuff should be tied securely to the plate after all screw fixation has been placed. This provides augmentation of the fixation by bypassing some the varus pull of the rotator cuff on the humeral head.

REHABILITATION

Patients are placed in a sling in the operating room. They are instructed on gentle self-directed pendulum exercises for the first two weeks. At the two-week point, formal physiotherapy is initiated, which includes passive shoulder motion exercises only. Hand, wrist, and elbow motion is also incorporated to minimize stiffness and distal swelling. At six weeks, if radiographs demonstrate that the reduction is maintained and early healing is present, active assisted exercises are added. When full healing has occurred, usually by the three-month visit, strengthening is begun.

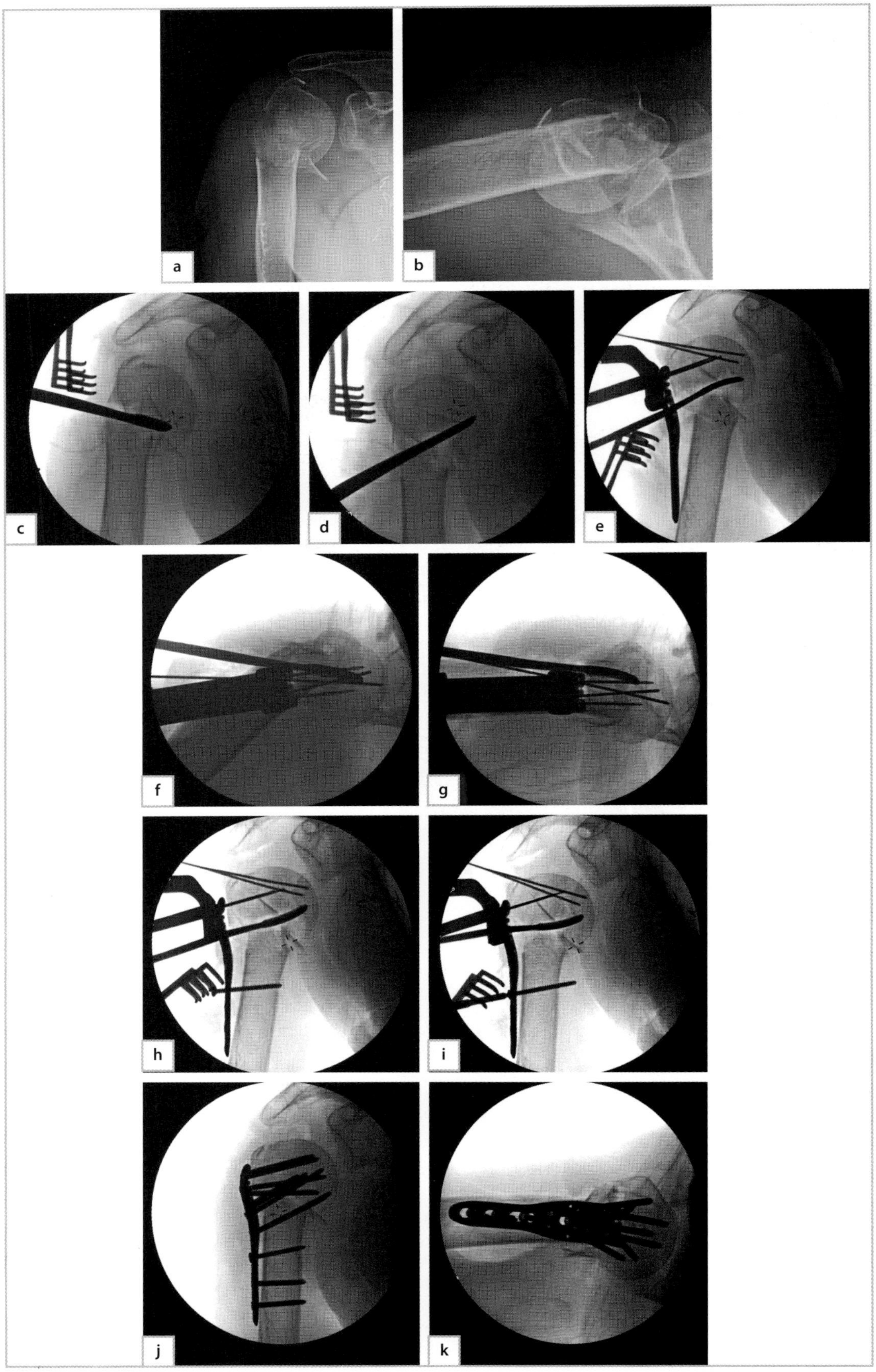

Figure 7.12 Treatment of a four-part fracture of the proximal humerus, with varus deformity. A 68-year-old woman sustained this fracture (a,b) when she tripped and fell while walking. Through an anterolateral acromial approach, an elevator was inserted at the base of the humeral head fragment (c), and used to partially reduce the varus displacement (d). The greater tuberosity was reduced with sutures and maintained with K-wires, and the plate was positioned laterally. The reduction was fine-tuned using arm abduction, K-wire joysticks in the humeral head, and an elevator (e). At this point, the sagittal plane was visualized on the axillary view, and the apex-anterior deformity was noted (f). Manual manipulation of the arm was used to correct the shaft relative to the plate; note the elevator in place anterior to the plate (g). The shaft remained translated medially, and a reduction screw was placed through the plate (h), and used to reduce the surgical neck component (i). Final fluoroscopic views show a reduced neck–shaft angle and stable fixation, with inferomedial calcar screws to support the comminuted medial column (j,k).

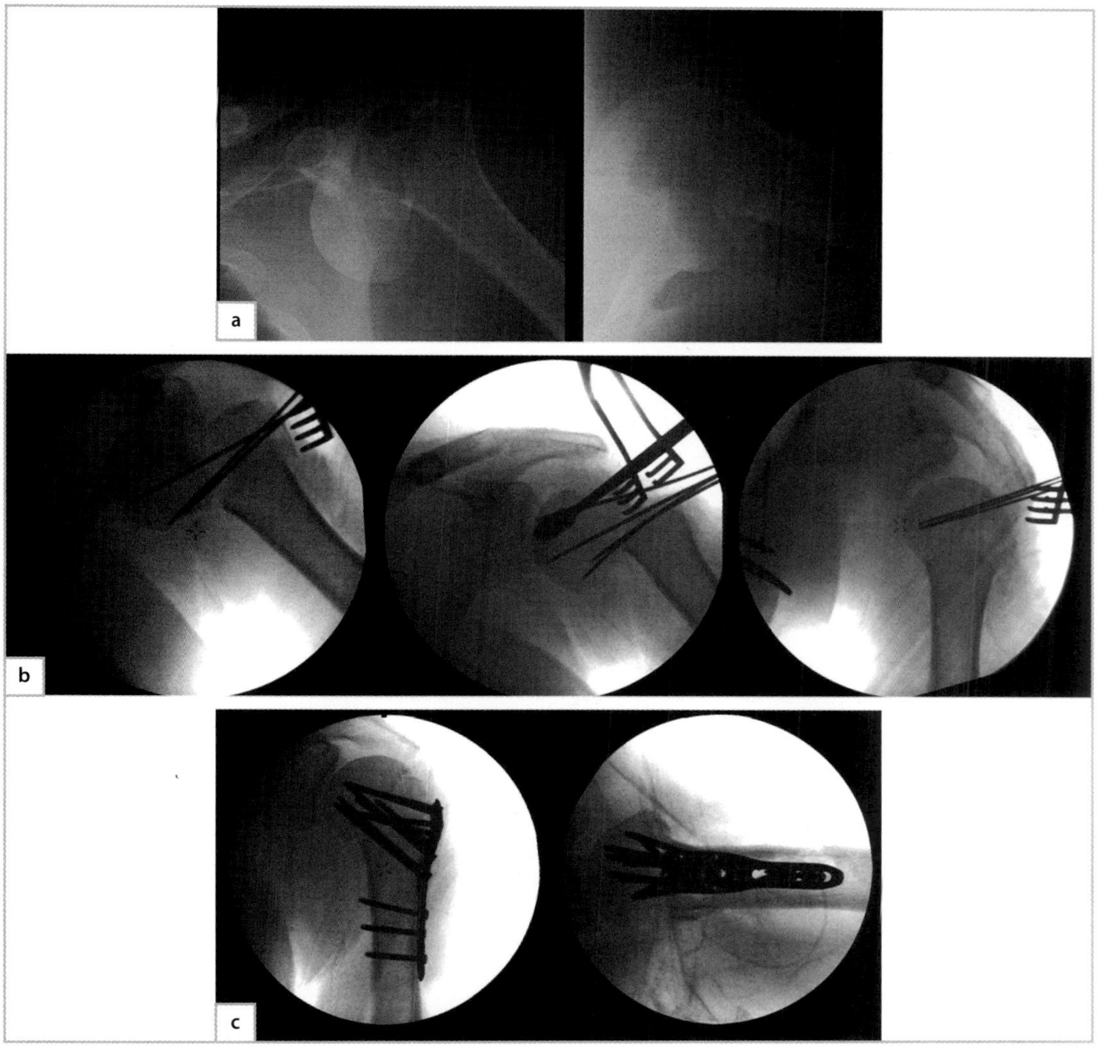

Figure 7.13 Treatment of a fracture dislocation of the proximal humerus. A 47-year-old man fell from a ladder and sustained this fracture (a). Multiple threaded Steinmann pins were placed in the cancellous surface of the humeral head, and an elevator was placed against the glenoid for counterforce to reduce the joint (b). Treatment of the fracture then proceeded using typical reduction and fixation techniques (c).

REFERENCES

Egol KA, Ong CC, Walsh M, et al. Early complications in proximal humerus fractures (OTA types 11) treated with locked plates. J Orthop Trauma 2008;22:159–164.

Gallo RA, Zeiders GJ, Altman GT. Two-incision technique for treatment of complex proximal humerus fractures. J Orthop Trauma 2005;19:734–740.

Gardner MJ, Griffith MH, Dines JS, et al. The extended anterolateral acromial approach allows minimally invasive access to the proximal humerus. Clin Orthop Relat Res 2005;434:123–129.

Gardner MJ, Voos JE, Wanich T, et al. Vascular implications of minimally invasive plating of proximal humerus fractures. J Orthop Trauma 2006;20:602–607.

Gardner MJ, Weil Y, Barker JU, et al. The importance of medial support in locked plating of proximal humerus fractures. J Orthop Trauma 2007a;21:185–191.

Gardner MJ, Lorich DG, Werner CM, Helfet DL. Second-generation concepts for locked plating of proximal humerus fractures. Am J Orthop 2007b;36:460–465.

Gardner MJ, Boraiah S, Helfet DL, Lorich DG. The anterolateral acromial approach for fractures of the proximal humerus. J Orthop Trauma 2008;22:132–137.

Gerber C, Schneeberger AG, Vinh TS. The arterial vascularization of the humeral head. An anatomical study. J Bone Joint Surg Am 1990;72:1486–1494.

Hertel R. Fractures of the proximal humerus in osteoporotic bone. Osteoporos Int 2005;16 Suppl 2:S65–72.

Owsley KC, Gorczyca JT. Displacement/screw cutout after open reduction and locked plate fixation of humeral fractures. J Bone Joint Surg Am 2008;90:233–240.

Solberg BD, Moon CN, Franco DP, Paiement GD. Locked plating of 3- and 4-part proximal humerus fractures in older patients: the effect of initial fracture pattern on outcome. J Orthop Trauma 2009;23:113–119.

Chapter 8 Percutaneous plate fixation of fractures of the proximal humerus

G. Yves Laflamme

INDICATIONS

Percutaneous plating of the proximal humerus was developed in an attempt to address two issues: humeral head necrosis associated with open reduction through an extensive approach; and insufficient primary stability associated with previous attempts at limited exposure and minimal internal fixation (Laflamme et al. 2008). A locking plate provides stable fixation for early establishment of range of motion, and also reduces soft-tissue scarring and loss of the gliding surfaces. Surgery is generally indicated when fracture instability prevents early motion or when fracture displacement is sufficiently great for functional impairment to be likely. Even among experts, controversy exists regarding the indications for surgical management, since evidence-based treatment guidelines are lacking (Gibson et al. 2001).

The fracture types that are ideally suited to reduction through a mini-incision are:

- displaced unstable two-part fractures of the surgical neck;
- isolated fractures of the greater tuberosity;
- valgus impacted (three- or four-part) fractures;
- fractures of the proximal third of the humeral shaft.

With increased experience, technically challenging fracture types can be tackled, like:

- three-part fractures;
- some four-part fractures, but sometimes extending this approach to a full anterolateral acromial incision as described by Gardner et al. (2005) is needed to obtain adequate reduction.

CONTRAINDICATIONS

With a minimally invasive approach, indirect reduction techniques are needed to achieve an acceptable reduction. A minimally invasive incision should not be an excuse for poor reduction. For this reason, we caution against the use of this approach for:

- fracture dislocations;
- head-splitting fractures;
- complex four-part fractures of the proximal humerus;
- non-unions and malunions.

TECHNIQUE

Patient positioning

Supine

Trauma surgeons prefer this positioning for multiply injured patients, especially if:

- cervical spines issues complicate head positioning;
- associated fractures to the extremities need simultaneous fixation (as there will be no need to reposition the patient).

The patient is placed in a supine position on a radiolucent table with a soft bump placed behind the chest. The entire upper extremity must be draped to allow free mobility for reduction maneuvers and for optimal imaging during surgery. The setup is checked before draping, with the C-arm unit brought to the opposite side to ensure complete visualization of the proximal humerus, including a modified axillary view (**Fig. 8.1**).

Beach chair

This alternative setup facilitates conversion to a hemiarthroplasty if the fracture proves not to be reconstructible. It also offers the best way to visualize the entire shoulder (axillary view), with the image intensifier placed parallel to the table at the patient's head on the injured side.

However, there are some disadvantages:

- The placement of the image intensifier at the patient's head limits access to the operating field. If it is placed on the opposite side, the axillary view is not possible.
- A specialized operating table that allows access to the shoulder is needed, with a head immobilizer, and (optionally) a hydraulic arm-holder.

Surgical approach

This minimally invasive technique allows limited disruption of soft tissue, with application of the plate on the lateral side of the humeral head, away from the primary vascular supply, the anterior humeral circumflex artery, which runs in the bicipital groove. A hypovascular bare spot, 3 cm wide, was identified by Gardner et al. on the greater tuberosity and application of the plate to this region may minimize iatrogenic vascular injury.

After proper positioning of the patient, we proceed with a direct minimally invasive lateral approach to the proximal humerus with two separate mini-incisions: the proximal window exposes the humeral head, and the distal window exposes the humeral shaft and distal part of the plate (**Fig. 8.2**). Internal or external rotation with abduction facilitates exposure through these mobile windows.

Proximal incision

The anterior edge of the acromion is palpated and used as a landmark (**Fig. 8.3a**). Starting 1 cm distal from this point, a direct lateral longitudinal incision is made distally for 4 cm in line with the middle of the humeral head. The subcutaneous tissue is incised, and the deltoid fascia is visualized and transected parallel to the underlying deltoid muscle fibers. The deltoid muscle fibers are bluntly split until the underlying subdeltoid bursa is exposed and incised (**Fig. 8.3c**).

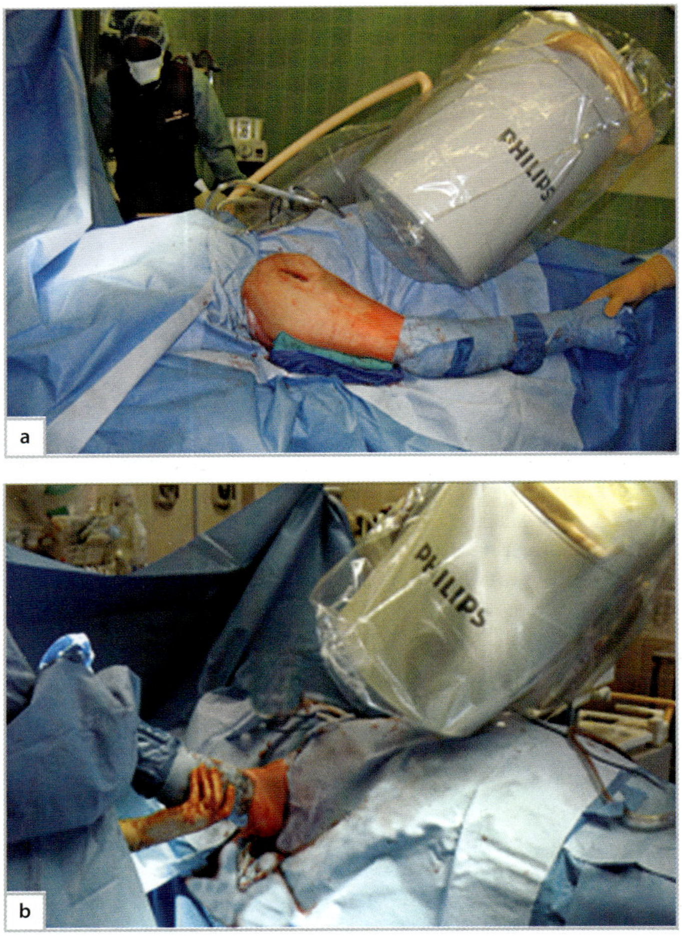

Figure 8.1 Patient positioning. (a) Our preferred setup is supine on a radiolucent table with the image intensifier on the opposite side. (b) Axillary view.

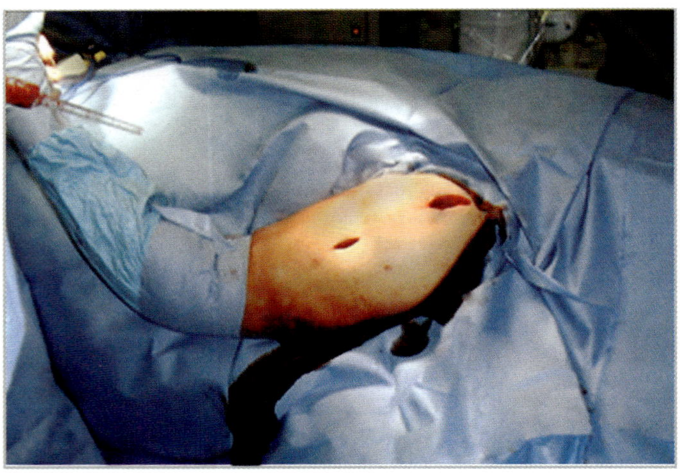

Figure 8.2 Direct minimally invasive lateral approach with two separate mini-incisions.

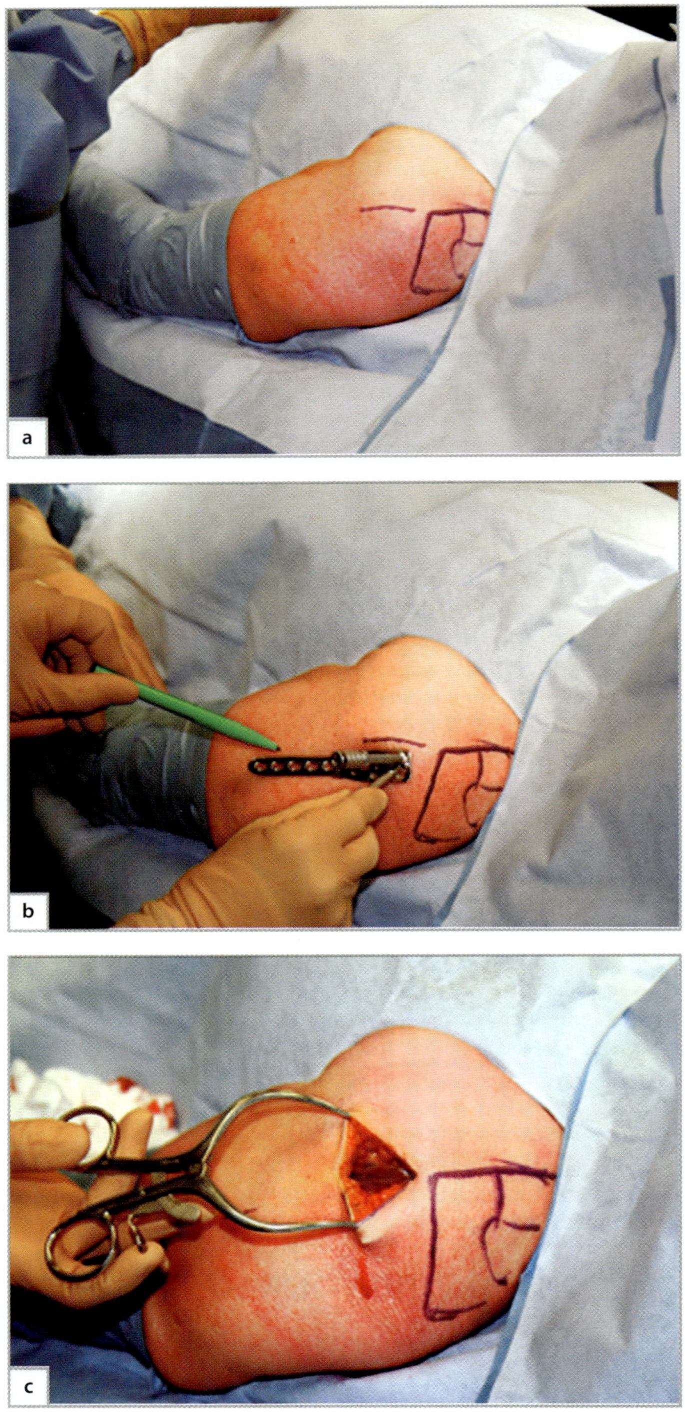

Figure 8.3 Surgical approach. (a) Landmarks. (b) Mapping of the distal incision with the plate. (c) Deltoid-splitting proximal incision.

Finger dissection is then needed to elevate the deltoid muscle from the proximal humerus to identify both the fracture and, especially, the axillary nerve (**Fig. 8.4**). (The surgeon should avoid pulling down on the bursa with a finger from top to bottom, as this may create a band of tissue that can be mistaken for the nerve.) The average distance from the lateral edge of the acromion to the axillary nerve is 7 cm (range 62–85 mm) (Smith et al. 2007). This cord-like band is first located in the posterior aspect of the wound as it exits the quadrangular space and then runs on the undersurface of the deltoid around the humerus as it supplies the deltoid muscle. If scarring or hematoma prevents palpation of the nerve, the surgeon should consider extending the incision and directly identifying the nerve using the extended lateral deltoid-splitting approach (Gardner et al. 2005).

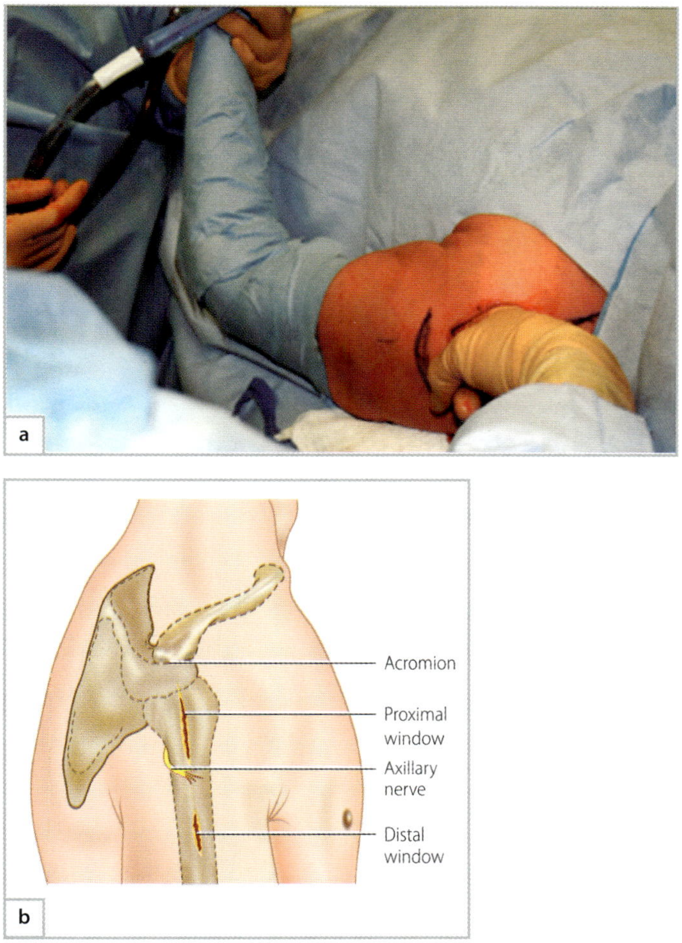

Figure 8.4 Identifying the axillary nerve. (a) Finger dissection to elevate the deltoid muscle from the humerus. (b) Location of the axillary nerve.

Distal incision

Mapping of the second window is done with the plate used as a template over the skin (see **Fig. 8.3b**). A 1–2 cm incision is made in-line and distal to the previous incision, and is centered over the distal three screw holes. Correct location is confirmed using fluoroscopy. The subcutaneous tissue and deltoid musculature are bluntly dissected. This incision is well below the course of the axillary nerve. It should be made wide enough for a finger to be inserted for inspection. If a radiolucent guide is available, an alternative for insertion of the distal screws is multiple stab wounds.

Reduction technique

The key to minimally invasive surgery is the ability to obtain acceptable reduction using indirect reduction techniques. As many surgeons have emphasized, normal anatomy is not crucial to normal function in the shoulder. However, optimizing stability by achieving adequate medial support is essential to prevent loss of reduction (Gardner et al. 2007). Varus reduction correlates with failure and should be avoided (Agudelo et al. 2007). The deforming forces on the fracture fragments must be understood for the selection of appropriate reduction maneuvers.

First step: humeral head and shaft

Reduction of the humeral head and shaft is the first step, whether the greater tuberosity is involved or not. The proximal window allows access, and is used to assist reduction of the tuberosities and humeral head. The humeral shaft always assumes a position of anteromedial displacement under the influence of the pectoralis major, with the humeral head assuming a retroverted position. As described for closed reduction, longitudinal traction with posterior directed force is applied to the arm to reduce the anterior apex deformity. To aid reduction, a small Cobb elevator (or a Hohmann retractor) is introduced in the fracture site anterolaterally between the overlapping fragments and tilted downward to correct the translational displacement, like a 'horseshoe maneuver', to lift the head over the shaft (**Fig. 8.5**). Placement of a Hohmann retractor anteromedial to the shaft may also help offset the deforming adduction force created by pectoralis major. Adequacy of the reduction is verified using the C-arm fluoroscope. Once the reduction is achieved with good medial calcar contact, a Kirschner wire (K-wire) can be inserted anteriorly from the shaft into the head (or from head to shaft) to stabilize the head–shaft fracture temporarily.

Second step: greater tuberosity

With the head–shaft segment reduced, the fragment of the greater tuberosity (if present) can be manually reduced. The displaced fragment is found posterosuperior to the humeral head, due to the external rotation and abduction imposed by supraspinatus, infraspinatus, and teres minor. External rotation and abduction of the arm are needed during this reduction technique. The greater tuberosity is caught with a Kocher forceps and pulled forward into the proximal window. Traction sutures are useful in the cuff to help control and manipulate the fragment into its appropriate space. It is then held with provisional K-wires directed away from the site of future plate placement (**Fig. 8.6a**). We like to secure (using non-absorbable fiberwire sutures) the rotator cuff attached to the greater and lesser tuberosities before plate insertion.

Valgus fractures

A valgus impacted fracture is reduced by applying a medial force to the superolateral aspect of the humeral head and using the medial soft tissues as a hinge. In the absence of lateral displacement of the fragment of the humeral head, the head is likely to remain viable. Precaution is needed in order to maintain the intact, medial, soft-tissue attachment often found between the humeral head and shaft.

Several instruments can be used for disimpaction, such as a blunt dissector (**Fig. 8.6b**). We usually prefer using a thumb to gently elevate the articular fragment onto the glenoid surface (used as a template). Lateral displacement must be avoided since the medial periosteal vessels that perfuse the articular segment may be ruptured, and avascular necrosis is more likely to result.

Once the humeral head is reduced to 130° of head–neck angle, the greater tuberosity is pulled out from the posterior aspect of the shoulder and brought back into its bed, after which it serves to maintain reduction of the humeral head. Temporary stabilization is achieved with 2 mm K-wires, which are driven from the fragment of the greater tuberosity, across the fracture, to end up in the calcar. High-density sutures are then added to secure the greater tuberosity.

The most common pitfall here is over-reducing the greater tuberosity into the void created by the severe impaction of the cancellous osteopenic bone. This leads to altered biomechanics of the rotator cuff, with reduced offset. Calcium phosphate cement may be a solution; it

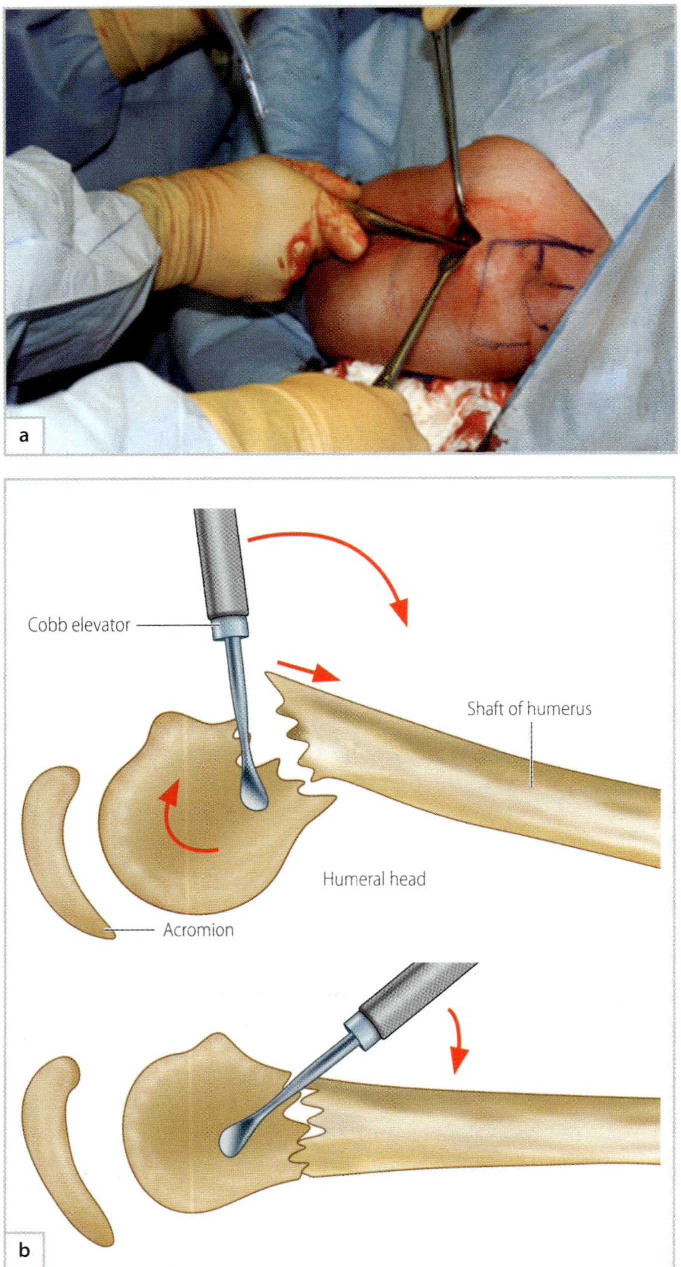

Figure 8.5 Reduction of the humeral head to the shaft. (a) Horseshoe maneuver. (b) Small Cobb elevator inserted in the fracture to correct the translational displacement of the shaft.

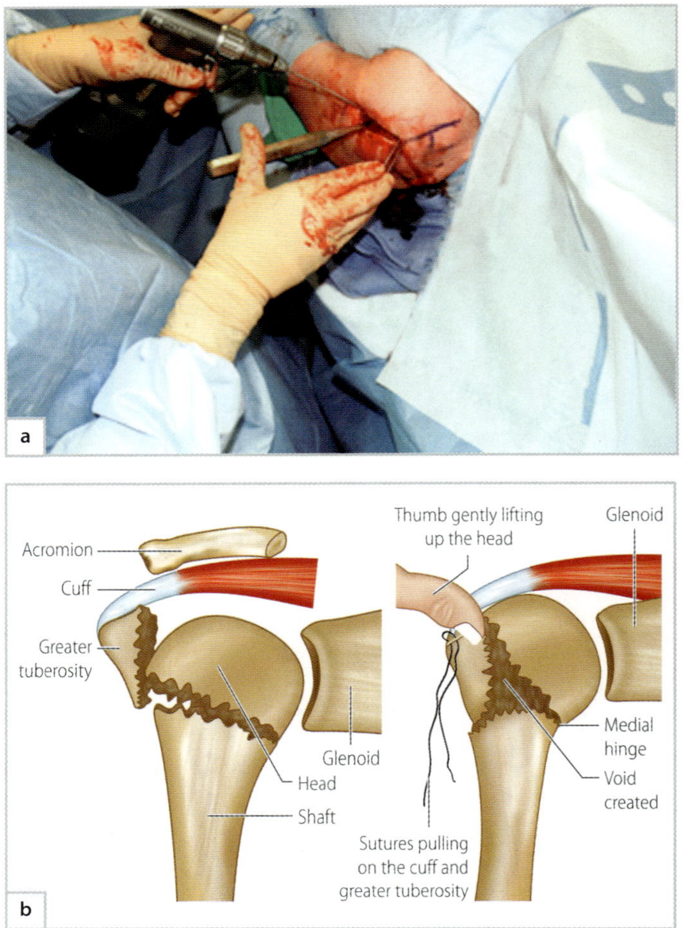

Figure 8.6 Reduction of the greater tuberosity. (a) The greater tuberosity is held with provisional K-wires directed away from future plate placement. (b) Valgus-type reduction technique.

can be used to fill the void, and offers good resistance to axial loading and head collapse. The two most proximal locking screws engaged in the superior aspect of the humeral head (the area with the best bone quality) are the most important to prevent collapse and loss of reduction in valgus.

Third step: plate insertion

During plate insertion, care is taken to keep the plate directly along the bone, to prevent trapping of the axillary nerve under the plate. (As mentioned above, the axillary nerve must be identified.) Keeping the index finger on the nerve during insertion of the plate on the proximal humerus is the best way to protect it from entrapment (**Fig. 8.7a**). If the nerve cannot be palpated, a separate deltopectoral approach or an extended anterolateral acromial approach should be used. The attachable insertion guide block cannot be safely used because the distal edge impinges directly on the axillary nerve when insertion is percutaneous. Our preferred implant is a five-hole Synthes (Paoli, Pennsylvania) 3.5 mm locking compression plate (LCP) for the proximal humerus. Two 3.5 mm locking screw sleeves are anchored into the proximal holes to act as a handle to aid insertion. Any similar low-profile, precontoured locking plate with multiple screw options can be used. Plates with targeting devices are available to facilitate insertion of the distal screws but are quite bulky and limit finger access (for tactile inspection).

The plate is positioned on the proximal lateral humerus with the inherent angulation of the plate sitting at the inferior portion of the greater tuberosity. To prevent acromial impingement, the plate should sit at least 5 mm lower than the greater tuberosity. To obtain purchase on and control of the articular head fragment, we like to fix two joysticks (2 mm K-wires) starting medial to the greater tuberosity. Once satisfactory plate placement is attained, the proximal fracture fragments are provisionally fixed by placing a K-wire, drill bit, or a fully threaded cancellous screw through any one of the proximal humeral head screw holes and into the humeral head (**Fig. 8.7b,c**). It is best not to fix the proximal locking screws before the final reduction is obtained, to allow fine-tuning (see below).

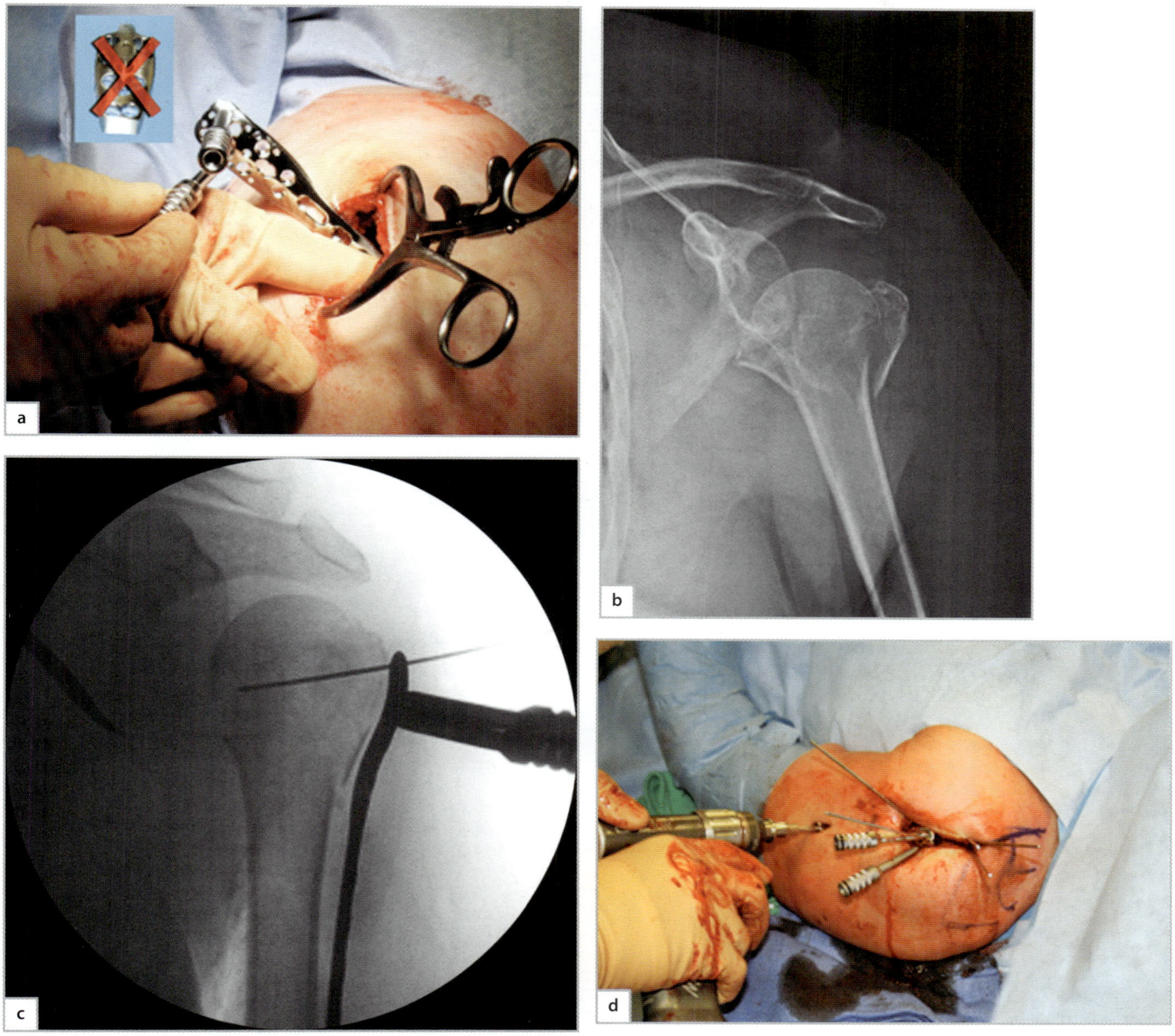

Figure 8.7 Plate insertion. (a) Finger protection to avoid entrapment of the axillary nerve. (b,c) Valgus impacted fracture and plate positioning to avoid acromial impingement. (d) plate reduction with push-pull device.

Fourth step: plate reduction

The anatomically contoured plate is used as a reduction tool to buttress the humeral head. Through the distal window, a conventional 3.5 mm screw or a push–pull device is tightened slowly to bring the diaphysis in close contact with the plate (**Fig. 8.7d**). This 'reduction screw' needs to be long enough to catch the far cortex and may need to be exchanged for a shorter one later on. The plate may slide on the diaphysis in the sagittal plane in this indirect reduction technique. Adding a K-wire (or a second cortical screw) in a distal hole will prevent rotation.

Fig. 8.8 shows the step-by-step reduction of a fracture of the surgical neck, with the humerus displaced in valgus.

Fifth step: fine-tuning

Readjustment and fine-tuning the position of the humeral head is possible with the K-wires (joysticks) fixed in the articular fragment before definitive fixation with locking screws. **Fig. 8.9** shows the step-by-step preliminarily reduction, and definitive reduction, of a varus fracture of the proximal humerus that was operated three weeks after failed conservative treatment. The 'reduction screw' can be untightened to readjust the head–neck angle with the joysticks, avoiding any varus (**Fig. 8.9e,f**).

If varus still persists, a pointed reduction forceps can be engaged between the superior aspect of the tuberosity and the plate to de-rotate the head by creating compression (**Fig. 8.9n**).

Tactile verification through both incisions and fluoroscopy must be used to confirm the plate position on the shaft and lateral surface of the head before proceeding to definitive fixation.

Placement of the plate too far anteriorly on the humeral head, with residual apex anterior angulation, is a common error. With a deltoid-splitting approach, the plate should sit on the lateral surface, and not the usual anterolateral surface close to the bicipital groove recommended for the deltopectoral approach.

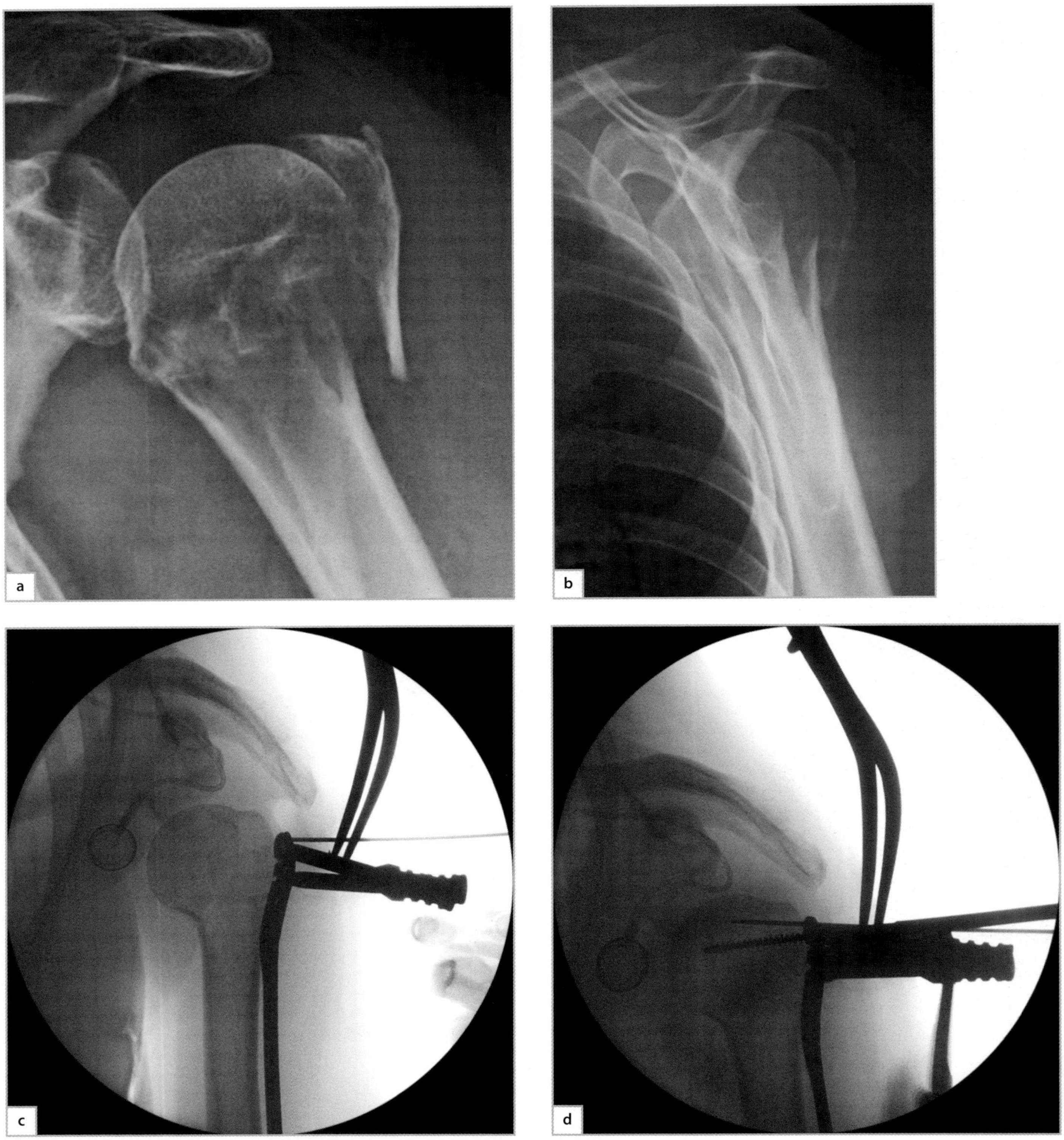

Figure 8.8 Step-by-step reduction and fixation of a valgus-type fracture. ***Contd...***

Definitive plate fixation

To prevent axillary nerve injury at this stage, we recommend that the plate is fixed with screws positioned in the safe zones as determined by the anatomic study of Smith et al. (2007). The most proximal six holes (A, B, C) and four most distal screws (i.e. distal to the slot hole) pose little danger to the axillary nerve (**Fig. 8.10**). In the proximal window, a minimum of four locking screws are inserted and tightened sequentially. Additional screws should be used with osteopenic bone or with comminution of the calcar. Arm abduction relieves tension from the deltoid on the lateral humerus and offers better visualization through this mobile window, especially for the screw in row D

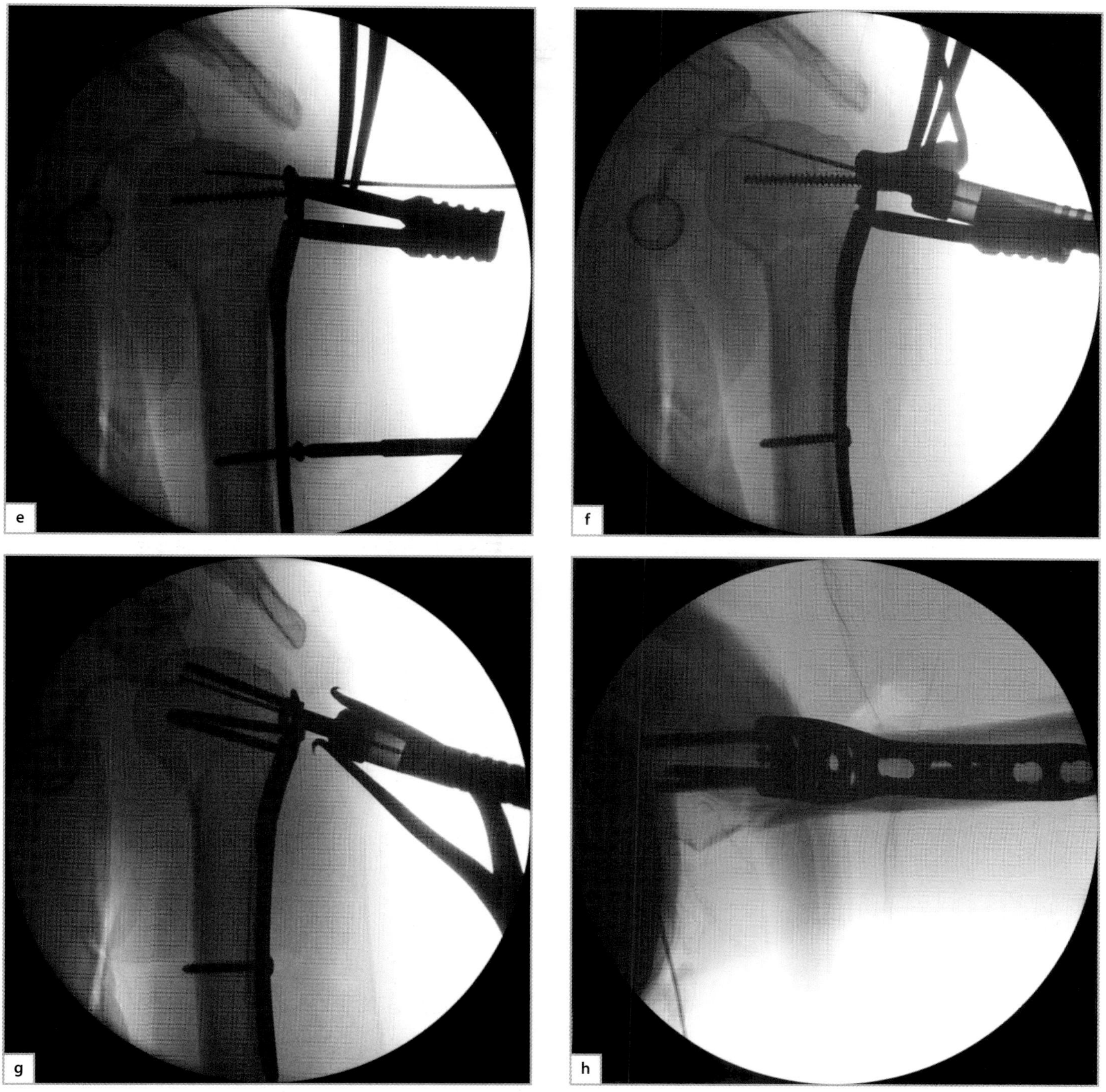

Figure 8.8 Step-by-step reduction and fixation of a valgus-type fracture. ***Contd...***

in **Fig. 8.10b**. A total of seven proximal locking screws can be safely secured if desired.

In the distal window, three 3.5 mm conventional screws (usually 26–28 mm long) are used to secure the plate distally. In osteopenic bone with thin cortices, one 3.5 mm locking screw may be added to protect the cortical screws from shear forces.

Once fixation is stable, dynamic fluoroscopy with full rotation confirms the correct placement and length of each screw. All temporary fixation devices are carefully removed and/or replaced. Tension-band sutures around both tuberosity fragments are anchored to the plate holes. The deltoid fascia and subcutaneous tissues are repaired with a non-absorbable suture (**Fig. 8.11**), and the skin edges reapproximated with staples or a running subcuticular stitch. A sterile dressing is applied, and the arm placed in a sling.

Pearls and pitfalls

Surgeons have long been cautioned regarding the axillary nerve when performing surgery around the shoulder. Injury to the axillary nerve can be avoided with this technique by observing the following precautions.

- The nerve must be identified.
- The attachable insertion guide block cannot be safely used because the distal edge impinges directly on the axillary nerve when insertion is percutaneous.

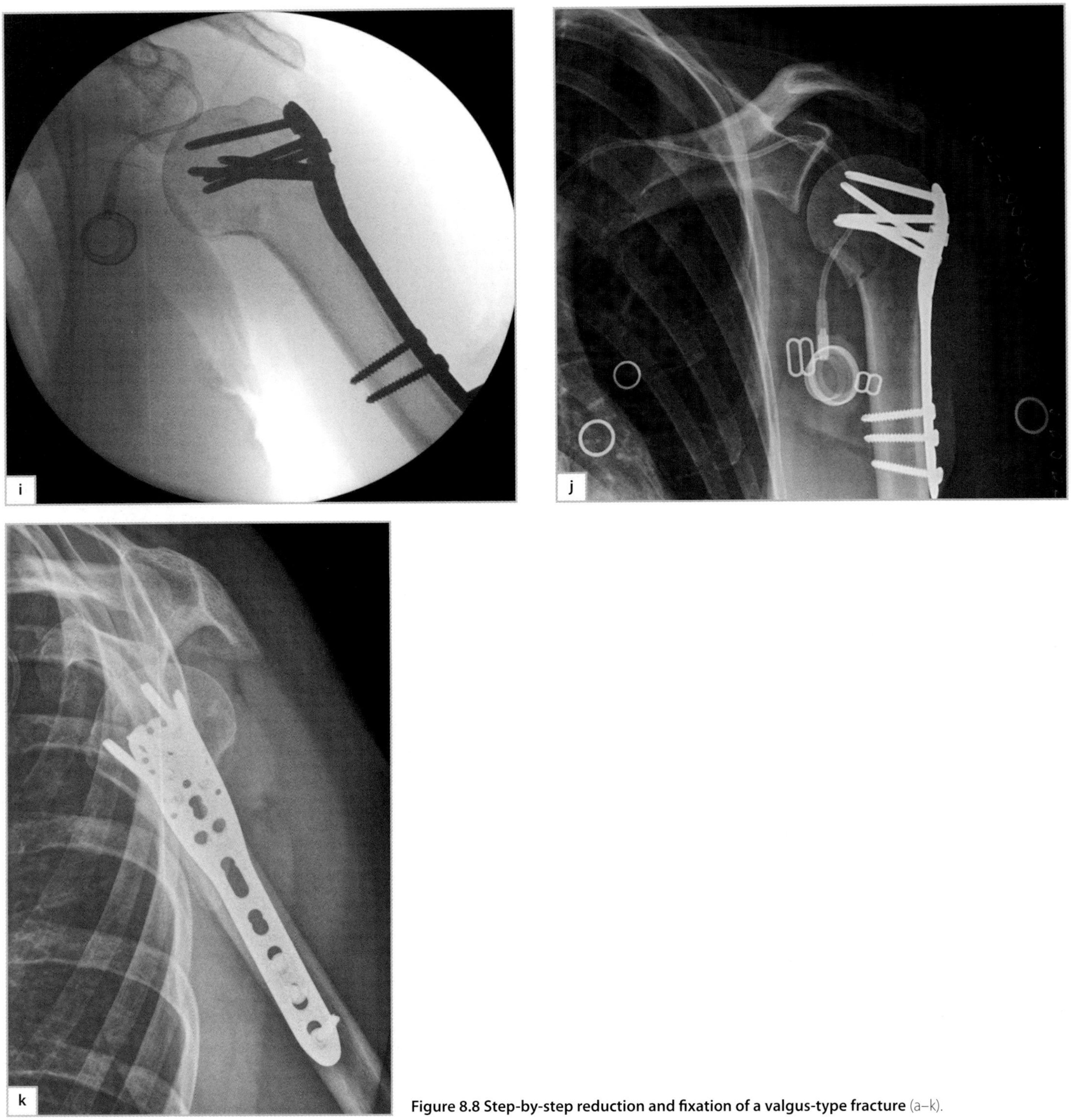

Figure 8.8 Step-by-step reduction and fixation of a valgus-type fracture (a–k).

- The index finger should be placed on the nerve during insertion of the plate on the proximal humerus.
- Screws should be positioned in the safe zone, away from the course of the axillary nerve.

The most common pitfall with the use of locking plates in the proximal humerus is screw penetration, which can be easily missed at the time of surgery. The following points will help to prevent the severe morbidity of such a complication.

- Exceptional vigilance is needed while placing proximal screws. Fluoroscopic imaging through a full range of motion is required. All the screw needs to be verified, one by one, especially the divergent screws in the third row.
- Tap drilling will enhance proprioceptive feedback and avoid damage to the subchondral bone. In osteopenic bone, we drill the proximal cortex and then use the depth gage with a twisting motion to advance up to the subchondral bone, eliminating the risk of joint perforation (**Fig. 8.12**).

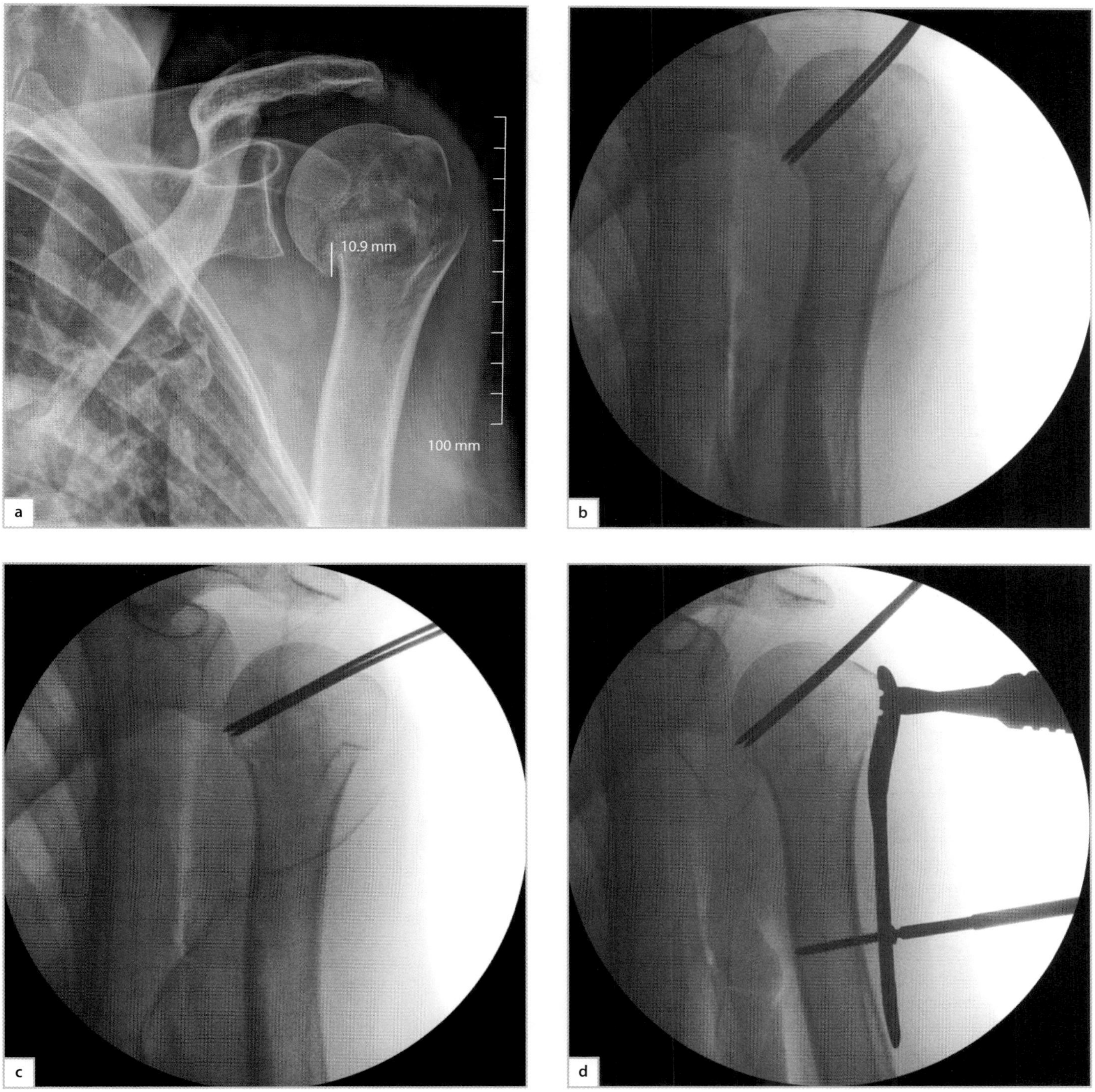

Figure 8.9 Step-by-step treatment of a fracture of the proximal humerus, displaced in varus. ***Contd...***

- Screws should be shortened by subtracting 3–5 mm from the measured screw length to allow for some fracture settling. Additional screws can be used to compensate for reduced stability.
- After surgery, fracture collapse can also lead to screw penetration. Optimizing stability by achieving adequate medial support and avoiding varus is essential.

REHABILITATION

Patients are started on immediate postoperative active range of motion of the shoulder and elbow. A standardized protocol begins with pendulum exercises and then active assisted exercises until there is clinical and radiographic evidence of healing. At this point (typically at about 8–12 weeks), the addition of strengthening and proprioception exercises is allowed.

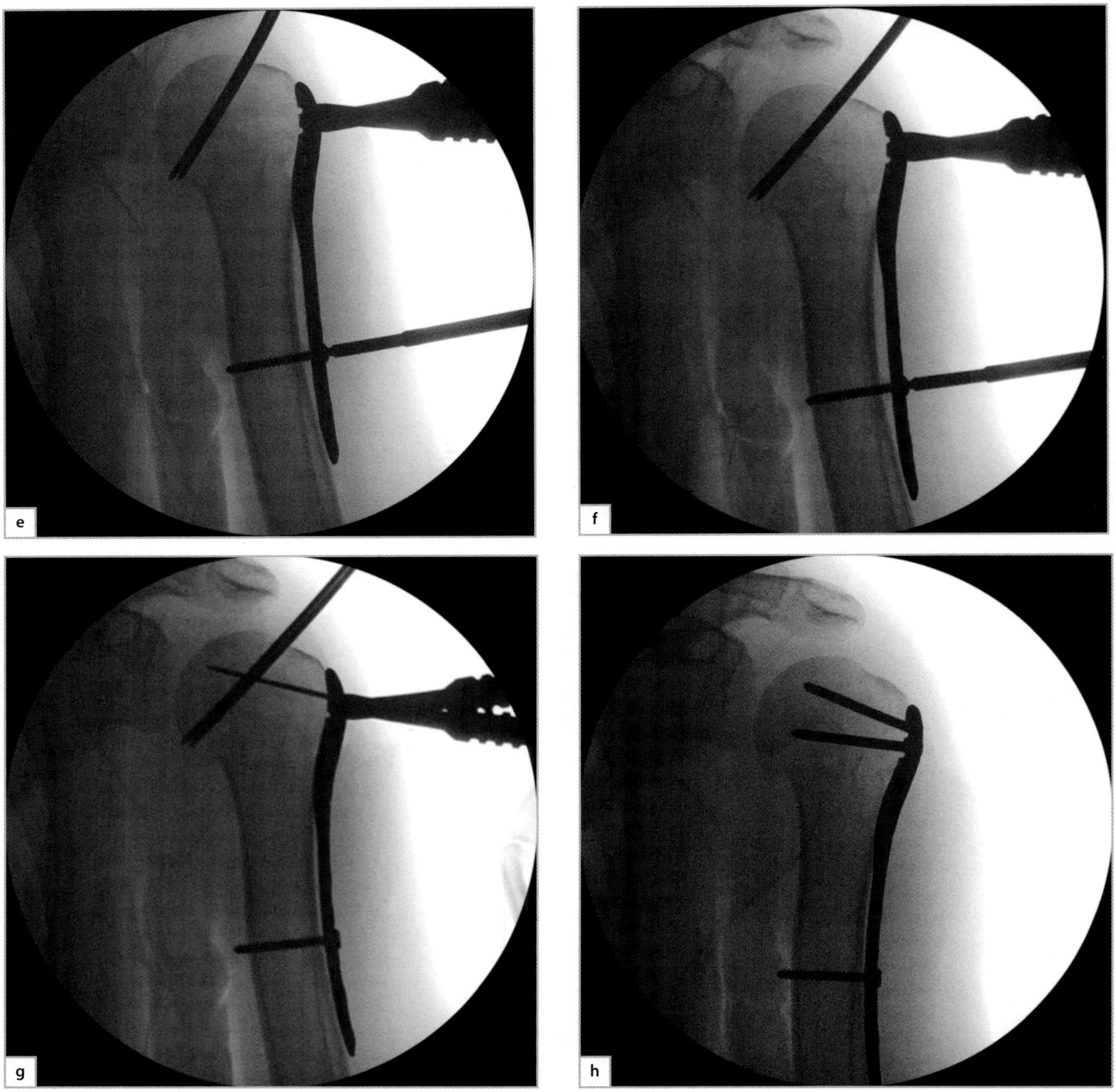

Figure 8.9 Step-by-step treatment of a fracture of the proximal humerus, displaced in varus. ***Contd...***

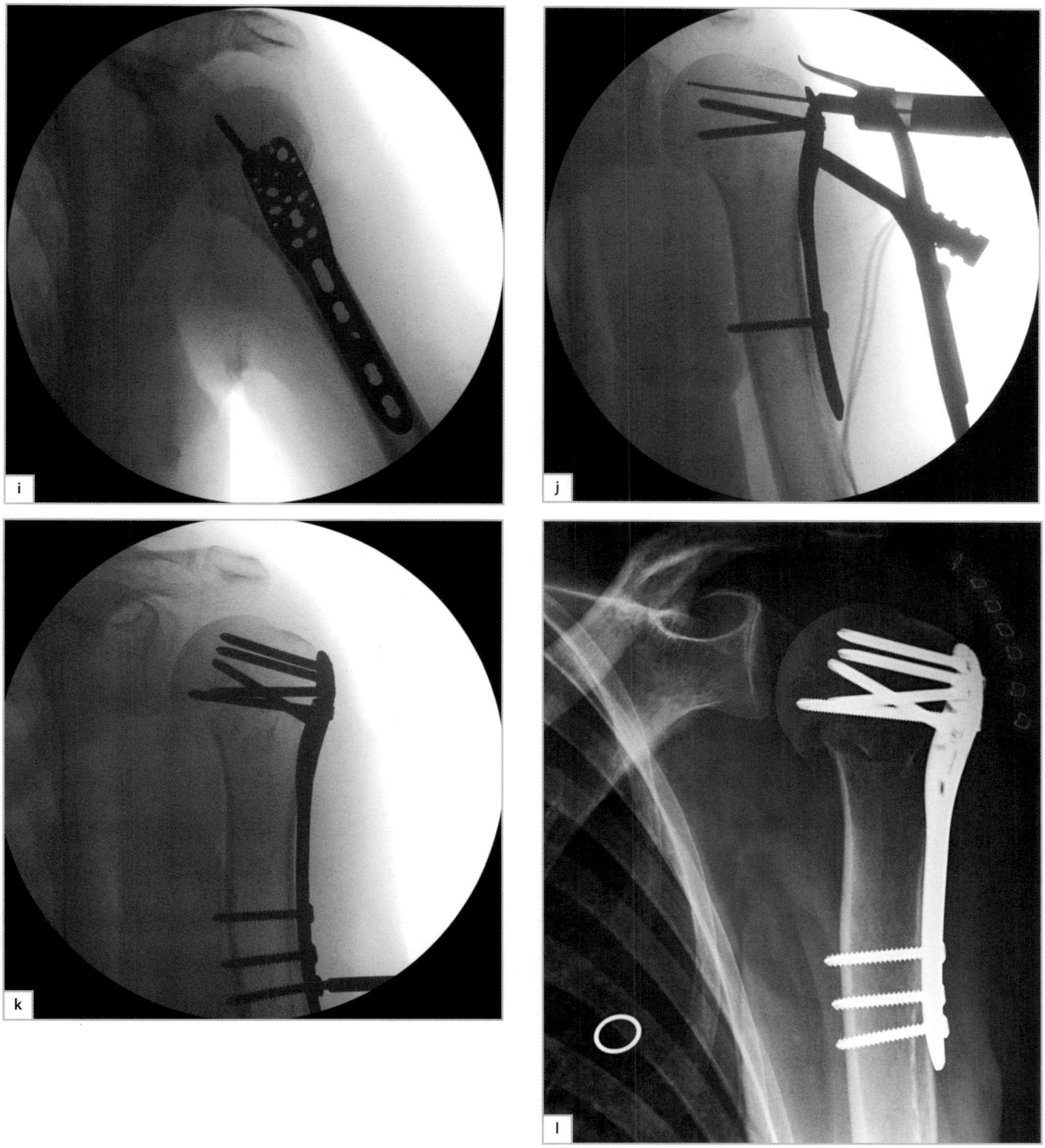

Figure 8.9 Step-by-step treatment of a fracture of the proximal humerus, displaced in varus. ***Contd...***

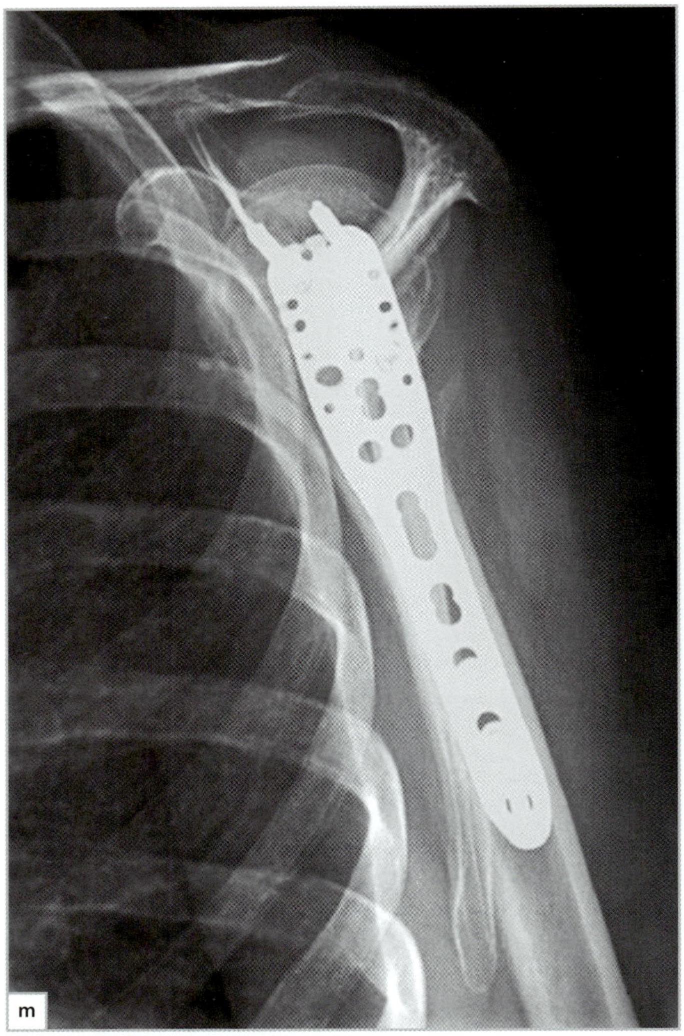

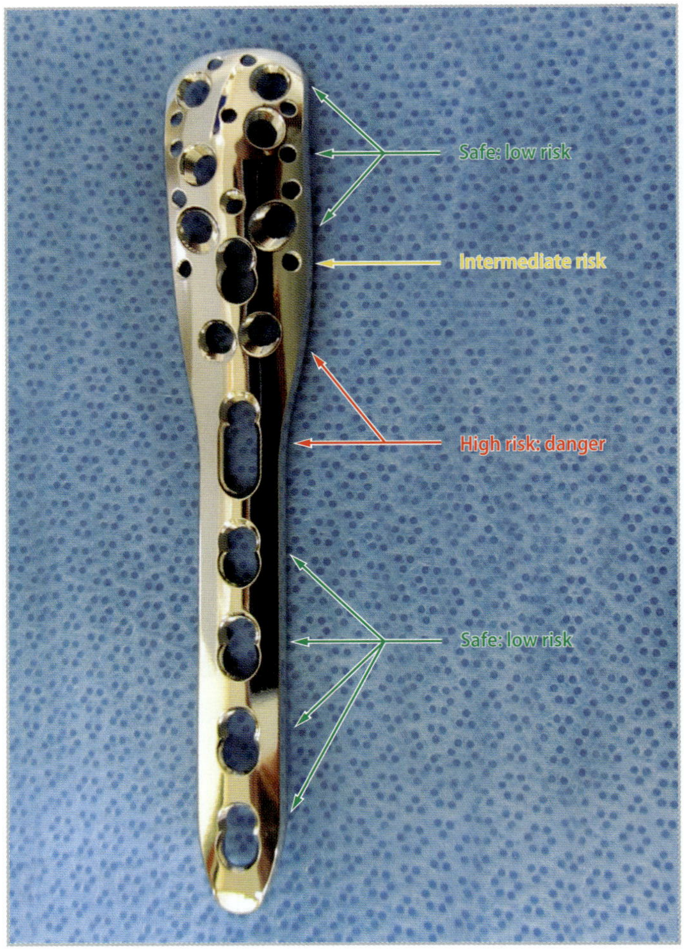

Figure 8.10 **Definitive fixation.** Safe zones for screw insertion.

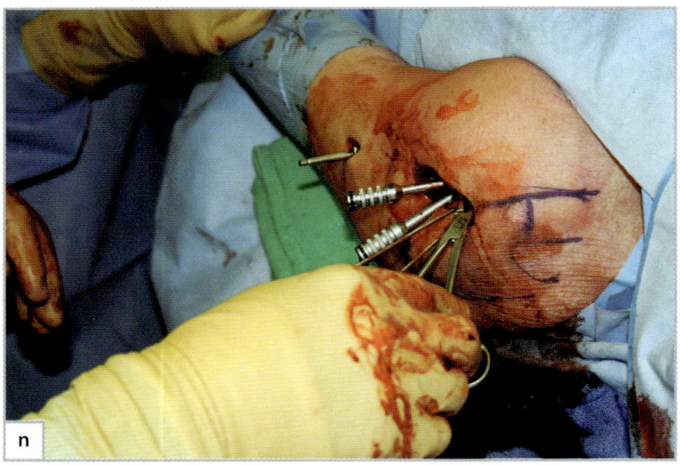

Figure 8.9 Step-by-step treatment of a fracture of the proximal humerus, displaced in varus (a–m). (n) Two joysticks with the addition of a pointed reduction forceps are used to readjust the reduction of the humeral head.

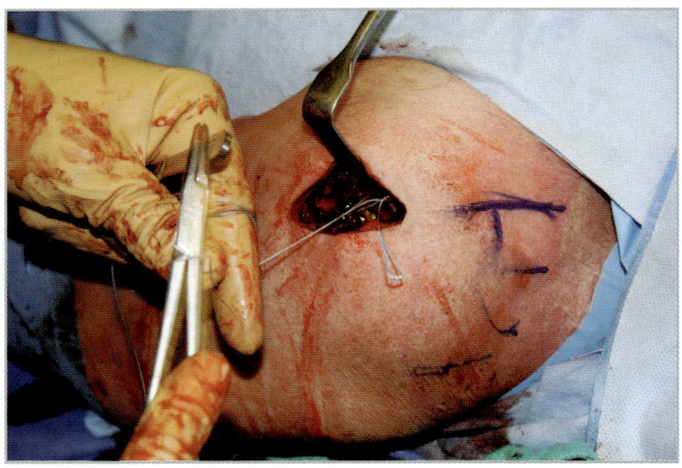

Figure 8.11 Suture augmentation.

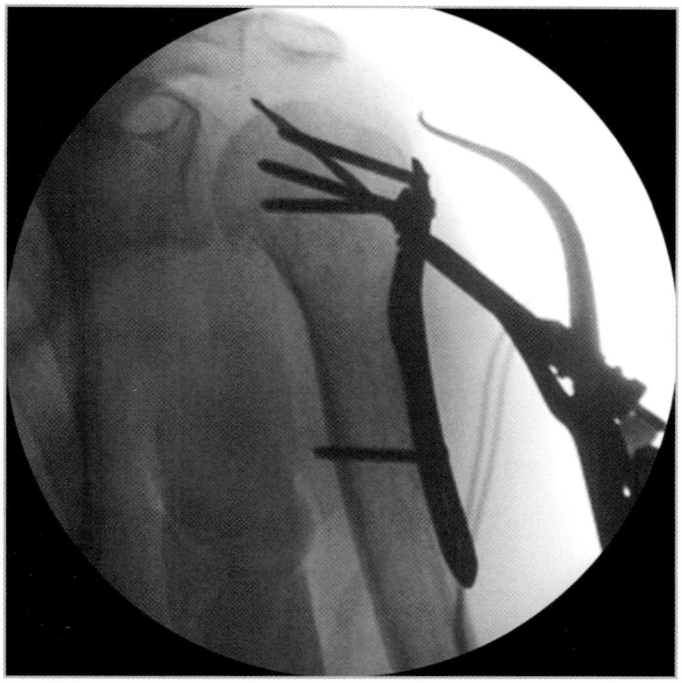

Figure 8.12 Perforation of the subchondral bone should be avoided.

REFERENCES

Agudelo J, Schürmann M, Stahel P, et al. Analysis of efficacy and failure in proximal humerus fractures treated with locking plates. J Orthop Trauma 2007;21:676–681.

Gardner MJ, Griffith MH, Dines JS, et al. The extended anterolateral acromial approach allows minimally invasive access to the proximal humerus. Clin Orthop Relat Res 2005;434:123–129.

Gardner M, Weil Y, Barker J, et al. The importance of medial support in locked plating of proximal humerus fractures. J Orthop Trauma 2007;21:185–191.

Gibson JN, Handoll HH, Madhok R. Interventions for treating proximal humerus fractures in adults. Cochrane Database Syst Rev 2001;(1):CD000434.

Laflamme GY, Rouleau DM, Berry GK, et al. Percutaneous humeral plating of fractures of the proximal humerus: results of a prospective multicenter clinical trial. J Orthop Trauma 2008;22:153–158.

Smith J, Berry G, Laflamme Y, et al. Percutaneous insertion of a proximal humeral locking plate: an anatomic study. Injury 2007;38:206–211.

Chapter 9 Intramedullary nail fixation of fractures of the proximal humerus

Clifford B. Jones, Jeffrey M. Bradley

INDICATIONS

Intramedullary nailing (IMN) of fractures of the proximal humerus is best suited to proximal diaphyseal fractures, two-, three-, and four-part fractures, fractures with diaphyseal extension, and segmental diaphyseal fractures.

CONTRAINDICATIONS

IMN is contraindicated for head-splitting fractures, marginal impaction fractures, isolated fractures of the greater or lesser tuberosity, fractures of the anatomical neck of the humerus, and where there is pre-existing humeral deformity or hardware. IMN is relatively contraindicated for patients with rotator cuff (RC) dysfunction (poor shoulder function), morbid obesity (due to inability to adduct arm for nail insertion), and elderly patients with severe osteoporosis (due to capacious canals and poor screw purchase), although the use of newer locking-screw technology in combination with nailing may assist fracture fragment stability with osteoporotic bone. In addition, smaller patients will have relatively smaller diaphyseal canals that may not accommodate manufactured or biomechanically feasible nail insertion.

TECHNIQUE

Positioning

The patient is positioned supine on a radiolucent 'diving board' table. To provide circumferential access, the patient should be placed in reverse relation to the table (i.e. head of patient at foot of table, and opposite the base plate). To allow for more room about the shoulder girdle, the table should be rotated about 20–30° away from the anesthesia machine. Too much rotation will impede fluoroscopy positioning (**Fig. 9.1**). A folded towel or radiolucent bump is then placed under the ipsilateral thorax and scapula, in order to stabilize and elevate the shoulder. This improves exposure, reduction, imaging, and implant insertion.

It can be best to avoid using a sand bag as a bump, as many are not radiolucent and will obscure the field of view. Large pannus folds or pendulous breasts are taped away from the affected arm so as not to impede adduction, subsequent nail insertion, and fluoroscopic visualization. The entire extremity is prepared and draped, up to and including the shoulder girdle and base of the neck. If the preparation is not extended to the neck area, the drapes may obscure or encroach on the operative field. Multiple towels or a folded blanket placed under the affected arm will assist with the fracture reduction, lessen the need for surgical assistants, and improve intraoperative fluoroscopic imaging. To avoid interference with the incoming fluoroscopy machine, the patient's contralateral arm is tucked under the sheets, with padding paralleling the trunk.

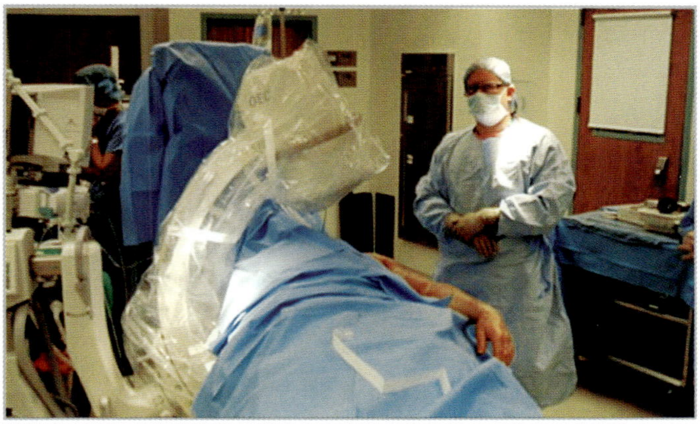

Figure 9.1 Prepped and draped patient in relation to surgeon, fluoroscopy imaging, and anesthesia machine. The photograph was taken from the end of the table next to the image-viewing unit.

The fluoroscopy unit is placed on the contralateral side of the table, while the viewing screen is placed at the end of the table. From the contralateral side, the fluoroscopy unit enters perpendicular and moves parallel to the patient. Scapular anteroposterior (AP) views (Grashey views) (**Fig. 9.2**) and lateral views (scapular Y and lateral diaphysis) (**Fig. 9.3**) are obtained by rotating the fluoroscopy unit 30–45° away from (backward rotation) and 45–60° toward (forward rotation) the surgeon, respectively. One disadvantage of IMN in relation to patient positioning is the inability to obtain a true axillary view without preliminary or final fixation. Therefore, the axillary view is obtained with abduction of the arm, in coordination with the fluoroscope tilting away from the head of the patient (**Fig. 9.4**). Distal interlocking is accomplished with distal translation of the fluoroscopy unit.

Surgical approach

The proximal humerus can be approached by splitting the deltoid muscle through the fascial junction of the anterior and middle heads, with the skin incision placed over the anterolateral portion of the acromion (**Fig. 9.5**). The deltoid is split in line with the muscular fibers up to, but not more than, 5 cm distal to the acromion. In order to decrease injury to the axillary nerve, a suture can be inserted into the musculature at 5 cm (Riemer and D'Ambrosia 1992, Lin et al. 1999, Albritton et al. 2003).

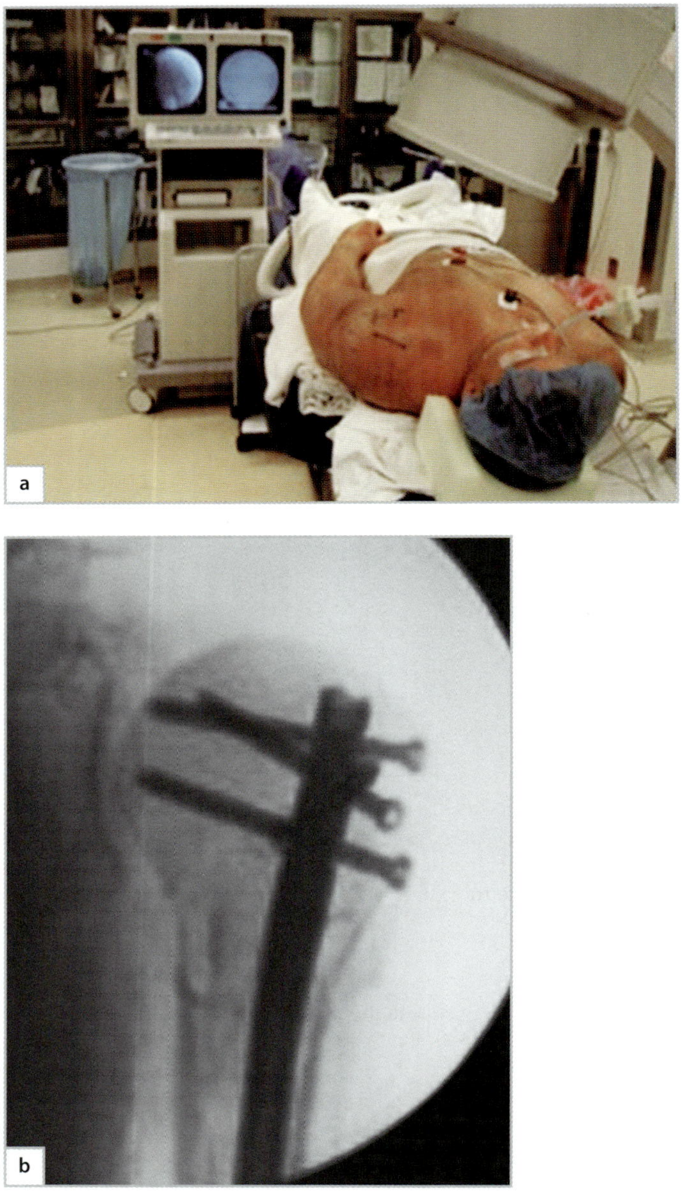

Figure 9.2 Setup for anteroposterior views. With a roll-back of about 30° (a), the image intensifier allows for scapular anteroposterior images (b).

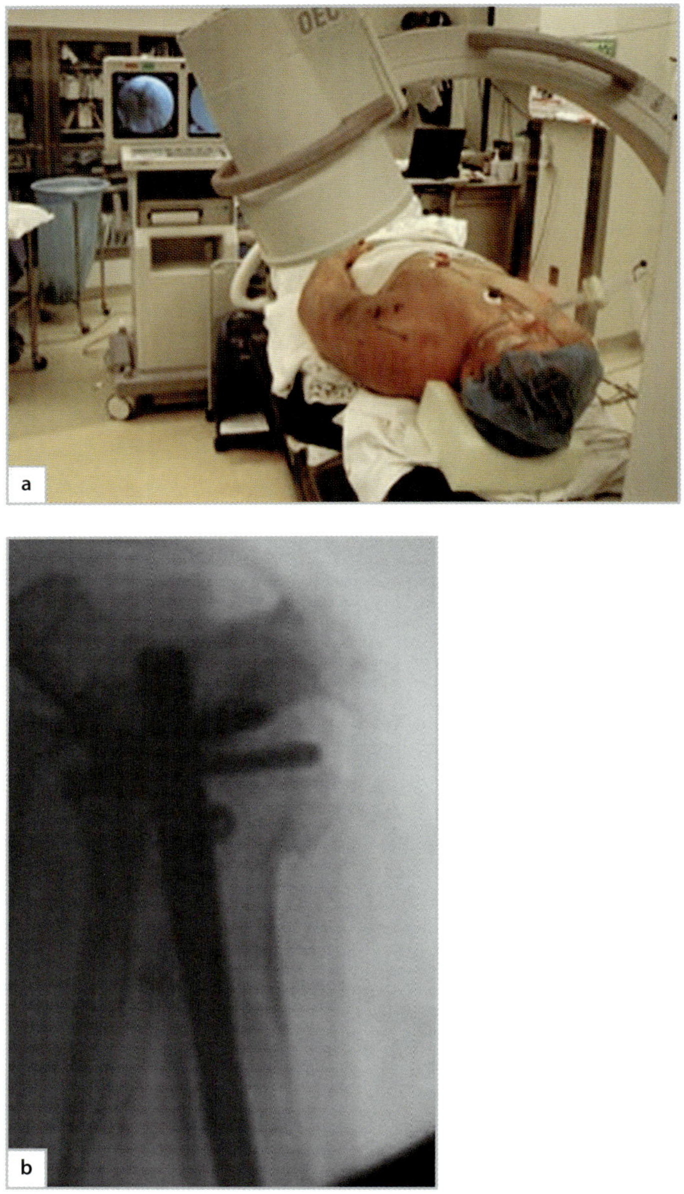

Figure 9.3 Setup for lateral views. With a roll-over of about 30° (a), the image intensifier allows for scapular Y images (b).

As an alternative, the lateral deltoid approach is via a split through the middle head of the deltoid, which can be extended after the axillary nerve is dissected (Gardner et al. 2004, Gardner et al. 2008). Once the deltoid has been gently retracted, the RC is visualized. Secondary to RC muscle forces, the head fragment is usually in a varus and flexed position (**Fig. 9.6a**). With the head fragment in a malrotated position, the correct starting point through the RC cannot be determined. The varus position and overlying acromion prevent proper visualization. An incision through the RC should not be made until the reduction has been completed. The middle of the humeral head is then determined, based on the lateral fluoroscopic view. The middle of the humeral head in this plane will determine the RC incision site. Since the ability to perform a reduction will determine whether a nail can be inserted, the RC incision should not be created yet. (For the RC incision, see under 'Two-part fractures', below.)

Reduction techniques

The reduction and realignment are achieved using joysticks. Orientation is aided by indirect identification of fracture fragments, the biceps tendon, and subsequent RC interval. The surgeon should not dissect deeply around the biceps tendon or distal to the RC interval. The anterolateral branch of the anterior circumflex artery, which is a prominent blood supply to the humeral head, is positioned within the bicipital groove (Laing 1956, Gerber et al. 1990, Riemer and D'Ambrosia 1992). Medial to this interval will be the lesser tuberosity and the subscapularis. Lateral to this interval will be the greater tuberosity and the supraspinatus, infraspinatus, and teres minor muscles. If the tuberosities are displaced, the displacement will occur in line with the muscular pull. The lesser tuberosity can displace under and medial to the conjoint tendon. The greater tuberosity will

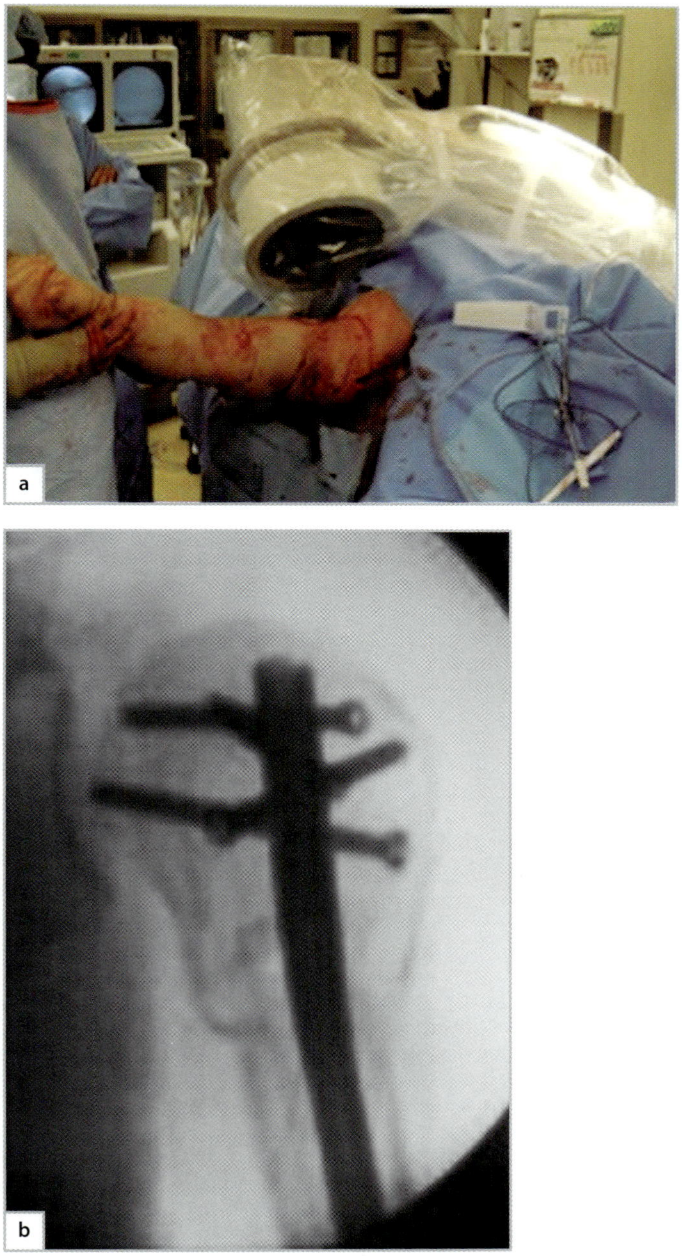

Figure 9.4 Setup for axillary views. With a roll-over of about 10° and caudal tilt of about 45° (a), the image intensifier allows for axillary images (b).

displace in a cephalad and posterior direction. Abduction of the arm, in order to release deltoid tightness, can assist visualization and reduction of the greater tuberosity. A Kocher clamp, dental pick, or shoulder hook will aid in rotating and translating the greater tuberosity anteriorly and caudally. Once all the components are in view, the reduction process can begin.

Two-part fractures

With two-part fractures, only de-rotation of the head is usually required. Initially, one or two 2.5 mm terminally threaded Schanz pins (TTSP) (Small External Fixator Set, Synthes, Paoli, PA) are placed into the head distally to the RC (**Fig. 9.6b**). TTSP are used

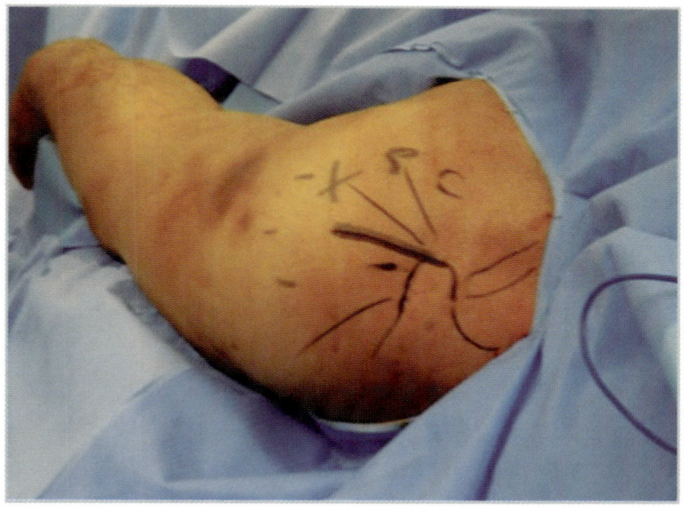

Figure 9.5 The approach to the rotator cuff. The approach is via the junction of the anterior and middle raphe of the deltoid muscle referenced to the anterolateral tip of the acromion.

instead of a Kirschner wire (K-wire) because they will avoid migration if contact occurs with a drill or reamer. With gentle distal force, the head is de-rotated out of varus, and the RC tendon is exposed (**Fig. 9.6 c, d**). The center position of the head is then confirmed fluoroscopically, on the scapular Y and Grashey views. A 3–4 cm opening is incised in line with the tendon fibers through the RC and 2–3 cm medial to the RC insertion. It is important not to dissect or reflect the RC attachment from the greater tuberosity. Another two 2.5 mm TTSP are then placed through the RC opening, along the anterior and posterior aspects, deep within the humeral head, in line with the diaphysis (**Fig. 9.7**). If applied correctly, the Schanz pins will hold the RC incision open, avoiding reamer injury to the RC, and in conjunction with the laterally overhanging acromion, will keep the head out of varus by resting along the lateral acromial border. Misaligned TTSP will interfere with reamer and nail insertion. The initial lateral TTSP can then be removed. The guide pin for the cannulated rigid reamed is then inserted within the mid-portion of the Schanz pins, in line with the diaphysis on the Grashey and scapular Y fluoroscopic images, and medial to the junction of the greater tuberosity and humeral head.

The starting point is intra-articular and within the articular cartilage of the humeral head. The orthopaedic surgeon should not ream laterally into the RC insertion on the greater tuberosity. In a sports analogy, the guide pin is the football and the Schanz pins are the football goalpost uprights. The surgeon should be hypercritical of the alignment and fracture reduction. Any varus will interfere with successful fracture healing, tuberosity impingement, and proximal screw insertion angles. In obese patients (problems with arm adduction) and osteoporotic fractures (problems with soft lateral bone), Poller (blocking) 2.5 mm TTSP or 3.5 mm bicortical screws can be used to guide the reaming in a central instead of a lateral direction. An intact lateral column of bone is important to anatomic reductions and improved humeral nail stability (Agel et al. 2004). Once an opening within the proximal humerus has been made and the fracture reduction maintained, a ball-tipped guide pin can be inserted through the proximal humeral segment and distally within the humeral diaphysis.

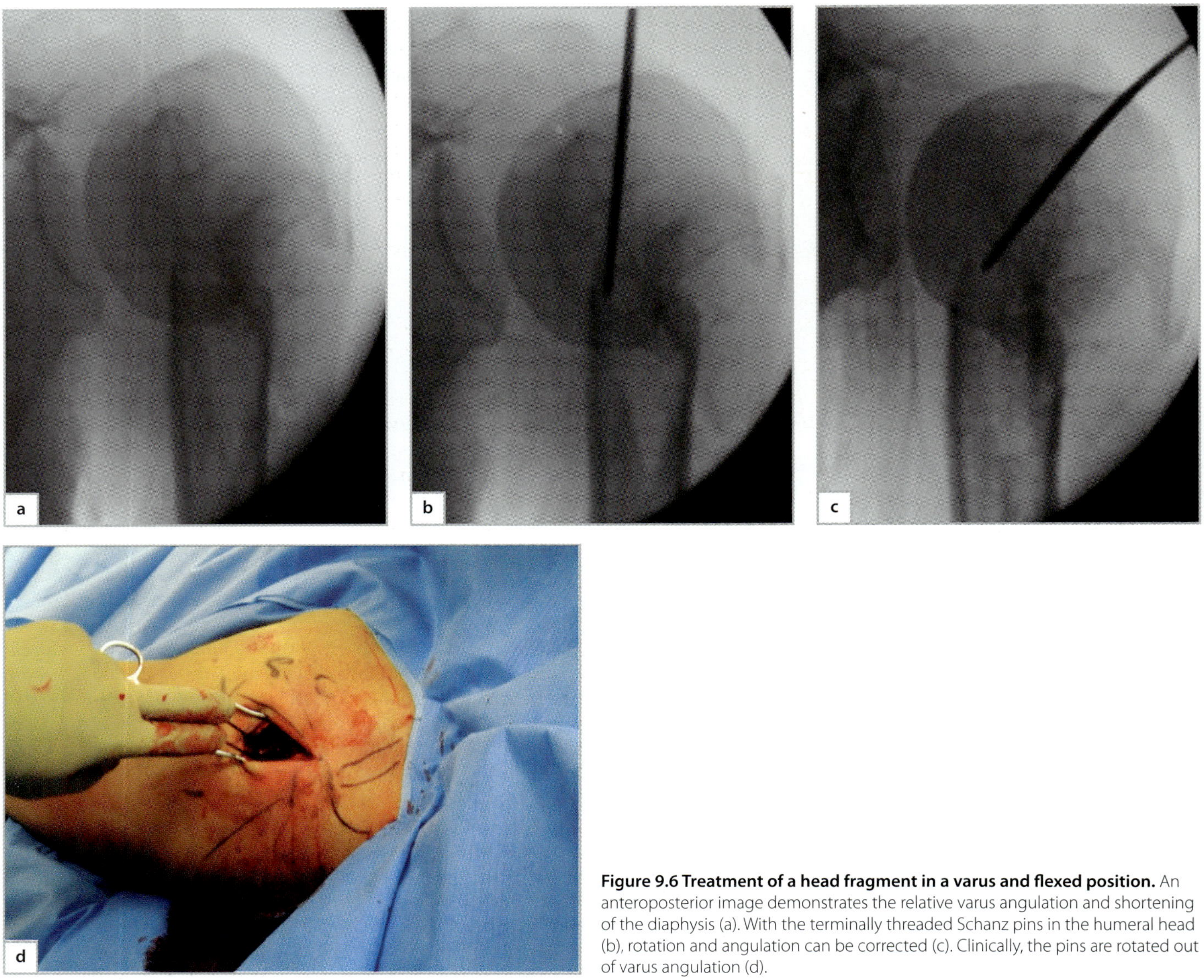

Figure 9.6 Treatment of a head fragment in a varus and flexed position. An anteroposterior image demonstrates the relative varus angulation and shortening of the diaphysis (a). With the terminally threaded Schanz pins in the humeral head (b), rotation and angulation can be corrected (c). Clinically, the pins are rotated out of varus angulation (d).

Three- and four-part fractures

With three- and four-part fracture patterns, the tuberosities require reduction initially. With a Webber clamp, the tuberosities are gently reapproximated anterolaterally and not overcompressed. Preliminary K-wire stabilization will aid in the temporary reduction. As in two-part fractures, initial and temporary TTSP are inserted into the head to remove the varus and improve RC visualization. The RC incision and TTSP insertion are performed. Usually through the RC opening and direct visualization, the greater tuberosity is reduced to the fracture lines on the articular surface of the humeral head. The reduction is maintained while lateral to medial 2.5 mm TTSP are inserted through the greater tuberosity, deep into the humeral head subchondral bone, to maintain the tuberosity reduction. Thinking ahead, the surgeon should diverge the greater tuberosity lateral to medial TTSP, in order to avoid problems with the guide pin, reamer, or nail alignment. Tuberosity reduction is maintained with tenaculum clamps while creating the proximal opening with the rigid reamer to create a hole or channel, and not displacement or widening ('blowout') of the tuberosities.

Pearls and pitfalls

Reduction of a fragment of the proximal humerus to the diaphysis

The head is reduced to the diaphysis in relation to length, rotation, and alignment. With comminuted fractures, length determination is difficult. Anterior humeral joystick insertion with a 2.5 mm or a 5.0 mm Schanz pin can improve control of the two fracture fragments (**Fig. 9.8**). Shortening of the humeral diaphysis by 2–3 cm should not affect the clinical result. Rotation parameters are based upon the humeral head in 30º of retroversion in relation to the diaphysis or humeral condyles. If the head is face on in the fluoroscopic image at 30º of retroversion, the humeral condyles will be face on with the fluoroscope on neutral rotation. Alignment is aided with unicortical TTSP within the proximal humeral diaphysis, to avoid reamer contact, or with the flat end of a mallet externally.

Reaming and nail insertion

The ball-tipped guide pin is placed distal to the humeral hourglass confluence. The surgeon then reams sequentially, without proximal

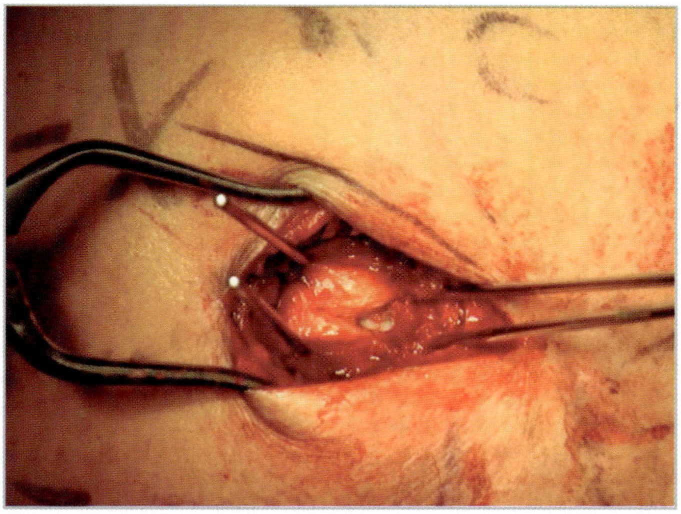

Figure 9.7 The temporary pins distal to the rotator cuff. The rotator cuff incision is performed within the tendinous portion proximal to the cuff insertion. The preliminary Schanz pins are noted within the humeral head and retracting the edges of the rotator cuff.

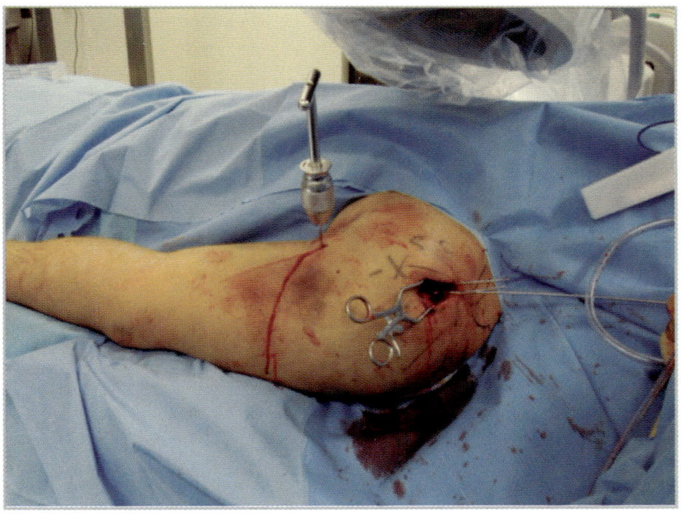

Figure 9.8 Joystick diaphyseal reduction aid with universal T-handle. The aid is placed anteriorly, and the intramedullary ball-tipped guide pin is in position.

lateral wall violation or thinning, without proximal varus alignment, and with the fracture reduced. Since fractures of the proximal humerus are metaphyseal, any errant reaming in varus or translation will result in similar deformities with nail insertion. If a reaming error is made, the surgeon should ream again with the fracture reduced, or with TTSP inserted as Poller (blocking) pins. The diaphysis should be reamed until appropriate audible chatter is felt, as this confirms that the medullary canal has been reamed down to the endosteal bone. More experienced orthopaedic surgeons will be comfortable with this. It is important not to over-ream in osteoporotic bone, as it will remove precious cortical bone, or in small tight canals, as there will be the potential for thermal necrosis. Once reaming is completed, a nail with a diameter 1 mm or less is selected, for ease of insertion, to decrease distal humeral hoop stresses, and to allow for nail rotation to give proper screw insertion angles. The surgeon should know nail demographics. If the nail is available only in 9 mm lengths, small canals will obviate nail insertion and reaming to a depth of more than 10 mm will be unnecessary.

With the guide pin inserted into the distal humeral diaphyseal confluence, the length of nail required can be determined. The orthopaedic surgeon should not penetrate the distal humeral cortex or olecranon fossa, especially with osteoporotic bone. On the roll-over lateral view, the appropriate length can be determined, based on the distal nail geometry, usual hourglass cortical confluence, and gradual flexion of the condyles. If deciding between two different nail lengths, the orthopaedic surgeon should choose the shorter one, to avoid distal cortex violation, distal humeral fracture, or proximal nail impingement/prominence. The nail is inserted through the RC opening and through the fracture site, and stops prior to the distal humeral confluence. Nail depth is finalized when the lateral (not medial) aspect of the nail is deep or flush with the humeral articular surface, to avoid impingement.

The nail is inserted with the fragments held reduced and the arm in adduction. To decrease the risk of fracture site extension or diaphyseal blow-out, the surgeon should avoid nail insertion with arm abduction, and should use the proximal joysticks to aid in a coordinated arm adduction as a single unit. The nail should be inserted without difficulty. Any resistance to nail insertion may arise from an improper starting site (anterior or posterior), inadequate diaphyseal reaming, or distal humeral hourglass encroachment. If an improper starting site was created, a smaller nail diameter or rereaming with Poller TTSP may afford some correction (**Fig. 9.9**). If inadequate reaming is noted, further reaming of 1 mm or downsizing of nail diameter should be done. If distal humeral impaction by the nail is noted, the surgeon should use a shorter nail, to avoid iatrogenic fracture or impingement proximally.

The correct rotation of the nail should be decided before its complete insertion. For a simple two-part fracture, the correct nail rotation is such that interlocking will not be through the bicipital groove. For a multipart fracture, the nail rotation is determined to optimally fix the greater tuberosity with interlocking screws. The nail at final insertion is 5–15 mm below the chondral surface. Prominent nails will create RC and/or subacromial irritation, as well as proximal impingement with abduction and forward elevation of the arm. Nails inserted too deep will place the proximal interlocking screws in suboptimal bone and increase the potential for injury to the axillary nerve (Riemer and D'Ambrosia 1992, Lin et al. 1999, Albritton et al. 2003). Drilling and screw insertion should be up to, but not through, the subchondral bone. Screw lengths of over 50 mm are likely to lead to chondral penetration. Head rotation and appropriate fluoroscopic imaging will assist the determination of screw length. If the screws have no purchase, alternative fixation options (locked screw implant or locking plates) should be considered. Maximal (i.e. three or four screws) instead of minimal screw fixation should be performed. After proximal screw insertion is completed, the TTSP can be removed. Premature TTSP removal can result in malreduction and tuberosity migration.

Once the surgeon is satisfied with proximal purchase and placement, the distal IMN interlocks should be performed through larger open instead of smaller percutaneous incisions. Anterior to posterior screws can injure the musculocutaneous nerve. Lateral-to-medial screws can injure the radial nerve, while overpenetration of the medial cortex places the ulnar nerve, median nerve, and brachial artery at risk (Rupp et al. 1996). The fluoroscopic imaging will determine the skin incision and approach. It is useful to remember that the 30° retroverted fluoroscopic image for the face-on head image will be neutral or straight up and down for the distal interlocking, to ensure relative anatomic humeral rotation. Furthermore, the fracture site should be anatomic or slightly impacted and not distracted, to avoid

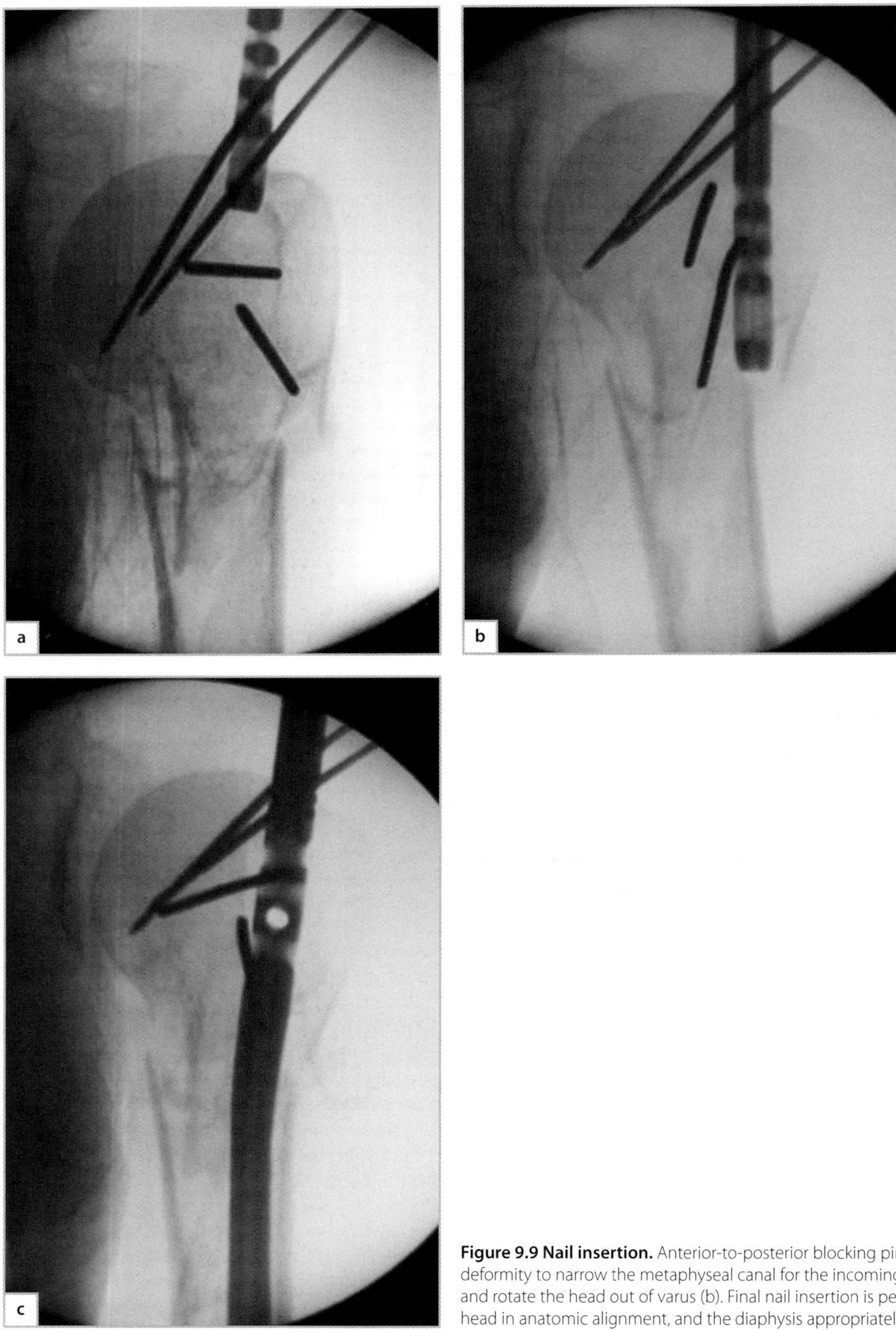

Figure 9.9 Nail insertion. Anterior-to-posterior blocking pins are inserted within the concavity of the deformity to narrow the metaphyseal canal for the incoming nail (a). The blocking pins deflect the nail and rotate the head out of varus (b). Final nail insertion is performed with the nail in proper position, head in anatomic alignment, and the diaphysis appropriately translated (c).

delayed healing. The author's preferred method is to utilize a hemostat to bluntly dissect the soft tissue until the anterior humeral surface is reached. Once on the surface of the bone, the hemostat ends are spread apart, advanced gently, and then the hemostat is relaxed on either side of the anterior humeral cortex (**Fig. 9.10**). This 'no hands' technique will retract the soft tissues without the need for an assistant, and will safely assist distal interlocking drilling and screw insertion. Osseous quality and fracture configuration will determine whether one or two distal interlock screws are used.

Nail fixation options

Three different types of nail system are available. The most commonly used is a nail system with multiple proximal screws specifically designed for the proximal humerus. The nail then narrows and allows

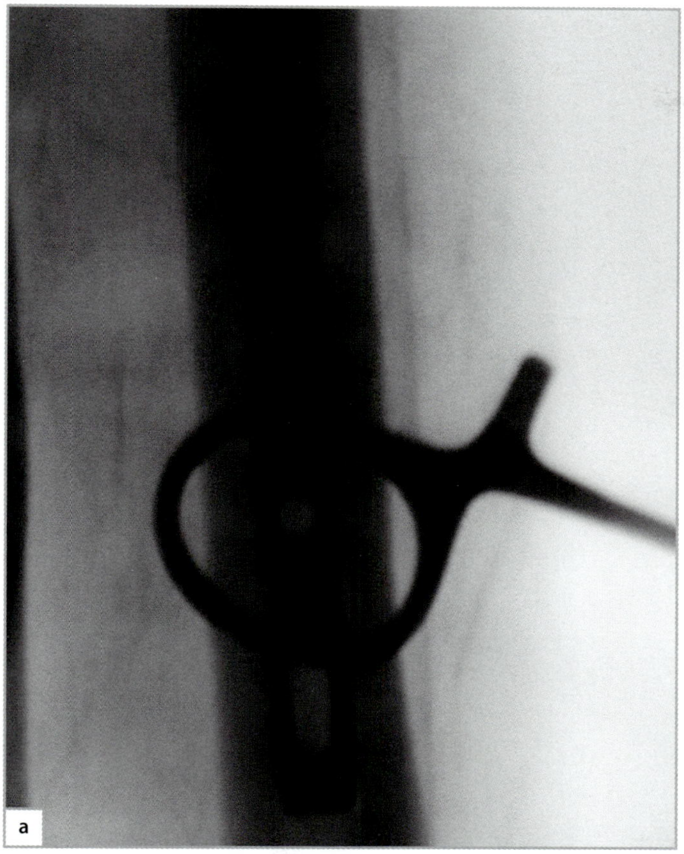
a

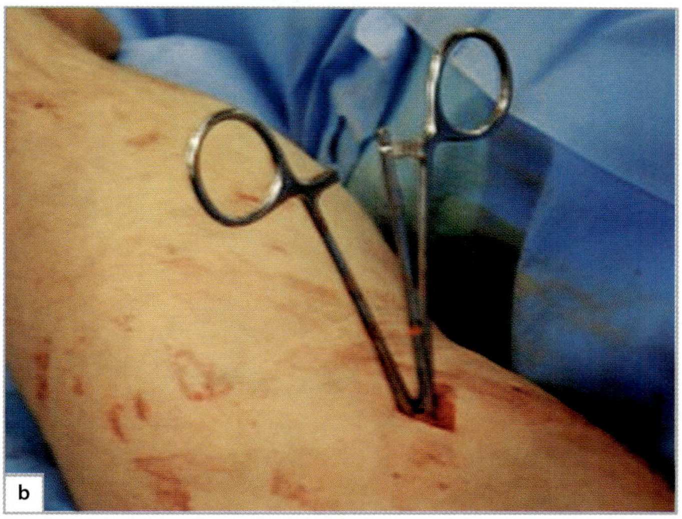
b

Figure 9.10 Use of a hemostat. The distal interlock position is confirmed with the circular portion of the hemostat along the skin (a). With the hemostat along the medial and lateral border of the distal humeral diaphysis, the distal interlock drill bit is inserted without soft-tissue entanglement (b).

for one or two screws to be inserted distally through the guide in a lateral-to-medial direction. Advantages of this type of nail include multiple screw options, the ability to stabilize the tuberosities, a narrowed distal stem that accommodates the hourglass distal humeral anatomy, insertion without distal reaming, and screw insertion via a guide. Its principal disadvantage is the need for inventory specifically for fractures of the proximal humerus, in additional to humeral diaphyseal nails. An additional disadvantage is the large flared portion of the nail that is required proximally for the larger multiple screws.

A second type of nail system utilizes a single modified blade or large screw for proximal stability. The proximal fixation is highly dependent on the optimal position of the device in relation to the head. This principle is very similar to the tip–apex distance (TAD) for lag screw placement in intertrochanteric hip fractures (Baumgaertner et al. 1995, Baumgaertner and Solberg 1997). These single proximal screws or blades are more rigid than other nail constructs, but provide only one site of fixation within the head.

The third type of implant is the standard humeral nail with additional proximal screw options. The proximal portion of these nails and the screw sizes are generally smaller than seen with the specialized nail systems. Some of these systems allow for locking of the most proximal screw using an end-cap. Other newer systems allow for locking-screw technology within the nail holes. A single humeral nail inventory for proximal and diaphyseal fractures is an advantage, but the smaller screws with fewer options is a disadvantage. Furthermore, longer nails allow for dissipation of forces distally along the diaphysis and reduce stress in comparison with shorter nails.

Additional fixation is usually necessary for severely osteoporotic bone or multiple fracture fragments. Suture fixation is excellent for the proximal humerus. The pull-out strength of sutures through the bone is usually less than that of the RC. Sutures placed through the RC will help neutralize cuff pull and facilitate early range of motion. Sutures placed from the subscapularis into the supraspinatus will help diminish tuberosity separation, and help to close down the rotator interval. This will allow for earlier range of motion during the healing process. Sutures placed into the diaphysis will neutralize the cephalad pull of the RC. Even if the tuberosities are not fractured or displaced, sutures into the cuff will help dissipate forces on the IMN proximal screws. In addition, screw washers or screws alone will help compress and maintain tuberosity reduction. Sutures can also be looped around the proximal interlocking screw head before the screw is seeded for additional back-up fixation. Problems with screw fixation consist of interference with nail placement, intra-articular insertion, or migration with early range of motion.

Closure

Closure of the approach is begun with the RC. Threaded non-absorbable sutures (number 2, Ethibond, Ethicon, Johnson & Johnson, San Angelo, TX) are inserted using a buried or simple interrupted technique (**Fig. 9.11**). Whether three or four sutures are used is the choice of the surgeon but they should be stable and watertight. The deltoid split is repaired with absorbable or non-absorbable sutures through the overlying deltoid fascia. The surgeon may choose to insert a Hemovac or pain pump drain into the subacromial space. Use of an elastic bandage from the patient's fingers to the humeral diaphysis will diminish dependent edema and enhance distal range of motion.

Complications

The treatment of fractures of the proximal humerus is complicated by a short fragment length, osteoporotic bone, and neurovascular structures (Svend-Hansen et al. 1998, Lin et al. 2003, Sperling et al. 2007, Vallier 2007). A common complication with IMN is loss of fixation. Newer nailing systems accommodate the insertion of locked proximal screws. This may diminish screw migration or fixation failure. Poor competency of the lateral wall (fracture communication) or too lateral a starting site, unbalanced screw fixation, and fixation failure may occur. Poller (blocking) screws or TTSP to medialize the nail will diminish this complication. Varus reductions result in higher rates of fixation failure and of tuberosity impingement. Nail prominence

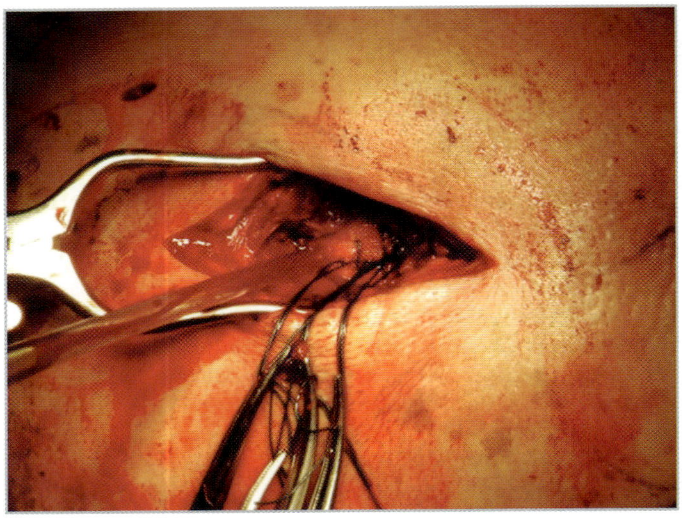

Figure 9.11 Watertight rotator cuff repair. This is performed with closely positioned number 2 inverted simple sutures.

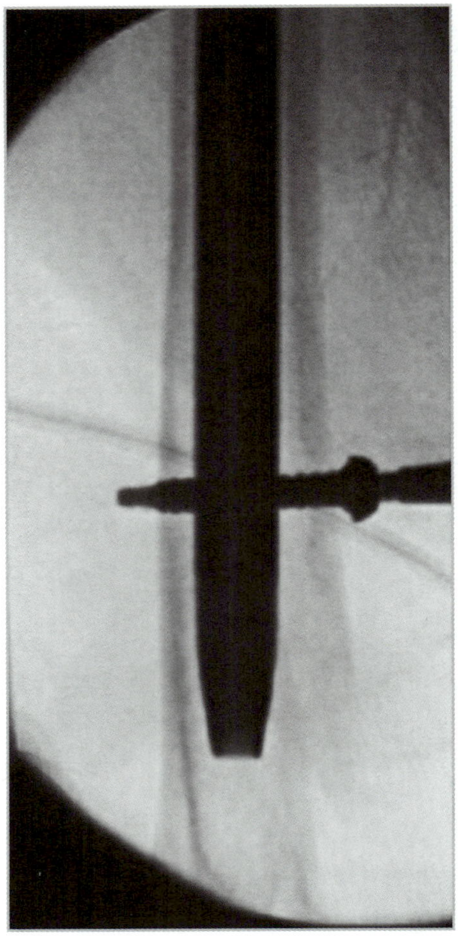

Figure 9.12 Overinsertion of the nail. On the lateral view, the distally inserted nail is inserted too deep in the gently anterior-sloping distal humerus, creating a posteriorly displaced metaphyseal fracture in osteoporotic bone.

can be avoided with direct visualization through the RC incision and recessing the tip 5 mm below the articular surface. Overinsertion of the nail will result in poor screw fixation angles and a higher risk of axillary nerve injury (Riemer and D'Ambrosia 1992, Lin et al. 1999, Albritton et al. 2003); it may also enhance iatrogenic or stress riser fractures at the nail tip (**Fig. 9.12**). Salvage of distal iatrogenic fracture displacement can be achieved with a larger distal incision, plate fixation, and incorporation of the distal interlock within the plate (**Fig. 9.13**). Proximal screws are usually 50 mm long or less, as longer ones have a higher risk of intra-articular penetration of the humeral head (Hernigou and Germany 2002). Over-exuberant dissection or nail malrotation with screw penetration into the bicipetal groove may increase the likelihood of osteonecrosis of the humeral head (Riemer and D'Ambrosia 1992).

Because nail insertion is performed through the RC, pre-existing cuff dysfunction can have adverse effects during rehabilitation. In the setting of concomitant RC arthropathy, a total shoulder or reverse total shoulder arthroplasty may be beneficial alternatives. Attempts at early range of motion with an irritable RC and adhesive capsulitis can lead to early fixation failure or a stiff, painful shoulder, or both. Revision options for a stiff, painful shoulder with cuff dysfunction are not associated with consistently good results.

Intraoperative fixation problems can occur if the fracture is displaced during nail insertion, or by the inability to obtain relatively stable fixation with proximal interlocking screws. In such instances, abandoning nail insertion and changing to plate fixation may be required, and can be performed through the same deltoid-splitting incision by sliding the plate submuscularly, or by extending the incision (Gardner et al. 2004, Gardner et al. 2008). The proximal screws can then be placed through the same proximal open incision, followed by percutaneous fixation of the diaphyseal component of the plate. Care must be taken not to injure the axillary nerve, which can occur if screws are placed distal to the deltoid-splitting incision and proximal to the diaphyseal screws. The other, more familiar and reliable approach is via a separate deltopectoral incision. The fracture is then re-reduced with standard methods.

For asymptomatic and symptomatic screw migration, screw removal can be performed. Head and tuberosity stability should be examined at the time of screw removal to avoid early fixation failure or non-union.

REHABILITATION

Protocol

A regional anesthetic block in conjunction with a general anesthesia is helpful to reduce postoperative pain. A formal physiotherapist-directed program is best suited for fractures of the proximal humerus. In order to protect the RC incision and tuberosity fixation, only passive motion for the first six weeks should be instituted. Full forward flexion (180°) and limited abduction (90°) should be initiated first. Frequent patient- and therapist-directed external rotation to neutral should be performed. Once the initial irritation is reduced, gradual increases in rotation should be advanced. Constant internal rotation associated with slings and shoulder immobilizers should be avoided. At six weeks postoperatively, once healing is noted, with resolution of the fracture lines and/or callus formation, unrestricted physiotherapist-directed strengthening, active range of motion, and weight bearing are allowed. RC rehabilitation is paramount, as trauma to the RC from the injury and surgery can result in overwhelming pain. Therapy sessions three times a week in conjunction with a home program performed two to three times a day are usually required for 12–16 weeks. The home program should be continued up to a year postoperatively, to avoid regression.

OUTCOME

Biomechanical studies suggest similar outcomes are achieved with IMN, with plates, and with enhanced fixation using pins. Balanced,

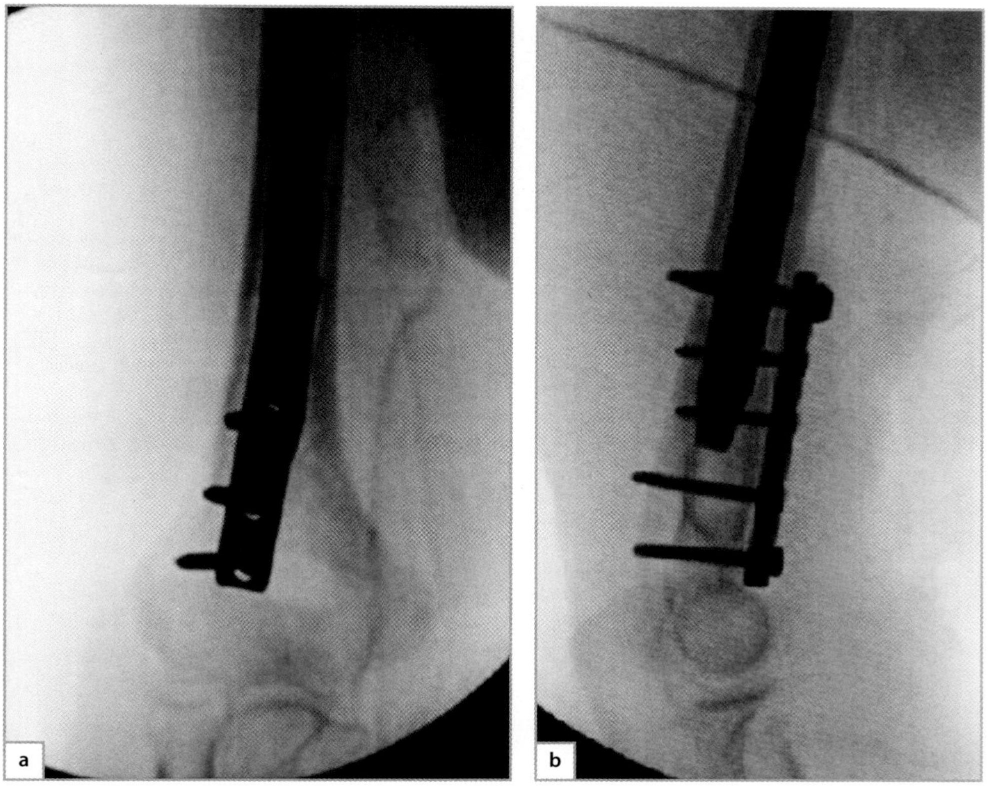

Figure 9.13 Salvage of distal iatrogenic fracture displacement. Anteroposterior (a) and lateral (b) views of the metaphyseal plate (four-hole 3.5 mm dynamic compression plate) utilized in conjunction with the nail to stabilize the iatrogenically created fracture.

stable fixation, especially with osteoporotic bone, is beneficial (Dalton et al. 1993, Koval et al. 1996, Ruch et al. 2000, Fernandez Dell'Oca 2002, Lill et al. 2003, Hou and Lin 2004, Durigan et al. 2005, Hessmann et al. 2005, Tamai et al. 2005, Wong et al. 2005, Edwards et al. 2006, Fuchtmeier et al. 2006, Fuchtmeier et al. 2007, Kitson et al. 2007). If fixation is too rigid, however, this can be detrimental. Newer locking-screw technology with or without plate utilization is an exciting option.

No outcome studies of the IMN fixation of fractures of the proximal humerus have been reported in the literature. Even though periosteal stripping is avoided, a load-sharing implant is inserted, and multiple screw fixation points are available, only results from small series have been reported (Fakler et al. 2008). Lin et al. have noted excellent results with standard locked nails for these fractures (Lin et al. 1998, Lin and Hou 2003, Lin et al. 2003, Lin 2006). No cases of fixation failure or revision were noted. Excellent or satisfactory results were obtained in 86% of patients (Lin et al. 1998, Lin 2006). While complications can be expected with a poor nail starting site and lateral comminution, Agel et al. (2004) found good results when nails were inserted properly. Adedapo and Ikpeme (2001) noted good function and results with the Polarus nail system. In order to introduce evidence-based medicine, more controlled, randomized studies are required.

REFERENCES

Adedapo AO, Ikpeme JO. The results of internal fixation of three- and four-part proximal humeral fractures with the Polarus nail. Injury 2001;32:115–121.

Agel J, Jones CB, Sanzone AG, et al. Treatment of proximal humeral fractures with Polarus nail fixation. J Shoulder Elbow Surg 2004;13(2):191–195.

Albritton MJ, Barnes CJ, Basamania CJ, Karas SG. Relationship of the axillary nerve to the proximal screws of a flexible humeral nail system: an anatomic study. J Orthop Trauma 2003;17:411–414.

Baumgaertner MR, Solberg BD. Awareness of tip–apex distance reduces failure of fixation of trochanteric fractures of the hip. J Bone Joint Surg Am 1997;79:969–971.

Baumgaertner MR, Curtin SL, Lindskog DM, Keggi JM. The value of the tip–apex distance in predicting failure of fixation of peritrochanteric fractures of the hip. J Bone Joint Surg Am 1995;77:1058–1064.

Dalton JE, Salkeld SL, Satterwhite YE, Cook SD. A biomechanical comparison of intramedullary nailing systems for the humerus. J Orthop Trauma 1993;7:367–374.

Durigan A Jr, Barbieri CH, Mazzer N, Shimano AC. Two-part surgical neck fractures of the humerus: mechanical analysis of the fixation with four Shanz-type threaded pins in four different assemblies. J Shoulder Elbow Surg 2005;14:96–102.

Edwards SL, Wilson NA, Zhang LQ, et al. Two-part surgical neck fractures of the proximal part of the humerus. A biomechanical evaluation of two fixation techniques. J Bone Joint Surg Am 2006;88:2258–2264.

Fakler JK, Hogan C, Heyde CE, John T. Current concepts in the treatment of proximal humeral fractures. Orthopedics 2008;31:42–51.

Fernandez Dell'Oca AA. The principle of helical implants. Unusual ideas worth considering. Injury 2002;33 Suppl 1:SA1–27.

Fuchtmeier B, May R, Fierlbeck J, Hammer J, Nerlich M. A comparative biomechanical analysis of implants for the stabilization of proximal humerus fractures. Technol Health Care 2006;14:261–270.

Fuchtmeier B, May R, Hente R, et al. Proximal humerus fractures: a comparative biomechanical analysis of intra and extramedullary implants. Arch Orthop Trauma Surg 2007;127:441–447.

Gardner MJ, Griffith MH, Dines JS, Lorich DG. A minimally invasive approach for plate fixation of the proximal humerus. Bull Hosp Jt Dis 2004;62:18–23.

Gardner MJ, Boraiah S, Helfet DL, Lorich DG. The anterolateral acromial approach for fractures of the proximal humerus. J Orthop Trauma 2008;22:132–137.

Gerber C, Schneeberger AG, Vinh TS. The arterial vascularization of the humeral head. An anatomical study. J Bone Joint Surg Am 1990;72:1486–1494.
Hernigou P, Germany W. Unrecognized shoulder joint penetration during fixation of proximal fractures of the humerus. Acta Orthop Scand 2002;73:140–143.
Hessmann MH, Hansen WS, Krummenauer F, Pol TF, Rommens PM. Locked plate fixation and intramedullary nailing for proximal humerus fractures: a biomechanical evaluation. J Trauma 2005;58:1194–1201.
Hou SM, Lin J. Biomechanical and clinical effects of adding interfragmentary wiring to locked nailing for humeral nonunions. J Formos Med Assoc 2004;103:836–843.
Kitson J, Booth G, Day R. A biomechanical comparison of locking plate and locking nail implants used for fractures of the proximal humerus. J Shoulder Elbow Surg 2007;16:362–366.
Koval KJ, Blair B, Takei R, et al. Surgical neck fractures of the proximal humerus: a laboratory evaluation of ten fixation techniques. J Trauma 1996;40:778–783.
Laing PG. The arterial supply of the adult humerus. J Bone Joint Surg Am 1956;38:1105–1116.
Lill H, Hepp P, Korner J, et al. Proximal humeral fractures: how stiff should an implant be? A comparative mechanical study with new implants in human specimens. Arch Orthop Trauma Surg 2003;123:74–81.
Lin J. Effectiveness of locked nailing for displaced three-part proximal humeral fractures. J Trauma 2006;61:363–374.
Lin J, Hou SM. Locked-nail treatment of humeral surgical neck nonunions. J Trauma 2003;54:530–535.
Lin J, Hou SM, Hang YS. Locked nailing for displaced surgical neck fractures of the humerus. J Trauma 1998;45:1051–1057.
Lin J, Hou SM, Inoue N, et al. Anatomic considerations of locked humeral nailing. Clin Orthop Relat Res 1999;(368):247–254.
Lin J, Shen PW, Hou SM. Complications of locked nailing in humeral shaft fractures. J Trauma 2003;54:943–949.
Riemer BL, D'Ambrosia R. The risk of injury to the axillary nerve, artery, and vein from proximal locking screws of humeral intramedullary nails. Orthopedics 1992;15:697–699.
Ruch DS, Glisson RR, Marr AW, et al. Fixation of three-part proximal humeral fractures: a biomechanical evaluation. J Orthop Trauma 2000;14:36–40.
Rupp RE, Chrissos MG, Ebraheim NA. The risk of neurovascular injury with distal locking screws of humeral intramedullary nails. Orthopedics 1996;19:593–595.
Sperling JW, Cuomo F, Hill JD, et al. The difficult proximal humerus fracture: tips and techniques to avoid complications and improve results. Instr Course Lect 2007;56:45–57.
Svend-Hansen H, Skettrup M, Rathcke MW. Complications using the Seidel intramedullary humeral nail: outcome in 31 patients. Acta Orthop Belg 1998;64:291–295.
Tamai K, Ohno W, Takemura M, et al. Treatment of proximal humeral fractures with a new intramedullary nail. J Orthop Sci 2005;10:180–186.
Vallier HA. Treatment of proximal humerus fractures. J Orthop Trauma 2007;21:469–476.
Wong MW, Chow DH, Li CK. Rotational stability of Seidel nail distal locking mechanism. Injury 2005;36:1201–1205.

Chapter 10 Hemiarthroplasty for four-part fractures of the proximal humerus

Todd C. Moen, Louis U. Bigliani

INTRODUCTION

The appropriate treatment for four-part fractures, selected three-part fractures, and fracture dislocations of the proximal humerus is controversial. Multiple surgical options exist, including open reduction and internal fixation (ORIF) with non-locking and locking plates and screws, ORIF with fixed-angle devices, suture fixation, percutaneous pinning, intramedullary nails, and prosthetic replacement with hemiarthroplasty. Of these techniques, ORIF with plate-and-screw constructs and hemiarthroplasty are the most often performed. There is current debate in the literature regarding the exact indications for ORIF versus hemiarthroplasty. The advent and refinement of locking-plate technology has expanded the indications for ORIF. However, ORIF can have considerable complications. Initially described by Neer et al. (1953), hemiarthroplasty has proven effective in providing pain relief for patients with complex fractures of the proximal humerus, although functional outcomes following hemiarthroplasty have been variable and unpredictable (Neer et al. 1953, Neer 1970a, Neer 1970b, Neer 1987, Mighell et al. 2003, Robinson et al. 2003, Kralinger et al. 2004, Robinson and Page 2004, Antuna et al. 2008). To achieve optimal function following hemiarthroplasty, proper surgical technique and postoperative rehabilitation are essential.

INDICATIONS AND CONTRAINDICATIONS

In his original series on fractures of the proximal humerus, Neer stated that three-part fractures were best treated with ORIF, while four-part fractures were best treated with hemiarthroplasty (Neer 1970a, Neer 1970b). This indication for hemiarthroplasty has been revised to include any fracture in which the humeral head is deemed unviable or not amenable to fixation with contemporary techniques. There is no consensus in the literature as to what precisely defines unviable or unreconstructable; however, broadly speaking, four-part fractures, comminuted osteoporotic three-part fractures, fracture dislocations of the humeral head, head-splitting fractures, and fractures involving impaction of greater than 40% of the humeral articular surface are considered best suited for hemiarthroplasty (Mighell et al. 2003, Robinson et al. 2003, Kralinger et al. 2004, Robinson and Page 2004, Antuna et al. 2008) (**Fig. 10.1**). Due to superior outcomes, it is best to perform hemiarthroplasty acutely as opposed to as a late salvage procedure for malunion (Norris et al. 1995, Mansat et al. 2004).

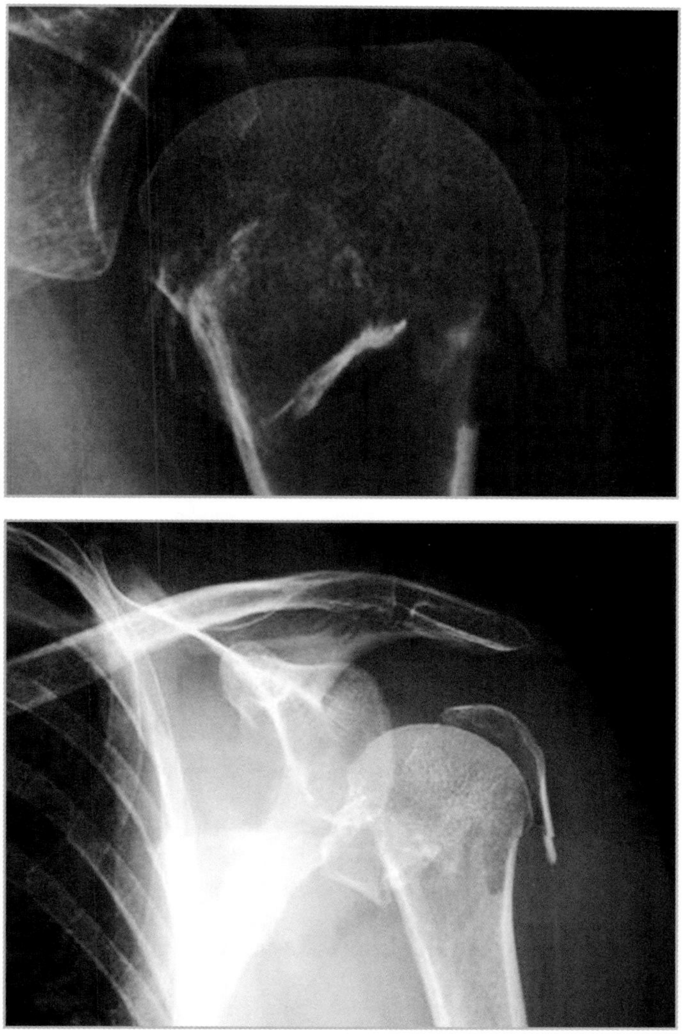

Figure 10.1 Radiographs showing a complex fracture of the proximal humerus. (Courtesy of Columbia Center for Shoulder, Elbow and Sports Medicine.)

TECHNIQUE

Hemiarthroplasty is a demanding procedure, and often complications are linked to surgical technique. Normal anatomic landmarks may be obscured or obliterated by the fracture, making restoration of the patient's native anatomy challenging. Nevertheless, with vigilance and meticulous attention to detail, it is possible to reliably reconstruct the proximal humerus, minimize complications, and ultimately improve results for patients.

Preoperative planning

As with all surgical procedures, it is imperative to have a thorough preoperative plan. Pursuant to this, appropriate radiographic studies are vital to completely delineate and understand the fracture pattern. In most cases, a standard shoulder trauma series is sufficient to characterize the fracture. This series includes: a true anteroposterior (AP) view of the scapula; a trans-scapular lateral Y view; and an axillary lateral view. The true AP view of the scapula is obtained with the x-ray beam angled 30–40° obliquely to the coronal plane of the body. The axillary view is obtained by abducting the arm 20–30°, with the tube directed into the axilla and the radiographic plate oriented above the shoulder; the arm does not need to be fully abducted. Often, the surgeon must position the arm, as the patient is unable to do so, due to pain. Alternatively, a Velpeau axillary view can be obtained. This is done by allowing the patient to have the affected arm in a sling for comfort, and then getting the patient to lean backward over a radiographic plate, with the tube positioned over the patient, directed downward. If plain radiographs leave questions as to the fracture pattern, a computerized tomography (CT) scan with three-dimensional reconstructions can be obtained. Finally, plain radiographs or a scanogram of the uninvolved arm can be obtained to aid in preoperative planning, and prosthetic sizing and templating.

Patient positioning

The patient is placed in a modified beach-chair position with the back of the operating table elevated to approximately 45°. A towel is placed under the medial border of the scapula, and a table with a cut-away section about the shoulder is used to allow global access to the shoulder. The entire arm is prepped and draped, beginning at the base of the neck and under the axilla, thus permitting the arm to be moved freely throughout surgery.

Procedure

A long deltopectoral incision is used. The incision begins inferior to the clavicle, just lateral to the coracoid, and extends laterally toward the deltoid insertion on the humeral shaft. The cephalic vein is identified in the deltopectoral interval, and the vein is retracted laterally as the interval is opened. To facilitate exposure, the proximal third of the pectoralis insertion is taken down and tagged with suture for later reattachment. A broad retractor is placed under the lateral border of the strap muscles, avoiding over-retraction, which could result in neurovascular injury. Another broad retractor is placed under the deltoid and this muscle is retracted laterally. The long head of the biceps brachii (LHB) is identified. With the LHB as the guide to the glenoid and the center of the shoulder, hemorrhagic bursae are carefully excised and the clavicopectoral fascia is incised. Typically, this dissection will reveal the fracture hematoma and fracture fragments.

At this point in the procedure, the fracture fragments must be identified and mobilized, and the LHB serves as a landmark to the individual parts. Typically, the lesser tuberosity lies medial to the LHB, the greater tuberosity lateral, with the head – in varying degrees of comminution – lying between the tuberosities. With the individual fragments identified, each tuberosity is tagged with number 2 non-absorbable suture. The suture is placed in cuff tendon, proximal to the tuberosity insertion, thereby avoiding further iatrogenic comminution to the fragment. Each tuberosity is mobilized sufficiently medially, laterally, superiorly, and inferiorly. The biceps is routinely tenodesed at the end of the operation.

With the tuberosities tagged and mobilized, attention is turned to the removal of the humeral head (**Fig. 10.2**). Removal of the head should be done carefully, without undue force. To accomplish this, the surgeon should follow the fracture line that typically lies in the bicipital groove to the rotator interval, and make a release in the rotator interval. It is important to release only what is necessary to remove the head, in an attempt to preserve as much of the soft-tissue attachment to the tuberosities as possible. Any loose fragments of cancellous bone as well as the humeral head should be preserved for use as autogenous bone graft.

There are two important further considerations here. First, if treatment has been delayed beyond 7–10 days after the initial injury, particular care must be taken in mobilizing the tuberosities and removing the humeral head, as scarring and adhesions make these tasks much more difficult. Second, if the head is dislocated anteriorly below the coracoid and medial to the strap muscles, caution must be exercised, given the proximity of neurovascular structures and hence the potential for neurovascular injury.

At this point in the procedure, attention is focused on preparing the humerus for the implant. This must be done gently, as the bone in patients who sustain these injuries is typically osteoporotic.

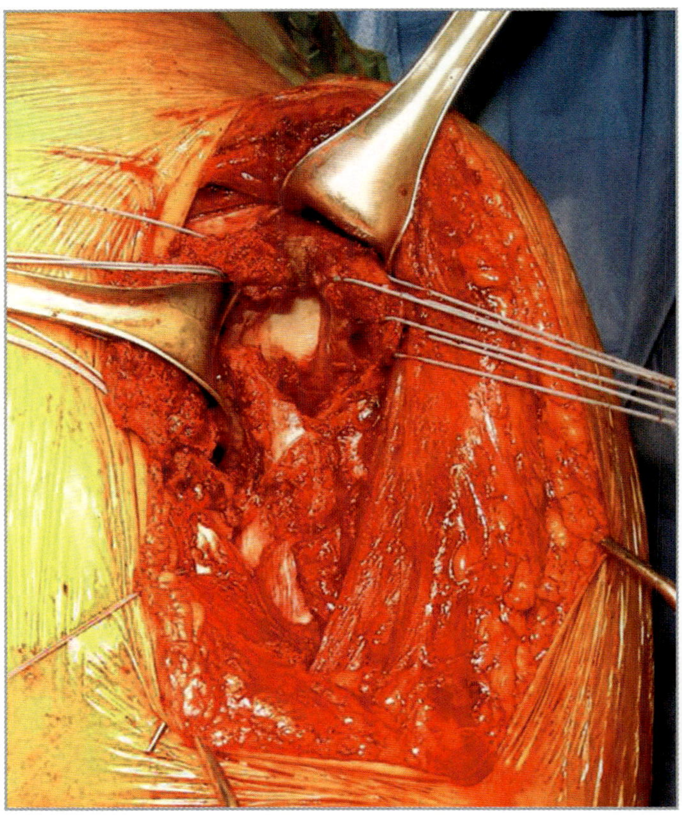

Figure 10.2 Tuberosities tagged with non-absorbable suture, and humeral head removed. The biceps tendon has been tenotomized. (Courtesy of Columbia Center for Shoulder, Elbow and Sports Medicine.)

To expose the humerus, the surgeon extends and externally rotates the arm, and then lifts the elbow in a distal-to-proximal direction. Medial and lateral Darrach retractors are placed posterior to the shaft for full exposure. Next, the surgeon opens and prepares the medullary canal with sequential reamers.

It is vitally important to determine the proper orientation, position, and size of the prosthesis. There are three aspects to this: retroversion, height, and head size. The prosthesis is the foundation on which the reconstruction is based, and the restoration of a patient's anatomy with the implant is vital to the success of the operation. A malpositioned implant leads to malpositioned tuberosities (Robinson et al. 2003), which will be subjected to greater stresses during healing (Frankle et al. 2001), impairing progression to union. Tuberosity malunion is well recognized as one of the most common and deleterious complications of arthroplasty for fractures of the proximal humerus, and ultimately leads to impaired functional outcomes (Smith et al. 1997, Boileau et al. 2002, Mighell et al. 2003, Robinson et al. 2003, Kralinger et al. 2004, Smith et al. 2007, Antuna et al. 2008). Fortunately, the current generation of modular prosthetic implants greatly increases the ability to recreate proximal humeral anatomy. In addition, improved instrumentation and jigs allow reproducible assessments of version and height. Furthermore, there is the ability to trial numerous head sizes and offsets that will maximize motion, stability, and tuberosity repair.

Version is initially assessed with the use of an intramedullary alignment system equipped with an outrigger that references the forearm (**Fig. 10.3**). Proximal humeral anatomy is variable, and studies have shown the humeral head to be retroverted between 0° and 40° (Roberts et al. 1991, Iannotti et al. 1992, Boileau and Walch 1997, Boileau et al. 2002, Iannotti et al. 2005). We typically position the implant in approximately 25–30° of retroversion. In the case of a chronic posterior fracture dislocation, we would decrease the amount of retroversion of the prosthesis. It is important to note that alternative techniques of determining version are available (Kontakis et al. 2001, Krishnan et al. 2008), and that this initial determination of version is preliminary; the final version is based on the trial reduction of the prosthesis and tuberosities, as discussed below.

The next step is to establish the height of the prosthesis. The trial stem is seated within the canal, with a sponge around the humeral stem. It is important not to seat the collar of the prosthesis so deeply that it is placed against the remaining proximal shaft (**Fig. 10.3**). A deep-seated prosthesis will decrease the length of the humerus and shorten the myofascial sleeve, compromising the mechanical advantage of the deltoid. We determine the height of the prosthesis based on the position of the tuberosities relative to the shaft and humeral head. When the greater tuberosity is reduced, its proximal portion should clear the head and overlap the proximal shaft by only a few millimeters. Also, the implant should be placed in a way that allows the greater and lesser tuberosities to be positioned below the level of the head. Alternative techniques for establishing height include referencing off the insertion of the pectoralis major insertion (Murachovsky et al. 2006, Greiner et al. 2008) and reconstruction of the 'Gothic arch' based off the medial calcar (Krishnan et al. 2008).

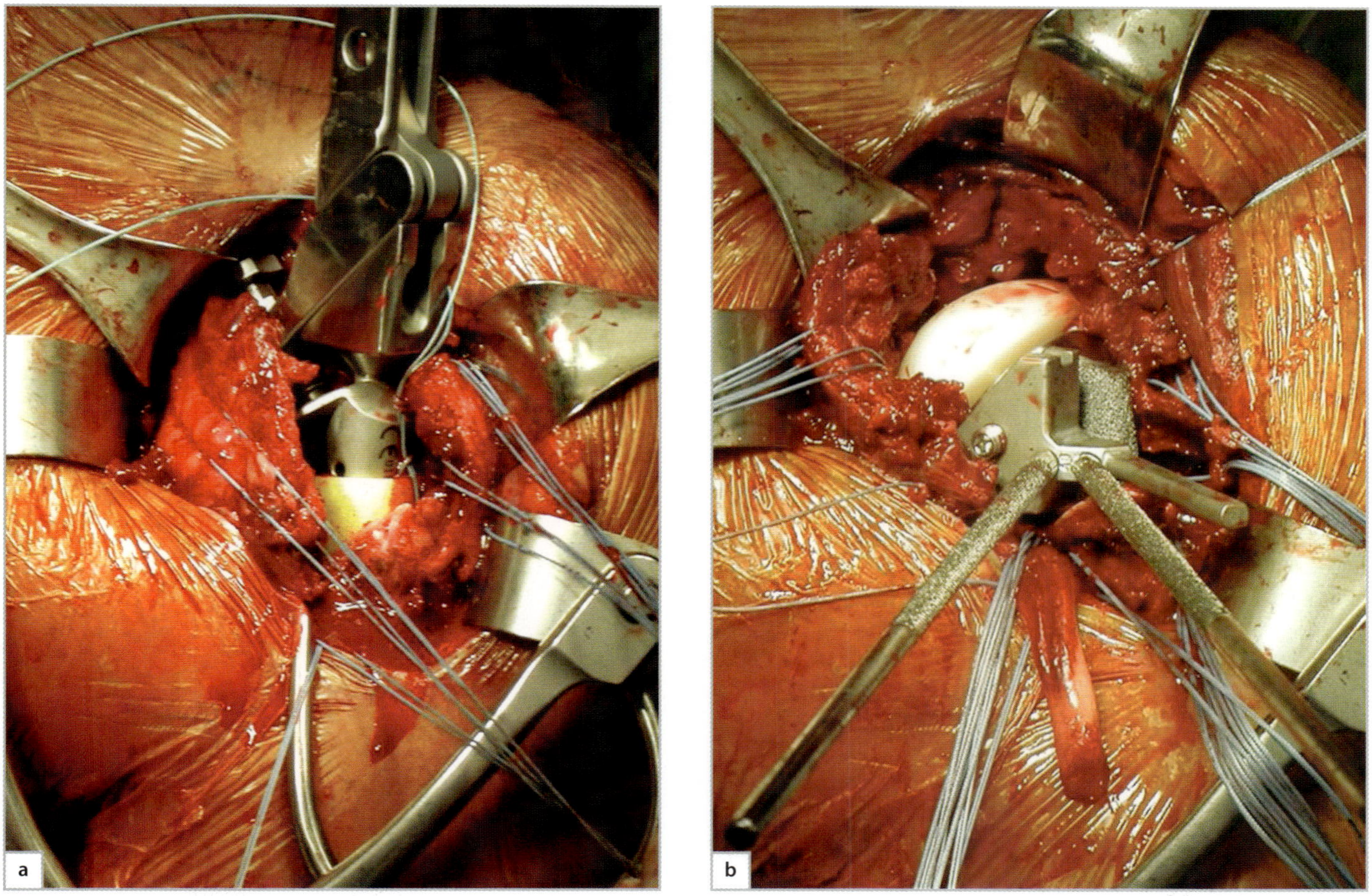

Figure 10.3 Trial implant in place. (a) Stem positioned to the proper height. (b) The jig can be used to establish appropriate version. A trial humeral head is attached. (Courtesy of Columbia Center for Shoulder, Elbow and Sports Medicine.)

Finally, a trial humeral head is selected and placed (**Fig. 10.3**). The choice of the correct head size can be facilitated by the use of templating radiographs of the uninvolved contralateral shoulder and/or by using for comparison the fractured head that was removed. We err toward undersizing the head, because overstuffing the joint increases the likelihood of postoperative stiffness. Generally, men require a larger head than women. We use an implant system that provides either concentric or offset heads in four different radii of curvature to optimize the restoration of anatomy and implant stability. With the appropriate head selected, the trial component is reduced by moving the tuberosities out of the way. Then the tagging sutures are used to reduce the tuberosities around the prosthesis.

Next, the position of the tuberosities is reassessed, as well as the alignment, height, and version of the prosthesis and tuberosities. The tuberosities should be below the head, such that there is no subacromial impingement, and the tuberosities are well apposed to the shaft. Then, height is assessed. The tension on LHB, if the tendon is intact, can be used as a guide to the appropriate tension for the entire myofascial sleeve. If the tendon is slack in its anatomic position, the prosthesis is implanted too deeply. If the tendon is tight, the prosthesis is proud. To evaluate version, the surgeon should assess the stability of the implant at 40–50° of internal and external rotation. If the prosthesis subluxes or dislocates posteriorly, there likely is too much retroversion, and this should be decreased. If the prosthesis is unstable anteriorly, this suggests that the retroversion should be increased. Finally, the surgeon should perform AP translation and push-pull assessments to assess the translational stability of the implant. Our goal is 50% translation in both the anterior-to-posterior and the superior-to-inferior directions. If there is any concern regarding alignment of the implant, intraoperative fluoroscopy can be used to confirm the appropriate position. When it is felt that the implant is in the ideal position, the distance from the lateral shaft to the lateral aspect of the collar is measured, to allow reproduction of appropriate height when the actual component is implanted.

The proximal humerus is then prepared with drill holes to allow for tuberosity fixation (**Fig. 10.4a**). We generally drill three or four holes in the area just distal to the tuberosities. Number 2 or number 5 heavy non-absorbable nylon sutures are passed with a swedged-on needle through the hole medial to the shaft, and tagged with a clamp.

Now attention is turned to implantation of the final prosthesis. In the vast majority of cases, the use of cement is suggested in the setting of this fracture, for two reasons. First, there is usually insufficient bone stock to allow adequate press-fit fixation. Secondly, cement restores the rotational stability of the implant that was lost via fracture of the tuberosities. The size of stem selected is close to that of the reamed canal, such that a minimum amount of cement will be required. An appropriately sized cement restrictor is placed within the canal, and the canal irrigated to remove excess blood and debris. After injection of the cement, the component is placed in position, using the previous measurements, anatomic landmarks, and instrumentation to assess

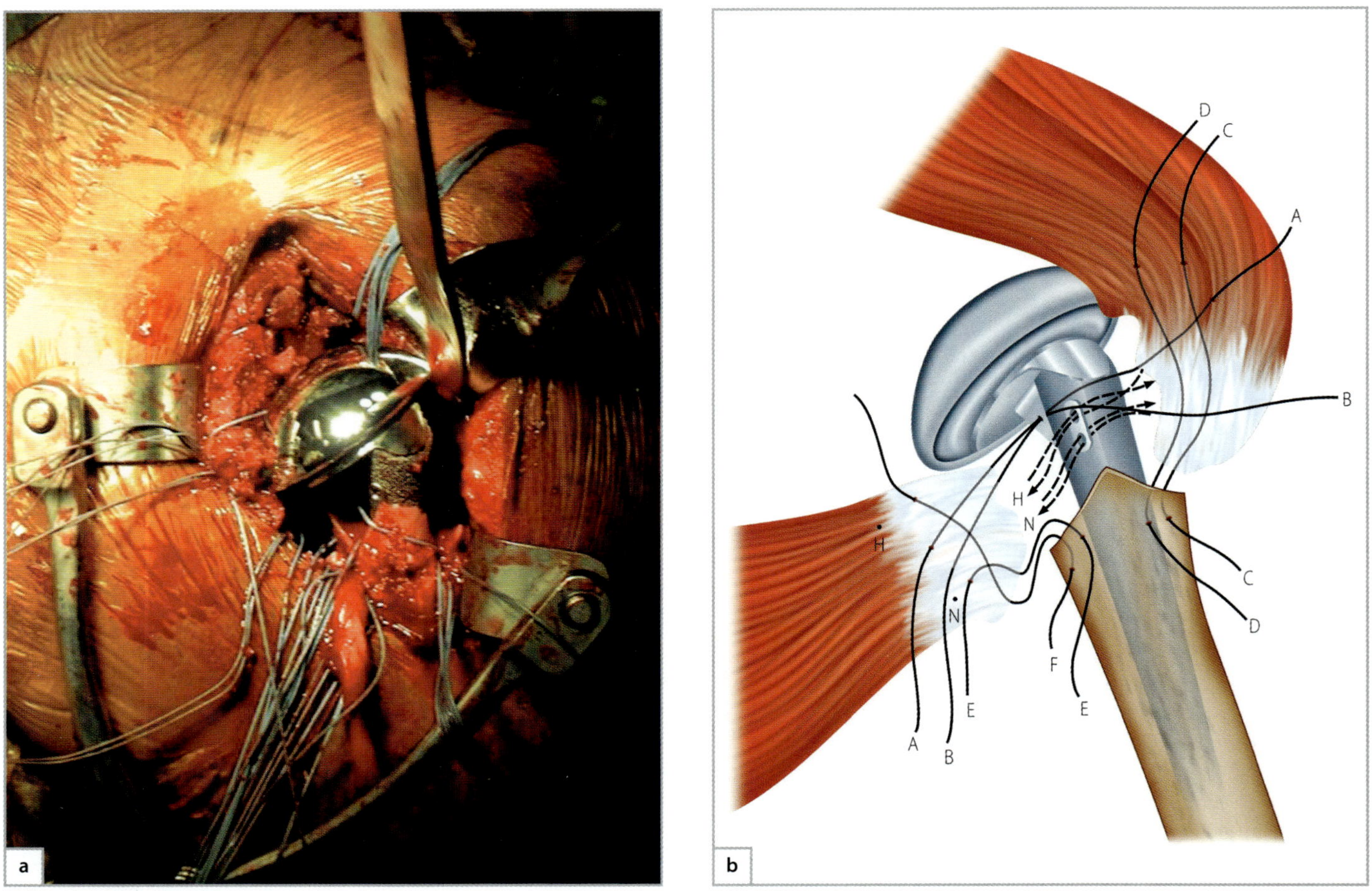

Figure 10.4 Preparation for tuberosity fixation. (a) Intraoperative photograph showing the final implant stem and humeral head in place, with suture prepared for tuberosity fixation. (b) Schematic of how the tuberosity sutures (A–N) are passed for final tuberosity fixation. (Courtesy of Columbia Center for Shoulder, Elbow and Sports Medicine.)

appropriate height and retroversion. Care should be taken to remove any excess cement from the proximal canal, because this could prevent tuberosity-to-shaft contact and impede healing. The actual head is then placed, and the prosthesis reduced.

Tuberosity repair is arguably the most important part of the procedure (**Fig. 10.4**). Tuberosity malposition and malunion are the most common and significant causes of functional failure in hemiarthroplasty for fracture (Smith et al. 1997, Mighell et al. 2003, Robinson et al. 2003, Smith et al. 2007). The surgeon should use the tagging sutures that have been previously placed to mobilize the tuberosities. The two number 5 non-absorbable sutures that are through the medial shaft hole and greater tuberosity are placed and tagged, but not tied until the sutures in the lesser and greater tuberosities are tied to bone. The surgeon should liberally apply cancellous bone as autogenous graft between the tuberosities and the shaft, and the tuberosities themselves. The greater tuberosity is reattached first, followed by the lesser tuberosity. The surgeon can use the number 2 and number 5 non-absorbable sutures previously passed through the shaft drill holes, with a total of three or four sutures of the greater tuberosity, and two or three for the lesser tuberosity. Then, the two sutures placed around the tuberosities are tied for compression. Then, with the arm supported in a slightly flexed and abducted position, the LHB should be tenodesed. Number 1 non-absorbable suture is used to repair the lateral aspect of the rotator interval above the biceps tendon, with the arm in neutral rotation so that the LHB comes out at the distal aspect of the interval. The surgeon should gently internally and externally rotate and flex the arm to test the stability of the tuberosity repair (**Fig. 10.5**). With gentle repositioning of the patient's arm, no movement of the repair should be seen (**Fig. 10.6**).

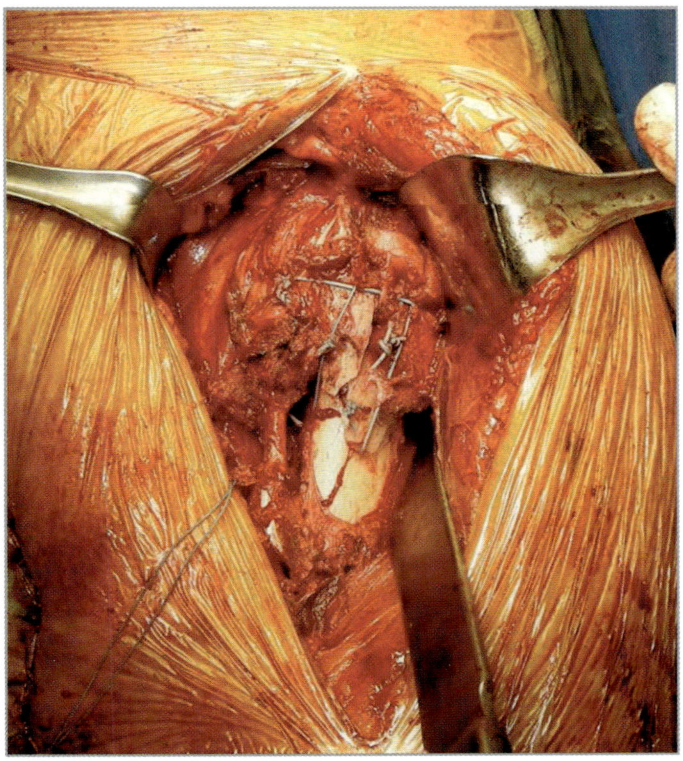

Figure 10.5 Final construct following tuberosity repair. (Courtesy of Columbia Center for Shoulder, Elbow and Sports Medicine.)

We routinely use a medium-suction drain placed in the deep interval for the first 12–24 hours to prevent initial hematoma formation. The drain should exit laterally in the proximal deltoid, avoiding injury to the axillary nerve. The insertion of the pectoralis major is repaired with number 2 non-absorbable suture. Multiple number 2 non-absorbable sutures are placed in the deltopectoral interval, and the interval is marked in the event of future revision surgery. The deep subcutaneous tissue is closed with 3-0 absorbable sutures. The skin is closed in a subcuticular fashion with 4-0 absorbable suture, and adhesive strips (e.g. Steri-Strips) are used to promote a cosmetic closure.

Pearls and pitfalls

- In the initial exposure of the fracture fragments, the LHB is a useful landmark. Typically, the lesser tuberosity lies medial to the tendon, the greater tuberosity lies lateral, while the head lies between the two tuberosities.
- If the operation is performed more than 7–10 days following injury, care must be exercised in exposing the fracture fragments. Post-traumatic scarring and adhesions obscure the identification of fragments and tissue planes.
- If the humeral head is dislocated anteriorly below the coracoids and medial to the strap muscles, extreme caution should be exercised in removing the head, to avoid damaging the neurovascular structures.
- Implant orientation is the foundation upon which this operation is built. Accurate restoration of the patient's native humeral head height, version, and head size is critical to achieving the proper orientation, tuberosity healing, and, in turn, a good functional result.
- Multiple landmarks and principles – such as the pectoralis insertion and restoration of the Gothic arch – exist to help establish proper orientation of the implant. Multiple methods should be used to double-check implant position.
- In choosing the size of the humeral head implant, it is best to err on the size of a smaller head, to avoid overstuffing the joint.
- If there is any concern over the alignment of the implant, intraoperative fluoroscopy can be used or an intraoperative radiograph obtained to confirm the appropriate position.
- Tuberosity repair is the most critical portion of the procedure. It is imperative to perform a secure, meticulous repair of the tuberosities.

REHABILITATION

In our rehabilitation protocol, a passive-motion program is begun on the first postoperative day. Range-of-motion limitations are determined based upon the intraoperative assessment of stability following tuberosity repair, taking into account the quality of bone, the status of the rotator cuff and deltoid, and the strength of tuberosity fixation to the shaft. On the morning after surgery, we usually raise the arm in the scapular plane to approximately 80–90°, to establish patient confidence. A therapist then gives gravity-assisted pendulum exercises to allow the patient to warm up. After this, assisted forward elevation (**Fig. 10.7**) and supine external rotation with a stick are performed. The goal ranges of motion prior to hospital discharge should be approximately 130° of forward elevation in the scapular plane, and 30° of external rotation, unless modified by the intraoperative assessment. Pulley and active exercises are not allowed in the first six weeks, after which, if there is radiographic evidence of tuberosity healing, resistive exercises are started (**Fig. 10.8**).

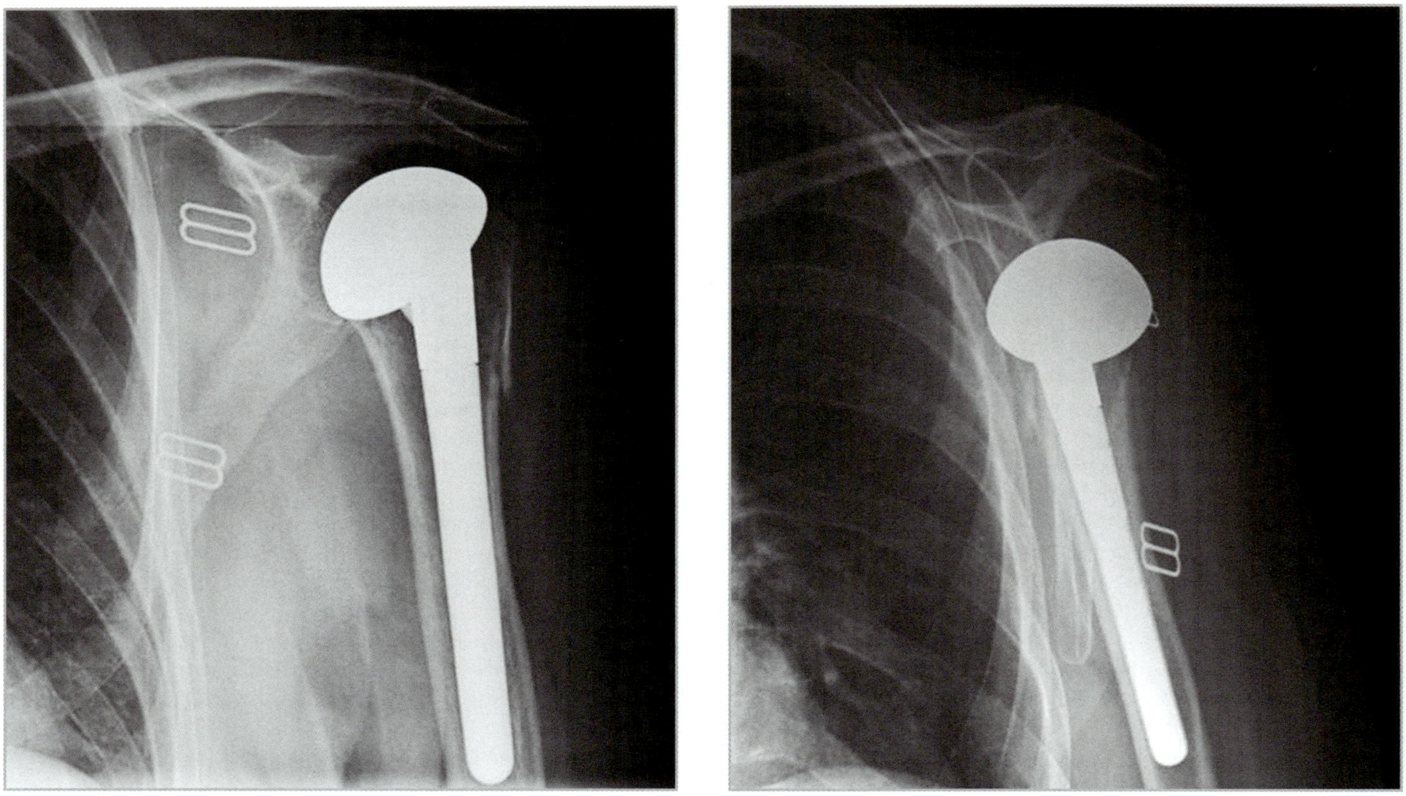

Figure 10.6 Postoperative radiographs demonstrating appropriate alignment of prosthesis and tuberosities. (Courtesy of Columbia Center for Shoulder, Elbow and Sports Medicine.)

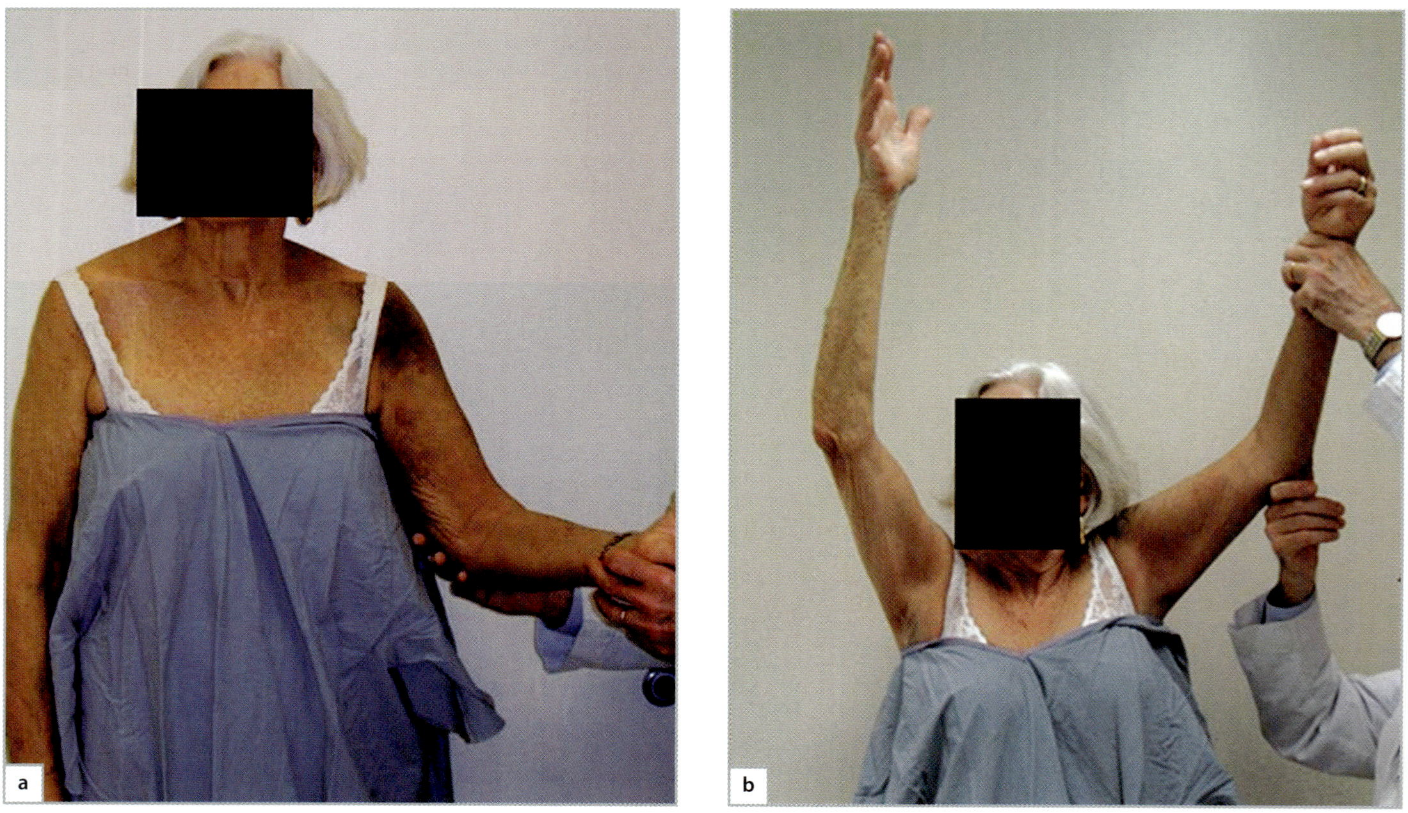

Figure 10.7 Assisted external rotation and forward elevation. Prior to evidence of union of the tuberosities, only assisted external rotation (a) and forward elevation (b) are permitted. No active motion is permitted. (Courtesy of Columbia Center for Shoulder, Elbow and Sports Medicine.)

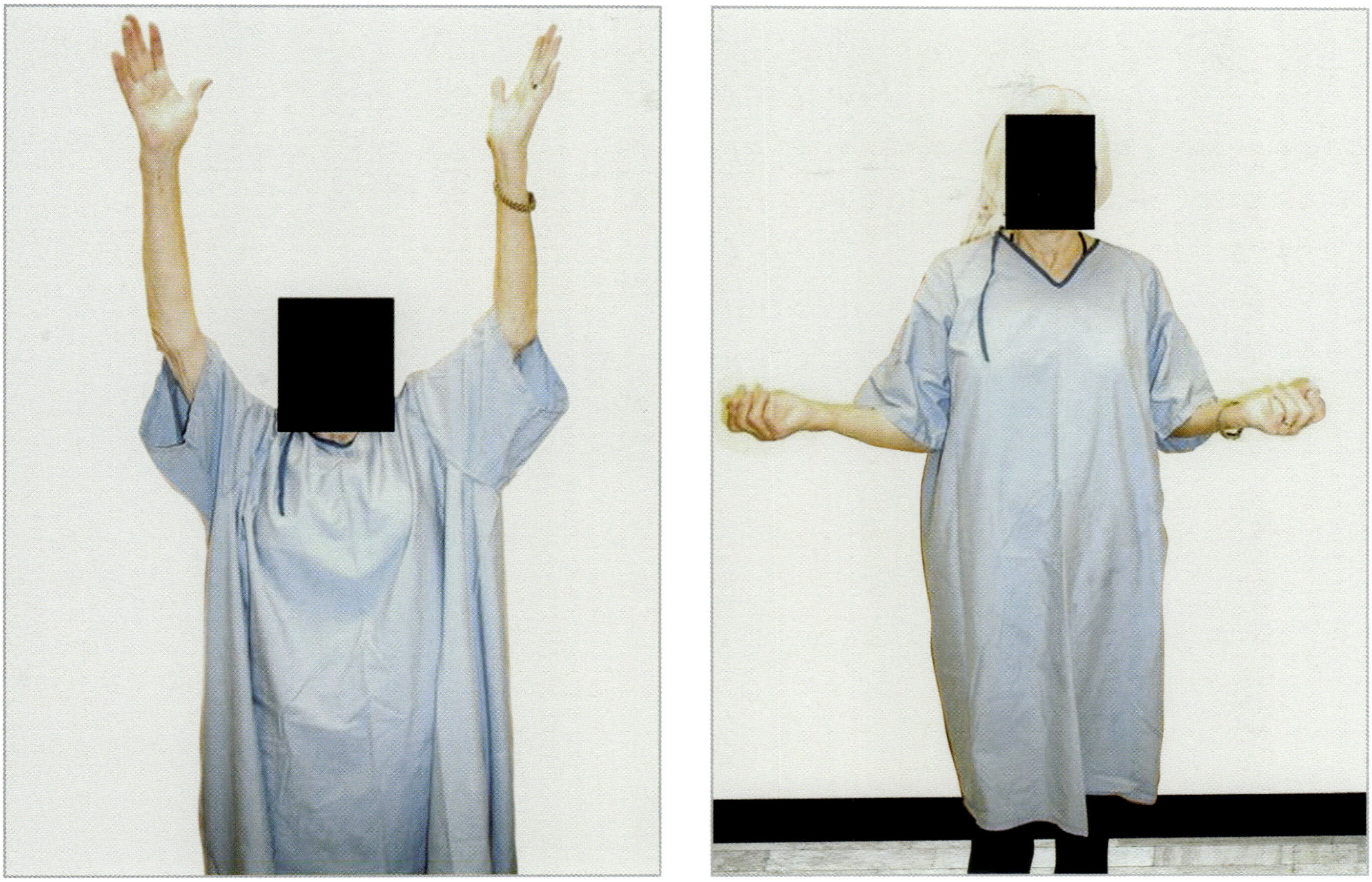

Figure 10.8 With evidence of union of the tuberosities, active exercises are allowed. (Courtesy of Columbia Center for Shoulder, Elbow and Sports Medicine.)

REFERENCES

Antuna SA, Sperling JW, Cofield RH. Shoulder hemiarthroplasty for acute fractures of the proximal humerus: a minimum five-year follow-up. J Shoulder Elbow Surg 2008;17:202–209.

Boileau P, Walch G. The three-dimensional geometry of the proximal humerus. Implications for surgical technique and prosthetic design. J Bone Joint Surg Br 1997;79:857–865.

Boileau P, Krishnan, SG, Tinsi L, et al. Tuberosity malposition and migration: reasons for poor outcomes after hemiarthroplasty for displaced fractures of the proximal humerus. J Shoulder Elbow Surg 2002;11:401–412.

Frankle MA, Greenwald DP, Markee BA, et al. Biomechanical effects of malposition of tuberosity fragments on the humeral prosthetic reconstruction for four-part proximal humerus fractures. J Shoulder Elbow Surg 2001;10:321–326.

Greiner SH, Kaab MJ, Kroning I, et al. Reconstruction of humeral length and centering of the prosthetic head in hemiarthroplasty for proximal humeral fractures. J Shoulder Elbow Surg 2008;17:709–714.

Iannotti JP, Gabriel JP, Schneck SL, et al. The normal glenohumeral relationships. An anatomical study of one hundred and forty shoulders. J Bone Joint Surg Am 1992;74:491–500.

Iannotti JP, Spencer EE, Winter U, et al. Prosthetic positioning in total shoulder arthroplasty. J Shoulder Elbow Surg 2005;14(1 Suppl S):111S–121S.

Kontakis GM, Damilakis J, Christoforakis J, et al. The bicipital groove as a landmark for orientation of the humeral prosthesis in cases of fracture. J Shoulder Elbow Surg 2001;10:136–139.

Kralinger F, Schwaiger R, Wambacher M, et al. Outcome after primary hemiarthroplasty for fracture of the head of the humerus. A retrospective multicentre study of 167 patients. J Bone Joint Surg Br 2004;86:217–219.

Krishnan SG, Bennion PW, Reineck JR, Burkhead WZ. Hemiarthroplasty for proximal humeral fracture: restoration of the Gothic arch. Orthop Clin North Am 2008;39:441–450.

Mansat P, Guity MR, Bellumore Y, Mansat M. Shoulder arthroplasty for late sequelae of proximal humeral fractures. J Shoulder Elbow Surg 2004;13:305–312.

Mighell MA, Kolm GP, Collinge CA, Frankle MA. Outcomes of hemiarthroplasty for fractures of the proximal humerus. J Shoulder Elbow Surg 2003;12:569–577.

Murachovsky J, Ikemoto RY, Nascimento LG, et al. Pectoralis major tendon reference (PMT): a new method for accurate restoration of humeral length with hemiarthroplasty for fracture. J Shoulder Elbow Surg 2006;15:675–678.

Neer CS 2nd. Displaced proximal humeral fractures. I. Classification and evaluation. J Bone Joint Surg Am 1970a;52:1077–1089.

Neer CS 2nd. Displaced proximal humeral fractures. II. Treatment of three-part and four-part displacement. J Bone Joint Surg Am 1970b;52:1090–1103.

Neer CS 2nd. Displaced proximal humeral fractures. Part I. Classification and evaluation. Clin Orthop Relat Res 1987;(223):3–10.

Neer CS, Brown TH Jr, McLaughlin HL. Fracture of the neck of the humerus with dislocation of the head fragment. Am J Surg 1953;85:252–258.

Norris TR, Green A, McGuigan FX. Late prosthetic shoulder arthroplasty for displaced proximal humerus fractures. J Shoulder Elbow Surg 1995;4:271–280.

Roberts SN, Foley AP, Swallow HM, et al. The geometry of the humeral head and the design of prostheses. J Bone Joint Surg Br 1991;73:647–650.

Robinson CM, Page RS. Severely impacted valgus proximal humeral fractures. J Bone Joint Surg Am 2004;86 Suppl 1 (Pt 2):143–155.

Robinson CM, Page RS, Hill RM, et al. Primary hemiarthroplasty for treatment of proximal humeral fractures. J Bone Joint Surg Am 2003;85:1215–1223.

Smith AM, Mardones RM, Sperling JW, Cofield RH. Early complications of operatively treated proximal humeral fractures. J Shoulder Elbow Surg 2007;16:14–24.

Smith ST, Cramer KE, Karges DE, et al. Early complications in the operative treatment of patella fractures. J Orthop Trauma 1997;11:183–187.

Chapter 11 Reverse shoulder arthroplasty for four-part fractures of the proximal humerus

Todd C. Moen, William N. Levine

INTRODUCTION

The appropriate treatment for complex three- and four-part fractures of the proximal humerus is controversial. Multiple surgical options exist, including open reduction and internal fixation (ORIF) with non-locking and locking plates and screws (Wijgman et al. 2002, Robinson and Page 2004), ORIF with fixed-angle devices (Ricchetti et al. 2010), suture fixation (Cornell et al. 1994), percutaneous pinning (Soete et al. 1999), intramedullary nails (Takeuchi et al. 2002), and prosthetic replacement with hemiarthroplasty. Of these techniques, ORIF with plate-and-screw constructs and hemiarthroplasty are the most often performed. However, there is current debate in the literature regarding the exact indications for ORIF versus hemiarthroplasty, as both procedures have characteristic complications (Lanting et al. 2008, Owsley and Gorczyca 2008, Solberg et al. 2009a, Solberg et al. 2009b, Guy et al. 2010). Successful ORIF is dependent upon a viable humeral head and fracture fragments, and adequate bone quality; if these conditions are not present, then humeral malunion, non-union, head avascular necrosis, and subsequent implant failure and migration are the likely results (Gorczyca et al. 2001, Solberg et al. 2009a, Südkamp et al. 2009, Ricchetti et al. 2010). On the other hand, hemiarthroplasty has proven to reliably relieve pain, but functional outcomes are less predictable; tuberosity comminution and/or osteopenia can lead to tuberosity non-union and, in turn, poor functional outcomes (Compito et al. 1994, Boileau et al. 2002, Mighell et al. 2003, Robinson et al. 2003, Kralinger et al. 2004, Antuna et al. 2008).

In response to the complications of ORIF and hemiarthroplasty, reverse shoulder arthroplasty has been proposed as an alternative treatment for complex fractures of the proximal humerus where the humeral head is at risk of avascular necrosis and the condition of the tuberosities is such that the osteosynthesis of these fragments would be challenging, if not impossible. The reverse shoulder prosthesis was designed for patients with a degenerative glenohumeral joint and an incompetent rotator cuff (Boileau et al. 2005). When used in the setting of a fracture of the proximal humerus, a reverse prosthesis is essentially addressing the complications of ORIF and hemiarthroplasty before they happen. This rationale is a relatively novel approach, and there is a paucity of data regarding the mid- to long-term outcomes of this procedure. However, early reports have described promising results, as well as directions for future research (Bufquin et al. 2007, Klein et al. 2008, Cazeneuve and Cristofari 2009, Gallinet et al. 2009, Cazeneuve and Cristofari 2010). This chapter describes the indications, contraindications, and surgical technique, and reviews the literature on reverse shoulder arthroplasty for complex fractures of the proximal humerus.

INDICATIONS

Reverse shoulder arthroplasty for fractures of the proximal humerus is indicated when the head is deemed unviable or unreconstructable, and the tuberosities are comminuted or osteopenic to a degree that would make successful tuberosity osteosynthesis difficult, if not impossible. What precisely constitutes an unviable or unreconstructable proximal humerus is controversial; however, broadly speaking, four-part fractures, comminuted osteoporotic three-part fractures, fracture dislocations of the humeral head, head-splitting fractures, and fractures involving impaction of over 40% of the humeral articular surface are considered best suited for proximal shoulder arthroplasty (Mighell et al. 2003, Robinson et al. 2003, Kralinger et al. 2004, Robinson and Page 2004, Antuna et al. 2008). The specific degree of osteopenia that puts the tuberosities at risk of malunion and/or non-union is also the subject of debate, but age can be used as an acceptable guideline. In general, reverse shoulder arthroplasty should be reserved for patients aged 70 and above. Although some authors are expanding the indications for reverse shoulder arthroplasty in terms of both patient age and condition (Mulieri et al. 2010), the procedure is best reserved as a salvage operation for older patients, given its technical complexity, potential for complications, and lack of a good alternative if the reverse arthroplasty itself fails (Boileau et al. 2006, Matsen et al. 2007, Rockwood 2007).

Although there are few long-term studies of reverse arthroplasty for fracture, there are certain principles regarding this procedure that have emerged in the literature, and it is important for the surgeon to be aware of these when electing to perform the operation. First of all, it is important to place reverse arthroplasty for fracture in context with the other common indications: cuff tear arthropathy, revision of a failed shoulder arthroplasty, or revision for failed fracture surgery. Broadly speaking, patients who have a reverse arthroplasty for any of these three indications can reliably expect to have pain relief. The functional performance will be superior for patients who have a reverse arthroplasty for cuff tear arthropathy, followed by those who have a reverse arthroplasty for a complex fracture of the proximal humerus, followed by those who have a revision reverse arthroplasty for a failed shoulder arthroplasty (Boileau et al. 2006, Wall et al. 2007, Klein et al. 2008, Cazeneuve and Cristofari 2009, Gallinet et al. 2009, Cazeneuve and Cristofari 2010). A comparison between reverse shoulder arthroplasty and hemiarthroplasty is also noteworthy. In general, the outcomes for patients who have a hemiarthroplasty for fracture have a bimodal distribution of excellent and poor functional scores (Mighell et al. 2003, Robinson et al. 2003, Kralinger et al. 2004, Antuna et al. 2008), while patients who have a reverse arthroplasty for fracture have more consistently average functional scores (Bufquin et al. 2007, Klein et al. 2008, Cazeneuve and Cristofari 2009, Cazeneuve and Cristofari 2010).

The final principle that must be kept in mind when indicating a patient for a reverse arthroplasty for fracture is caution. Although preliminary reports have been promising, longer-term studies are disclosing complications such as loosening of the glenoid component, and significant deterioration of functional scores (Cazeneuve and Cristofari 2009, Cazeneuve and Cristofari 2010). The scope of these initial reports remains unclear. Nevertheless, based on the available information, it is best to view reverse shoulder arthroplasty as a salvage-type procedure reserved for elderly patients.

CONTRAINDICATIONS

The contraindications include a fracture pattern with a viable and reconstructable humeral head, and tuberosities that can be reliably expected to progress to osteosynthesis with appropriate fixation, as these are better treated with ORIF or hemiarthroplasty.

TECHNIQUE

Reverse shoulder arthroplasty is a demanding procedure, and often complications can be linked to surgical technique. Normal anatomic landmarks may be obscured or obliterated by the fracture, making implantation of the prosthetic components in the appropriate alignment challenging. Nevertheless, vigilance and meticulous attention to detail can reliably allow for an adequate reconstruction, minimize complications, and ultimately improve results for patients.

The patient is placed in a modified beach-chair position with the back of the operating table elevated to approximately 45°. A towel is placed under the medial border of the scapula, and a table with a cut-away section about the shoulder is used to allow global access to the shoulder. The entire arm is prepped and draped, beginning at the base of the neck and under the axilla, thus permitting the arm to be moved freely throughout surgery.

A deltopectoral incision is used. At most centers in Europe (Bufquin et al. 2007, Cazeneuve and Cristofari 2009, Gallinet et al. 2009, Cazeneuve and Cristofari 2010, Sirveaux et al. 2010), and some in the United States (Klein et al. 2008), a superolateral approach is used, because it reportedly enhances stability (Sirveaux et al. 2010). We prefer a deltopectoral approach, as it is extensile, familiar, and allows adequate exposure of all the relevant anatomy. More importantly, a deltopectoral approach is potentially less harmful than a superolateral approach to the deltoid; we feel this is vitally important for an operation so critically dependent on the deltoid for function.

The incision begins just inferior and lateral to the coracoid, and extends laterally toward the deltoid insertion on the humeral shaft (**Fig. 11.1**). The cephalic vein is identified in the deltopectoral interval, and the vein is retracted medially or laterally as the interval is opened. With the deltoid retracted laterally and the pectoralis major retracted medially, the clavicopectoral fascia is exposed. The coracoid process and conjoined tendon (confluence of the coracobrachialis and short head of the biceps) are identified. The clavicopectoral fascia is incised at the lateral border of the conjoined tendon. Typically, this dissection will reveal the fracture hematoma and fracture fragments (**Fig. 11.2**). A self-retaining retractor is then placed with one limb under the deltoid, and one limb under the lateral border of the conjoined tendon (**Fig. 11.3**). Care is taken to avoid over-retraction, as this could result in a tension neurapraxia of the musculocutaneous nerve.

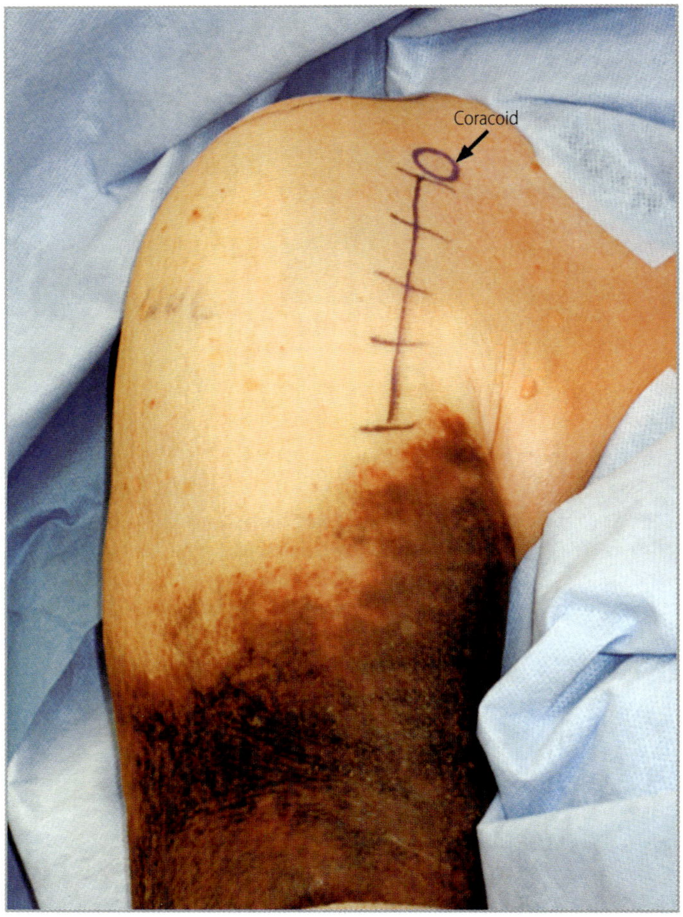

Figure 11.1 The planned deltopectoral interval, beginning adjacent to the coracoid process and extending just lateral to the anterior axillary crease. Note the ecchymosis from the acute injury: this 76-year-old woman tripped and fell, suffering a four-part fracture of the proximal humerus. (Courtesy of the Center for Shoulder, Elbow and Sports Medicine.)

The long head of the biceps brachii (LHB) is identified, and it serves as a landmark to guide further dissection and recognition of individual fracture fragments. Tracing the LHB proximally leads to the glenoid, and allows further identification of the tuberosities and fracture fragments. The lesser tuberosity lies medial to the LHB, while the greater tuberosity will be lateral. The articular surface – in varying degrees of comminution – lies between the tuberosities.

With the fragments identified, the hemorrhagic bursa and the clavipectoral fascia are resected. Each tuberosity is then tagged with two heavy non-absorbable sutures. Each suture should be placed in the rotator cuff tendon–tuberosity junction, to avoid further damage to the already comminuted tuberosities. Each tuberosity is sufficiently mobilized circumferentially. Tuberosity mobilization should be performed cautiously, particularly if surgery has been delayed beyond 7–10 days after the injury, as scarring and adhesions can make dissection difficult, and increase the risk of iatrogenic neurovascular injury. The biceps is then tenotomized near its origin on the supraglenoid tuberosity, and tagged for later tenodesis (**Fig. 11.4**). A biceps tenotomy greatly enhances exposure, with minimal morbidity given the later tenodesis.

Attention is now turned to removing the humeral head (**Fig. 11.5**). It should be removed carefully, without excessive force. The potential

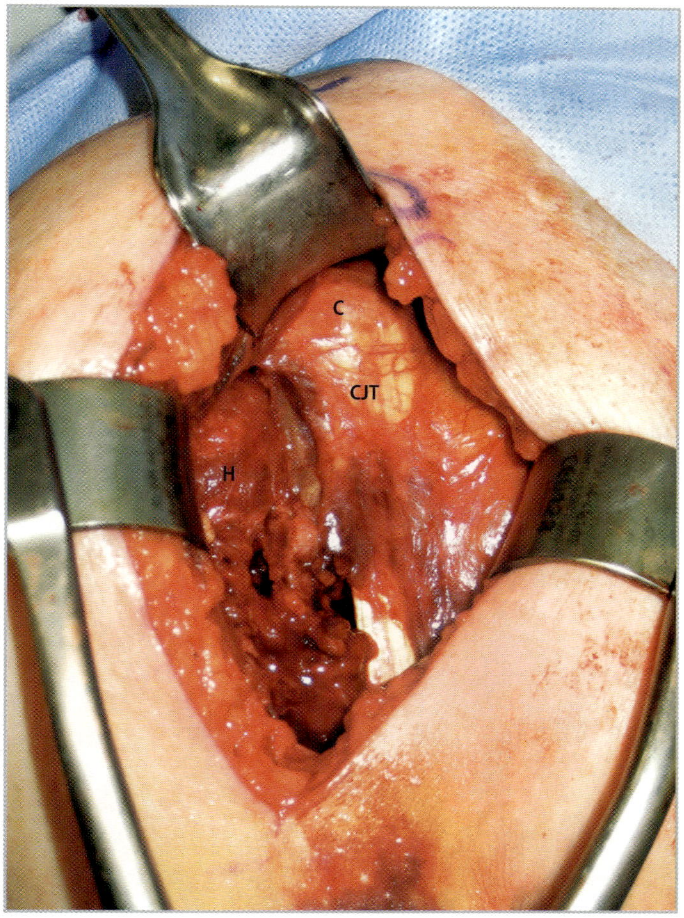

Figure 11.2 The clavipectoral fascia has been incised, exposing the underlying hematoma (H). The coracoid (C) is identified and the conjoined tendon (CJT) of the coracobrachialis and short head biceps is readily identified. (Courtesy of the Center for Shoulder, Elbow and Sports Medicine.)

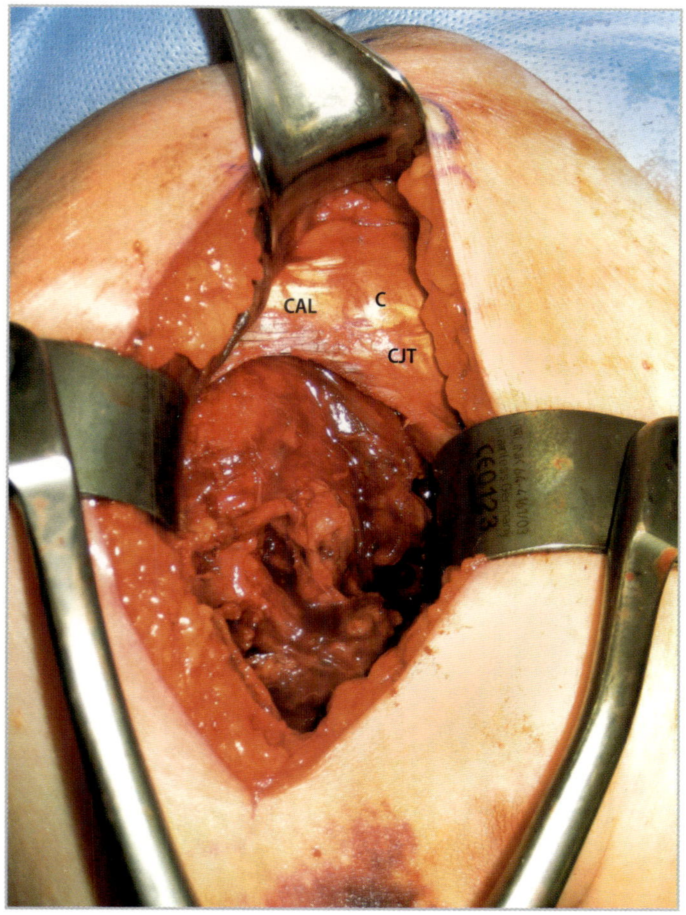

Figure 11.3 A self-retaining retractor is placed with the lateral blade beneath the deltoid and the medial blade beneath the conjoined tendon. CJT = conjoined tendon, C = coracoid, CAL = coracoacromial ligament. (Courtesy of the Center for Shoulder, Elbow and Sports Medicine.)

for iatrogenic neurovascular injury is greatest when surgery has been delayed beyond 7–10 days from the initial injury, and when the humeral head is dislocated anteriorly below the coracoid and medial to the strap muscles. In either of these situations, it is appropriate to schedule the surgery in a location and at a time when a vascular surgeon is readily available, in the event of an intraoperative emergency.

The humeral head is then removed and attention is turned to preparation of the glenoid. This is a departure from the technique used in a primary reverse arthroplasty for cuff tear arthropathy, in which the humerus is provisionally prepared in advance of the glenoid. Preparing the glenoid first allows the humerus to be prepared, and the prosthesis to be implanted, in the correct alignment, with adjustments for optimum stability (Van Seymortier et al. 2006). In comparison with most primary shoulder arthroplasty operations, achieving adequate exposure of the glenoid in the case of a reverse arthroplasty for fracture is considerably less challenging, as the mobilization and removal of some of the fracture fragments allow for excellent visualization (**Fig. 11.6**).

The glenoid is prepared as it is for a primary reverse arthroplasty. Any articular cartilage is removed. The ideal location for the glenoid component is identified (slightly inferior to the glenoid center), and a guide pin oriented with a 10° inferior tilt with respect to the glenoid face is placed (**Fig. 11.7**) (Frankle et al. 2006, Gutierrez et al. 2007). When the orientation of the guide pin is judged to be satisfactory, the glenoid is reamed over the guide pin. What bone is removed should be from the inferior glenoid, in order to preserve the 10° inferior tilt. A properly prepared glenoid will leave a 'subchondral smile' of a small amount of exposed subchondral bleeding bone on the inferior margin of the glenoid (**Fig. 11.8**). The final glenoid component is then implanted. We prefer a base-plate (Zimmer, Warsaw, Indiana) that uses two holes for locking screws oriented along the diameter of the base-plate. The base-plate is implanted such that the diameter through these two screw holes points just anterior to the mid-axillary line, toward the base of the coracoid process (**Fig. 11.9**). With the glenoid base-plate implanted, it is then secured with two locking screws. The screws are inserted in a standard fashion by drilling and perforating the far cortex of the scapula, measuring the length, and then inserting the screw (**Fig. 11.10**). The screws are converted from standard screws to locking screws with the use of locking caps over the screw holes. The glenosphere is then inserted onto the base-plate (**Fig. 11.11**). A vacuum effect will be felt when the glenosphere slides over the base-plate.

Attention is then turned to humeral preparation. In preparing the humerus, two principles are critical to achieve a successful outcome. First, the humerus must be aligned at the appropriate height and the correct version to optimize prosthetic stability. Secondly, the tuberosities should be repaired. Some authors argue that the tuberosities should be excised, as they limit adduction, and generate instability (Cazeneuve and Cristofari 2009, Cazeneuve and Cristofari 2010), and

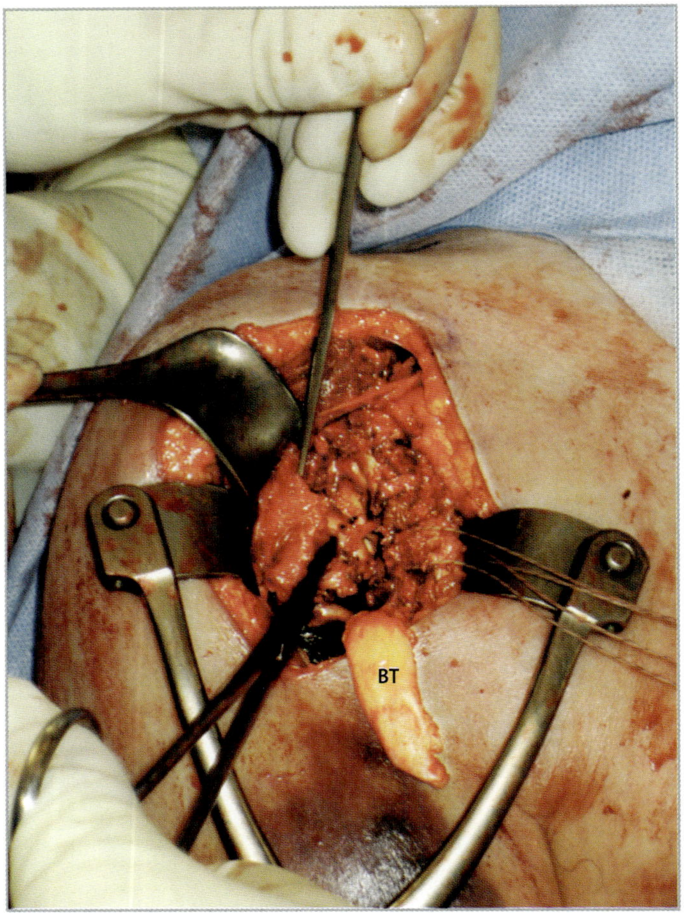

Figure 11.4 The biceps tendon (BT) has been tenotomized at the supraglenoid tuberosity and will be tenodesed at the conclusion of the case. This step in the procedure is critical to improve visualization, and to easily identify the lesser tuberosity (medial) and the greater tuberosity (lateral). (Courtesy of the Center for Shoulder, Elbow and Sports Medicine.)

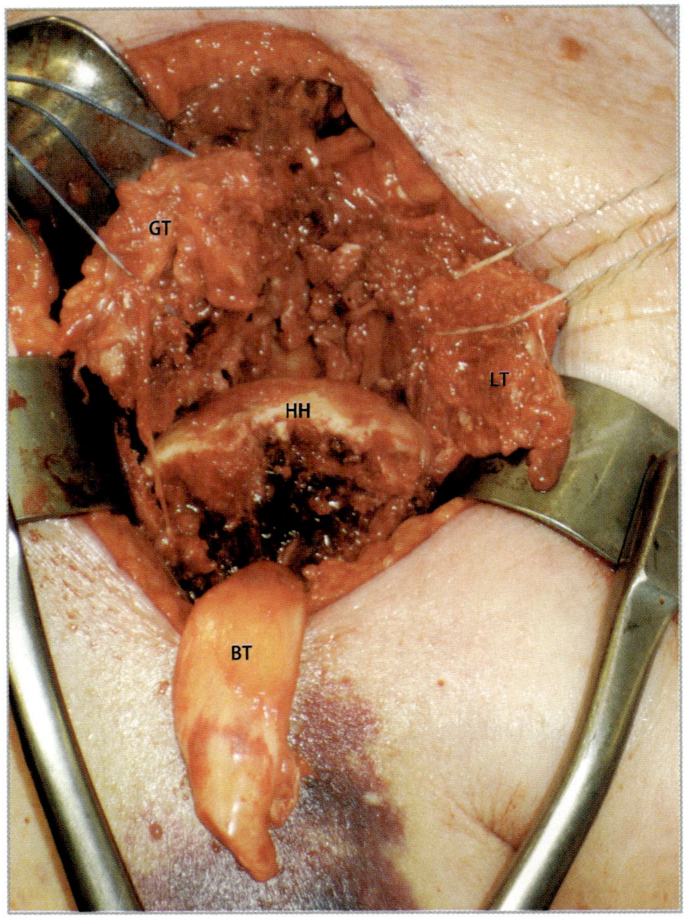

Figure 11.5 The humeral head (HH) is identified between the tuberosities. Note that different color sutures are placed in the greater tuberosity (GT) and lesser tuberosity (LT) to aid in suture management. BT = biceps tendon. (Courtesy of the Center for Shoulder, Elbow and Sports Medicine.)

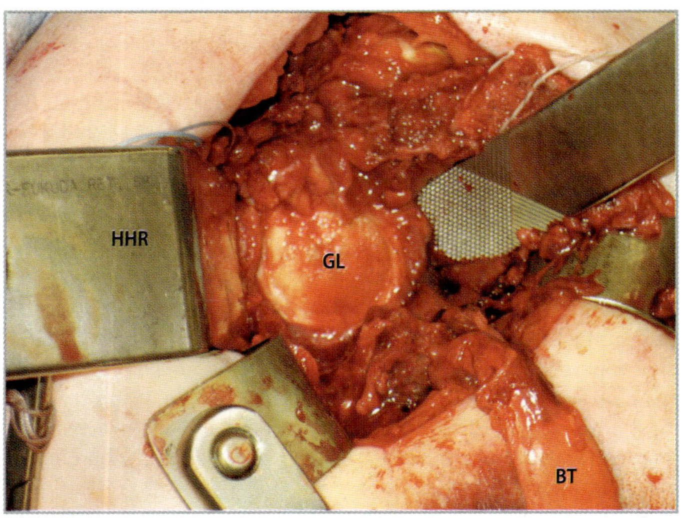

Figure 11.6 A humeral head retractor is placed laterally, allowing excellent exposure to the glenoid for base-plate and glenosphere implantation. BT = biceps tendon, HHR = humeral head retractor, GL = glenoid. (Courtesy of the Center for Shoulder, Elbow and Sports Medicine.)

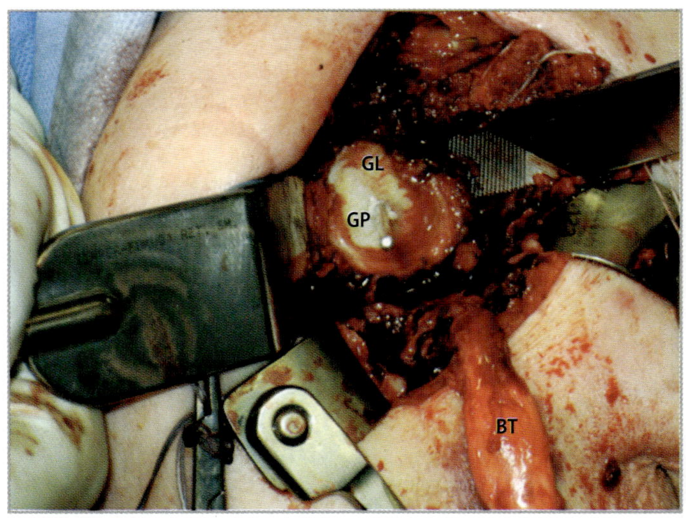

Figure 11.7 A guide pin has been placed (slightly posterior and inferior to the glenoid center) and is angled 10° inferiorly to prevent against future scapular notching. GL = glenoid, BT = biceps tendon, GP = guide pin. (Courtesy of the Center for Shoulder, Elbow and Sports Medicine.)

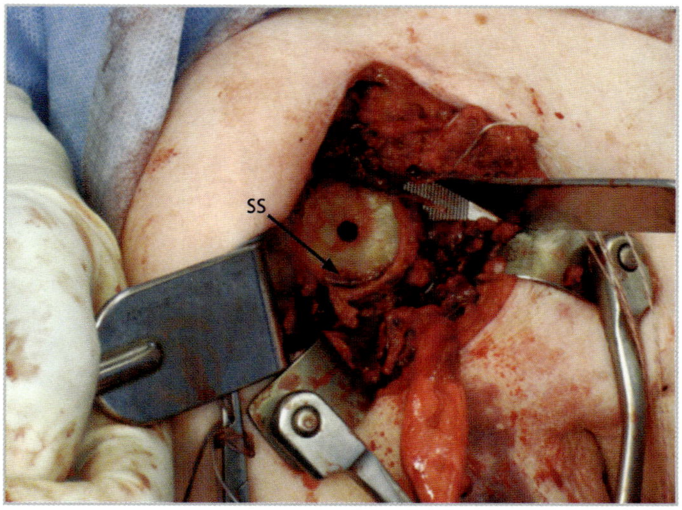

Figure 11.8 The glenoid has been prepared by reaming over the previously placed guide pin. Note the center hole for the base-plate and the 'subchondral smile' (SS), indicating appropriate preparation. (Courtesy of the Center for Shoulder, Elbow and Sports Medicine.)

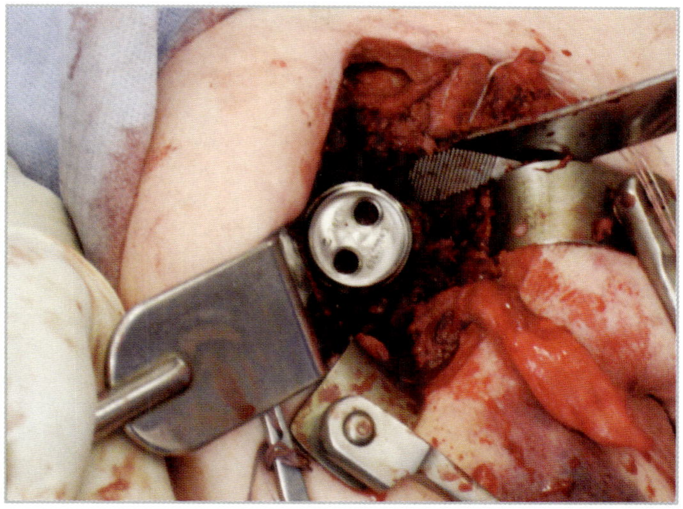

Figure 11.9 The base-plate has been implanted after glenoid preparation. The porous ingrowth metal design of this prosthesis affords excellent early stability. (Courtesy of the Center for Shoulder, Elbow and Sports Medicine.)

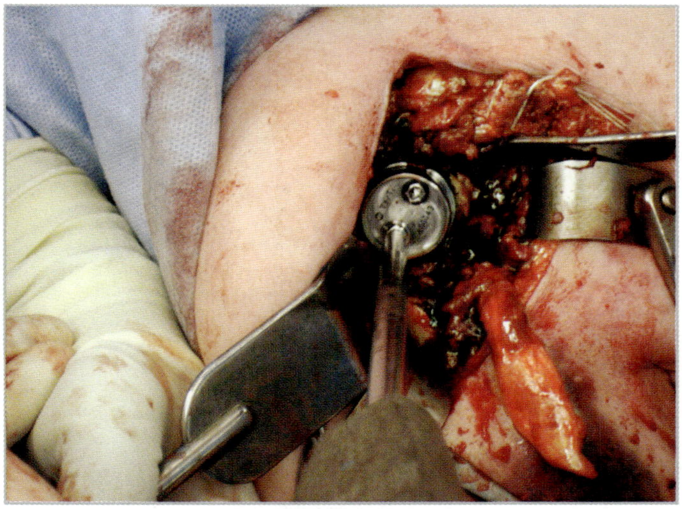

Figure 11.10 The variable-angle screws are placed in the best bone available. They are angled 15° off the perpendicular in all planes. A locking cap is placed over the screw, securing it in position. (Courtesy of the Center for Shoulder, Elbow and Sports Medicine.)

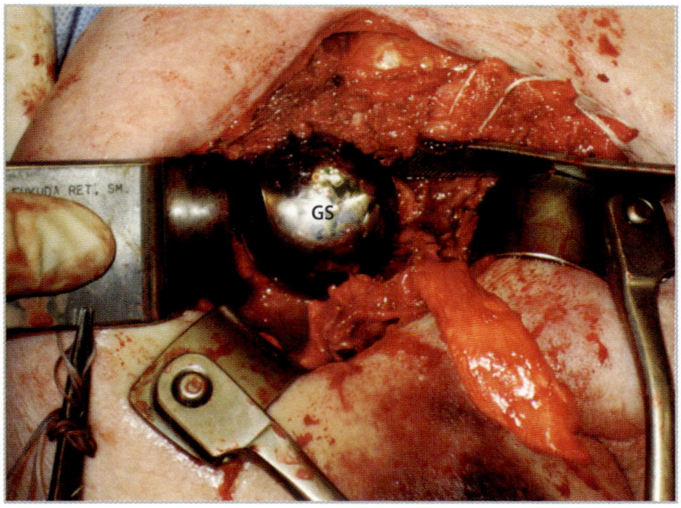

Figure 11.11 The glenosphere has been placed onto the base-plate. There is no central locking set screw in this design. A vacuum sensation is experienced when the glenosphere (GS) is placed on the base-plate. If this vacuum phenomenon is not experienced, it is possible to asymmetrically impact the glenosphere onto the base-plate. An axillary radiograph will demonstrate appropriate positioning of the glenosphere on the base-plate. (Courtesy of the Center for Shoulder, Elbow and Sports Medicine.)

that repair or resection of the tuberosities has no bearing on outcome (Klein et al. 2008). However, the impact of tuberosities on stability remains unclear, and tuberosity repair in reverse arthroplasty for fracture has been shown to improve external rotation (Bufquin et al. 2007). Therefore, we recommend that the tuberosities are repaired whenever possible.

The humerus is then delivered into the wound by extension and adduction. To facilitate later tuberosity repair, two drill holes are made in the lateral humeral shaft, and two heavy non-absorbable sutures are passed through these drill holes (**Fig. 11.12**). The humeral shaft is then sequentially reamed (**Fig. 11.13**) until light cortical chatter is achieved, or to the predetermined size based on preoperative templating. A trial implant based on the reaming of the canal is then placed. It is critical to establish the proper version and height when placing the trial implant. While no consensus exists regarding appropriate version, we typically place the humeral component in 10° of retroversion. Version is determined utilizing alignment rods on the implant inserter that reference off the forearm (**Fig. 11.14**). The appropriate height of the prosthesis is referenced off the medial calcar of the humerus. The prosthesis should be placed such that it rests on the medial calcar. If the calcar is fractured or otherwise unrecognizable, then the remaining fracture fragments should be used to reapproximate the calcar, and the prosthetic height should be referenced accordingly. Corresponding marks are made on the humeral shaft and prosthesis to record the appropriate height.

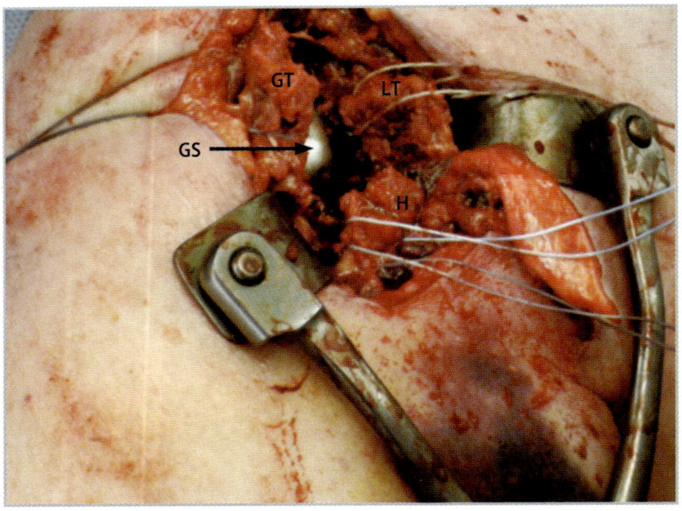

Figure 11.12 Two drill holes have been placed in the humeral shaft, and heavy non-absorbable sutures are placed for tuberosity to shaft fixation. GS = glenosphere, GT = greater tuberosity, LT = lesser tuberosity, H = humeral shaft. (Courtesy of the Center for Shoulder, Elbow and Sports Medicine.)

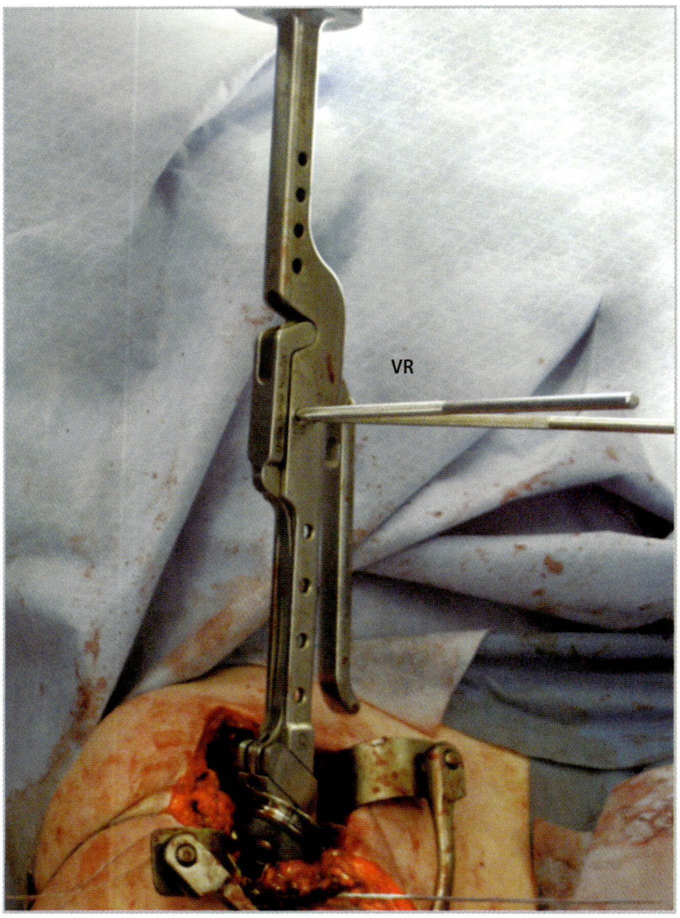

Figure 11.14 The final humeral component version is determined by using the version rods on this system. The version rods (VR) are aligned at 0° and 20° of retroversion, respectively. The forearm and transepicondylar axis are used to align the humeral retroversion at 10° ('splitting the goal posts' of the 0° and 20° positions). (Courtesy of the Center for Shoulder, Elbow and Sports Medicine.)

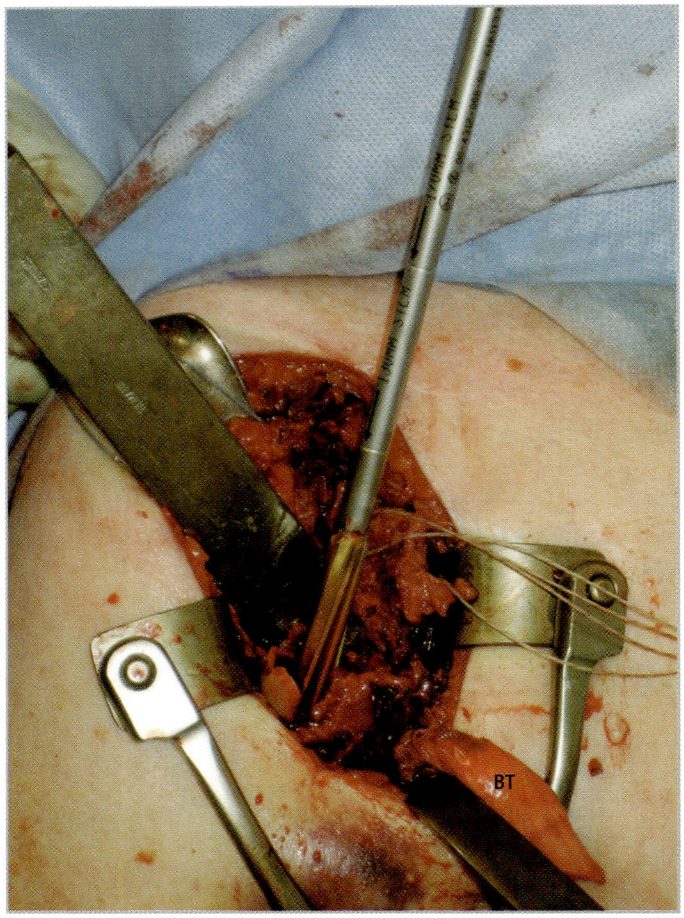

Figure 11.13 A humeral reamer is placed into the canal. As the humeral prosthesis will be cemented in all fracture cases, line-to-line fit is not necessary, and in fact in most situations contraindicated, given the osteoporotic bone. BT = biceps tendon. (Courtesy of the Center for Shoulder, Elbow and Sports Medicine.)

Next, the prosthesis is trialed. If the humeral stem is loose in the intramedullary canal, a sponge can be wrapped around the implant to maintain the trial stem's position. A trial polyethylene liner is placed on the stem. The tuberosities around the stem are gently reduced. Then the humeral component on the glenosphere is gently reduced via adduction and internal rotation. Prosthetic stability is tested through a range of motion of flexion, extension, and internal and external rotation. The size of the humeral polyethylene, as well as the overall height of the humeral stem, can be adjusted until sufficient stability is achieved.

In most cases, the humeral component will be cemented, given the typical osteopenia and capacious intramedullary canal. The trial component is removed, and the humeral intramedullary canal is irrigated. A cement restrictor is placed to the appropriate height, based on the size of the humeral implant. The cement is mixed, and the canal is filled with cement when the cement has reached the desired consistency. The humeral stem is then placed in the canal, during which process the surgeon should keep in mind the correct version of the implant, as well as the height marked on the humeral shaft and stem (**Fig. 11.15**). As the stem is being placed, two heavy non-absorbable sutures are placed around the stem of the implant for later cerclage

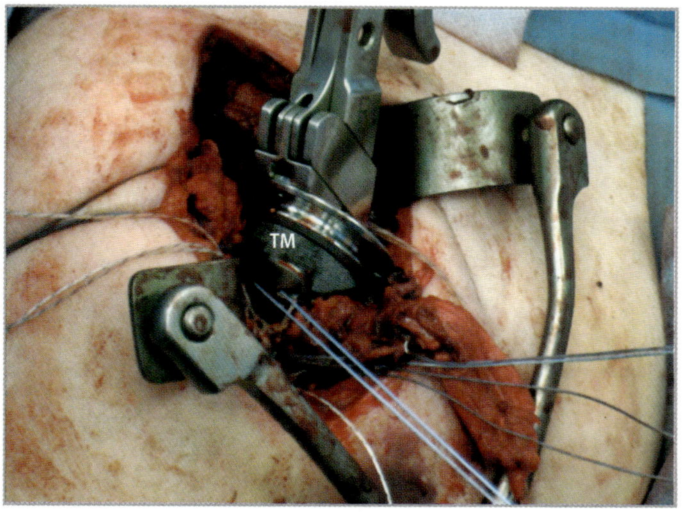

Figure 11.15 The final humeral prosthesis has been placed after intramedullary preparation and methylmethacrylate insertion. Care is taken to remove all proximal cement to allow tuberosity healing. The prosthesis demonstrated has tantalum (TM) proximally to enhance bone healing of the tuberosities to the prosthesis itself, as well to the surrounding bone. Note also the sutures in the prosthesis, which allow 'around the world' placement around the prosthesis and through both tuberosities to enhance tuberosity stability and ultimately healing. (Courtesy of the Center for Shoulder, Elbow and Sports Medicine.)

fixation of the tuberosities. After the cement has sufficiently cured and hardened, implant stability is retested with trial polyethylene liners. When the most stable size of polyethylene liner, with or without metal augments, has been determined, the final liner is securely implanted on the humeral stem (**Fig. 11.16**). The humeral component is then reduced on the glenoid.

Finally, the tuberosities are repaired. Tuberosity repair for a reverse arthroplasty for fracture follows analogous steps for tuberosity repair for a hemiarthroplasty as described by Boileau and Frankle (Boileau et al. 2002, Frankle et al. 2001, Frankle et al. 2002, Frankle and Mighell 2004). The tuberosities are repaired with sutures, allowing for horizontal, vertical, and cerclage fixation. Two additional heavy non-absorbable sutures are placed at the tendon-bone interface of the fragment of the greater tuberosity.

Two of the four sutures from the greater tuberosity are passed around the neck of the humeral stem; these are suture group 1. Next, the two cerclage sutures around the humeral stem are each passed through the tendon-bone interface of the greater and lesser tuberosities, respectively; these are suture group 2. Then one limb of one suture of those passed through the humeral diaphysis is passed through the greater tuberosity, at the superior aspect of the tendon. Then one limb of the other suture passed through the humeral diaphysis is passed through the fragment of the lesser tuberosity, at the superior aspect of the tendon. These are suture group 3. Finally, the remaining two sutures in the fragment of the greater tuberosity are passed through the tendon-bone interface of the fragment of the lesser tuberosity; these are suture group 4. The tuberosities are gently reduced, and the sutures are then sequentially tightened and tied. The first suture group tied is group 1, the second is group 4, the third is group 2, and the last group to be tied is group 3.

The wound is then thoroughly irrigated with a pulse lavage. A medium hemovac is placed, exiting just lateral to the acromion. The deltopectoral interval is reapproximated with non-absorbable sutures to help identify the interval in the event of a revision operation.

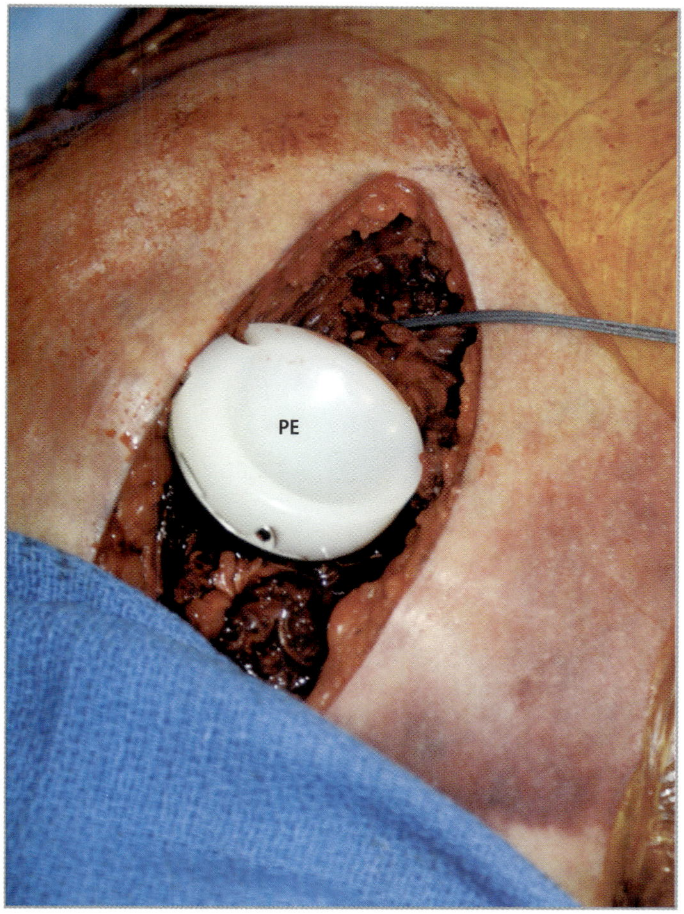

Figure 11.16 The polyethylene liner is tapped into final position. Stability is rechecked through a full range of motion, especially in extension and external rotation (a vulnerable position for dislocation). (Courtesy of the Center for Shoulder, Elbow and Sports Medicine.)

The subcutaneous tissues are closed with interrupted absorbable 3-0 sutures, and the skin is closed with a running 4-0 absorbable suture. A sterile dressing is applied.

Pearls and pitfalls

The current indications for reverse shoulder arthroplasty for fractures of the proximal humerus are a fracture pattern in which the head is deemed unviable or unreconstructable, and the tuberosities are comminuted or osteopenic to a degree that would make successful tuberosity osteosynthesis difficult, if not impossible

Reverse shoulder arthroplasty for fracture is best viewed as a salvage operation, reserved for older patients, given its technical complexity, the associated complications, and lack of a salvage operation if the procedure fails.

A patient who has a reverse arthroplasty for a fracture of the proximal humerus will do better than one undergoing revision surgery, but not as well as one has it for a degenerative cuff-deficient shoulder.

Patients who have a hemiarthroplasty for a complex fracture of the proximal humerus have the possibility of a spectacular success or a spectacular failure, while patients who have a reverse shoulder arthoplasty for such a fracture will likely have a more middling result.

A deltopectoral approach is the preferred approach, as it is extensile, familiar, and allows adequate exposure of all the relevant anatomy.

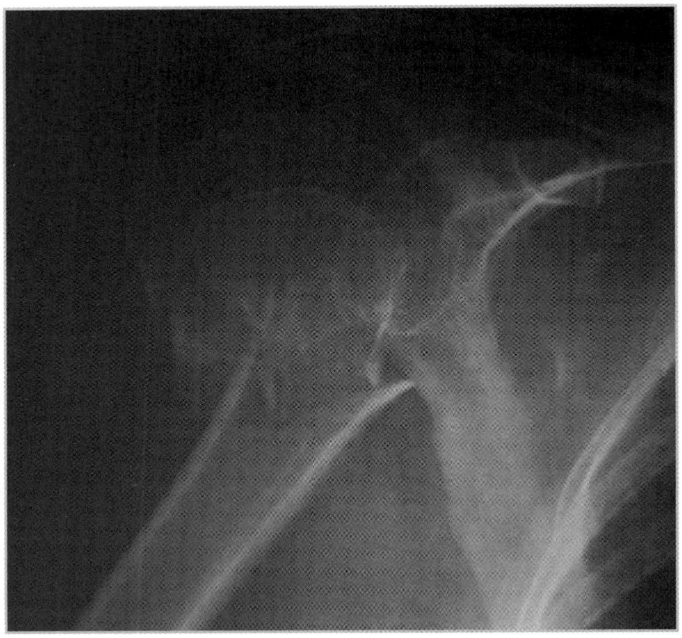

Figure 11.17 Preoperative anteroposterior radiograph demonstrating a four-part comminuted fracture of the proximal humerus. (Courtesy of the Center for Shoulder, Elbow and Sports Medicine.)

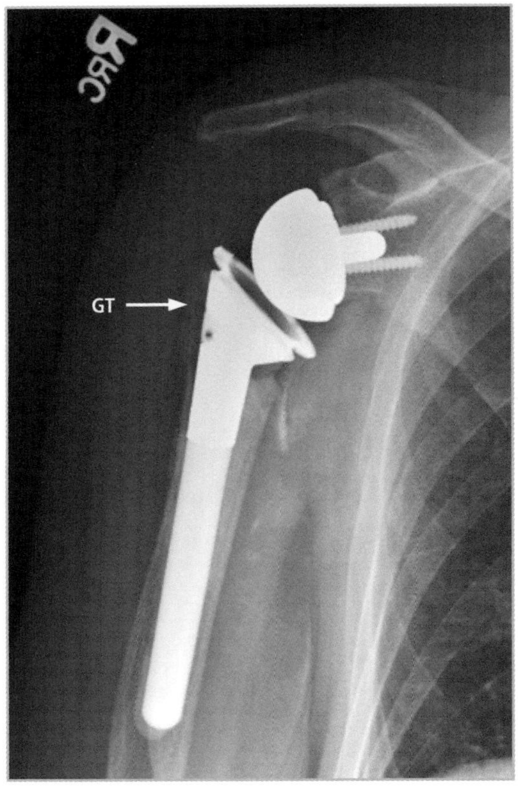

Figure 11.18 Three-month postoperative anteroposterior radiograph demonstrating healing of the greater tuberosity (GT). (Courtesy ofthe Center for Shoulder, Elbow and Sports Medicine.)

More importantly, it is potentially less harmful than a superolateral approach to the deltoid; we feel this is vitally important for an operation so critically dependent on the deltoid for function.

The LHB is a useful surgical landmark during the surgical exposure, as it guides further dissection and recognition of individual fracture fragments. Following the LHB proximally leads to the glenoid and the center of the shoulder, and serves to orient the fracture fragments. Typically, the lesser tuberosity lies medial to the LHB, the greater tuberosity lateral, with the head - in varying degrees of comminution - lying between the tuberosities.

Tuberosity mobilization and removal of the humeral head should be performed cautiously, particularly if surgery has been delayed beyond 7–10 days after the injury, as scarring and adhesions can make dissection difficult, and increase the risk for iatrogenic neurovascular injury. If surgery has been delayed, it is prudent to perform the procedure at a time and in a location where a vascular surgeon is readily available should there be an intraoperative emergency.

Prosthesis height should be referenced off the medial calcar of the humerus. If the calcar has been fractured or is otherwise unrecognizable, the calcar should be reapproximated with the use of fracture fragments.

The tuberosities should be repaired. Tuberosity repair can help to improve postoperative external rotation. The tuberosities should be repaired with a combination of horizontal, cerclage, and vertical sutures.

The use of a postoperative drain is critical. Given the large dead space and potential for postoperative hematoma formation, the drain should be kept in place for longer than would be done for a standard total shoulder arthroplasty.

REHABILITATION

Given the increased risk of postoperative hematoma formation due to the excessive dead space (Matsen et al. 2007, Wierks et al. 2009), the drain is left in place for longer than would be customary following traditional total shoulder replacement. The patient is given an abduction sling, and instructed to wear it at all times for the first six weeks following surgery. No shoulder motion is permitted. However, the patient is instructed to perform elbow, wrist, and finger range-of-motion exercises multiple times per day. At six weeks, formal physiotherapy is begun. The rehabilitation program consists of deltoid strengthening, scapular stabilization and strengthening, and modification of activities of daily living to avoid positions that place the shoulder at risk of dislocation.

REFERENCES

Antuna SA, Sperling JW, Cofield RH. Shoulder hemiarthroplasty for acute fractures of the proximal humerus: a minimum five-year follow-up. J Shoulder Elbow Surg 2008;17:202–209.

Boileau P, Krishnan SG, Tinsi L, et al. Tuberosity malposition and migration: reasons for poor outcomes after hemiarthroplasty for displaced fractures of the proximal humerus. J Shoulder Elbow Surg 2002;11:401–412.

Boileau P, Watkinson DJ, Hatzidakis AM, Balg F. Grammont reverse prosthesis: design, rationale, and biomechanics. J Shoulder Elbow Surg 2005;14 (1 Suppl S):147S–161S.

Boileau, P, Watkinson D, Hatzidakis AM, et al. The Grammont reverse shoulder prosthesis: results in cuff tear arthritis, fracture sequelae, and revision arthroplasty. J Shoulder Elbow Surg 2006;15:527–540.

Bufquin T, Hersan A, Hubert L, Massin P. Reverse shoulder arthroplasty for the treatment of three- and four-part fractures of the proximal humerus in the elderly: a prospective review of 43 cases with a short-term follow-up. J Bone Joint Surg Br 2007;89:516–520.

Cazeneuve JF, Cristofari DJ. Delta III reverse shoulder arthroplasty: radiological outcome for acute complex fractures of the proximal humerus in elderly patients. Orthop Traumatol Surg Res 2009;95:325–329.

Cazeneuve JF, Cristofari DJ. The reverse shoulder prosthesis in the treatment of fractures of the proximal humerus in the elderly. J Bone Joint Surg Br 2010;92:535–539.

Compito CA, Self EB, Bigliani LU. Arthroplasty and acute shoulder trauma. Reasons for success and failure. Clin Orthop Relat Res 1994;(307):27–36.

Cornell CN, Levine D, Pagnani MJ. Internal fixation of proximal humerus fractures using the screw-tension band technique. J Orthop Trauma 1994;8:23–27.

Frankle MA, Greenwald DP, Markee BA, et al. Biomechanical effects of malposition of tuberosity fragments on the humeral prosthetic reconstruction for four-part proximal humerus fractures. J Shoulder Elbow Surg 2001;10:321–326.

Frankle MA, Ondrovic LE, Markee BA, et al. Stability of tuberosity reattachment in proximal humeral hemiarthroplasty. J Shoulder Elbow Surg 2002;11:413–420.

Frankle MA, Mighell MA. Techniques and principles of tuberosity fixation for proximal humeral fractures treated with hemiarthroplasty. J Shoulder Elbow Surg 2004;13:239–247.

Frankle M, Levy JC, Pupello D, et al. The reverse shoulder prosthesis for glenohumeral arthritis associated with severe rotator cuff deficiency: a minimum two-year follow-up study of sixty patients surgical technique. J Bone Joint Surg Am 2006;88 Suppl 1 Pt 2:178–190.

Gallinet D, Clappaz P, Garbuio P, et al. Three or four parts complex proximal humerus fractures: hemiarthroplasty versus reverse prosthesis: a comparative study of 40 cases. Orthop Traumatol Surg Res 2009;95:48–55.

Gorczyca JT, Davis RT, Hartford JM, Brindle TJ. Open reduction internal fixation after displacement of a previously nondisplaced acromial fracture in a multiply injured patient: case report and review of literature. J Orthop Trauma 2001;15:369–373.

Gutierrez S, Greiwe RM, Frankle MA, et al. Biomechanical comparison of component position and hardware failure in the reverse shoulder prosthesis. J Shoulder Elbow Surg 2007;16 (3 Suppl):S9–S12,.

Guy P, Slobogean GP, McCormack RG. Treatment preferences for displaced three- and four-part proximal humerus fractures. J Orthop Trauma 2010;24:250–254.

Klein M, Juschka M, Hinkenjann B, et al. Treatment of comminuted fractures of the proximal humerus in elderly patients with the delta III reverse shoulder prosthesis. J Orthop Trauma 2008;22:698–704.

Kralinger F, Schwaiger R, Wambacher M, et al. Outcome after primary hemiarthroplasty for fracture of the head of the humerus. A retrospective multicentre study of 167 patients. J Bone Joint Surg Br 2004;86:217–219.

Lanting B, MacDermid J, Drosdowech D, Faber KJ. Proximal humeral fractures: a systematic review of treatment modalities. J Shoulder Elbow Surg 2008;17:42–54.

Matsen FA 3rd, Boileau P, Walch G, et al. The reverse total shoulder arthroplasty. J Bone Joint Surg Am 2007;89:660–667.

Mighell MA, Kolm GP, Collinge CA, Frankle MA. Outcomes of hemiarthroplasty for fractures of the proximal humerus. J Shoulder Elbow Surg 2003;12:569–577.

Mulieri P, Dunning P, Klein S, et al. Reverse shoulder arthroplasty for the treatment of irreparable rotator cuff tear without glenohumeral arthritis. J Bone Joint Surg Am 2010;92:2544–2556.

Owsley KC, Gorczyca JT. Fracture displacement and screw cutout after open reduction and locked plate fixation of proximal humeral fractures [corrected]. J Bone Joint Surg Am 2008;90:233–240.

Ricchetti ET, Warrender WJ, Abboud JA. Use of locking plates in the treatment of proximal humerus fractures. J Shoulder Elbow Surg 2010;19 (2 Suppl):66–75.

Robinson CM, Page RS. Severely impacted valgus proximal humeral fractures. J Bone Joint Surg Am 2004;86 Suppl 1 (Pt 2):143–155.

Robinson CM, Page RS, Hill RM, et al. Primary hemiarthroplasty for treatment of proximal humeral fractures. J Bone Joint Surg Am 2003;85:1215–1223.

Rockwood CA Jr. The reverse total shoulder prosthesis. The new kid on the block. J Bone Joint Surg Am 2007;89:233–235.

Sirveaux F, Roche O, Mole D. Shoulder arthroplasty for acute proximal humerus fracture. Orthop Traumatol Surg Res 2010;96:683–694.

Soete PJ, Clayson PE, Costenoble VH. Transitory percutaneous pinning in fractures of the proximal humerus. J Shoulder Elbow Surg 1999;8:569–573.

Solberg BD, Moon CN, Franco DP, Paiement GD. Locked plating of 3- and 4-part proximal humerus fractures in older patients: the effect of initial fracture pattern on outcome. J Orthop Trauma 2009a;23:113–119.

Solberg BD, Moon CN, Franco DP, Paiement GD. Surgical treatment of three and four-part proximal humeral fractures. J Bone Joint Surg Am 2009b;91:1689–1697.

Südkamp N, Bayer J, Hepp P, et al. Open reduction and internal fixation of proximal humeral fractures with use of the locking proximal humerus plate. Results of a prospective, multicenter, observational study. J Bone Joint Surg Am 2009;91:1320–1328.

Takeuchi R, Koshino T, Nakazawa A, et al. Minimally invasive fixation for unstable two-part proximal humeral fractures: surgical techniques and clinical results using j-nails. J Orthop Trauma 2002;16:403–408.

Van Seymortier P, Stoffelen D, Fortems Y, Reynders P. The reverse shoulder prosthesis (delta III) in acute shoulder fractures: technical considerations with respect to stability. Acta Orthop Belg 2006;72:474–477.

Wall B, Nove-Josserand L, O'Connor DP, et al. Reverse total shoulder arthroplasty: a review of results according to etiology. J Bone Joint Surg Am 2007;89:1476–1485.

Wierks C, Skolasky RL, Ji JH, McFarland EG. Reverse total shoulder replacement: intraoperative and early postoperative complications. Clin Orthop Relat Res 2009;467:225–234.

Wijgman AJ, Roolker W, Patt TW, et al. Open reduction and internal fixation of three and four-part fractures of the proximal part of the humerus. J Bone Joint Surg Am 2002;84:1919–1925.

Chapter 12 Operative treatment of non-union of the proximal humerus

Peter S. Johnston, Matthew L. Ramsey

INTRODUCTION

In the vast majority of cases, fractures of the proximal humerus are minimally displaced and heal uneventfully with non-operative treatment. Non-union is rare, and Neer stated that there were only 29 cases reported in the literature up to 1983 (Neer 1983). Non-union of the proximal humerus can be functionally debilitating and painful for the patient, and the decision to pursue operative management is based on the severity of symptoms and functional disability, viewed against the known results of surgery. To date, the results of operative management of this difficult problem are mixed, and present a difficult challenge to both surgeon and patient.

Factors complicating the management of non-union of the proximal humerus include poor bone quality as a result of shaft resorption, head cavitation, osteoporosis, and communication with synovial fluid from the glenohumeral joint. Additionally, capsular contracture due to post-traumatic scarring, positional shortening of rotator cuff and capsular tissues, and disuse contribute to the challenge of successful management of proximal humeral non-union.

ETIOLOGY

Approximately 40% of fractures of the humerus occur in the proximal region. These are distributed in a bimodal fashion, with higher-energy injuries occurring in younger patients, and lower-energy injuries in the elderly. Non-union of the proximal humerus is predominantly seen in elderly women, mostly after displaced two-part fractures (Norris et al. 1995) or after failure of open reduction and internal fixation (ORIF), as a result of inadequate fixation or poor bone stock (Jupiter and Mullaji 1994). Non-union is less frequent than malunion.

Factors contributing to the incidence of non-union include patient age, degree of displacement and comminution, osteoporosis, nutritional status, medical comorbidities, alcohol use, and a history of smoking. Neer (1983) reported an incidence as high as 23% in the elderly, debilitated patient with osteoporosis. Healy et al. (1990) reported that of 25 patients with non-union of the proximal humerus, nearly 65% possessed at least one serious medical comorbidity, and this significantly correlated with a poor outcome, regardless of treatment modality. Other factors predisposing to non-union are the use of hanging arm casts (which ultimately increase displacing forces due to the weight of the arm), soft-tissue interposition, the institution of range-of-motion exercises prior to sufficient healing, and inadequate ORIF.

CLINICAL EVALUATION

Evaluation of the patient with proximal humeral non-union begins with a careful history and physical examination. A clear understanding of the mechanism of injury provides insight into the energy of the injury, which, in turn, correlates with the degree of fracture displacement, comminution, and soft-tissue trauma. If the fracture was initially treated non-operatively, the duration and type of immobilization used are important considerations. Additionally, the patient's comorbidities, nutritional status, alcohol use, and functional disabilities are an important part of the history that will assist in decision making.

If the patient has had surgery, any history of postoperative wound complications and a need for irrigation and debridement and antibiotics is established. Deep infection should be considered in all cases of non-union after attempted surgical reconstruction. Baseline laboratory studies include a complete blood count (CBC), C-reactive protein, and erythrocyte sedimentation rate (ESR). Aspiration of the shoulder is performed if the clinical suspicion of infection is high.

Physical examination begins with a general inspection of the shoulder girdle. Previous surgical incisions, overlying skin changes, and gross deformity, including atrophy, should be noted. Active and passive arcs of motion are evaluated. The active range of motion in elevation, external rotation at the side and overhead, and internal rotation up the back is assessed and compared with the passive range of motion in the same planes. Range of motion is often severely limited as a result of pain and stiffness (Neer 1983). Manual muscle testing is performed in order to evaluate the functional strength of the rotator cuff and deltoid, as strength may be compromised by the non-union.

A careful neurologic examination should focus on the axillary, suprascapular, spinal accessory, long thoracic, musculocutaneous, median, radial, and ulnar nerves.

Radiographic evaluation begins with plain radiographs. A trauma series is typically all that is required and includes an anteroposterior (AP) view in internal and external rotation in the scapular plane, a scapular Y view, and an axillary view. A Velpeau axillary view is obtained if the patient is unable to tolerate positioning for a standard axillary radiograph. Plain radiographs allow evaluation of the location of fracture, type of non-union, bone quality, previous fixation, and viability of the humeral head. They are also important in determining the adequacy of the native bone stock, which can help guide the surgeon to reconstructive options or ORIF.

Computerized tomography (CT) can assist in establishing non-union of the surgical neck. However, the true value of CT is in establishing the relationship of the tuberosities to the humeral head, and whether they are non-united or malunited (**Fig. 12.1**). The severity of bone loss and the degree of cavitation of the humeral head can also be assessed. Three-dimensional reconstructions are occasional helpful in establishing the degree of deformity.

Magnetic resonance imaging (MRI) is rarely required to establish the diagnosis of non-union. However, it does allow assessment of any concomitant rotator cuff pathology, and the presence and location of avascular necrosis (AVN) of the humeral head (**Fig. 12.2**).

NON-UNION BY LOCATION

The most frequent location of a non-union in the proximal humerus is at the surgical neck (**Fig. 12.3**). Muscle forces from the rotator cuff combined with difficulty with immobilization contribute to non-union. The vascularity of the humeral head is also quite vulnerable, and any disruption of the medial soft tissues secondary to fracture displacement can increase rates of AVN.

Non-union of the greater tuberosity is uncommon. More commonly this fracture results in malunion. When non-union is present, posterior superior displacement of the fragment can lead to rotator cuff dysfunction and subacromial impingement, which will cause pain and limit function.

TREATMENT OPTIONS

Although, non-union of the proximal humerus is often associated with pain and severe functional limitation (Neer 1983, Rockwood and Pearce 1989, Healy et al. 1990, Norris et al. 1990) 50% of patients may be relatively asymptomatic, with satisfactory range of motion, and functional use of the arm. Non-operative treatment should be considered in these patients, as the risks of surgery outweigh the potential marginal outcomes that have been reported. In addition, patients with multiple medical comorbidities, who are unfit for surgery, should be treated non-operatively. There is little information on the non-operative management of non-unions. Healy et al. in their series of 25 proximal humeral non-unions reported that the four patients managed non-operatively all had an unsatisfactory outcome, with an average of 85° of elevation, 28° of external rotation, and internal rotation to the ipsilateral buttock (Healy et al. 1990).

Indications for surgical treatment include significant pain, deformity, and functional limitations. The decision for operative fixation versus reconstructive options is based on the age of the patient, the degree of displacement, and the viability of the humeral head. The goals of surgical treatment are twofold: pain resolution and improved function of the extremity.

Many approaches to the treatment of non-unions of the proximal humerus have been described, including intramedullary rods, rods with tension bands, ORIF, prosthetic replacement, and use of intramedullary cortical bone grafts, all with varying rates of success (Kristiansen and Christensen 1987, Healy et al. 1990, Jupiter and Mullaji 1994, Nayak et al. 1995, Norris et al. 1995, Duralde et al. 1996, Ring et al. 2001). When evaluating these retrospective studies and comparing outcomes, one must appreciate the bias that exists with regard to the heterogeneity of the groups and treatments. Prosthetic replacement is usually performed in more elderly, debilitated patients, or patients with more severe bone loss and deformity, in contrast to ORIF, which is reserved for younger patients with a viable humeral head, no underlying arthritis, and adequate bone stock for osteosynthesis.

Open reduction and internal fixation

Numerous techniques have been used for ORIF, each with its own advantages and disadvantages. Plate fixation, either with a blade plate or with a proximal humeral plate in association with bone grafting, requires sufficient bone stock, and relies on screw or blade fixation in the often osteoporotic humeral head. Walch et al. (1996) described a technique using harvested intramedullary cortical bone peg autograft taken from the iliac crest, anterior tibial crest, or middle

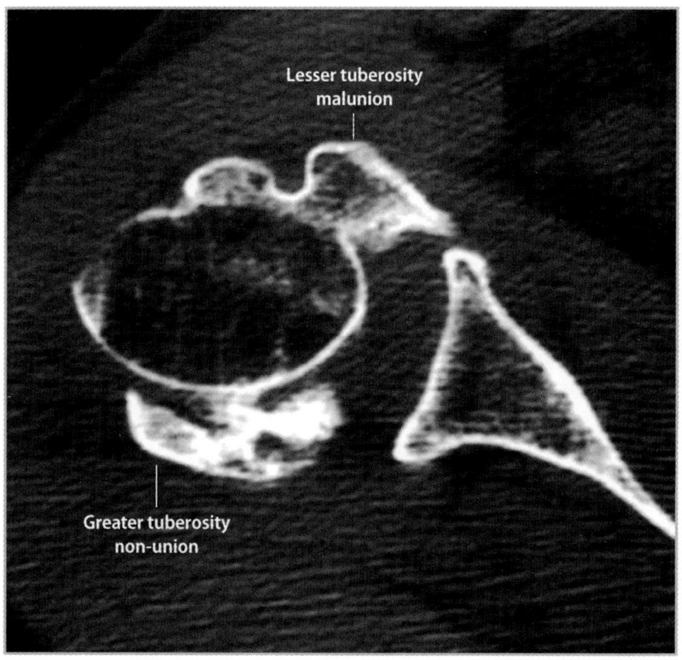

Figure 12.1 A computerized tomography scan demonstrating malunion of the lesser tuberosity, and non-union of the greater tuberosity. Computerized tomography offers the ability to establish the relationship of the tuberosities to the head and shaft fragments.

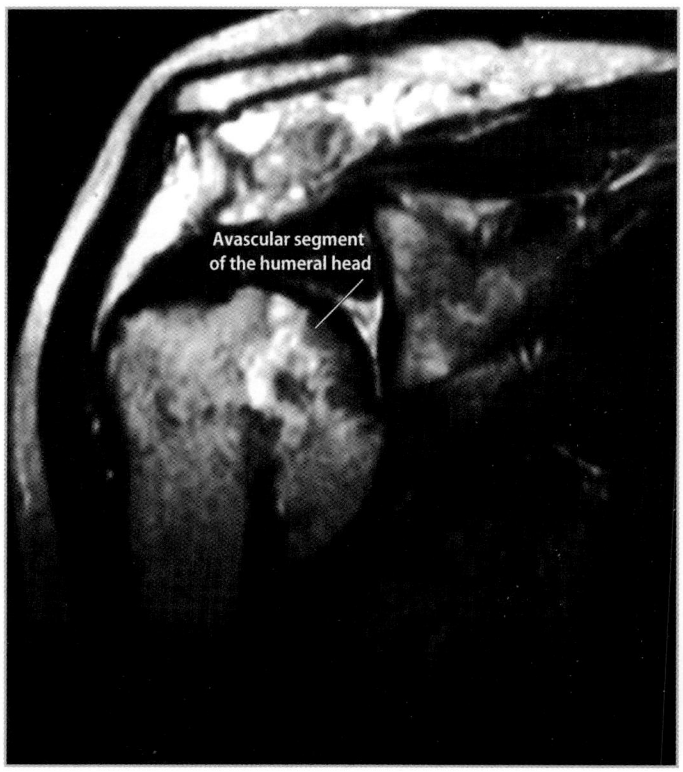

Figure 12.2 Coronal oblique magnetic resonance scan demonstrating avascular necrosis of a portion of the humeral head following a fracture of the proximal humerus.

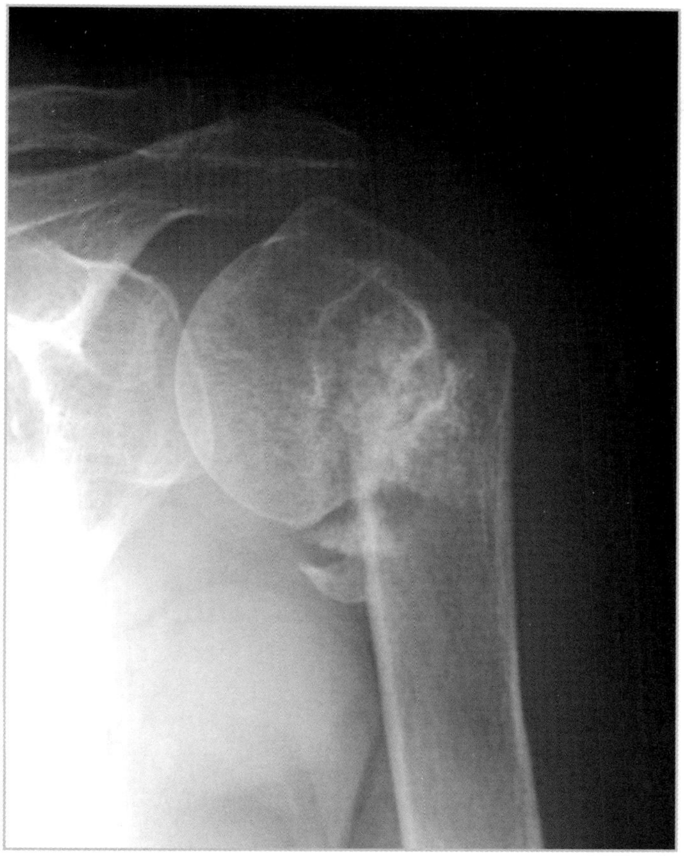

Figure 12.3 Anteroposterior (AP) radiograph demonstrating a non-union of the surgical neck following a fracture with associated medial comminution.

third of the fibula in combination with blade or T-plate fixation in 20 patients with an average age of 58 years. Ninety-six per cent of the patients went on to union, with an average of 131° of forward elevation, and a 95% overall satisfaction rate. Galatz and Iannotti (2000) reported on 13 patients, mean age 61, treated with ORIF with either a blade plate or T-plate in combination with iliac crest bone grafting. All patients had a united bone at final follow-up and improved pain scores, as well as a significantly improved range of motion postoperatively: 24° preoperatively compared with 144° postoperatively. Range-of-motion exercises were initiated for all patients in the early postoperative period.

Intramedullary fixation either with locked nailing or in combination with tension banding through the rotator cuff has been described with good results but also has limitations. Removal of hardware secondary to painful mechanical impingement is often required after union. Lin and Hou (2003) reported on 15 patients, mean age 55.1 years, treated for painful non-union with locked intramedullary nailing; 14 of these patients went on to union, with an average forward elevation of 152°. More recently, Yamane et al. (2008) reported on 14 patients treated with locked intramedullary nailing and bone grafting for non-union of the surgical neck. All but two patients had undergone a failed course of non-operative management prior to surgery. With a follow-up of 38 months, all the lesions were united, with mean forward elevation of 122° and external rotation to 35°. They concluded that locked intramedullary nailing was a successful method for stable fixation and allowed early range of motion postoperatively.

Shoulder arthroplasty

Reconstructive options include hemiarthroplasty, anatomic total shoulder arthroplasty, and reverse total shoulder arthroplasty. Arthroplasty is indicated in patients with severe osteoporosis, head cavitation, AVN, inadequate bone stock, and/or degenerative joint changes usually seen in the setting of non-union of a three- or four-part fracture, or after failed previous fixation. Studies have demonstrated that arthroplasty can reliably provide pain relief, but less reliably functional restoration, and is usually considered a 'salvage' operation. These surgeries are technically demanding, and have generally yielded poor results (Antuna et al. 2002, Boileau et al. 2006, Neyton and Boileau 2006).

Experience with hemiarthroplasty or total shoulder arthroplasty for non-union of the proximal humerus has established several key principles. The most significant has been to avoid performing an osteotomy of the greater tuberosity, and to adapt the implant to the deformed anatomy. Boileau et al. (2001) reported on six patients with non-union of the proximal humerus treated with hemiarthroplasty who underwent osteotomy of the greater tuberosity. None of the patients was able to elevate the arm above 90°. Antuna et al. (2002) investigated management of the tuberosity further in their series of 27 patients who were treated with hemiarthroplasty or total shoulder arthroplasty for non-union. Almost half of the patients experienced complications associated with tuberosity healing, resorption, or malunion. The lack of postoperative range of motion was attributed to complications with the tuberosity, and these authors recommended meticulous care with tuberosity fixation. They concluded that, despite functional limitations, they were able to achieve good pain relief and high levels of subjective patient satisfaction. Lin et al. (2006) attributed gains of 64° from preoperative levels to a forward elevation of 113° to preservation of the anatomy of the proximal humerus and avoidance of osteotomy of the greater tuberosity. Almost 80% of their patients experienced complete pain relief in addition to functional range of motion, gains which had not been previously demonstrated in this difficult treatment group. The authors also pointed out the need for extensive soft-tissue releases and the addition of medial calcar bone grafting.

In cases of non-union with distorted proximal humeral anatomy or rotator cuff deficiency, a reverse total shoulder arthroplasty has been demonstrated to be a viable option. Boileau et al. (2006) reported the mid-term results of reverse shoulder arthroplasty for proximal humeral non-union, which included improved function and restored active elevation to 122°, although with limited external rotation. When compared with patients who underwent reverse shoulder arthroplasty for cuff tear arthropathy or malunion with severe distortion of anatomy, the results in patients with non-union of the proximal humerus were less reliable. The authors reported fairly high rates of complication, including instability, infection, and stiffness, which required five re-operations in their series of seven patients. The authors recommended that a non-arthroplasty option be considered initially. Only in the presence of severe humeral head cavitation, associated non-union of the tuberosities, and glenohumeral arthritis should reverse shoulder arthroplasty be considered as a salvage operation.

TECHNIQUE

Patient positioning

The patients are positioned in the beach-chair position, with the head of the table elevated approximately 30°. The patient needs to be positioned on the operating table such that the arm can be freely manipulated, and adduction to the side is unencumbered by encroachment from the table. Intraoperative fluoroscopy is frequently required, especially if ORIF of the non-union is planned. It is important to establish the ability to acquire AP and axillary images of the shoulder prior to proceeding with surgery.

The arm is prepped and draped, allowing for access to the anterior aspect of the shoulder. The arm can be supported with a sterile arm-holder (**Fig. 12.4**) or on a modified Mayo stand.

Surgical approach

Incisions from previous surgery should be noted and utilized whenever possible. However, extensile exposure to the shoulder may be required, and previous incisions should not be used if they compromise visualization or the ability to progressively extend the exposure.

An extended deltopectoral approach to the shoulder is utilized (**Fig. 12.5**). The cephalic vein defines the deltopectoral interval (**Fig. 12.6**). If previous surgery was undertaken, the cephalic vein may have been compromised and is not a useful marker of the deltopectoral interval. In this case, the coracoid process in the proximal extent of the wound identifies this interval, and can be used to begin deep exposure.

The coracoid marks the origin of the short head of the biceps and the coracobrachialis. The lateral border of the conjoint tendon is dissected, and the axillary and musculocutaneous nerves are identified visually and by digital palpation (**Fig. 12.7**). The subacromial and subdeltoid spaces need to be established. Scarring from the non-union and from previous surgical manipulation can make identification of this space challenging. Identification is most easily achieved by beginning the dissection proximally and distally. Proximally, the origin of the coracoacromial (CA) ligament on the coracoid is identified, and followed to the insertion on the acromion. Dissection under the anterior leading edge of the CA ligament defines the subacromial space. Distally, the deltoid insertion is defined. The humeral shaft is identified just proximal to the deltoid insertion. A periosteal elevator is used to tease the scarred deltoid away from the humerus, establishing the distal extent of the subdeltoid space.

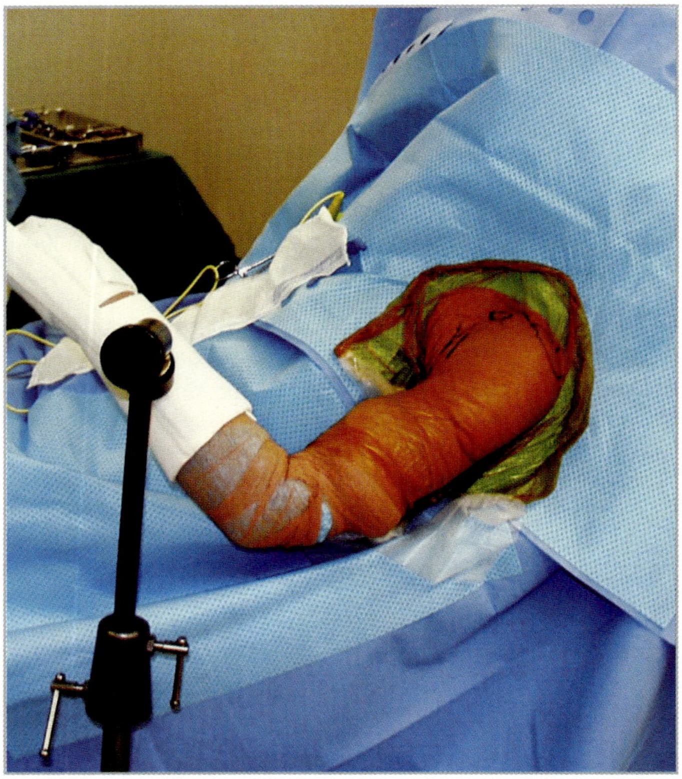

Figure 12.4 Sterile arm-holder. This allows the arm to be maintained in any position, thereby eliminating the need for an assistant to hold the arm.

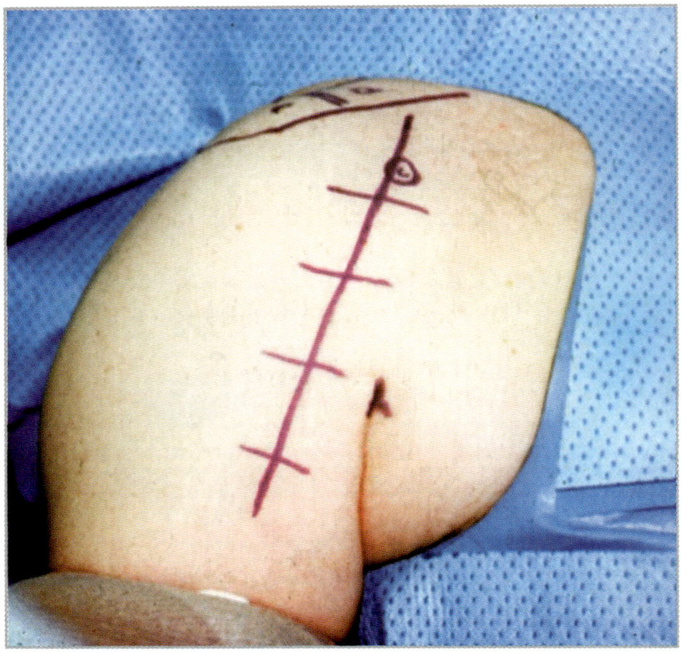

Figure 12.5 The incision marked for an extended deltopectoral approach to the shoulder. The deltopectoral interval runs obliquely from the tip of the coracoid to the middle of the arm at the deltoid insertion. The length of the incision is determined by the need for surgical exposure.

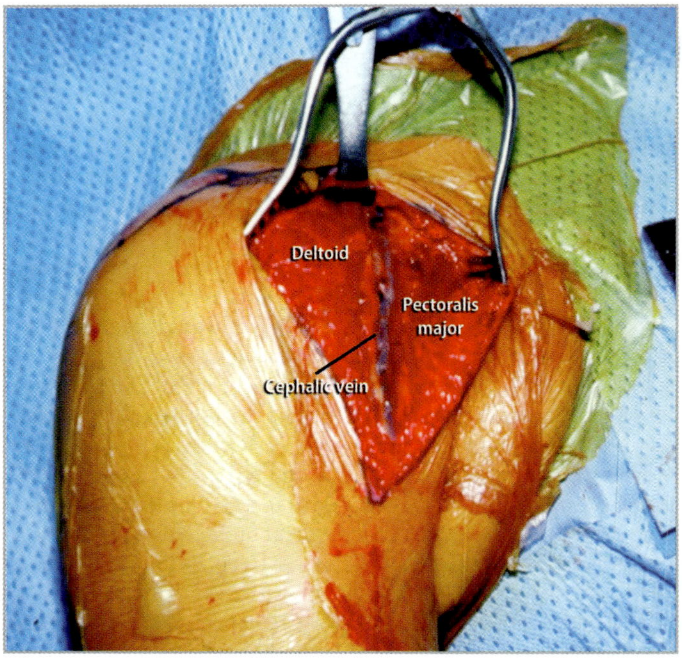

Figure 12.6 The cephalic vein defines the deltopectoral interval. The vein is dissected and retracted laterally with the deltoid muscle or medially with the pectoralis major muscle.

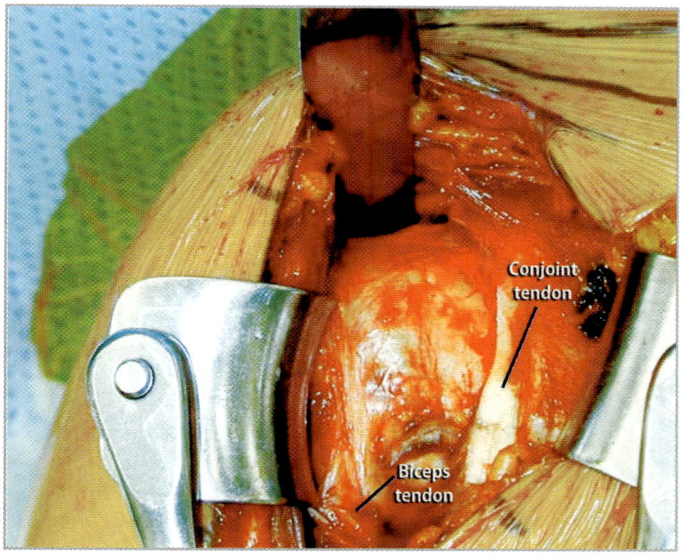

Figure 12.7 The lateral border of the conjoint tendon is identified. There is often a muscular portion of the short head of the biceps that lies lateral to the tendon. Dissection must be carried out lateral to this muscle, to avoid denervating this portion of the biceps.

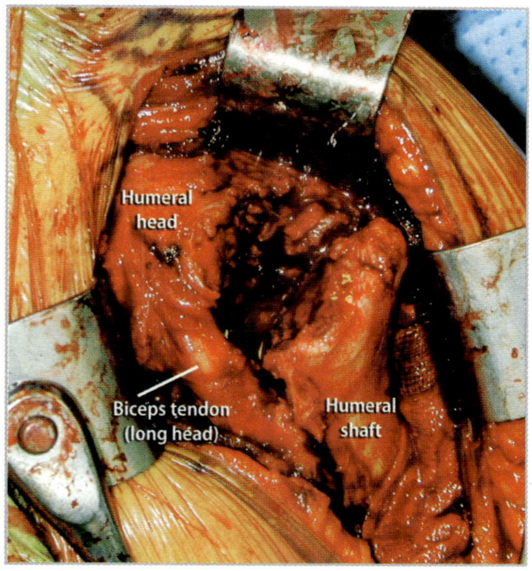

Figure 12.8 The non-union is identified and any interposed scar tissue is removed. The ends of the non-union are freshened and contracted soft tissues are released.

Working from proximally and distally toward the center, the subacromial and subdeltoid spaces are established.

The long head of the biceps serves as the lighthouse to deeper dissection, and is the branch point for each of the surgical techniques described below.

Open reduction and internal fixation

The biceps tendon sheath is unroofed up to and including the rotator interval. The superior rotator cuff and capsular tissues are typically contracted as a result of the varus and retroverted position of the humeral head. The biceps tendon is released from the attachment at the superior glenoid, and tenodesed to the pectoralis major tendon. A superior capsular release between the supraspinatus and labrum is performed. Additionally, the coracohumeral ligament is released, completing the soft-tissue releases required to get the humeral head out of varus and retroversion. Traction stitches are placed at the tendon–bone junction of the subscapularis, supraspinatus, and infraspinatus/teres minor in order to control the humeral head fragment.

The non-union site is identified, and any interposed soft tissue and scar are excised (**Fig. 12.8**). The bone ends at the non-union site are freshened to bleeding bone, and bone quality and quantity are assessed. If structural bone graft is not required, the non-united surfaces are impacted, and the non-union is stabilized with a fixed-angle plate (blade plate or proximal humeral locking plate) (**Fig. 12.9**). Currently, most surgeons prefer proximal humeral locking plates. The head fragment is positioned, and the plate is affixed to the distal fragment through a slotted hole on the implant that allows minor adjustments to the height of the plate. The height of the plate relative to the top of the greater tuberosity is dependent on the specific type of plating system to be used. With more proximally based plating systems, care must be taken not to place the plate too high, in order to avoid impingement against the acromion in elevation. In more distally placed implant systems, care must be taken not to place the plate too distally, in order to guarantee that the most inferior locking screws engage the humeral head instead of exiting inferior to it.

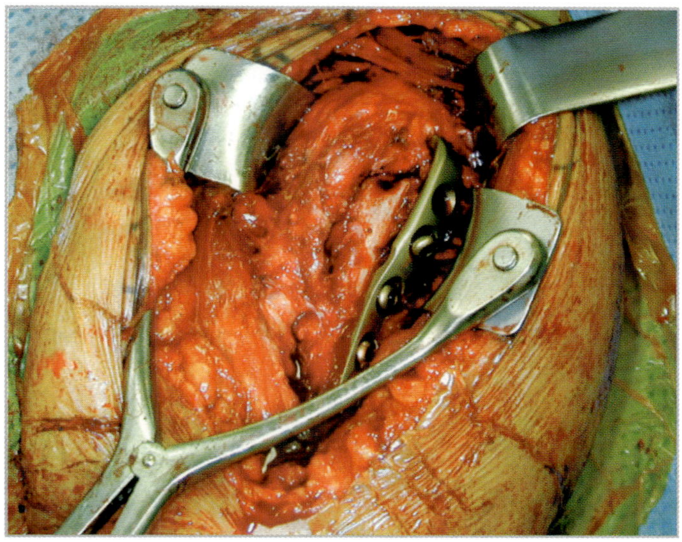

Figure 12.9 Stable fixation is obtained once the non-union is reduced. Currently, proximal humeral locking plates are preferred. In this example, a fixed-angle blade plate was used to obtain rigid fixation.

Once the height of the plate is established, the plate if definitively fixed to the humeral shaft. The traction sutures are passed through the plate and tied, reducing the head to the plate. Intraoperative fluoroscopy confirms the reduction of the non-union. Once confirmed, locked screws are placed into the humeral head, completing fixation.

If there is enough bone for plate fixation of the non-union, but there is some attritional loss of bone from the humeral head, an intramedullary autograft or allograft is utilized (**Fig. 12.10**). Currently, the authors prefer fibular allograft, since it fits well within the intramedullary canal and allows support of the lateral humeral head or medial calcar, depending on the position of the graft. If graft is felt to be required, the location of attritional bone loss is assessed so that the graft can be appropriately positioned. The fibular allograft is positioned in the intramedullary canal, medially or laterally. The head fragment is positioned over the allograft such that the bone deficiency is supported by the graft. The remainder of the technique for plate fixation is as described above.

Hemiarthroplasty, with or without tuberosity takedown

Hemiarthroplasty for non-union of the proximal humerus is considered when salvage of the articular surface is deemed impossible (**Fig. 12.11**). The surgical approach is similar to that described above. Once the non-union has been identified, the decision on how to manage the tuberosities must be made. Traditionally, they are isolated with their rotator cuff attachments, and repaired about the humeral implant after its insertion. The head fragment, if intact, is split from the bicipital groove toward the articular surface. The remnant articular surface is then removed from within the joint, leaving the tuberosities isolated with their cuff attachments.

The humeral trial component is inserted in the appropriate height and version (**Fig. 12.12**). Version is most easily established by placing the arm in neutral rotation and directing the implant head toward the glenoid. Implant height is determined by using the size of the tuberosity as a guide. The tuberosities should be placed under the humeral head to re-establish the tuberosity-to-head height at between 8 and 10 mm and still allow contact with the humeral shaft. Before the humeral stem is implanted, sutures are placed in the shaft and at the bone–tendon junctions of the tuberosities in order to allow vertical and horizontal fixation of the tuberosities to the shaft and to each other.

The humeral implant is then cemented into the prepared canal at the predetermined height and version. Once the cement is hardened, tuberosity reconstruction is completed by tying first the horizontal sutures, followed by the vertical sutures. Tuberosity reconstruction is

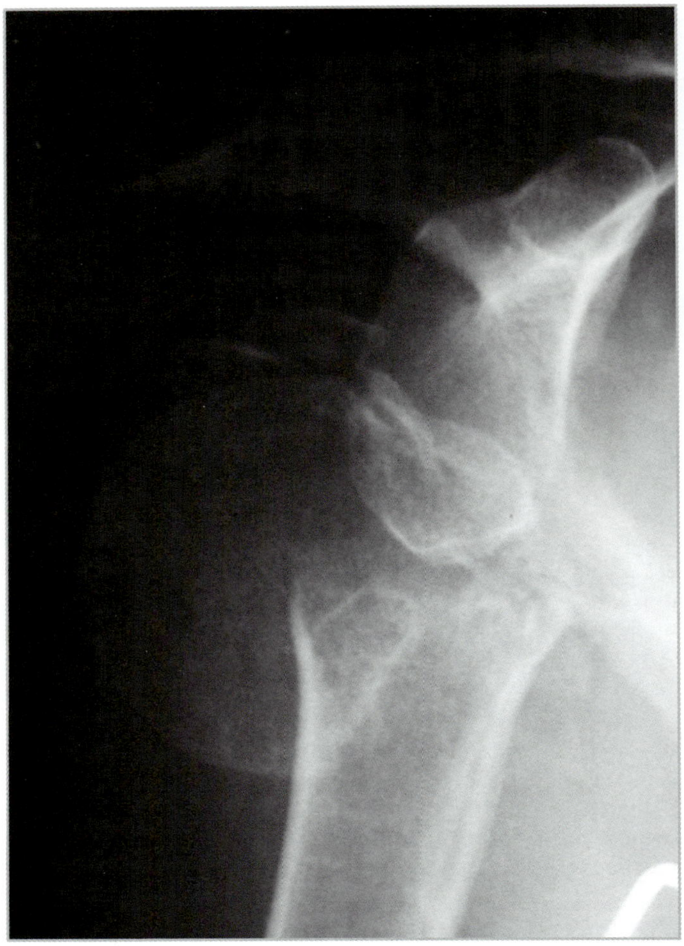

Figure 12.11 Non-union of the surgical neck, with cavitation of the humeral head. This is an indication for hemiarthroplasty.

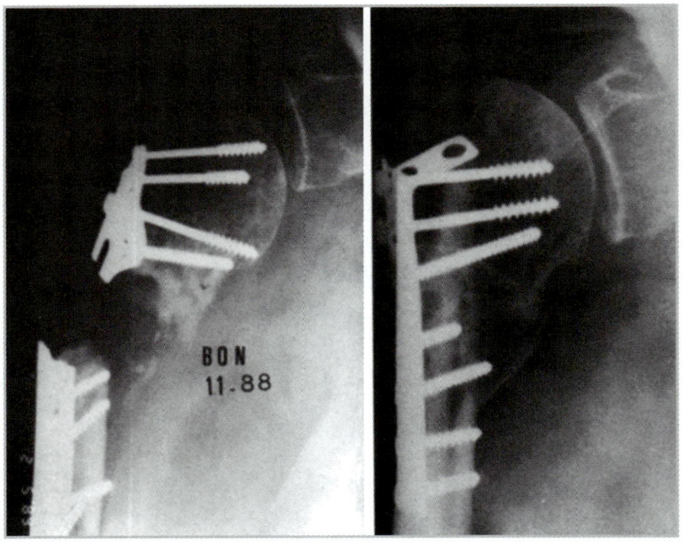

Figure 12.10 Management of the non-union of a fracture of the surgical neck of the humerus. (a) Failure of the open reduction and internal fixation. (b) Management includes the use of an intramedullary fibular allograft. (Reprinted from Walch G, Badet R, Nove-Josserand L, et al. Nonunions of the surgical neck of the humerus: surgical treatment with an intramedullary bone peg, internal fixation, and cancellous bone grafting. J Shoulder Elbow Surg 1996;5:161–168.)

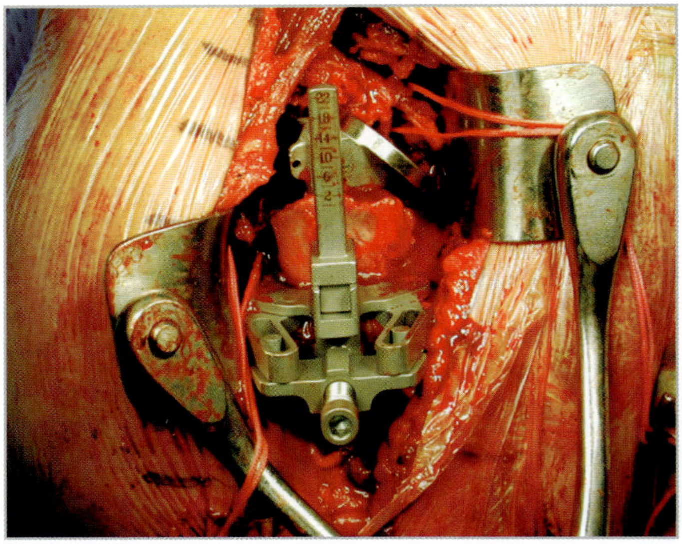

Figure 12.12 The humeral stem is inserted in an appropriate height and version. The height of the tuberosity can be used to help establish the appropriate height of the implant.

confirmed via intraoperative fluoroscopy before the surgeon leaves the operating room.

The results of hemiarthroplasty for non-union of the proximal humerus when the tuberosities are reconstructed has led to a modification for the management of the humeral head segment. Alternatively, the proximal head fragment is isolated and the subscapularis is released from the lesser tuberosity. A cut is made in the anatomic neck at an appropriate angle in order to prepare for implantation of the humeral stem. If there has been attritional bone loss of the medial calcar at the non-union site, the greater and lesser tuberosities remain as a C-fragment. If there is no medial erosion, a ring-shaped piece of bone remains, including thetuberosities and intact medial calcar. Sutures are placed in the tuberosities for repair to the shaft. The humeral stem is inserted through the tuberosity ring of bone into the shaft (**Fig. 12.13**). The sutures passed through the tuberosity are tied, securing the tuberosity ring to the shaft. The subscapularis is repaired to the lesser tuberosity to complete the repair.

Reverse total shoulder arthroplasty

Reverse total shoulder arthroplasty is the treatment of choice for many surgeons for older patients with non-union of the proximal humerus, either with or without previous surgery (**Fig. 12.14**). The critical aspect of reverse total shoulder arthroplasty following non-union is maintenance of the integrity of the rotator cuff attachments to the fragments of tuberosity. The functional results are related to the ability to re-establish the external rotation of the posterior rotator cuff (**Fig. 12.15**). If reconstruction of the greater tuberosity is not possible, some authors advocate latissimus transfer to the posterior humerus to re-establish external rotation.

Reverse total shoulder arthroplasty for non-union of the proximal humerus is performed through a deltopectoral approach (as above). A superior approach does not provide exposure to the humeral shaft, which may be required. The deltopectoral approach is described above but some key points should be made here. In the absence of previous surgery, the non-union is typically at the surgical neck and the tuberosities, if involved, are malunited. After previous surgery, the ttuberosities

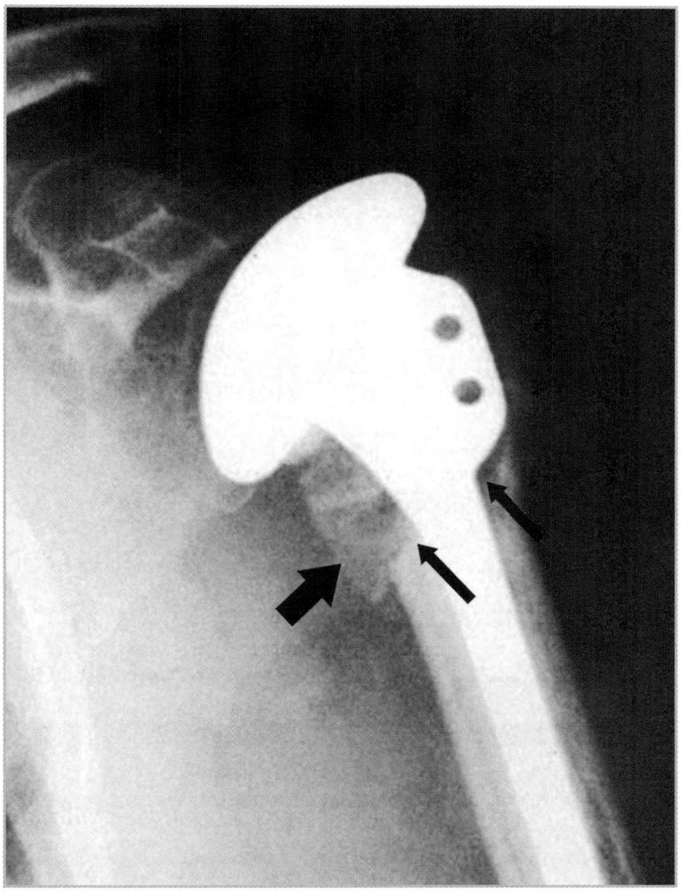

Figure 12.13 Anteroposterior radiograph demonstrating a ring graft consisting of the greater and lesser tuberosities. (Reprinted from Lin JS, Klepps S, Miller S, Cleeman E, Flatow EL. Effectiveness of replacement arthroplasty with calcar grafting and avoidance of greater tuberosity osteotomy for the treatment of humeral surgical neck nonunions. J Shoulder Elbow Surg 2006;15:12–18.)

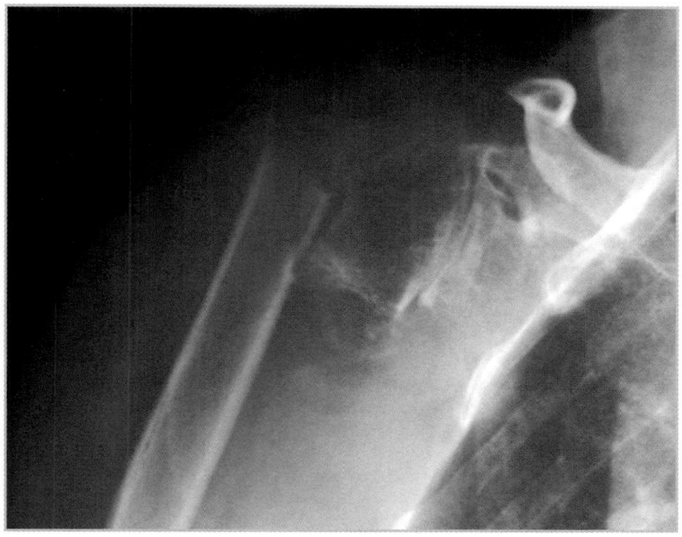

Figure 12.14 Anteroposterior radiograph from an elderly woman, demonstrating a non-union of the surgical neck. Note the associated degenerative arthritis in the glenohumeral joint.

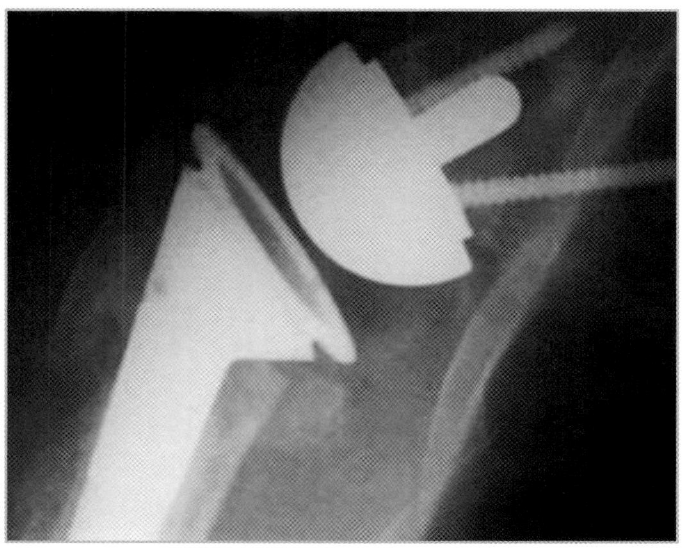

Figure 12.15 Radiograph following reverse total shoulder replacement. The greater and lesser tuberosity are reconstructed around the humeral component in order to re-establish the function of the rotator cuff.

are often non-united. The tuberosities are identified. If the non-union is at the level of the surgical neck, the head is split at the bicipital groove, yielding a fragment of the lesser tuberosity with the anterior portion of the humeral head. The greater tuberosity, with cuff attachments, is included with the posterior portion of the humeral head. If the supraspinatus remains attached to the greater tuberosity superiorly, it is released. The anterior and posterior portions of the humeral head are removed, leaving the tuberosities with their cuff attachments. Sutures are placed at the bone–tendon junctions of the lesser and greater tuberosities.

Removal of the humeral head provides excellent visualization to the glenoid. The glenoid is prepared for the base-plate of the glenoid sphere. It is critical to place the glenoid base-plate as low as possible, so that the glenoid sphere will clear the inferior aspect of the glenoid, to avoid notching. Once the base-plate is placed, the glenoid sphere is placed definitively.

Attention is then directed to the humerus. The intramedullary canal is reamed and sized. An appropriate-sized stem and body are inserted. In the face of deficiency of the proximal humerus, the challenge is to tension the soft tissues adequately. With the humeral implant in place, the smallest polyethylene trial is inserted and the shoulder is reduced. Longitudinal traction is applied to the arm to establish the height of the implant. The trial components are removed and a cement restrictor is placed. The intramedullary canal is lavaged and packed with a thrombin-soaked sponge. The canal is dried, and cement is injected into the canal and pressurized. The implant is inserted at the previously trialed height in neutral version and held while the cement hardens. Once the cement has hardened, trial reduction is performed. The final polyethylene insert with any necessary spacers is impacted.

The greater tuberosity is positioned prior to reduction, to facilitate retrieval after the joint is located. The intra-articular portions of the sutures are passed around the medial aspect of the humerus prior to reduction. Once the shoulder is reduced, the joint is irrigated and the sutures from the greater tuberosity are passed through the lesser tuberosity. Vertical sutures are also passed to fix the tuberosities to the shaft. All sutures are tied.

Closure is performed in routine fashion.

CONCLUSIONS

The surgical management of non-union of the proximal humerus continues to challenge the treating surgeon. In general, several important points have been established. First, ORIF with bone grafting is the preferred treatment in patients with sufficient bone stock for fixation who are deemed appropriate surgical candidates. Humeral head replacement, particularly when tuberosity osteotomy is required, typically yields limited functional gains. If hemiarthroplasty is considered, avoiding osteotomy of the greater tuberosity appears to improve the results. Reverse shoulder arthroplasty yields improved function but carries a significant risk of complication.

REFERENCES

Antuna SA, Sperling JW, Sanchez-Sotelo J, Cofield RH. Shoulder arthroplasty for proximal humeral nonunions. J Shoulder Elbow Surg 2002;11:114–121.

Boileau P, Trojani C, Walch G, et al. Shoulder arthroplasty for the treatment of the sequelae of fractures of the proximal humerus. J Shoulder Elbow Surg 2001;10:299–308.

Boileau P, Watkinson D, Hatzidakis AM, Hovorka I. Neer Award 2005: The Grammont reverse shoulder prosthesis: results in cuff tear arthritis, fracture sequelae, and revision arthroplasty. J Shoulder Elbow Surg 2006;15:527–540.

Duralde XA, Flatow EL, Pollock RG, et al. Operative treatment of nonunions of the surgical neck of the humerus. J Shoulder Elbow Surg 1996;5:169–180.

Galatz LM, Iannotti JP. Management of surgical neck nonunions. Orthop Clin North Am 2000;31:51–61.

Healy WL, Jupiter JB, Kristiansen TK, White RR. Nonunion of the proximal humerus. A review of 25 cases. Journal Ortho Trauma 1990;4:424–431.

Jupiter JB, Mullaji AB. Blade plate fixation of proximal humeral non-unions. Injury 1994;25:301–303.

Kristiansen B, Christensen SW. Proximal humeral fractures. Late results in relation to classification and treatment. Acta Orthop Scand 1987;58:124–127.

Lin JS, Hou SM. Locked-nail treatment of humeral surgical neck nonunions. J Trauma 2003;54:530–535.

Lin JS, Klepps S, Miller S, et al. Effectiveness of replacement arthroplasty with calcar grafting and avoidance of greater tuberosity osteotomy for the treatment of humeral surgical neck nonunions. J Shoulder Elbow Surg 2006;15:12–18.

Nayak NK, Schickendantz MS, Regan WD, Hawkins RJ. Operative treatment of nonunion of surgical neck fractures of the humerus. Clin Orthop Relat Res 1995;(313):200–205.

Neer CS. Nonunion of the surgical neck of the humerus. Orthop Trans 1983;7:389.

Neyton L, Boileau P. Results of reverse shoulder arthroplasty in proximal humeral fracture sequelae. In: Walch G, Boileau P, Favard L, et al., eds. Reverse Shoulder Arthroplasty: Clinical Results, Complications, Revisions. Montpellier: Sauramps Medical, 2006: 81–102.

Norris TR, Turner JA, Bovill DF. Nonunion of the upper humerus: an analysis of etiology and treatment: 28 cases. In: Post M, Morrey BF, Hawkins RJ, eds. Surgery of the Shoulder. St Louis: Mosby, 1990: 63–67.

Norris TR, Green A, McGuigan FX. Late prosthetic shoulder arthroplasty for displaced proximal humerus fractures. J Shoulder Elbow Surg 1995;4:271–280.

Ring D, McKee MD, Perey BH, Jupiter JB. The use of a blade plate and autogenous cancellous bone graft in the treatment of ununited fractures of the proximal humerus. J Shoulder Elbow Surg 2001;10:501–507.

Rockwood CA, Pearce JC. Management of proximal humerus nonunions. Orthop Trans 1989;13:644.

Walch G, Badet R, Nove-Josserand L, Levigne C. Nonunions of the surgical neck of the humerus: surgical treatment with an intramedullary bone peg, internal fixation, and cancellous bone grafting. J Shoulder Elbow Surg 1996;5:161–168

Yamane S, Suenaga N, Oizumi N, Minami A. Interlocking intramedullary nailing for nonunion of the proximal humerus with the straight nail system. J Shoulder Elbow Surg 2008;17:755–759.

Chapter 13 Operative management of malunions of the proximal humerus

Jason D. Doppelt, Eric T. Ricchetti, Peter J. Evans, Joseph P. Iannotti

INTRODUCTION

While some degree of anatomical malalignment after a fracture of the proximal humerus can be well tolerated, more significant malunions can be disabling injuries, associated with pain and loss of motion. The goal of treatment is avoidance of this condition by appropriate evaluation of the initial fracture, and early and effective surgical invention when displacement of the fracture fragments is significant. However, in some cases, despite proper management, patient factors such as osteoporotic bone or inadequate immobilization of the limb, or too high an activity level, or lack of adherence to the rehabilitation program can result in fracture malunion. Realistic goals must be established when correction of the deformity is planned, as full restoration of function is often not possible in the setting of severely distorted osseous and soft-tissue anatomy.

Symptomatic malunions of the proximal humerus can be the result of inadequate or misinterpreted imaging following the patient's injury. The fracture fragments often demonstrate predictable patterns of displacement, due to their soft-tissue attachments; however, the degree of displacement can easily be misinterpreted. Non-operative management for what was assumed to be a minimally displaced fracture can easily result in pain and dysfunction secondary to the malunion of fracture fragments. Patients managed operatively can also present with a symptomatic malunion if an acceptable initial reduction was not obtained, or if there was subsequent displacement due to inadequate or loss of fixation (this most commonly occurs when fixation was through the weaker cancellous bone of the proximal humerus). Associated soft-tissue pathology must also be considered, as it can play an equally important role in the patient's symptoms (Beredjiklian et al. 1998).

A detailed history of the injury and prior treatment is required to comprehend the nature of the initial injury, as well as the reasons why the previous management failed. Comorbidities such as osteoporotic bone and tobacco use should be clearly documented, as they have negative impacts on proper fracture union. Loss of fixation may also be related to aggressive therapy. Understanding the patient's goals and expectations for functional demand is a major factor in determining surgical management. Low-demand patients with minimal pain may not benefit from surgical intervention.

Physical examination must include a careful assessment of the patient's neurologic function, to rule out injury to the axillary nerve or brachial plexus, which may occur in this patient population. Displacement of a fracture fragment medial to the coracoid process increases the risk of nerve injury. If an injury to the axillary nerve is suspected, the radiographic examination may demonstrate inferior subluxation of the humeral head, due to decreased deltoid tension. Electromyographic examination should be performed to confirm neurologic injury if the physical examination is abnormal. An electromyogram (EMG) should be undertaken before any further surgical care is performed, approximately 4-6 weeks after the clinical diagnosis of an acute neurological injury without signs of early nerve recovery over that period of time.

Loss of shoulder motion is typically present, and it is important to distinguish between deficiencies in passive versus active arcs of motion. Weakness in the setting of good passive motion can be due to an unrecognized rotator cuff tear or tuberosity non-union. Loss of both active and passive motion can be due to mechanical impingement in the setting of bony malalignment, as well as to soft-tissue pathology such as capsular contracture. In most cases both factors contribute to severe loss of passive motion.

An accurate assessment of the osseous malalignment requires a thorough radiographic evaluation. Plain radiographs in at least two orthogonal planes should be obtained to determine whether advanced imaging is necessary. The true anteroposterior radiograph will demonstrate the alignment of the articular surface relative to the humeral shaft. Superior malalignment of the greater tuberosity can also be appreciated. The position of the lesser tuberosity is better assessed on an axillary lateral radiograph. A trans-scapular lateral view is beneficial in the setting of a fracture of the greater tuberosity, to assess the degree of combined superior and posterior displacement. Restoration of alignment in the sagittal plane is critical to regaining forward elevation, and the typical apex anterior angulation with the humeral head displaced posteriorly can be appreciated on the transcapular lateral and axillary views.

Computerized tomography (CT) is indicated when plain radiographs incompletely characterize the bony anatomy. With plain radiographs, the degree of displacement of the tuberosities and humeral head can be underestimated, and the presence of an articular impression fracture can be missed. Three-dimensional CT reconstructions may further aid the assessment of tuberosity malposition. Magnetic resonance imaging (MRI) will help characterize the soft-tissue abnormalities such as rotator cuff tears, deltoid deficiency, and labral pathology, but artifact may limit the usefulness of this modality if metallic implants are present.

Several classification systems have been proposed for malunions of the proximal humerus, although no one is universally accepted and consistently utilized. Neer's classification of acute fractures of the proximal humerus (Neer 1970) is known by most surgeons (see Chapter 1) and has been modified to describe malunions. The classification system described by Beredjiklian et al. (1998) takes both osseous and soft-tissue abnormalities into consideration. Three types of osseous abnormalities are recognized: type I is malposition of the greater or lesser tuberosity by more than 1 cm; type II is incongruity or step-off of the articular surface by more than 5 mm; and type III is malalignment of the articular segment by more than 45° of rotation in any plane. Additionally, the presence of soft-tissue contractures, rotator cuff tears, and subacromial impingement are documented as part of the classification system and should be considered and identified when evaluating the patient. The presence of such characteristics helps to reinforce the concept that bony abnormalities are typically not the sole cause of the patient's symptoms.

INDICATIONS

Two-part malunion of the greater tuberosity

Fractures involving the greater tuberosity are commonly encountered. As an isolated injury the humeral head remains centered relative to the glenoid; in contrast, the greater tuberosity may be pulled superiorly and posteriorly, due to the unopposed pull of the supraspinatus, infraspinatus, and teres minor muscles. If the fragment is allowed to heal in a superiorly displaced position, there can be a mechanical block to motion, due to impingement with the acromion on attempted abduction. Attrition of the rotator cuff can occur with this type of impingement. Posterior malposition of the greater tuberosity may cause impingement between the tuberosity and the posterior glenoid on attempted external rotation (**Fig. 13.1**). Instability can result from this impingement, as the humeral head is forced to translate anteriorly. Additionally, malposition of the tuberosity will compromise rotator cuff function, requiring generation of a greater abduction force by the deltoid to achieve motion (Bono et al. 2001).

The specific surgical indications have not been clearly defined for malunions of the greater tuberosity. Neer used 1 cm as the criterion for significant displacement in the acute setting. With a malunion this same distance can be used; however, in patients with greater functional demand, a malunion of only 5 mm may cause dysfunction that warrants surgical intervention (Iannotti and Williams 2007). Mechanical impingement or rotator cuff dysfunction attributed to the malunion is unlikely to improve with non-operative modalities, making surgical intervention advisable.

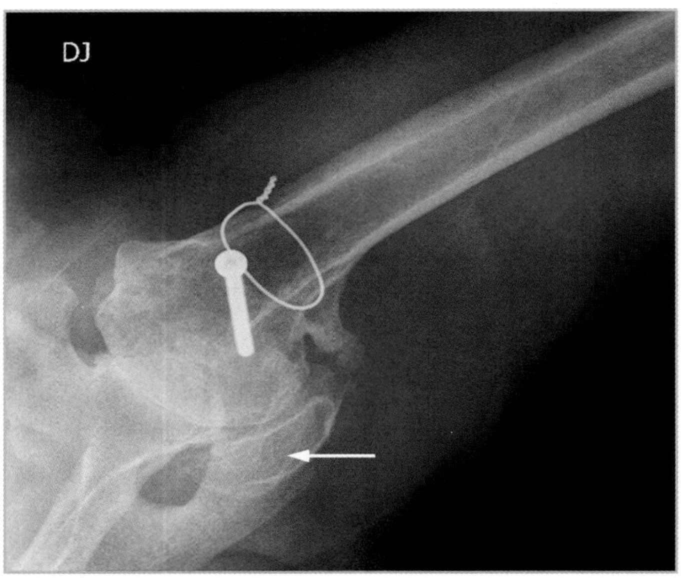

Figure 13.1 Malunion of the proximal humerus. Axillary radiograph demonstrating posterior malposition of the greater tuberosity (arrow) which will prevent external rotation due to impingement with the glenoid.

Two-part malunion of the lesser tuberosity

Isolated fracture of the lesser tuberosity is rare. It has been reported in the pediatric population as an isolated injury (Paschal et al. 1995). In adults it may be seen in association with a posterior shoulder dislocation (Hayes et al. 2003). If union occurs in a medialized position there can be impingement on attempted internal rotation. This can also result in subscapularis weakness, due to the decreased musculotendinous length.

The initial injury can easily be missed on plain radiographs if the axillary lateral view is not obtained or is not carefully examined (van Laarhoven et al. 1995). Advanced imaging is helpful in characterizing the size and displacement of the fragment. Chronic posterior dislocation must be carefully ruled out, as it can often be missed on anteroposterior and scapular Y radiographs. Surgery is indicated if clinically significant impingement or subscapularis weakness is present.

Malunion of the surgical neck

Displaced fractures of the surgical neck typically demonstrate medial displacement of the shaft and apex anterior angulation at the fracture site, due to pull of the pectoralis major (Duralde et al. 1996). The head assumes a varus position relative to the shaft, due to the unopposed tension of the superior rotator cuff (Neer 1970). The most common cause of decreased forward elevation is apex anterior angulation, and the head is frequently more than 45° malrotated (**Fig. 13.2**).

Orthogonal plain radiographs will demonstrate the alignment of the humeral head to the shaft. The degree of varus (**Fig. 13.3**) and sagittal plane (**Fig. 13.4**) malalignment should be calculated. Comparison radiographs of the contralateral proximal humerus should be obtained to assess the patient's normal neck-shaft angle and humeral head version, as this can be variable (Jeong et al. 2009). Malalignment in either the coronal or the sagittal plane of over 45° is likely to cause dysfunction and warrant surgical intervention (Beredjiklian and Iannotti 1998, Beredjiklian et al. 1998).

Three- and four-part malunions

Patients with three- and four-part malunions may present with significant dysfunction. The abnormal osseous anatomy will be a combination of the above-mentioned fracture patterns, and significant displacement is typically present (**Fig. 13.5**). An adequate understanding of the malunion pattern may not be possible with plain radiographs, making three-dimensional CT reconstructions helpful in most cases. The indications for two-part malunions (see above) also apply in this setting; however, additional factors must also be considered. The congruity of the glenohumeral joint can be compromised, due to either the acute injury itself or the subsequent development of avascular necrosis of the humeral head. If joint incongruity is present, the patient is unlikely to benefit from non-operative measures, making arthroplasty the best management option.

CONTRAINDICATIONS

The decision to proceed with surgery is based on patients' degree of discomfort and disability, while taking their functional demands into consideration. Minor deficits are unlikely to be completely corrected, making surgery inadvisable unless patients are unable to tolerate

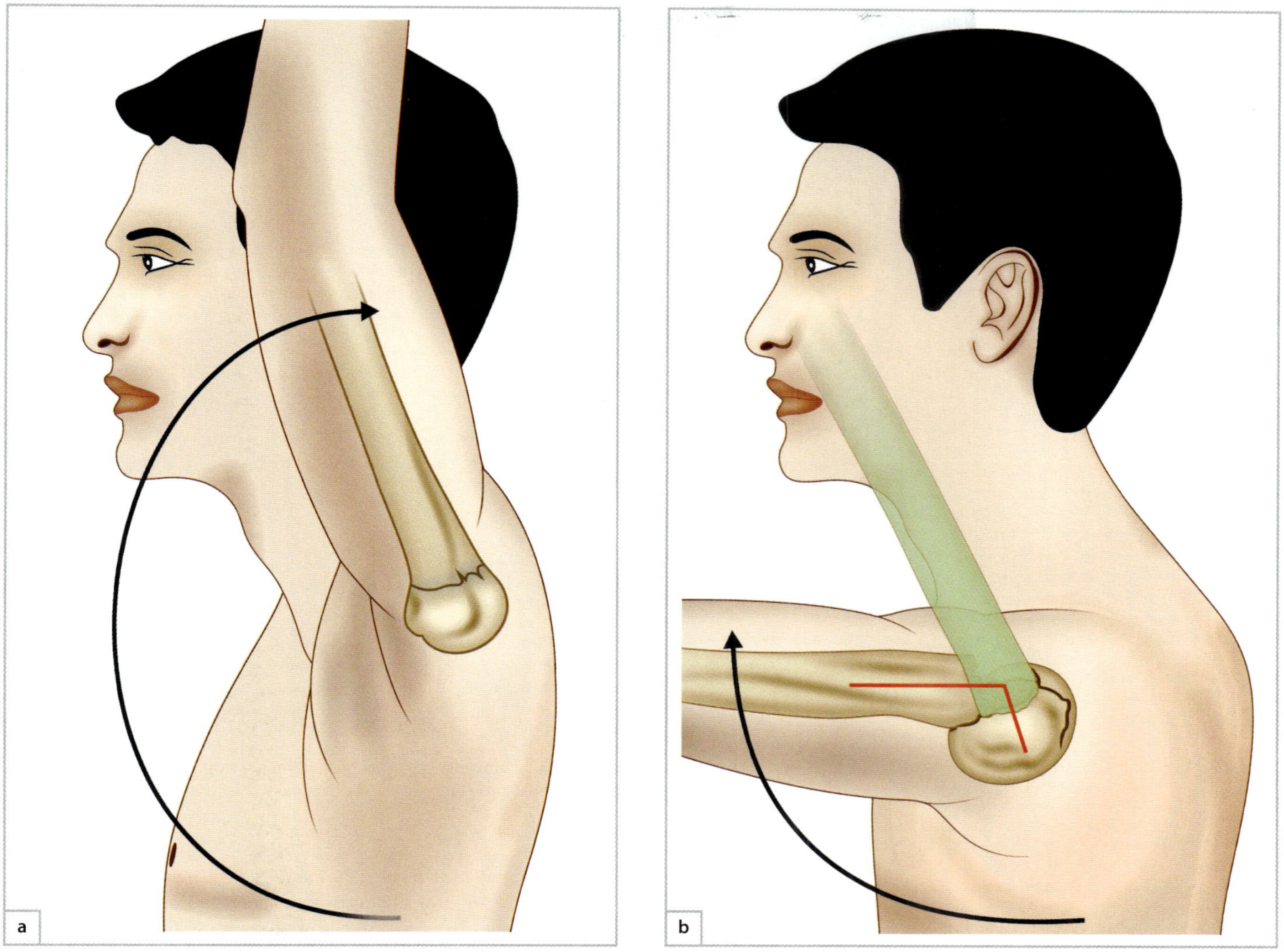

Figure 13.2 Malunion of the surgical neck. (a) Full range of motion is possible when anatomic aligment is achieved following a fracture of the surgical neck. (b) Apex anterior angulation (outlined angle) at the surgical neck will result in decreased forward elevation compared to normal, the latter shown in green.

their present condition. Low-demand patients with dysfunction but minimal pain may not benefit from extensive surgery to correct the bony anatomy.

In the setting of prior surgery, the presence of an undiagnosed infection must be ruled out carefully. An ongoing infection is a contraindication to definitive management of the malunion. Preoperative blood work, including a complete blood count with differential test, erythrocyte sedimentation rate, and C-reactive protein should be performed. If a fluid collection or joint effusion is present or suspected, an attempt to obtain an aspirate should be made, with the fluid sent for Gram stain, culture, and cell count. If the patient is taking antibiotics it will not be possible to obtain a reliable fluid sample. All cultures should be observed for 10–14 days to allow for growth of low-virulence organisms, such as *Propionibacterium acnes*. If a diagnosis of infection remains unclear, but is suspected, intraoperative frozen sections should be obtained before definitive management of the malunion. An extensive irrigation and debridement should be performed, followed by a six-week course of intravenous antibiotics, if infection is proven or highly suspected.

Other relative contraindications include malunions in severely debilitated patients, or patients with multiple medical comorbidities, patients with minimal ability to benefit from surgery because of neurologic or other functional impairment, and patients at high risk for local complications because of deficient soft tissues.

TECHNIQUE

Two-part malunion of the greater tuberosity

The size and position of the malunited fragments of the greater tuberosity will dictate the appropriate surgical approach. Arthroscopic techniques which include mobilization and reduction of a relatively small fragment with suture anchor fixation have been described (Ji et al. 2009). The patient can be positioned in either the beach-chair or lateral decubitus position, depending on surgeon preference. The malunited tuberosity is visualized from the subacromial space, and mobilized with a small osteotome placed through a lateral portal. The original fracture bed is abraded with a bur to remove fibrous tissue and to promote healing. Provisional reduction of the fragment is performed with a grasper to ensure excessive tension is not present due to adhesions. Fixation can be accomplished with a number of different suture configurations. We prefer a suture bridge, double-row repair technique, in order to create compression at the fracture site with the suture

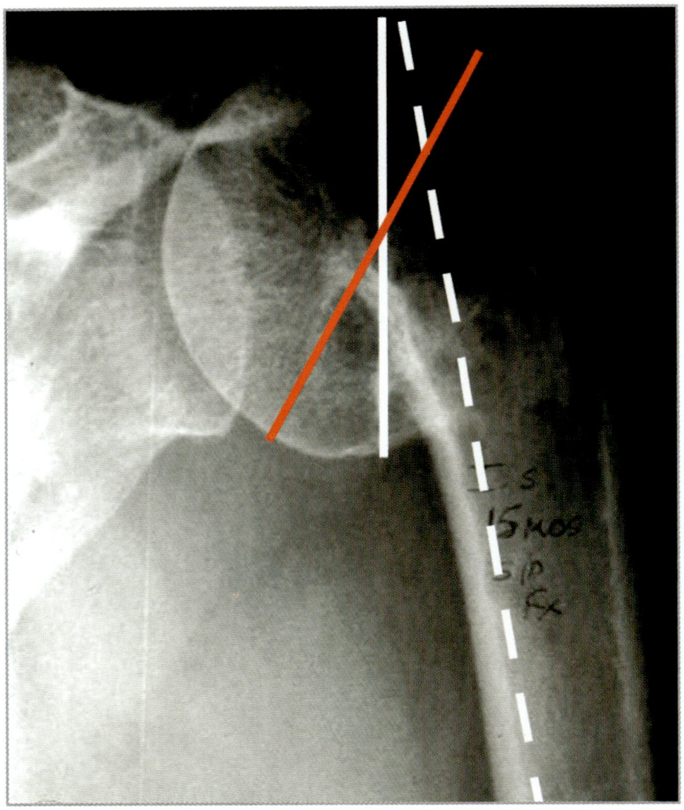

Figure 13.3 Varus malalignment. The degree of malalignment is determined by calculating the angle between the anatomic neck (white line) and the shaft of the humerus (dotted white line). This can be compared with the expected anatomic position of the surgical neck (red line).

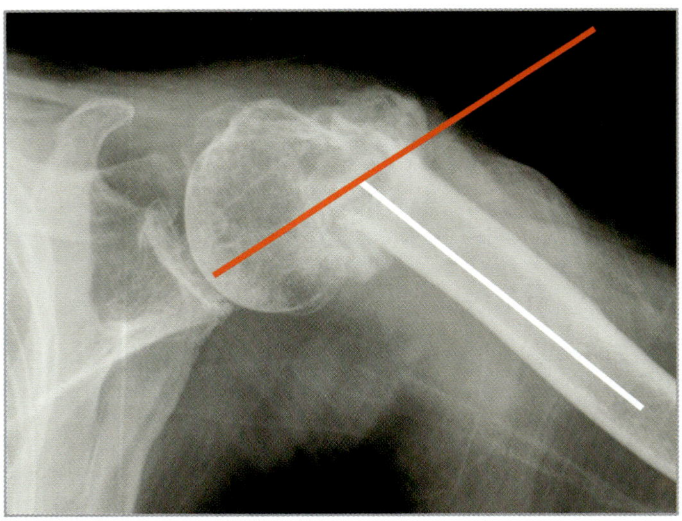

Figure 13.4 Sagittal plane deformity. The degree of deformity is determined calculating the angle between the alignment of the humeral head (red line) and the shaft of the humerus (white line).

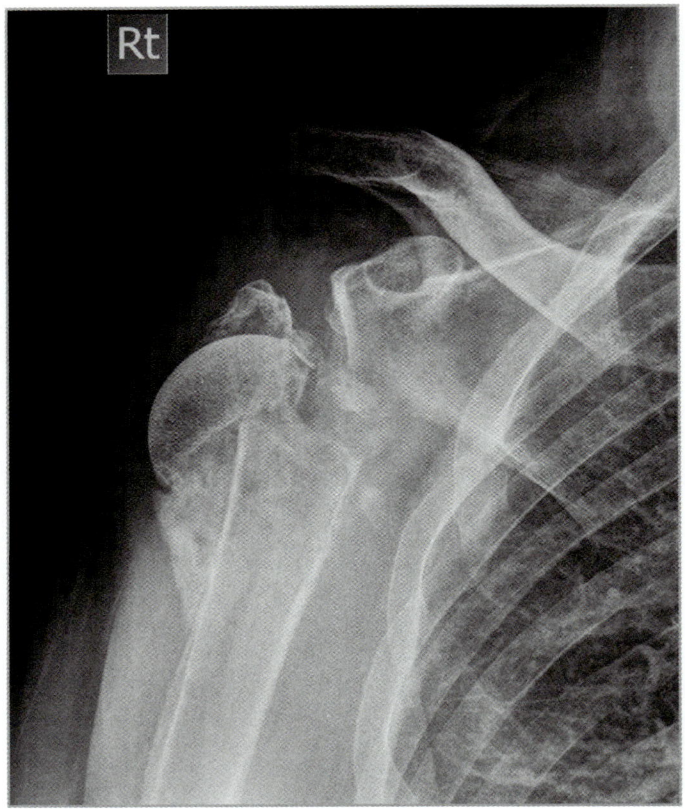

Figure 13.5 Four-part proximal humeral malunion. These can be associated with significant fracture displacement and abundant new bone formation.

fixation. A medial row of double-loaded suture anchors is first placed adjacent to the articular margin. The sutures are passed in a horizontal mattress fashion at the bone–tendon junction of the mobilized fragment and tied down, providing medial fixation of the tuberosity fragment. The suture limbs from these anchors can then be passed through and incorporated into a set of lateral row anchors that are placed approximately 5 mm distal to the lateral aspect of the reduced fracture fragment. This creates a compressive suture bridge over the fracture fragment, similar to more traditional open techniques. Additional fixation may be provided, if necessary, by passing and tying rotator interval sutures to better secure the anterior edge of the fracture. After fixation, the stability of the construct should be assessed under fluoroscopy and direction visualization through a full passive range of motion of the shoulder.

An alternative arthroscopic technique that may provide symptomatic relief in certain situations involves performing an isolated tuberoplasty, in order to avoid take-down of the malunion (Martinez et al. 2010). This typically requires elevation and subsequent reattachment of the rotator cuff insertion; however, transtendinous abrasion techniques have been described which minimize disruption of the cuff footprint (Calvo, Merino-Gutierrez et al. 2010).

Regardless of the chosen arthroscopic technique, all associated soft-tissue abnormalities should be addressed during arthroscopy, including performing a capsular release and lysis of adhesions if soft-tissue contractures are contributing to the patient's loss of motion, and subacromial decompression if impingement complaints are contributing to the patient's dysfunction.

Open techniques to manage malunions of the greater tuberosity are required for larger fragments with significant displacement and lateral extension of the fracture fragment. A superior approach is indicated for fragments of moderate size. The incision is made within the Langer's lines, and centered on the anterolateral corner of the acromion. The deltoid is detached from the anterior acromion for fracture exposure, and split no more than 4 cm distal to the acromion, to avoid injury to the axillary nerve. This limitation makes fixation of larger fragments or those with metaphyseal–diaphyseal extension difficult. For these fractures, the deltopectoral interval is preferred, owing to its extensile nature. This approach is also beneficial if an open capsular release and/or mobilization of subscapularis is required.

Mobilization of the greater tuberosity will typically require combined soft-tissue and bony dissection. The original fracture bed must be properly exposed, which may necessitate removal of both fibrous tissue and new bone formation. Tuberosity osteotomy may be needed if the fracture is well healed. When the malunion plane is adequately visualized, it can be marked with several drill holes, to ensure an osteotomy incorporates the entire malunited fragment (Craig 2004). Once the fragment has been freed up, temporary traction sutures placed at the bone–tendon junction of the rotator cuff insertion will assist the surgeon in translating the fragment anteriorly and inferiorly, to assess reduction and the need for further soft-tissue releases. The bicipital groove is a useful landmark to determine where the anterior aspect of the tuberosity should be reduced. In some cases where the greater tuberosity is severely displaced posterior to the humeral head, the posterior rotator cuff is retracted and scarred such that mobilization of the tendon and bone cannot be accomplished.

Fixation of the tuberosity will depend on the size of the fragment and the quality of the patient's bone. One or two interfragmentary screws with washers can be used if the tuberosity fragment is large and of good bone quality. Use of an anatomically contoured proximal humerus locking plate may even be indicated if it will provide better fixation than screw fixation alone. In either situation, supplemental suture fixation may still be advisable, and can be secured to the locking plate. Fixation with heavy non-absorbable suture alone should be utilized if screw placement is likely to cause fragmentation of the tuberosity fragment due to small size or poor bone quality. A combination of transosseous, simple horizontal and figure-of-eight vertical sutures will provide adequate compression of the fracture fragment, and minimize motion of the fragment postoperatively (**Fig. 13.6**). Sutures should be passed through the tendon–bone junction, to maximize fixation strength. This type of fixation avoids placement of sutures through the bone fragment itself, in order to decrease the risk of fragmentation of the tuberosity. As with the arthroscopic technique, additional fixation may be provided by repairing the rotator interval to improve stability. After fixation, the stability of the construct should be assessed under fluoroscopy and direction visualization through a full passive range of motion of the shoulder.

A proximal humerus locking plate may also be utilized for additional fixation in the setting of a small fragment of the tuberosity or a fragment with poor bone quality. In this situation, the plate is used as a buttress over the fragment (**Fig. 13.7**). The plate is secured distally by passing screws through the shaft holes, but screws holes are not filled to capture the tuberosity fragment, in order to avoid fragmentation of the piece. Suture fixation is still used in combination with the plate to secure the tuberosity, but can be passed through drill holes in bone, through the screw or suture holes in the plate, or through a combination of both.

Anatomic reduction of the fragment should eliminate subacromial impingement; however, the subacromial space should be assessed at the end of the case, and a decompression can be performed if necessary.

Two-part malunion of the lesser tuberosity

The deltopectoral approach provides excellent exposure for this malunion. The fragment is mobilized with techniques similar to those utilized with the greater tuberosity. Release of the underlying anterior capsule is required for mobilization when chronic retraction is present; however, care should be taken to avoid damage to the subscapularis tendon. The fragment of the lesser tuberosity should be carefully inspected after mobilization, as it can involve a portion of the articular surface. As with the greater tuberosity, fixation is accomplished with either interfragmentary screws or transosseous, heavy non-absorbable sutures passed through the tendon–bone junction, in order to maximize construct strength and to avoid fragmentation of the tuberosity. Gerber et al. (2006) advocated the use of a button plate to prevent suture cut-out through the cortical bone of the lateral proximal humerus when performing an osteotomy on the lesser tuberosity for shoulder arthroplasty. This may also be an option in the setting of a malunion, if bone quality is poor and there is concern about suture cut-out.

Two-part malunion of the surgical neck

Adequate surgical exposure can again be obtained with the deltopectoral approach. The malunion site should be exposed and mobilized with techniques similar to those utilized with the greater and lesser tuberosities. The commonly encountered varus malunion can be managed with a laterally based valgus closing-wedge osteotomy, supplemented with a neutralization T-plate (**Fig. 13.8**) (Solonen and Vastamaki 1985, Benegas et al. 2007). We prefer application of a precontoured proximal humerus locking plate for improved fixation. The osteotomy can be biplanar if correction of apex anterior angulation is also necessary. Traction sutures passed through the bone–tendon junction of the greater and lesser tuberosities can again assist with fracture reduction prior to definitive fixation and plate placement, and can be sutured to the proximal humerus plate at the end of the operation to provide additional fixation. If bone from the osteotomy is insufficient for adequate bony contact and grafting, iliac crest autograft should be obtained to enhance healing.

An alternative technique has been used to correct congenital varus deformity (Gill and Waters 1997). A closing-wedge osteomy is performed, with care to ensure the medial periosteal hinge is not disrupted. Closing wedge osteotomy requires pre-operative templating and planning that is best accomplished with 3D CT scan modeling. 3D surgical planning software, custom patient-specific models for pre-operative planning and patient-specific guides are currently available to assist the surgeon in the execution of the operative procedure. These methods aid in the 3D correction of the deformity and are preferred over biplanar 2D radiographs. Fixation is achieved with two retrograde Kirschner wires (K-wires) passed into the humeral head and a figure-of-eight tension band with heavy non-absorbable suture. This fixation may not be adequate in an adult patient.

If post-traumatic arthritis or avascular necrosis is present, hemiarthroplasty or reverse total shoulder arthroplasty is indicated, depending on bone loss and the status of the tuberosity. In either case, an open capsular release performed at the start of the surgery will likely be necessary to restore passive motion.

Three- and four-part malunions

The deltopectoral approach is again the preferred surgical approach, as it allows adequate exposure to all elements of the malunion. Release of subacromial and subdeltoid adhesions should be performed, followed by an assessment of the degree of capsular contracture. An extensive capsular release is typically required to permit adequate

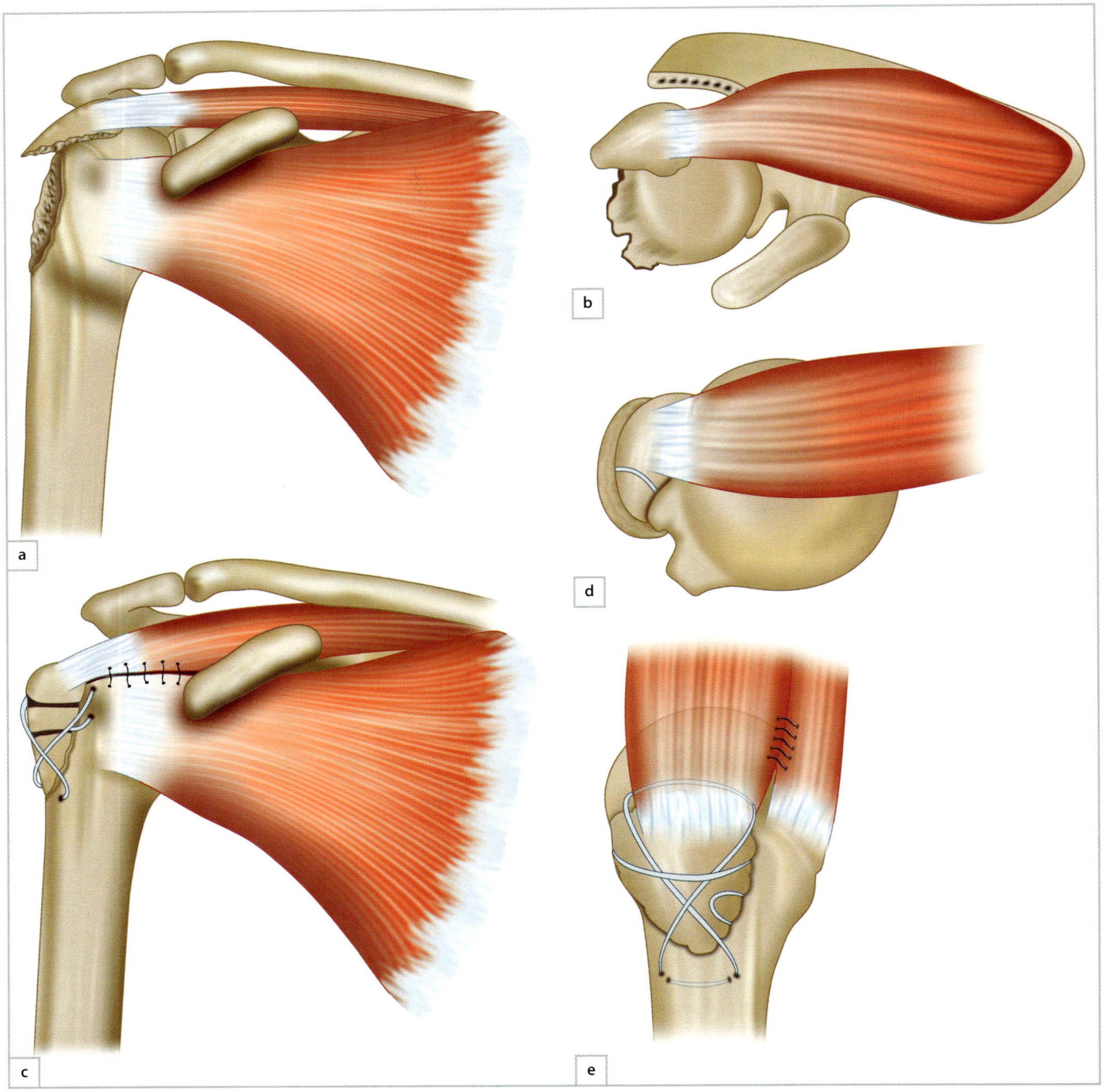

Figure 13.6 Fixation of a malunion of the greater tuberosity. (a,b) Superior and posterior displacement is seen with isolated fractures of the greater tuberosity. (c–e) Fixation of the reduced fragment can be achieved with transosseus horizontal sutures and vertical figure-of-eight sutures. (Redrawn from Warner JJP, Iannotti JP, Flatow EL, eds. Complex and Revision Problems in Shoulder Surgery, 2nd edn. Philadelphia: Lippincott, Williams and Wilkins, 2005.)

range of motion. The condition of the rotator cuff must be carefully inspected, and, if necessary, the cuff repaired.

Mobilization of the malunited fragments and subsequent fixation with a precontoured proximal humerus locking plate is possible when excellent bone stock is present, utilizing the techniques described above. However, some form of prosthetic replacement is commonly required for treatment of three- and four-part malunions, particularly if post-traumatic arthritis or avascular necrosis is present. The malposition of the tuberosities can occasionally be tolerated by adjusting the level of the humeral osteotomy (**Fig. 13.9**). Additionally, the use of an eccentric head component or an eccentrically cemented humeral stem will help accommodate the distorted anatomy. Resurfacing of the humeral head can also be performed if placement of a stemmed implant is not desired (**Fig. 13.10**). Osteotomy of the tuberosities is required if modified placement of the humeral component does not adequately recreate the patient's anatomy (**Fig. 13.11**); however, poor functional results have been reported when osteotomy of the greater tuberosity is required in the setting of severe malunion (Boileau et al. 2006). The bicipital groove is an important anatomic landmark for tuberosity osteotomy, and care

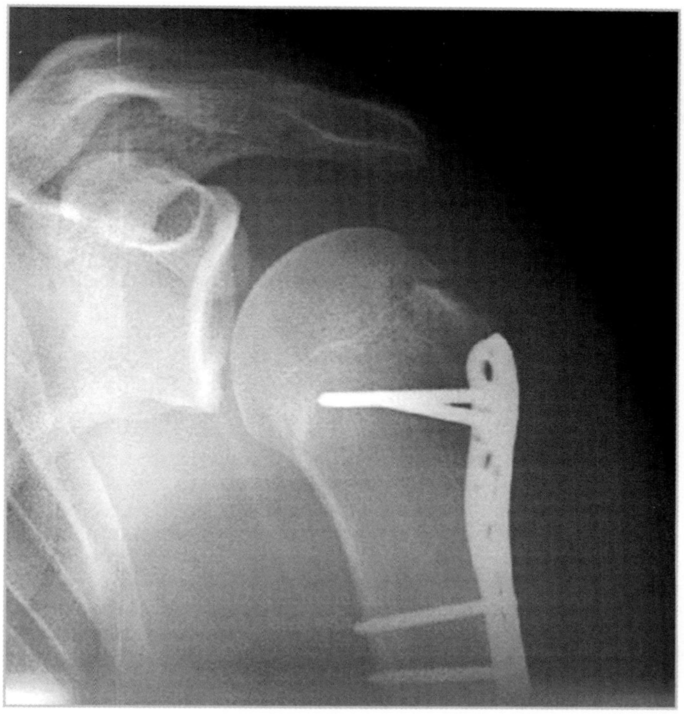

Figure 13.7 Fixation of the greater tuberosity. The greater tuberosity can be secured with buttress plate fixation, augmented with non-absorbable sutures placed through the tendon–bone junction.

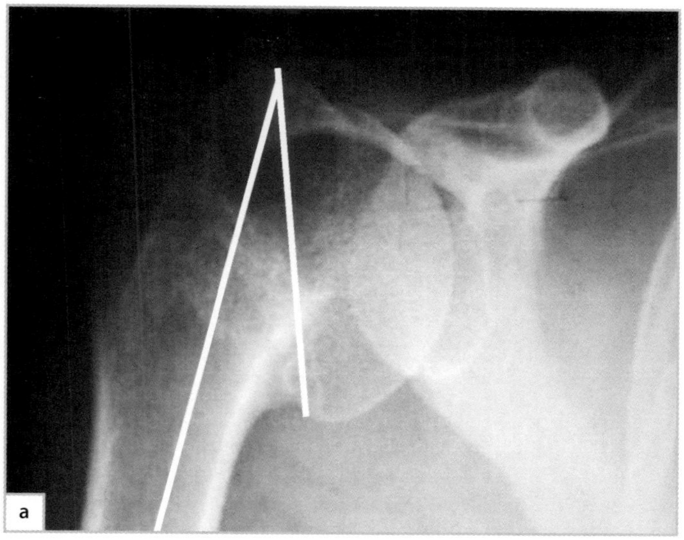

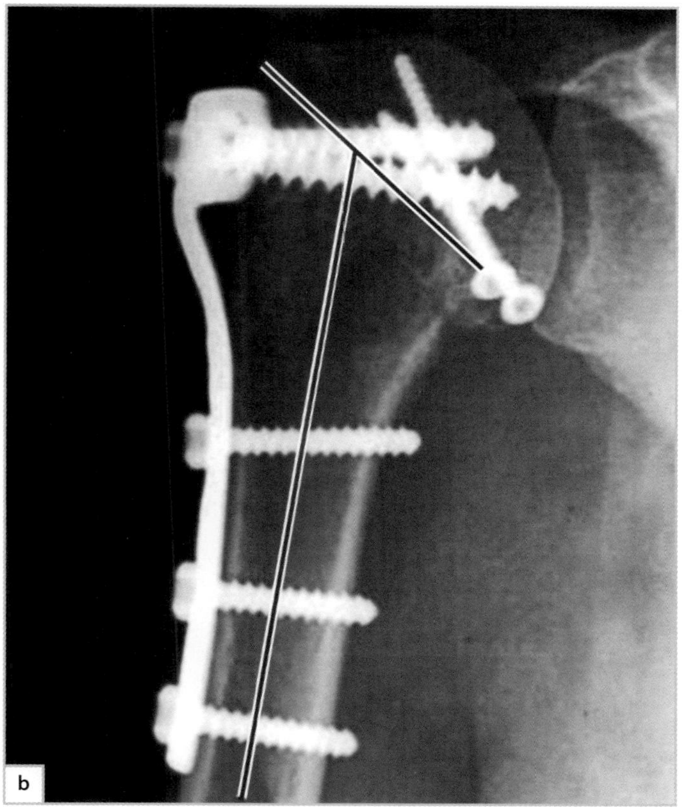

Figure 13.8 Varus malunion can be corrected with a laterally based closing-wedge osteotomy to restore anatomic alignment. (a) Preoperative and (b) postoperative radiographs.

should be taken to err on the side of producing large fragments of tuberosity. Creation of small fragments should be avoided, as there will be only small bony surface areas for healing. Complete release of scar tissue around the rotator cuff tendons is essential to restore the tuberosities to their anatomic position, and to allow a tension-free tuberosity repair. Fixation of the mobilized tuberosities is similar to that performed for acute fractures, as described elsewhere in this book (see also Mighell et al. 2003). Placement of a glenoid component is indicated prior to fixation of the tuberosities if significant glenoid arthrosis is present, and can be performed more easily by displacing the greater tuberosity posteriorly and the shaft anteriorly, giving a direct view of the glenoid.

Reverse shoulder arthroplasty should be performed when adequate mobilization of the tuberosity fragments is not possible, or if irreparable cuff defects are present (**Fig. 13.12**) (Martin and Iannotti 2008). Reverse shoulder arthroplasty may also be indicated when osteotomy of the greater tuberosity is required, when the tuberosity cannot be mobilized sufficiently to place it in anatomic position, or when there are premorbid tears in the rotator cuff. In these settings, a reverse total shoulder replacement will yield better functional results than non-constrained shoulder arthroplasty (Boileau et al. 2006). Careful attention should be paid to the bony anatomy of the glenoid preoperatively, to ensure adequate fixation of the glenoid sphere is possible. External rotation will be improved if the posterior rotator cuff or greater tuberosity is reattached, and stability is enhanced if the subscapularis or lesser tuberosity is repaired; however, this may not be possible, due to contracture.

Pearls and pitfalls

Pearls

- The operative shoulder should be positioned off the side of the table, and supported with a mechanical arm-holding device, to ensure that appropriate arm positioning and access to all components of the deformity are possible.
- Knowledge of the location of neurovascular structures is critical. Failure to identify the axillary nerve, musculocutaneous nerve, and humeral circumflex vessels may lead to neurovascular injury, particularly if dissection strays too far medially.
- Muscle paralysis may improve visualization, mobilization, and reduction of the fracture fragments; however, the risk of iatrogenic neurologic injury may be increased.
- Intraoperative fluoroscopy is necessary to confirm adequate correction of the malunion; the unit should be positioned to allow orthogonal views of the proximal humerus.

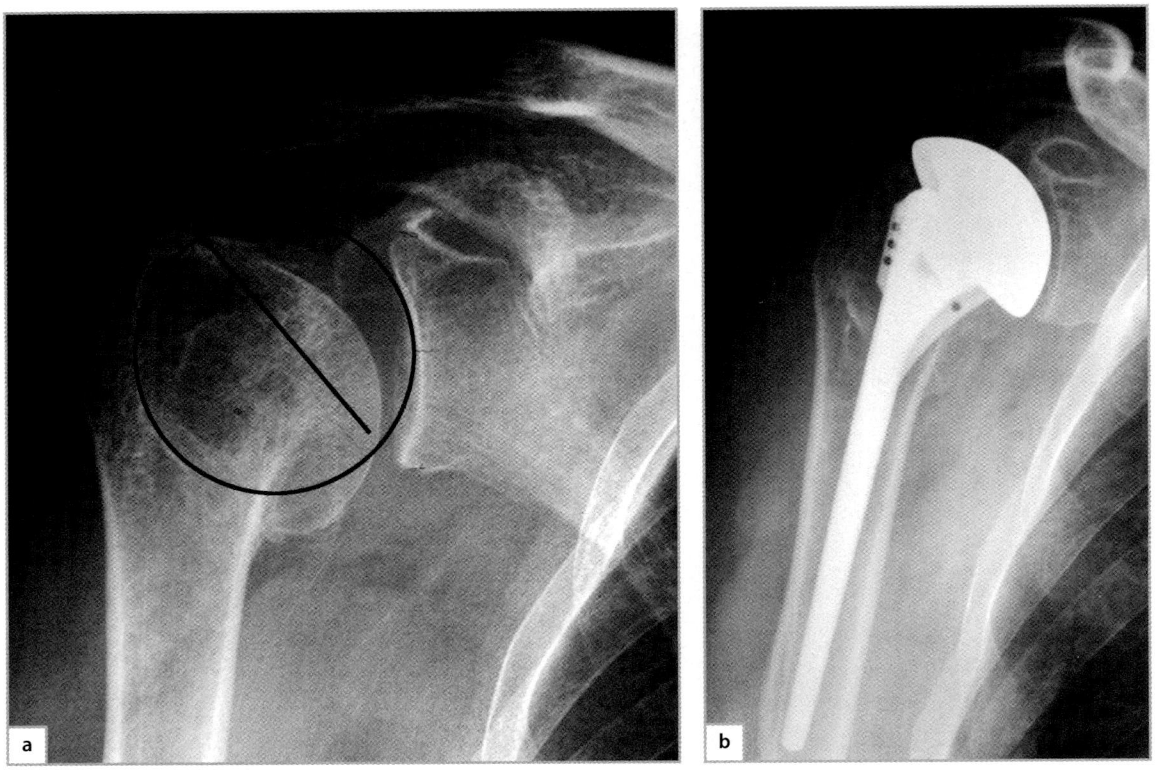

Figure 13.9 Hemiarthroplasty for malposition of the tuberosities, performed with an adjusted humeral osteotomy. (a) Preoperative planning for a hemiarthroplasty will require an adjusted humeral osteotomy to place the prosthetic humeral head in a more anatomic position relative to the tuberosities and humeral shaft. (b) Postoperative radiograph of a hemiarthroplasty performed with an adjusted humeral osteotomy without mobilization of the tuberosities.

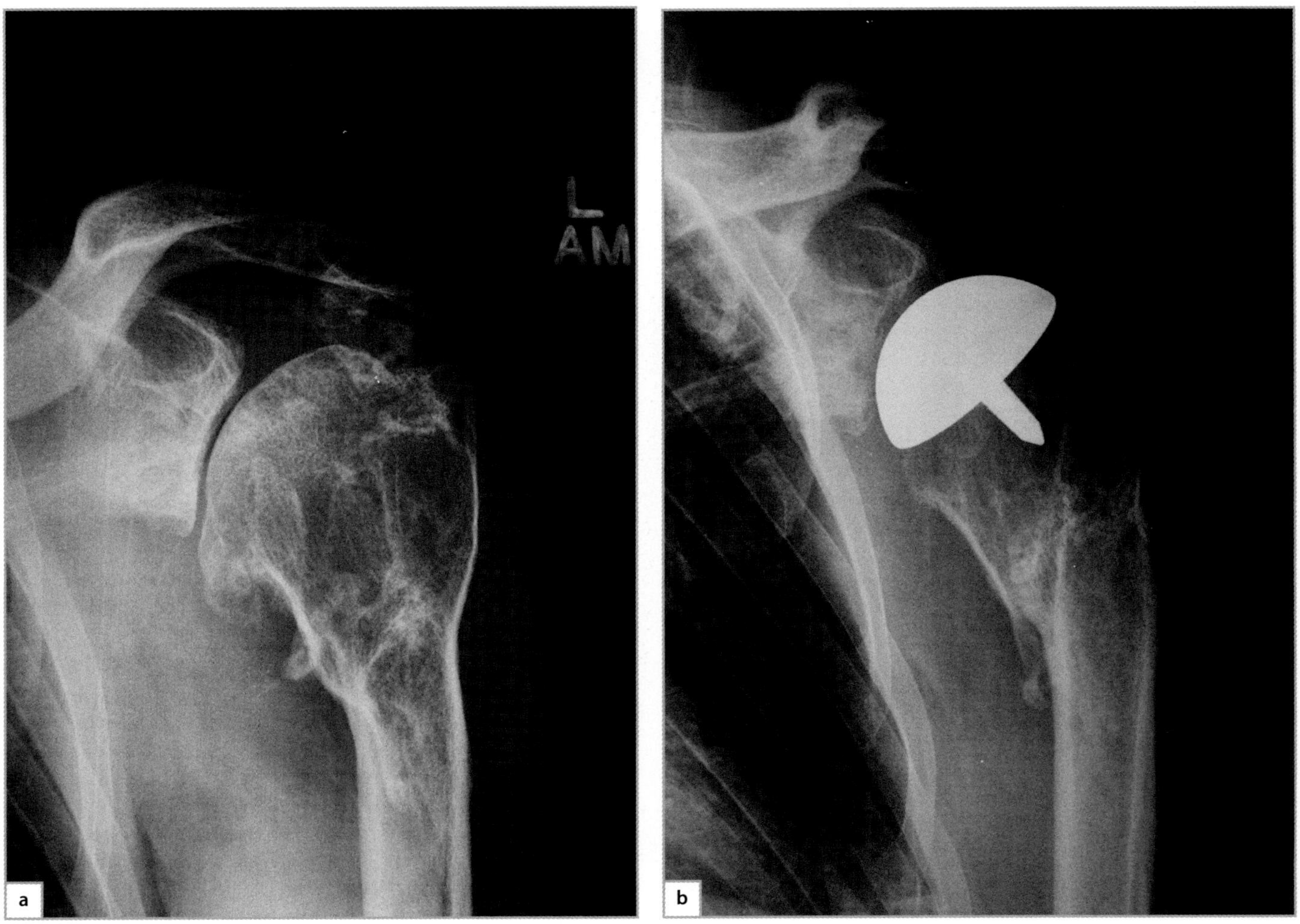

Figure 13.10 Malunion of the proximal humerus managed with humeral head resurfacing. (a) Preoperative and (b) postoperative anteroposterior radiographs.

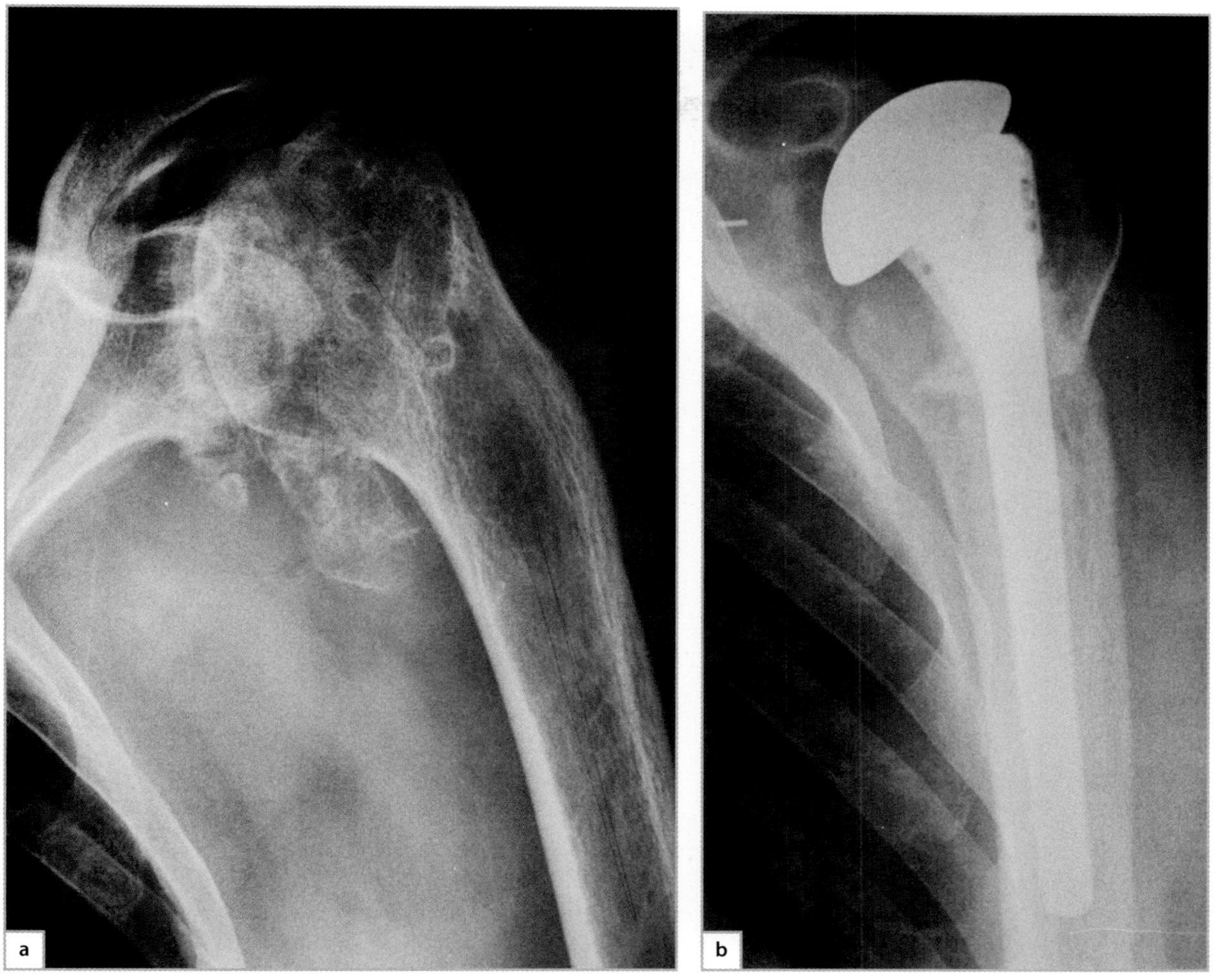

Figure 13.11 Management of a malunion of the proximal humerus with malposition of the greater tuberosity. (a) Preoperative radiograph of proximal humerus malunion, demonstrating complete loss of joint space with malposition of the greater tuberosity. (b) Postoperative radiograph of total shoulder arthroplasty performed with osteotomy of the greater tuberosity secured with heavy non-absorbable suture placed around the stem of the prosthesis.

- The bicipital groove is an important anatomic landmark for defining the greater and lesser tuberosity prior to performing tuberosity osteotomy.
- Rotator cuff sutures can be utilized for fracture mobilization and reduction, as well as for definitive fixation. Heavy non-absorbable sutures should be passed through the bone–tendon junction of the rotator cuff, to avoid cut-out through bone and tuberosity fragmentation. These sutures can also be used in combination with a proximal humerus locking plate for added construct stability. The sutures can be tied down through the peripheral holes in the locking plate to help neutralize the deforming forces of the rotator cuff.
- Fracture fixation should be assessed during shoulder range of motion prior to wound closure, under both direct visualization and fluoroscopy, to ensure adequate fixations with no motion across the fracture site(s).
- Shoulder arthroplasty may be required for treatment of proximal humerus malunions, particularly if post-traumatic arthritis, avascular necrosis, or significant bone loss is present. A reverse shoulder arthoplasty should be available when adequate mobilization of tuberosity fragments is not possible, tuberosity osteotomy is needed, or irreparable cuff defects are present.

Pitfalls

- Inadequate preoperative imaging will compromise surgical planning.
- Low-grade infections can easily be missed in patients with a prior surgical history and inadequate work-up.
- Creation of small fragments of tuberosity during mobilization results in minimal surface contact for bony healing, and should be avoided.
- Unless shoulder arthroplasty is performed, the blood supply to the humeral head must be preserved. Excessive exposure and soft-tissue stripping of the fracture fragments may result in interruption of the blood supply to the fragments, particularly if the posteromedial soft-tissue sleeve is disrupted.
- Failure to address all soft-tissue contractures during surgical intervention may result in poor functional results, from limited range of motion, even if the bony malunion has been adequately corrected.
- Prolonged postoperative immobilization may lead to recurrence of soft-tissue contractures despite correction of the osseous abnormalities.

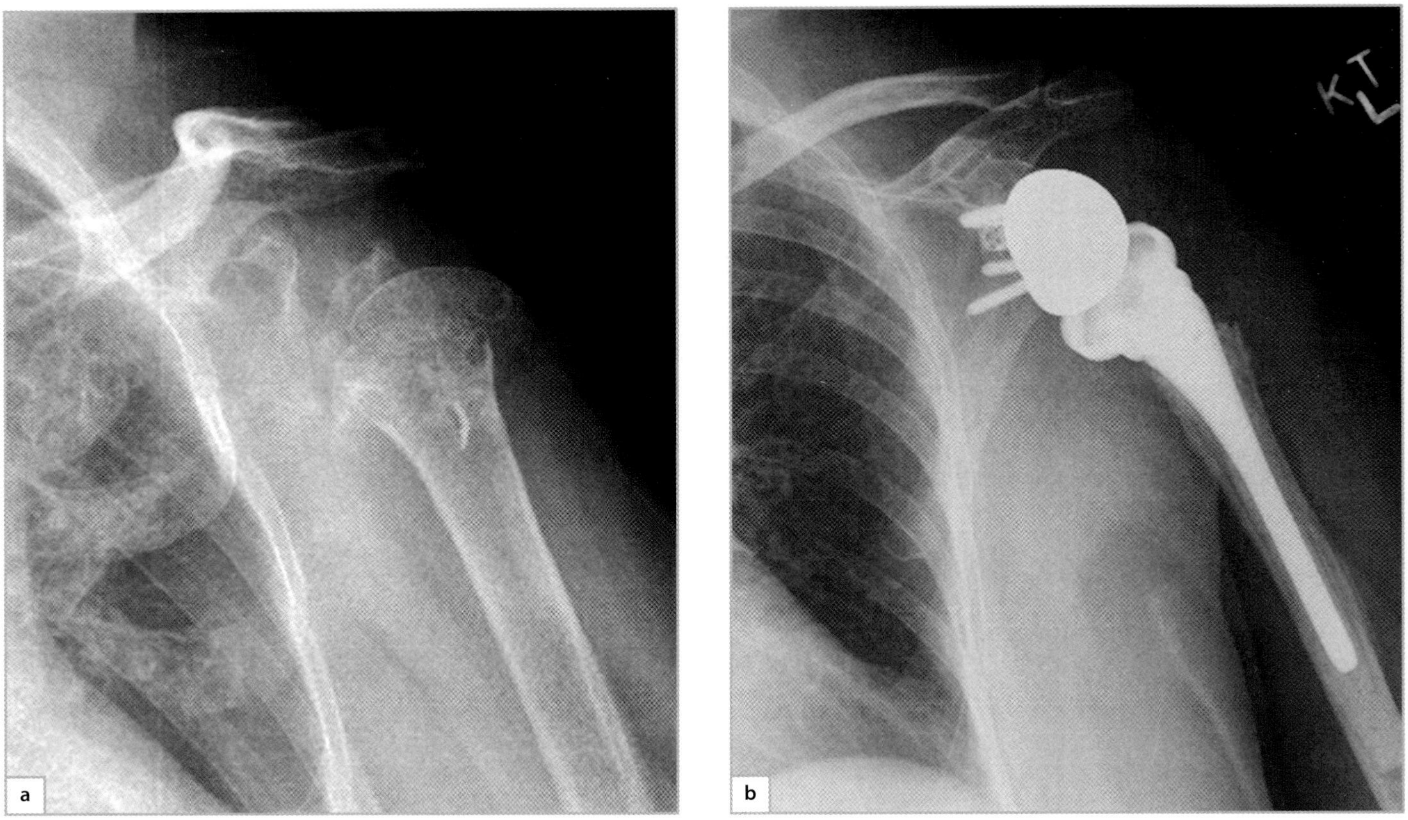

Figure 13.12 Management of a four-part valgus impacted malunion of the proximal humerus with medial malposition of the greater and lesser tuberosities. (a) Anteroposterior radiograph. (b) Postoperative radiograph following reverse shoulder arthroplasty.

REHABILITATION

Rehabilitation begins with passive and active assisted range-of-motion (ROM) exercises in forward flexion and external rotation, typically performed supine initially and started within the first two weeks postoperatively. Patients can usually be taught how to perform these exercises on their own at home. Overaggressive formal physiotherapy should be avoided during this early postoperative period, as it may lead to loss of fracture reduction or construct failure. Active ROM of the elbow, wrist, and hand can also be started in the early postoperative period, to avoid the development of stiffness in the distal part of the extremity. If reduction of the greater tuberosity was difficult due to soft-tissue contracture, the patient may be placed in an abduction orthosis to prevent excessive internal rotation and adduction. In this situation, internal rotation to the abdomen is delayed for four weeks.

Active shoulder ROM exercises begin at approximately four to six weeks postoperatively, and include stretching exercises in all planes (forward flexion and extension, external and internal rotation, abduction and adduction). Strengthening or resistive exercises are not initiated on the shoulder until approximately 10–12 weeks postoperatively, when significant bony consolidation is confirmed on plain radiographs and adequate coordination of the extremity has been achieved. Shoulder ROM should be maximal or near maximal at that point. Comparison of active versus passive ROM will help identify the presence of either muscle weakness or soft-tissue contractures. Resistive exercises are used to strengthen the rotator cuff, deltoid, and scapula, and are advanced as tolerated. Return to unrestricted activity with the operative extremity occurs five or six months postoperatively.

Serial radiographs, including standard anteroposterior, axillary, and scapular Y radiographic views of the shoulder, should be obtained during the rehabilitation to follow fracture healing, to rule out loss of fixation, to evaluate for signs of post-traumatic arthritis or avascular necrosis, and to detect signs of implant loosening if a shoulder arthroplasty was performed.

CONCLUSION

The ideal treatment for malunions of the proximal humerus is prevention by proper management of acute injuries. The expected result from operative intervention for a malunion depends on the ability of the surgeon to restore the patient's bony anatomy and correct all associated soft-tissue pathology. The best outcomes can be expected when the malunion involves a single tuberosity and all soft-tissue abnormalities are corrected. In this setting, pain relief is reliably achieved, and functional capacity is improved in 75% of patients (Beredjiklian et al. 1998). More complex malunions requiring arthroplasty are associated with an increased complication rate and poorer functional outcomes; however, reverse shoulder arthroplasty holds promise for improved outcomes with these conditions (Boileau et al. 2006). Prior to any surgical intervention for a malunion of the proximal humerus, the surgeon must establish realistic goals with the patient, as this population does not uniformly achieve complete recovery following surgery.

REFERENCES

Benegas E, Zoppi Filho A, Ferreira Filho AA, et al. Surgical treatment of varus malunion of the proximal humerus with valgus osteotomy. J Shoulder Elbow Surg 2007;16:55–59.

Beredjiklian PK, Iannotti JP. Treatment of proximal humerus fracture malunion with prosthetic arthroplasty. Instr Course Lect 1998;47:135–140.

Beredjiklian PK, Iannotti JP, Norris TR, Williams GR. Operative treatment of malunion of a fracture of the proximal aspect of the humerus. J Bone Joint Surg Am 1998;80:1484–1497.

Boileau P, Chuinard C, Le Huec JC, et al. Proximal humerus fracture sequelae: impact of a new radiographic classification on arthroplasty. Clin Orthop Relat Res 2006;442:121–130.

Bono CM, Renard R, Levine RG, Levy AS. Effect of displacement of fractures of the greater tuberosity on the mechanics of the shoulder. J Bone Joint Surg Br 2001;83:1056–1062.

Calvo E, Merino-Gutierrez I, Lagunes I. Arthroscopic tuberoplasty for subacromial impingement secondary to proximal humeral malunion. Knee Surg Sports Traumatol Arthrosc 2010;18:988–991.

Craig EV. The Shoulder. Philadelphia, PA: Lippincott, Williams & Wilkins, 2004.

Duralde XA, Flatow EL, Pollock RG, et al. Operative treatment of nonunions of the surgical neck of the humerus. J Shoulder Elbow Surg 1996;5:169–180.

Gerber C, Pennington SD, Yian EH, et al. Lesser tuberosity osteotomy for total shoulder arthroplasty. Surgical technique. J Bone Joint Surg Am 2006;88 Suppl 1 Pt 2:170–177.

Gill TJ, Waters P. Valgus osteotomy of the humeral neck: a technique for the treatment of humerus varus. J Shoulder Elbow Surg 1997;6:306–310.

Hayes PR, Klepps S, Bishop J, et al. Posterior shoulder dislocation with lesser tuberosity and scapular spine fractures. J Shoulder Elbow Surg 2003;12:524–527.

Iannotti JP, Williams GR. Disorders of the Shoulder: Diagnosis and Management. Philadelphia, PA: Lippincott, Williams & Wilkins, 2007.

Jeong J, Bryan J, Iannotti JP. Effect of a variable prosthetic neck–shaft angle and the surgical technique on replication of normal humeral anatomy. J Bone Joint Surg Am 2009;91:1932–1941.

Ji JH, Moon CY, Kim YY, Shafi M. Arthroscopic fixation for a malunited greater tuberosity fracture using the suture-bridge technique: technical report and literature review. Knee Surg Sports Traumatol Arthrosc 2009;17:1473–1476.

Martin TG, Iannotti JP. Reverse total shoulder arthroplasty for acute fractures and failed management after proximal humeral fractures. Orthop Clin North Am 2008;39:451–457.

Martinez AA, Calvo A, Domingo J, et al. Arthroscopic treatment for malunions of the proximal humeral greater tuberosity. Int Orthop 2010;34:1207–1211.

Mighell MA, Kolm GP, Collinge CA, Frankle MA. Outcomes of hemiarthroplasty for fractures of the proximal humerus. J Shoulder Elbow Surg 2003;12:569–577.

Neer CS 2nd. Displaced proximal humeral fractures. I. Classification and evaluation. J Bone Joint Surg Am 1970;52:1077–1089.

Paschal SO, Hutton KS, Weatherall PT. Isolated avulsion fracture of the lesser tuberosity of the humerus in adolescents. A report of two cases. J Bone Joint Surg Am 1995;77:1427–1430.

Solonen KA, Vastamaki M. Osteotomy of the neck of the humerus for traumatic varus deformity. Acta Orthop Scand 1985;56:79–80.

van Laarhoven HA, te Slaa RL, van Laarhoven EW. Isolated avulsion fracture of the lesser tuberosity of the humerus. J Trauma 1995;39:997–999.

Chapter 14 Operative management of locked anterior and posterior dislocations

Clayton Riley, Arnaldo I. Rodríguez-Santiago, T. Bradley Edwards

INTRODUCTION

Locked or fixed shoulder dislocations are uncommon. They may be anterior or posterior (**Figs 14.1, 14.2**) and usually occur within two distinct subsets of patient. Younger patients (< 60 years) may present with a chronically dislocated shoulder because the diagnosis was missed. Often these patients have sustained multiple traumatic injuries, and the shoulder dislocation was not recognized until concomitant injuries had been stabilized.

The second subset includes elderly patients who have dislocated their shoulder and usually sustained a concomitant massive rotator cuff tear, contributing to the instability. The dislocation may have been initially reduced, but later recurred, with the shoulder remaining dislocated for an indeterminate amount of time. In addition to the massive rotator cuff tear often sustained by the elderly patient, rapidly appearing osteoarthritis may occur with or without glenoid erosion. This chapter details the management of chronic anterior and posterior glenohumeral dislocations in both of these patient populations.

INDICATIONS

Anterior dislocations

Chronic anterior dislocations can have a constellation of associated injury components. The varied presentation and lack of distinctly superior treatment options make these dislocations difficult to manage. Although the length of time necessary to define a dislocation as chronic (locked, fixed, neglected) has ranged from several days to six months, we generally use three weeks as a guide (Sahajpal and Zuckerman 2008). Once there has been a prolonged duration of dislocation, attempts at closed reduction will most likely be unsuccessful, and can actually cause further damage, such as fracture.

Younger patients

It is rare to see a chronic anterior dislocation in young patients. Treatment options are directed at the underlying pathology. Open reduction

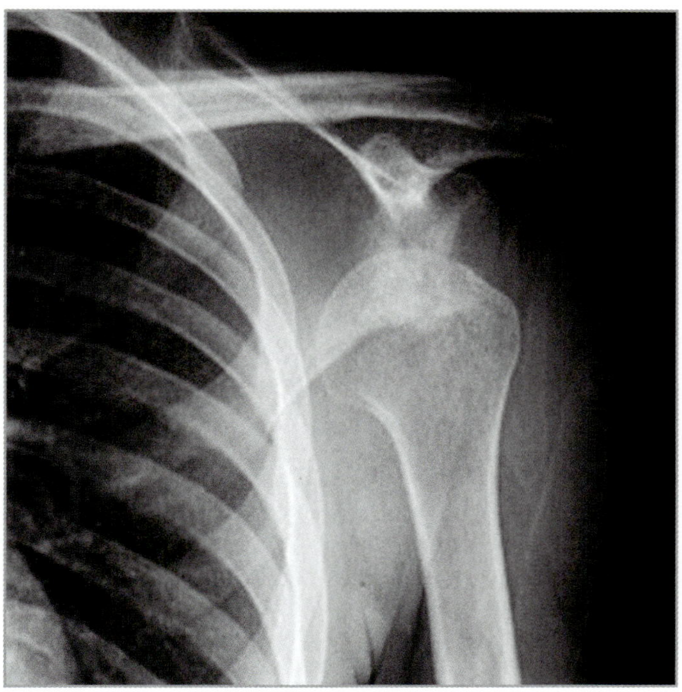

Figure 14.1 Radiograph depicting a chronic anterior shoulder dislocation.

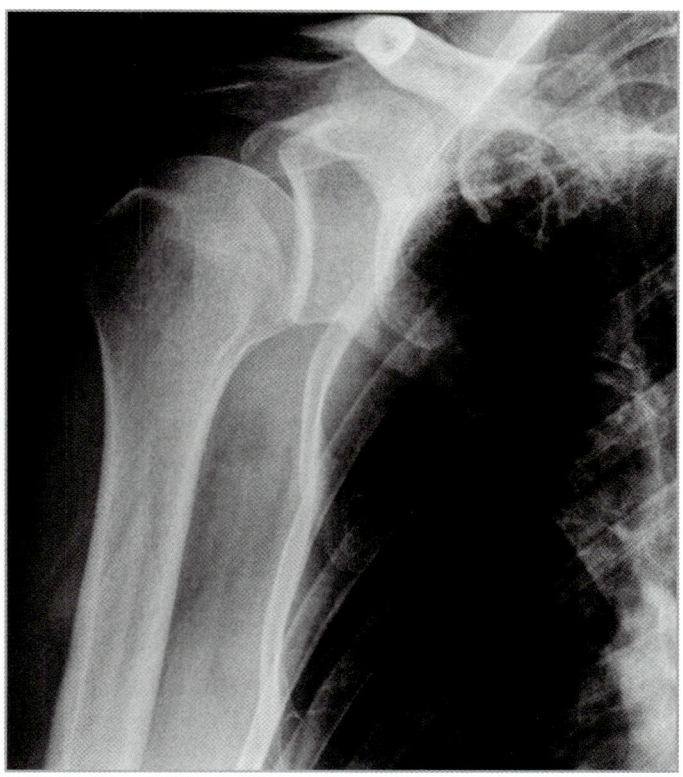

Figure 14.2 Radiograph depicting a chronic posterior dislocation. Note the overlap of articular surfaces of the humeral head and glenoid, confirming the dislocation.

alone with appropriate postoperative immobilization may be all that is necessary if no significant concomitant injuries are identified that will compromise stability, in which case additional procedures are indicated to ensure stability.

Soft-tissue disruption and contracture will be encountered in most cases of chronic anterior dislocation (Oyston 1964). Disruption of the anterior inferior capsulolabral structures (the Bankart lesion) is an indication for open capsulolabral repair. Concomitant posterior capsular contractures should be released at the time of open reduction. Rotator cuff tears are rare in younger patients, but should be repaired at the time of open reduction when they do occur. These tears may involve the subscapularis, but can also involve the posterior superior rotator cuff.

Anteroinferior glenoid deficiency is commonly seen with chronic anterior dislocations. When this occurs, capsulolabral repair alone is insufficient, and a procedure to restore glenoid surface area will be required (Griggs et al. 1999). This can be accomplished with a coracoid transfer procedure or iliac crest bone graft. We prefer the Latarjet-type coracoid transfer to address most cases of glenoid bone loss. In situations in which the glenoid bone defect is greater than one third of the normal glenoid anteroposterior diameter, we perform a capsulolabral repair combined with a glenoid reconstruction using extracapsular iliac crest bone graft.

Impression fractures of the humeral head cause defects that will inevitably need to be addressed once they compromise over 20% of the articular surface. Defects over 40% will most often require replacement of the head. In patients with small defects of the humeral head (less than 20% of the articular surface), we prefer use of the Latarjet procedure to increase the anteroposterior diameter of the glenoid, as this makes it more difficult for the lesion to engage on the anterior glenoid and dislocate the glenohumeral joint. For larger defects, we opt for some type of arthroplasty. In patients under the age of 40, we prefer an allograft replacement of the defect. In patients older than 40 years, we perform a prosthetic replacement of the humeral head.

Older patients

While many of the same procedures described for younger patients can be utilized in a select group of older patients, most will require prosthetic replacement. The older population tends to present with longer duration of dislocation and, often, significant articular degeneration. Massive rotator cuff tears frequently accompany the dislocation. Severe bone loss of the glenoid and/or humerus may also occur. These conditions, along with other indications for arthroplasty, such as age and activity level, make prosthetic replacement the best choice for older patients. Prosthetic options include hemiarthroplasty, unconstrained total shoulder arthroplasty, and reverse shoulder arthroplasty. It has been our experience that unconstrained shoulder arthroplasty leads to a high rate of recurrent instability (Matsoukis et al. 2006). This high rate of recurrent instability, the frequent presence of massive rotator cuff tears, and the occasional need for glenoid bone grafting have led us to use a reverse prosthesis as the implant of choice in this population of patients (Gartsman and Edwards 2008a).

Posterior dislocations

Like chronic anterior dislocations, locked posterior dislocations can have a constellation of associated injuries. Furthermore, once there has been a prolonged duration of dislocation, attempts at closed reduction will most likely be unsuccessful, and can actually cause further damage. Several operative treatment options are available for the patient with a locked posterior glenohumeral dislocation; multiple factors will influence the selection of preferred procedure. Factors that must be assessed include patient age, duration of the dislocation, presence of associated bony lesions (humerus and glenoid), presence of associated soft-tissue lesions (rotator cuff, capsuloligamentous structures, labrum), and the presence of glenohumeral arthritis. In general, patients with fixed posterior dislocations tend to be younger than patients with fixed anterior dislocations.

Younger patients

Open surgical treatment is usually necessary for posterior glenohumeral dislocations that have been present for more than three weeks. When the joint remains unstable after open reduction, a specific procedure to restore stability must be undertaken. A residual large impression fracture of the humeral head is characteristic following open reduction of a fixed posterior dislocation. Stability is compromised when the impression fracture approaches 20% of the humeral articular surface, and so a stabilization procedure will be required. We prefer transfer of the subscapularis tendon into the osseous void for cases in which the humeral head defect is between 20% and 40% of the articular surface (McLaughlin 1952). Alternatively, Neer's modification with transfer of the lesser tuberosity into the defect can be performed. Prosthetic replacement is indicated when more than 40% of the articular surface is involved, or when there is significant cartilage degeneration of the remaining articular surfaces (regardless of the defect size).

Older patients

Fixed posterior dislocations in older patients are similar to fixed anterior dislocations, in that massive rotator cuff tears and glenohumeral arthritis often accompany the dislocation. In this scenario, as in cases of fixed anterior dislocations in older patients, we prefer to use a reverse prosthesis to address the instability, rotator cuff pathology, and glenohumeral arthritis.

CONTRAINDICATIONS

Contraindications to surgical treatment of locked shoulder dislocation using the procedures described include presence of significant medical comorbidities presenting an unacceptable surgical risk, patients unable to participate in the required postoperative rehabilitation program, neurologic impairment preventing use of the shoulder, active infection, and insufficient bone stock to allow performance of the prescribed procedure.

TECHNIQUE

General principles

Room setup and patient positioning

Proper patient positioning is crucial during shoulder surgery. We use a standard operating table with the patient positioned sufficiently to the operative side to allow extension of the arm. If an arthroplasty procedure is planned, a rolled sheet is placed between the scapulae, to slightly elevate the shoulder off the operating table and to allow proper preparation of the posterior aspect of the shoulder. If a coracoid transfer is planned, a flat sheet is placed beneath the ipsilateral scapula, to make the coracoid process more readily palpable.

The patient is placed in the modified beach-chair position, with the back of the table elevated approximately 45–60° relative to the floor. The position of the patient's head and neck is checked to ensure neutral alignment before they are secured.

The area included in the surgical preparation extends medially to the midline, distally to the level of the nipple, and proximally to the level of the mandible, and encompasses the entire upper extremity, including the hand. Draping of the patient must ensure full access to both anterior and posterior aspects of the shoulder. The anterior iliac crest region must also be prepped and draped in cases in which use of an autogenous iliac crest bone graft is planned.

Surgical approach

A deltopectoral approach is used for exposure in cases of chronic shoulder dislocation. For cases involving arthroplasty or subscapularis transfer, the skin incision is started at the tip of the coracoid, and extends distally and laterally approximately 10–15 cm, depending on the size of the patient. For cases involving coracoid transfer, anterior glenoid bone grafting, or open capsulolabral repair, a more limited skin incision is performed, starting at the tip of the coracoid and extending inferiorly toward the axilla, provided a large soft-tissue release is unnecessary. A needle-tip electrocautery is used for deep dissection throughout the procedure, to minimize hemorrhage. The interval between the deltoid and the pectoralis major is identified by locating the cephalic vein. If difficulty is encountered in locating the cephalic vein, the deltopectoral interval can be readily detected proximally by identifying a small triangular area devoid of muscle tissue between the proximal portions of the deltoid and pectoralis major muscle. We prefer to retract the cephalic vein laterally with the deltoid because most of the branches of the cephalic vein are based on the deltoid. A self-retaining deltopectoral retractor is placed to maintain exposure during the procedure. Release of the upper 1 cm of pectoralis major tendon is performed during arthroplasty cases to facilitate exposure. The conjoined tendon is identified and traced to its insertion on the coracoid process. The tip of a Hohmann-type retractor is placed behind the base of the coracoid process, to provide proximal retraction. The apex formed by the insertion of the coracoacromial ligament and the conjoined tendon onto the coracoid process is identified. The conjoined tendon is retracted medially.

Special considerations

Long-standing glenohumeral dislocations are often accompanied by severe soft-tissue contracture. These contractures must be released during the surgical exposure. Subcoracoid, subdeltoid, and subacromial adhesions are carefully released. Performance of these releases may necessitate exposure of vulnerable neurovascular structures, such as the axillary nerve and musculocutaneous nerve.

Anterior dislocations

Open reduction with capsulolabral repair

The limited deltopectoral approach is the same for both capsulolabral repairs and glenoid augmentation procedures. The subscapularis is exposed and divided in line with its fibers at the junction of the middle and inferior thirds of the muscle. The underlying capsule is exposed and a 1 cm vertical capsulotomy is performed at the glenohumeral articulation. A humeral head retractor is placed into the glenohumeral joint. When capsular redundancy is observed, a capsular shift will likely be necessary. When a capsular shift is to be performed, a separate capsular incision is made, extending medially at the midportion of the capsule. This forms a T-type capsular incision. Corner sutures are placed for traction to facilitate exposure.

When a Bankart lesion is noted, it is mobilized from the glenoid rim medially to the glenoid neck. An anterior glenoid rim retractor is placed deep to the lesion, exposing the anterior glenoid rim. The bone on the anterior glenoid is abraded to enhance healing of the labral tissue. Suture anchors are placed at the margin of the glenoid rim, oriented in a posteromedial direction (Griggs et al. 2007). The surgeon must avoid placing the anchors too medially on the glenoid neck. Depending on the extent of labral detachment, two or three suture anchors are typically required (**Fig 14.3**). Anchor placement proceeds in an inferior to superior direction. The capsule is pulled laterally, and the anterior glenoid rim retractor is placed between the subscapularis and the capsule. Sutures are then passed through the labrum–capsule junction, at a point that brings the labrum to its anatomic insertion site on the glenoid. The torn labrum is usually displaced medially and inferiorly; therefore, the labrum is pierced with the suture, such that when the knot is tied the labrum is translated superiorly and laterally.

After the labrum repair is complete, the patient's arm is placed in 45° of external rotation, 10° of flexion, and 20° of abduction. If no capsular redundancy is present, anatomic repair of the capsule is performed using non-absorbable sutures. When capsular redundancy is present at this arm position, a capsular shift is performed using a 'pants over vest' suturing technique. The wound is irrigated and closed in layers, as usual.

Open reduction with Latarjet coracoid transfer

The Latarjet procedure (**Figs 14.4** and **14.5**) is performed through a limited deltopectoral approach (Edwards and Walch 2002). The coracoacromial ligament is transected 1 cm lateral to its insertion on the coracoid. The arm is placed in an internally rotated position, and the pectoralis minor is identified and released from its coracoid insertion. A periosteal elevator is used to expose the flexure of the coracoid medially. The coracoid is osteotomized at the flexure using a microsagittal saw equipped with a 90° angled blade. The coracohumeral ligament is released, and the coracoid is reflected inferiorly, exposing its deep surface. Grasping forceps are used to hold the coracoid process, and any remaining soft tissue is removed from the deep surface of the coracoid, taking care not to disrupt the stump of the coracoacromial

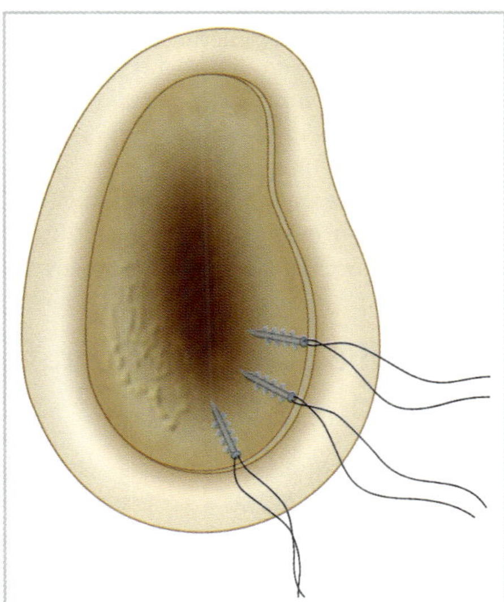

Figure 14.3 Anchor position for anterior capsulolabral repair following open reduction for a fixed anterior dislocation.

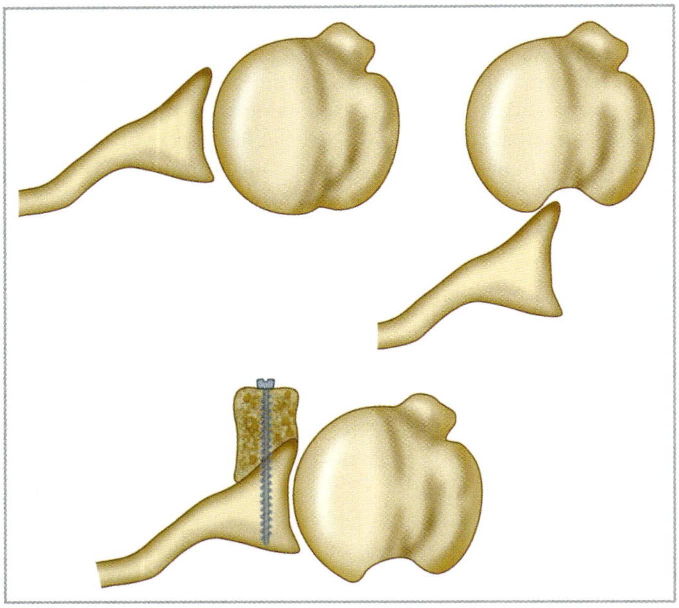

Figure 14.4 Mechanism by which a Latarjet coracoid transfer increases the anteroposterior diameter of the glenoid, thereby preventing engagement of a humeral head lesion. The humeral head must translate a greater distance for the humeral head lesion to engage.

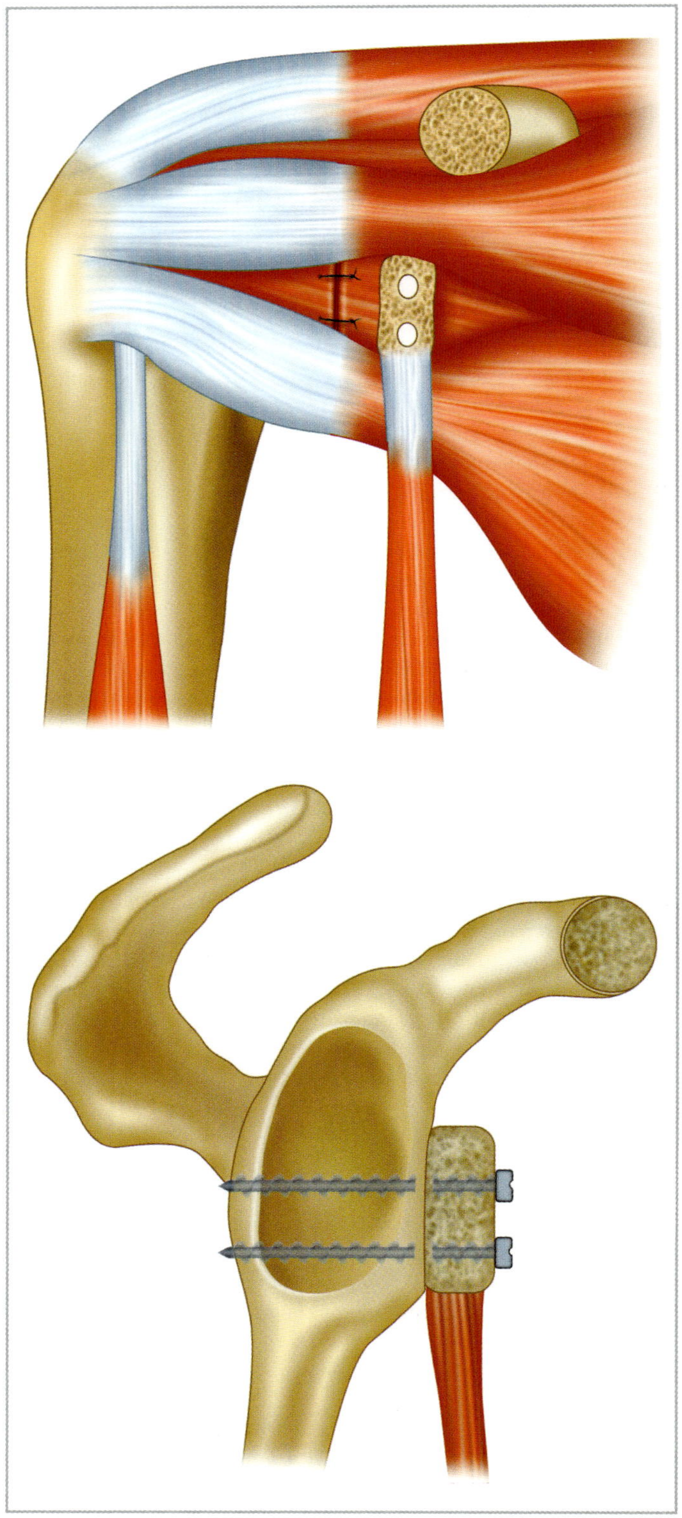

Figure 14.5 Final construct following Latarjet coracoid transfer for a fixed anterior dislocation with glenoid bone loss.

ligament. The deep surface of the coracoid process is decorticated using the microsagittal saw. Two 3.2 mm holes are drilled in the coracoid process perpendicular to its long axis, and centered with respect to its width.

The subscapularis is exposed and divided in line with its fibers at the junction of the middle and inferior thirds of the muscle. The underlying capsule is exposed, and a 1 cm vertical capsulotomy is performed at the glenohumeral articulation. A humeral head retractor is placed into the glenohumeral joint, and the anteroinferior glenoid labrum, Bankart lesion, and periosteum are excised. The bone on the anterior scapula is roughened, to stimulate healing of the coracoid. A 3.2 mm drill is used to make an anterior-to-posterior hole in the scapula at approximately the 5 o'clock position for the right shoulder, or 7 o'clock position for the left shoulder. An appropriately sized, partially threaded malleolar screw is inserted. The goal is to position the coracoid flush with the articular surface of the glenoid. It is acceptable for the coracoid to be positioned slightly medial to the articular border of the glenoid, but no lateral overhang should be accepted. A second screw is inserted in the same manner, using the superior hole in the coracoid as a template.

Repair of the coracoacromial ligament stump to the inferior glenohumeral ligament and capsule is performed using a number 2 nonabsorbable braided suture. It is not necessary to suture the horizontal split in the subscapularis. The wound is irrigated and close in layers.

Open reduction with iliac crest bone graft glenoid reconstruction

Surgical exposure, subscapularis dissection, and lateral capsulotomy are performed as described above. A tricortical iliac crest autograft of appropriate size is harvested. The glenoid defect is burred to a flat surface. Suture anchors are placed at the glenoid rim. Sutures are passed through the labrum and capsule, as described for repair of a Bankart lesion. The tricortical iliac crest bone graft is placed flush with the articular surface of the glenoid, with its cancellous surface against the cancellous bone of the defect, and the cortical table of the graft facing laterally (**Fig. 14.6**). The bone graft is fixed to the anterior glenoid using two 4.0 mm partially threaded cancellous screws. The sutures passed through the labrum and capsule are now tied. The wound is irrigated and closed in layers.

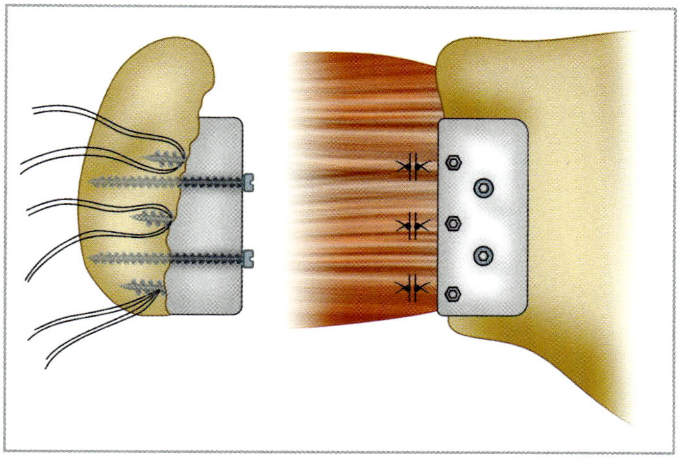

Figure 14.6 Final construct following anterior glenoid reconstruction using iliac crest bone graft for a fixed anterior dislocation with glenoid bone loss of greater than 30% of the anteroposterior glenoid diameter.

Reverse shoulder arthroplasty

Chronic anterior shoulder dislocations in older patients often result in chondrolysis, rotator cuff tear, and anterior glenoid bone loss. Reverse shoulder arthroplasty is indicated in treating this combination of lesions in the elderly patient (Gartsman and Edwards 2008b). When no native glenoid bone is present to support the anterior portion of the base, anterior glenoid reconstruction with bone graft is required. The need for a bone graft is usually determined from the preoperative computerized tomography scan. A bone graft (either from the humeral head or a tricortical segment of iliac crest, depending on the size of the defect) is harvested and shaped with a small oscillating saw to fill the glenoid defect. The bone graft is positioned anteriorly and fixed with two or three guide pins for 4.0 mm cannulated screws. Care is taken to place the pins so that they will not interfere with the post of the glenoid base-plate. Partially threaded 4.0 mm cannulated screws of appropriate length with washers are inserted after overdrilling the guide pins. After restoration of the glenoid bone stock with the bone graft, the glenoid is prepared and the glenoid component is inserted (**Fig. 14.7**).

When glenoid reconstruction with iliac crest bone graft is necessary, then, before insertion of the glenoid component, every effort should be made to have a portion of the central post of the base-plate placed in native glenoid bone. Some companies manufacture base-plates with a longer central post to address this problem. If the central post cannot be placed within the native glenoid bone, or if the glenoid component does not seem securely fixed, staged arthroplasty should be performed. In staged arthroplasty, the glenoid component is inserted, and the humerus, after being prepared for the humeral component, is left without a humeral implant for six months, to allow the glenoid bone graft to incorporate. The patient is allowed to use the arm as tolerated, although function will be limited. After six months, the second stage is completed by inserting the humeral component.

Posterior dislocations

Open reduction with subscapularis tendon transfer

Following exposure, the long head of the biceps is identified and followed to the rotator interval proximally. The rotator interval is opened. Retraction of the supraspinatus superiorly and subscapularis inferiorly allows for visualization and palpation of the joint. Information regarding the size and location of both the impression fracture of the humeral head and the glenoid articular surface can be obtained.

The subscapularis is elevated off its insertion into the lesser tuberosity, to allow for tendon transfer into the defect. The subscapularis tendon is tagged with number 2 non-absorbable suture and release of the coracohumeral ligament, anterior capsule, and subscapularis is performed.

Once the glenohumeral joint is exposed, any intra-articular fibrous tissue is excised, with care not to damage the articular surfaces. Fibrous tissue within the humeral head defect should also be removed. Proper visualization must be obtained before any attempted reduction. The humeral head, which is displaced medially and posteriorly relative to the glenoid, is carefully disengaged using a blunt-ended flat elevator. With gentle internal rotation, the elevator is inserted between the humeral head and the posterior glenoid. The elevator is used to 'shoehorn' the humeral head laterally into the joint (Zuckerman 2004) while gentle external rotation with anterior translation is applied to the humerus.

Once the humeral head is reduced (**Fig. 14.8**) the anteromedial impression fracture can be fully appreciated, and any fibrous tissue is debrided from the defect. Under direct visualization the patient's arm is internally rotated to identify the position at which posterior dislocation occurs. This information will allow assessment of stability after subscapularis tendon transfer. The subscapularis is transferred into the defect and fixed with three double-loaded suture anchors (**Fig. 14.9**). Sutures are passed though the tendon using a horizontal mattress technique. The horizontal mattress sutures from each anchor are passed through the tendon in a cruciform pattern, with the first suture passed vertically to act as a 'rip stop' to the horizontal component. It is important that the transferred subscapularis tendon is in close contact with the articular edge of the humeral head defect, as this is the most critical area to achieve a buttress effect (**Fig. 14.10**). The wound is irrigated and closed in layers.

Humeral head replacement

Prosthetic replacement is indicated for humeral impression defects involving over 40% of the articular surface, as well as for smaller defects in the presence of significant articular degeneration (Hawkins et al. 1987). If prosthetic replacement is to be undertaken, a subscapularis tenotomy 1 cm medial to its insertion on the lesser tuberosity is performed. Again, alternatively the lesser tuberosity can be taken off instead of subscapularis tenotomy. After humeral head reduction on the glenoid, further external rotation and extension are performed, progressively dislocating the humeral head anteriorly. Humeral head resection is performed along the anatomic neck. The glenoid is inspected to evaluate the presence or degree of bone loss and integrity of the remaining articular cartilage. If there is significant bone loss or the remaining cartilage is compromised, bone grafting and/or glenoid resurfacing may be required. When no glenoid changes are observed, hemiarthroplasty is the treatment of choice. In young patients with significant wear of the glenoid articular cartilage, biologic resurfacing may be considered. Our outcomes using unconstrained shoulder arthroplasty for the treatment of fixed glenohumeral dislocations in elderly patients have been disappointing, in that we have observed a high rate of recurrent instability and a high rate of rotator cuff insufficiency. For these reasons, we now use a reverse prosthesis as our implant of choice for fixed glenohumeral dislocations in elderly patients.

Pearls and pitfalls

- Appropriate preoperative imaging should be obtained. A computerized tomography scan is most helpful to assess bone loss for

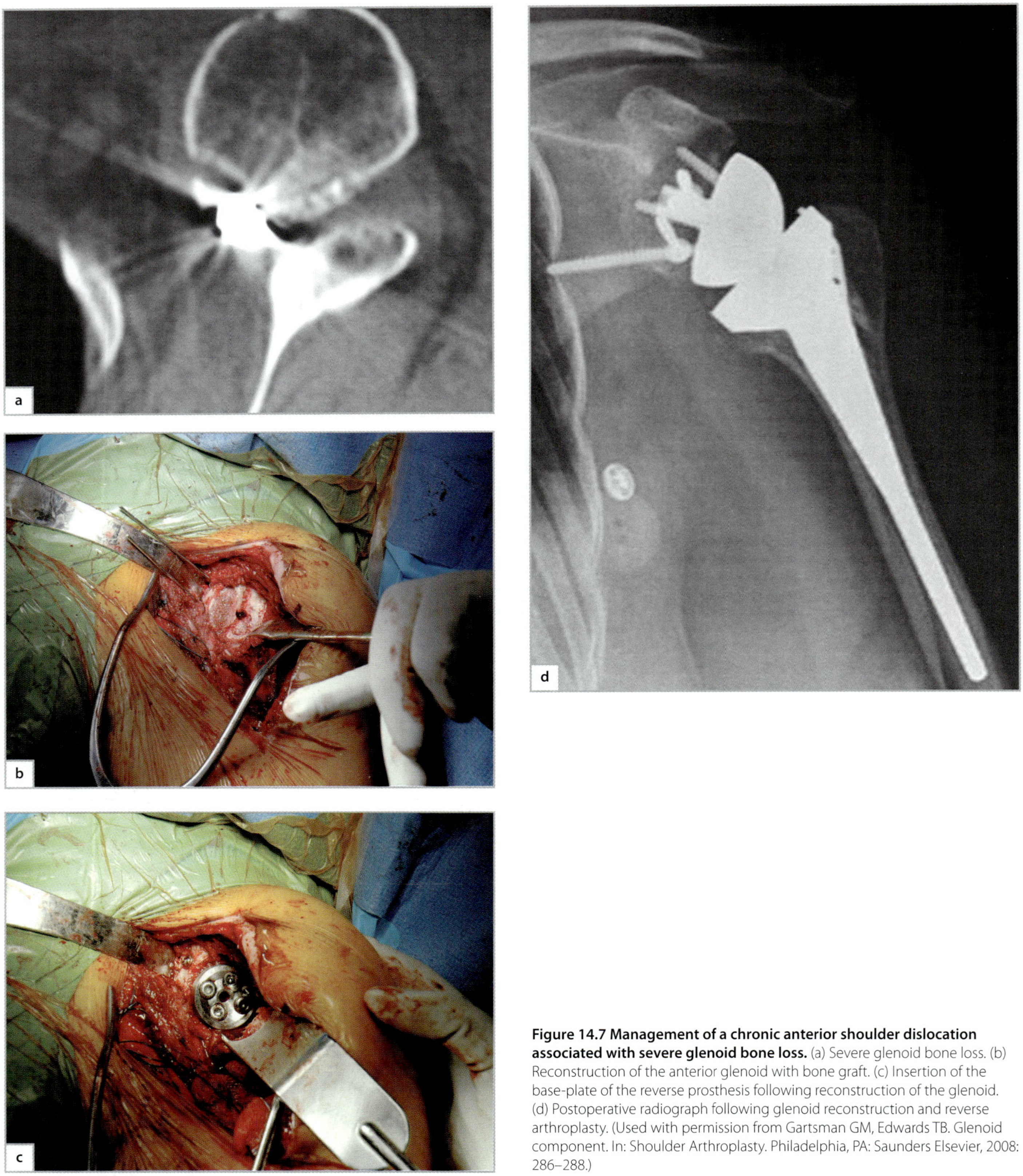

Figure 14.7 Management of a chronic anterior shoulder dislocation associated with severe glenoid bone loss. (a) Severe glenoid bone loss. (b) Reconstruction of the anterior glenoid with bone graft. (c) Insertion of the base-plate of the reverse prosthesis following reconstruction of the glenoid. (d) Postoperative radiograph following glenoid reconstruction and reverse arthroplasty. (Used with permission from Gartsman GM, Edwards TB. Glenoid component. In: Shoulder Arthroplasty. Philadelphia, PA: Saunders Elsevier, 2008: 286–288.)

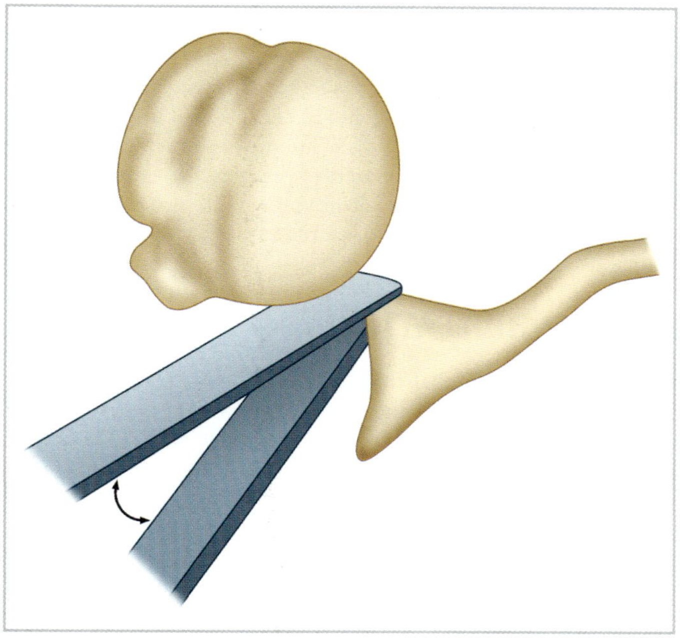

Figure 14.8 Open reduction maneuver utilized for a fixed posterior shoulder dislocation.

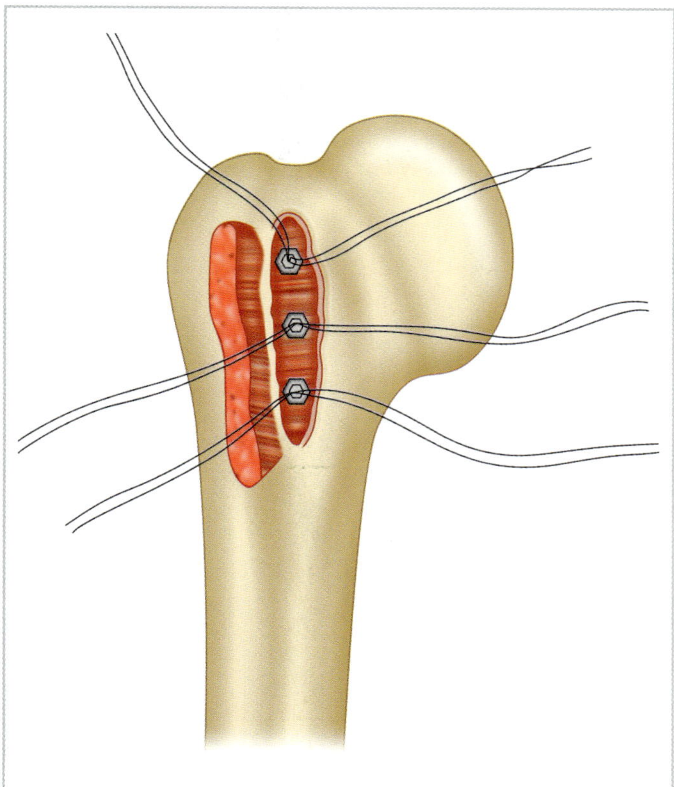

Figure 14.9 Anchor position within the humeral head defect for subscapularis tendon transfer for a locked posterior shoulder dislocation.

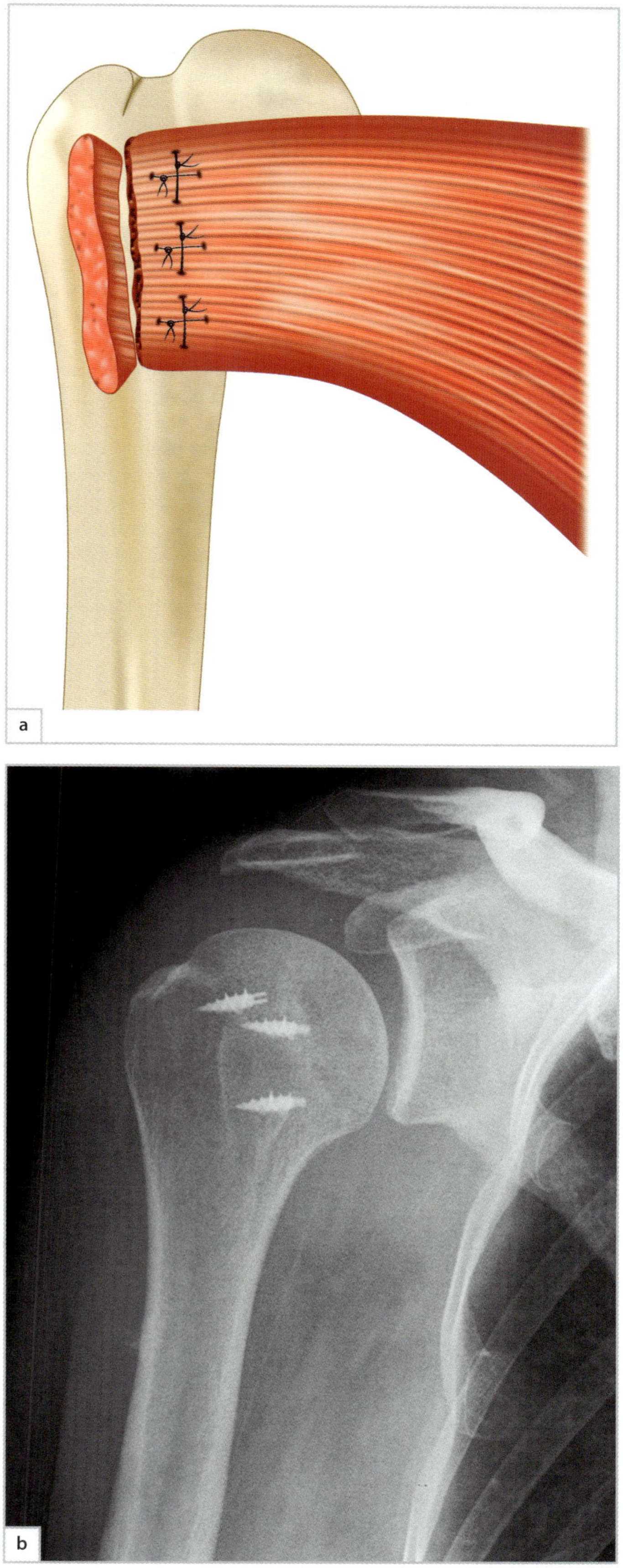

Figure 14.10 Subscapularis tendon transfer for a locked posterior shoulder dislocation. (a) Final construct. (b) Postoperative radiograph.

both the humerus and the glenoid. Magnetic resonance imaging is most helpful in assessing the rotator cuff.

- The preoperative imaging studies should be used to establish a surgical plan. The surgeon should be fairly certain of which procedure is to be performed preoperatively.
- Heroic efforts at closed reduction should be avoided. Closed reduction is rarely successful in dealing with chronic shoulder dislocations, and may actually cause more damage (fracture).
- The surgeon should always be prepared to perform a generous release of soft-tissue contractures, usually requiring release of the superior, middle and inferior glenohumeral ligaments. Long-standing dislocations usually have a large amount of scar tissue present that must be addressed at the time of surgery.
- The surgeon should have a plan for dealing with bone loss. The patient must be informed about the possible need to use an autogenous iliac crest bone graft.
- The Latarjet coracoid transfer can be very useful in the treatment of patients with large impression fractures of the humeral head with a fixed anterior dislocation. The increase of glenoid diameter created by this procedure can prevent the humeral head lesion from engaging the anterior glenoid and dislocating the shoulder.
- Posterior dislocations with loss of up to 40% of the humeral head can be effectively treated using a subscapularis tendon transfer. The surgeon should not be quick to perform an arthroplasty in these patients.
- Older patients with chronic dislocations usually have complete glenohumeral chondrolysis. The articular surfaces in older patients do not tolerate prolonged dislocation. It is difficult to evaluate the articular surfaces preoperatively because the joint space cannot be assessed, as the articular surfaces are not opposed. The surgeon should always be prepared to perform an arthroplasty in these cases.

REHABILITATION

All patients are instructed in hand, wrist, and elbow mobility exercises on postoperative day 1. Patients are instructed how to perform pendulum exercises as soon as they feel comfortable, while maintaining the shoulder in a neutral position. Abduction, passive elevation in the scapular plane, and external rotation, as determined intraoperatively after tendon transfer, are also allowed. At four weeks, the orthosis is removed and the patient is allowed full active motion of the shoulder without resistance. Also at four weeks, an aquatic-based therapy program is initiated, to assist in obtaining mobility (Liotard et al. 2003). Patients who have undergone prosthetic replacement are permanently restricted from performing contact sports, but otherwise unrestricted activity is allowed after six months.

REFERENCES

Edwards TB, Walch G. The Latarjet procedure for recurrent anterior shoulder instability: rationale and technique. Op Tech Sports Med 2002;10:25–32.

Gartsman GM, Edwards TB. Glenoid component. In: Shoulder Arthroplasty. Philadelphia, PA: Saunders Elsevier, 2008a: 271–289.

Gartsman GM, Edwards TB. Results and complications. In: Shoulder Arthroplasty. Philadelphia, PA: Saunders Elsevier, 2008b: 305–321.

Griggs S, Holloway B, Williams G. Treatment of locked anterior and posterior dislocations of the shoulder. In: Iannotti J, Williams G, eds. Disorders of the Shoulder: Diagnosis and Management. Philadelphia, PA: Lippincott, Williams and Wilkins, 1999: 335–359.

Griggs SM, Holloway GB, Williams GR, Iannotti JP. Chronic dislocations. In: Iannotti JP, Williams GR, eds. Disorders of the Shoulder: Diagnosis and Management, 2nd edition. Philadelphia, PA: Lippincott, Williams and Wilkins, 2007: 461–486.

Hawkins RJ, Neer CS, Pianta RM, Mendoza FX. Locked posterior dislocation of the shoulder. J Bone Joint Surg Am 1987;69:9–18.

Liotard JP, Edwards TB, Padey A, et al. Hydrotherapy rehabilitation after shoulder surgery. Tech Shoulder Elbow Surg 2003;4:44–49.

Matsoukis J, Tabib W, Guiffault P, et al. Primary unconstrained shoulder arthroplasty in patients with a fixed anterior glenohumeral dislocation: results of a multicenter study. J Bone Joint Surg Am 2006;88:547–552.

McLaughlin H. Posterior dislocations of the shoulder. J Bone Joint Surg Am 1952;34:584–590.

Oyston JK. Unreduced posterior dislocation of the shoulder treated by open reduction and transposition of the subscapularis tendon. J Bone Joint Surg Br 1964;46:256–259.

Sahajpal DT, Zuckerman JD. Chronic glenohumeral dislocation. J Am Acad Orthop Surg 2008;16:385–398.

Zuckerman JD. McLaughlin procedure for acute and chronic posterior dislocations. In: Craig EV, ed. Master Techniques in Orthopaedic Surgery: The Shoulder, 2nd edition. Philadelphia, PA: Lippincott, Williams and Wilkins, 2004: 289–305.

Chapter 15 Operative management of fractures of the scapula

Peter A. Cole, Aaron R. Jacobson

CLASSIFICATION

Several classifications have been developed for fractures of the scapula. However, its unique anatomy and the usual high-energy mechanism of fracture have presented a challenge in developing a classification that is both comprehensive and prognostic. The most widely used classifications include those of the Hardegger et al. (1984), Ada and Miller (1991), and the Orthopaedic Trauma Association (OTA) (Marsh et al. 2007). The first two of these were developed through a review of fractures observed in a clinical setting. They therefore benefit from the fact that their subclassifications reflect patterns commonly encountered in practice, and the fractures are organized by anatomic location (**Fig. 15.1**). Neither, though, takes into account important associated lesions of the superior shoulder suspensory complex; thus, they may be limited in value regarding operative decision making.

The OTA classification is an alphanumeric system which classifies both intra- and extra-articular variants. It was modified in 2007 to improve its utility. It follows the long-bone classification in which fractures are categorized as articular, partial articular, and extra-articular. Its main weakness is that it was not developed by correlating patterns of injury from either clinical observation or radiographic analysis, or patterns of combined injuries, which are common.

Ogawa et al. proposed a classification system specific to the acromion and coracoid (Ogawa and Naniwa 1997, Ogawa et al. 1997). They recommended that coracoid fractures be classified based on whether the fracture line runs anterior or posterior to the coracoclavicular ligaments, while the acromion is classified based on the fracture's proximity

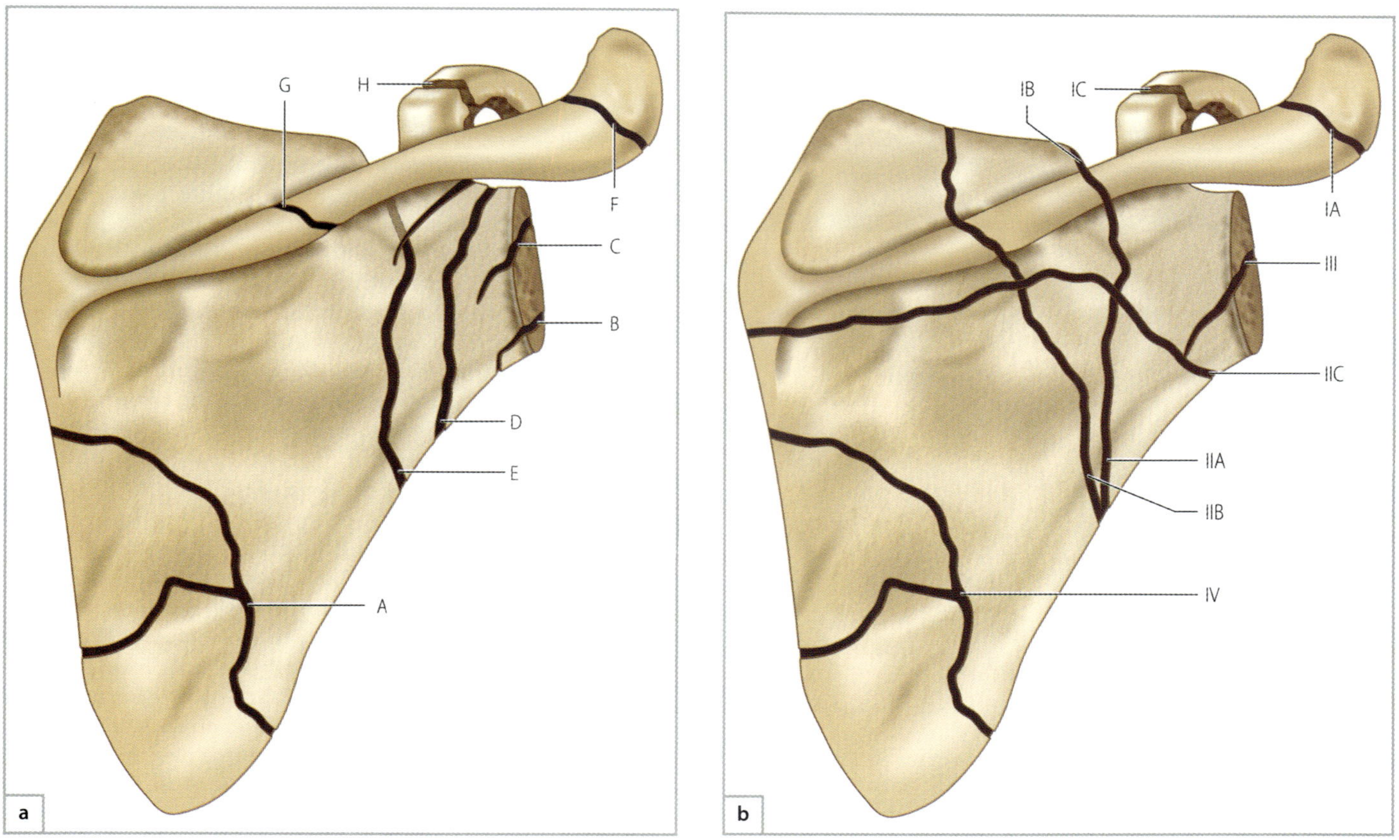

Figure 15.1 Two classification systems for fractures of the scapula. (a) The classification proposed by Hardegger. The eight anatomic categories are. A, body; B, glenoid rim; C, glenoid fossa; D, anatomical neck; E, surgical neck; F, acromion; G, spine; H, coracoid. (Adapted from Hardegger FH, Simpson LA, Weber BG. The operative treatment of scapular fractures. J Bone Joint Surg Br 1984;66:725–731.) (b) The classification proposed by Ada and Miller. The system stratifies fractures into four categories, based on anatomic location. Type I includes fractures of the acromion, coracoid, and spine. Type II are fractures of the scapula neck, which are commonly encountered in clinical practice. Type III are intra-articular fractures, including of both the glenoid rim and fossa. Type IV include all extra-articular fractures of the scapular body. (Adapted from Ada JR, Miller ME. Scapular fractures. Analysis of 113 cases. Clin Orthop Relat Res 1991;(269):174–180.)

to the spinoglenoid notch (**Fig. 15.2a**). More recently, Anavian et al. (2009) reported and mapped fractures of 26 operatively treated process fractures. They noted a higher prevalence of coracoid base fractures and acromion fractures that extended to the region of the spinoglenoid notch that met their operative indications compared to coracoid fractures located anterior to the coracoclavicular ligaments and far lateral acromion fractures (**Fig. 15.2b**).

Recently, scapula fractures have been mapped from analysis of three-dimensional (3D) reconstructions to clearly illustrate the true nature of fracture patterns, and perhaps this mapping should serve as a basis for a comprehensive classification scheme (Armitage et al. 2009). In addition, 3D computerized tomography (CT) has recently been shown to afford superior interobserver and intraobserver reliability over plain films (Anavian et al. 2011).

Glenoid fractures which involve the articular surface have been distinguished by their own classification schemes. That developed by Mayo et al. (1998) for intra-articular fractures is a reorganized version of the Ideberg classification, and was based on the imaging and operative findings for 27 intra-articular glenoid fractures (**Fig. 15.3**). This classification is helpful in directing surgical decision making, and it takes into account the fractures of the scapular body and of the acromion or coracoid process with which glenoid fractures frequently occur.

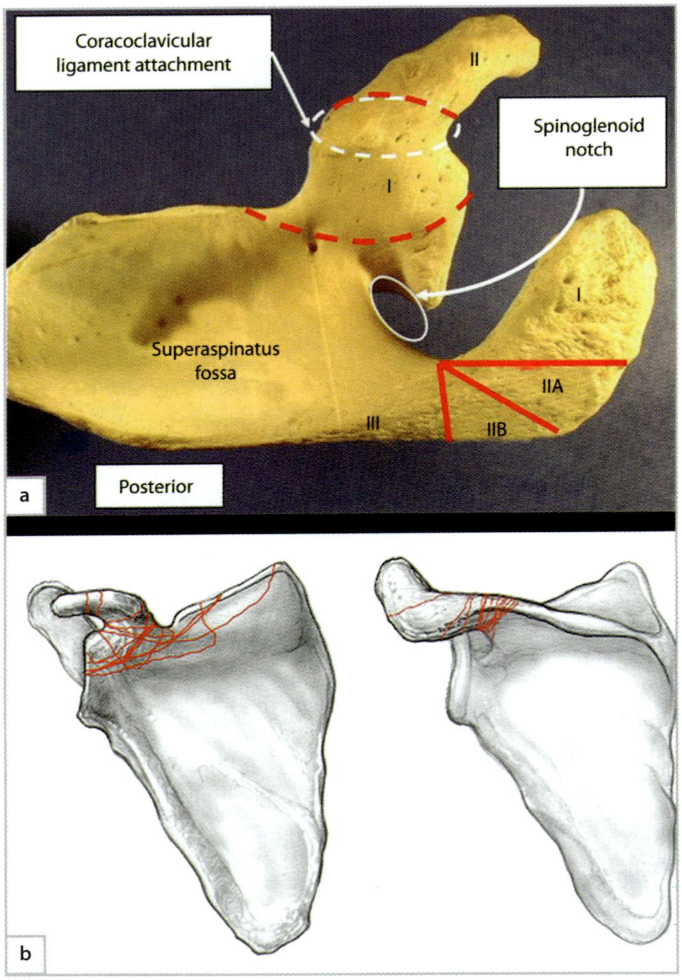

Figure 15.2 Classification and incidence of fractures of the scapula. (a) The classification proposed by Ogawa et al. (Ogawa and Naniwa 1997, Ogawa et al. 1997). They recommended that coracoid fractures be classified based on whether the fracture line runs anterior or posterior to coracoclavicular ligaments, while fractures of the acromion are classified based on their proximity to the spinoglenoid notch. (b) The fracture lines of 26 operatively treated process fractures. There was a higher prevalence of coracoid base fractures and acromion fractures that extended to the region of the spinoglenoid notch that met their operative indications. (From Anavian J, Wijdicks CA, Schroder LK, et al. Surgery for scapula process fractures. Acta Orthop 2009;80:344–350, with permission.)

INDICATIONS

The proximal forequarter is a complex anatomic region: 18 muscles originate, insert, or cross the scapula and glenohumeral joint, more than in any other articulation of the body. The shoulder's extensive musculature and universal motion can often provide significant compensation for alterations in morphology following fracture of the scapula. Scapula malunions do, however, have the potential to compromise normal stability and motion. Glenohumeral stability is maintained by compressive loading of the humeral head against the glenoid and a balanced interplay of shoulder muscles, in addition to stability offered by the labrum, which serves to deepen the glenoid fossa. Fractures of the glenoid rim and fossa disrupt shoulder stability by decreasing the surface area of the joint as well as disrupting the labrum. Malunions of the scapular neck have been shown in a biomechanical model to shorten the resting length of the rotator cuff muscles, which results in a loss of force as well as altered normal muscle activation during abduction (Chadwick et al. 2004). Patient-based outcomes have shown that results are not uniformly good for non-operatively treated fractures of the scapula. Cole et al. (2011) identified a group of patients who developed highly symptomatic malunion following an extra-articular fracture of the scapula. These patients underwent revision surgery, which improved function to near normal levels. Multiple authors have suggested operative criteria based on personal experience, but there is little objective data on which to judge the need for surgery based on displacement, angulation, or glenoid version. Hardegger et al. (1984), Ada and Miller (1991), Nordqvist and Petersson (1992), and Romero et al. (2001) found a significant relationship between persistent shoulder disability and residual radiographic deformity. Their work helped shape the operative criteria currently utilized.

Clear evidence-based operative guidelines have yet to be developed and thus it is our opinion that all operative indications, except for unstable and displaced fractures of the glenoid fossa, should be regarded as relative. Judgment must be rendered for each case, taking into consideration the age, health, and shoulder function of the patient.

Extra-articular fractures

Extra-articular fractures of the glenoid neck and body are the most commonly encountered. These fractures provide the most controversial area in surgical decision making. However, increased recognition of shoulder morbidity following forequarter trauma and increasing familiarity with surgical approaches have provided greater acceptance of the surgical treatment of such scapula fractures, particularly given the low complication rates reported. More surgeons seem to be applying equivalent surgical principles utilized for all other fractures, to the treatment of fractures of the scapula, with the goal of restoration of alignment, length, and rotation, as well as anatomic articular reduction. The deforming force that fractures the scapula is commonly one that drives the head of the humerus into the glenoid. This force pushes the glenoid medially, and the resulting fracture and displacement most often occur at the level of the inferior glenoid neck. Shortening, medialization, and lateral border

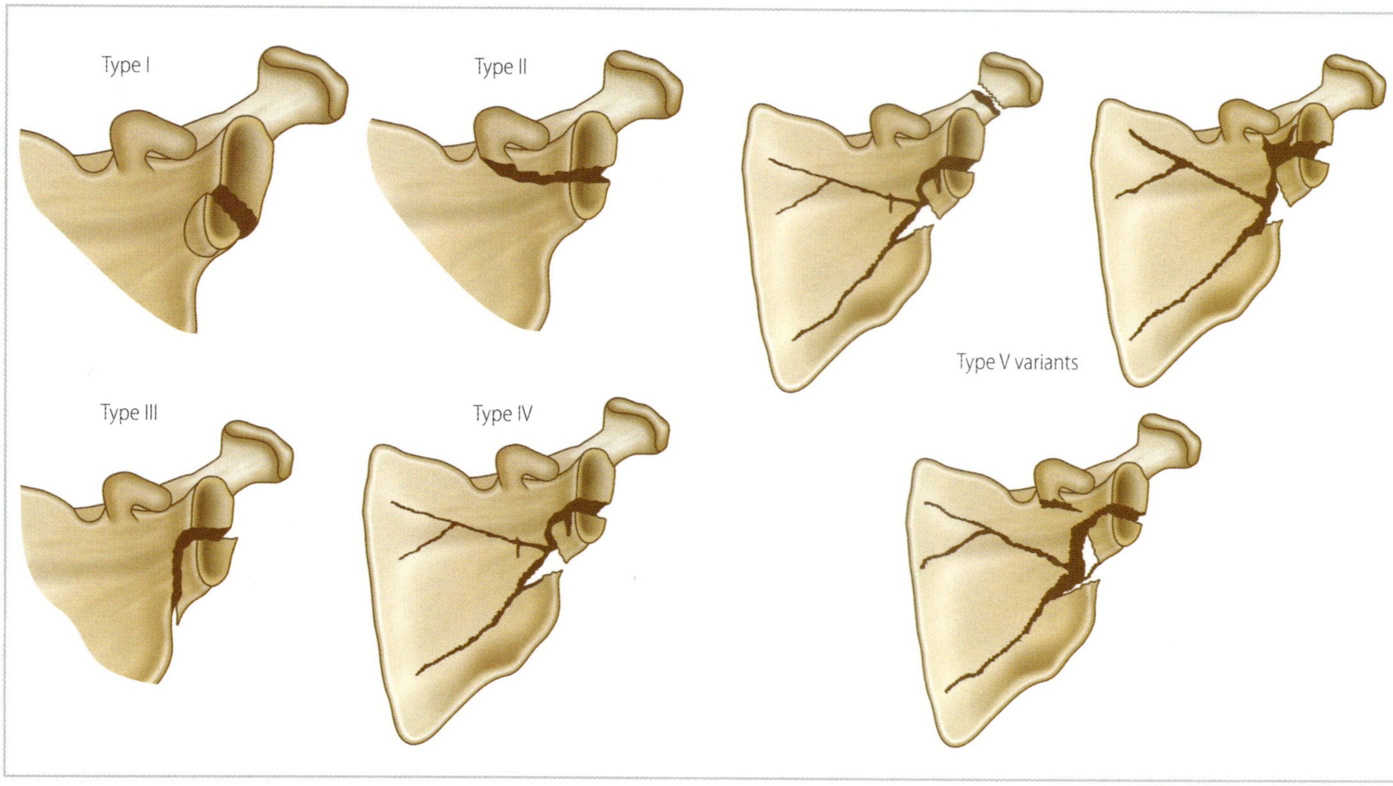

Figure 15.3 Classification of fractures of the glenoid fossa. This classification, proposed by Mayo, is commonly referred to as the modified Ideberg. (Adapted from Mayo KA, Benirschke SK, Mast JW. Displaced fractures of the glenoid fossa. Results of open reduction and internal fixation. Clin Orthop Relat Res 1998;(347):122–130.)

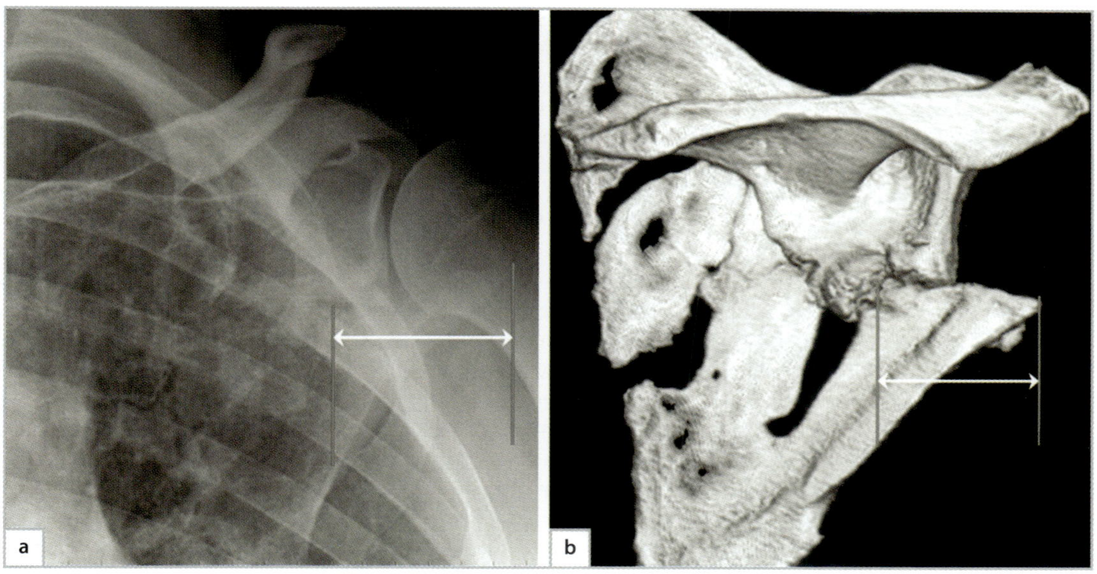

Figure 15.4 The method used to measure lateral border offset on radiographs and on three-dimensional computerized tomography (3D CT). (a) Radiographically, this measurement is performed on a Grashey x-ray view. (b) The scapula is rotated to see the largest scapula diameter on 3D CT. Measurement on 3D CT has been shown to have higher inter- and intrarater reliability than measurement on radiographs. (From Anavian J, Conflitti JM, Khanna G, Guthrie ST, Cole PA. A reliable radiographic measurement technique for extra-articular scapular fractures. Clin Orthop Relat Res 2011;469:3371–3378, with permission.)

offset are all terms used to describe this displacement observed on a true anteroposterior (Grashey) x-ray view (**Fig. 15.4**). We prefer the term 'lateral border offset' (LBO), as it offers less confusion when describing the fracture pattern, since some surgeons have interpreted medialization to be relative to the spine rather than the proximal versus distal lateral border. Opinions on what is considered significant enough LBO to warrant surgery varies among contemporary authors. Ranges of 10–25 mm have been reported as the threshold for surgery. Glenopolar angle (GPA) is also measured on the true anteroposterior (Grashey) shoulder x-ray view (**Fig. 15.5**). GPA reflects the orientation of the glenoid in relation to the scapular body. Multiple authors have noted less favorable patient outcomes when this angle is less than 20–22°. This measurement is perhaps the most validated prognostic indicator for extraarticular fractures. Angulation (**Fig. 15.6**), which is measured on a scapula Y x-ray, also has prognostic value. Most recent studies publishing operative results use 45° as their criteria.

Our current guidelines for operative management of isolated extraarticular fractures are as follows:

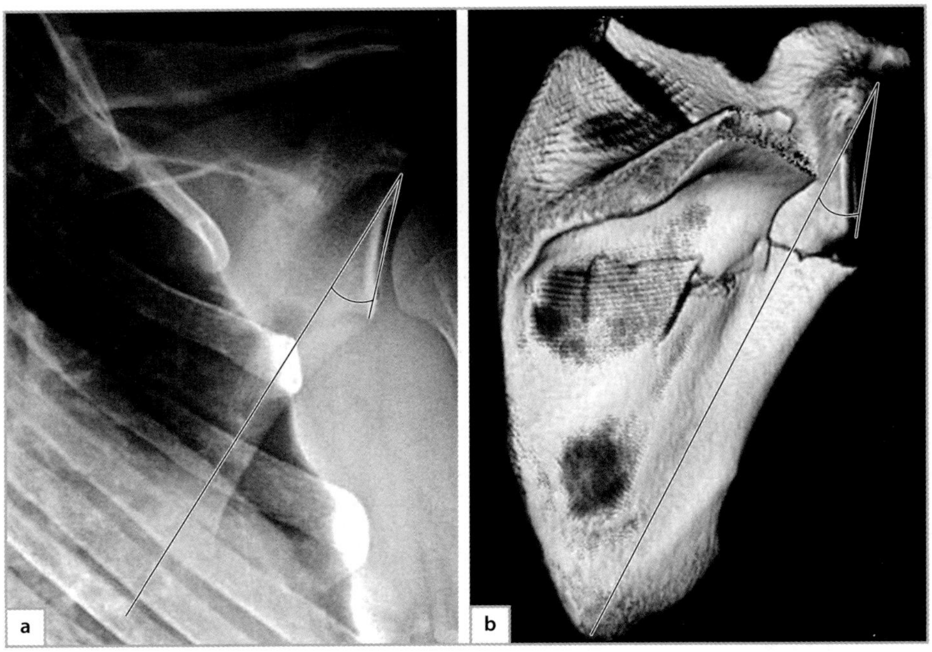

Figure 15.5 The method used to measure glenopolar angle on radiographs and on three-dimensional computerized tomography (3D CT). (a) Radiographically, this measurement is performed on a Grashey view. (b) The scapula is rotated to see the largest scapula diameter on 3D CT. Measurement on 3D CT has been shown to have higher inter- and intrarater reliability than measurement on radiographs. (From Anavian J, Conflitti JM, Khanna G, Guthrie ST, Cole PA. A reliable radiographic measurement technique for extra-articular scapular fractures. Clin Orthop Relat Res 2011;469:3371–3378, with permission.)

- GPA < 22°
- LBO > 20 mm
- angular deformity > 45°
- LBO > 15 mm + angular deformity > 30°.

These indications must be placed in the context of the patient's functional demands. The patient's age, occupation, hand dominance, and activity levels should be weighed in determining appropriate management.

Double lesions of the superior shoulder suspensory complex

Goss (1993) theorized that if two or more 'breaks' in the superior shoulder suspensory complex (SSSC) occur, they will create an unstable shoulder girdle, as a result of the discontinuity between the axial and appendicular skeleton (**Figs 15.7, 15.8**). There have been numerous case series looking at the outcomes of both operatively and non-operatively treated double disruptions. Goss's theory has been challenged by some authors (Edwards et al. 2000, Ramos et al. 1997), who point out that not all double disruptions warrant operative intervention. Based on these two clinical studies and the experience of the senior author, we have modified the original 'double disruption' indication by stating that both the lesions must be unstable, as indicated by displacement greater than 10 mm in both disruptions.

Articular fractures

Fractures of the glenoid rim, commonly referred to as bony Bankart lesions, are associated with anterior shoulder dislocations. If shoulder instability is present (demonstrated either by a luxation on radiographic examination, or by a positive apprehension or 'jerk test' on clinical examination), then operative intervention is indicated, given an appropriate surgical candidate. These criteria are likely to be met by patients with fractures involving more than 20% of the articular surface.

Our current indications for the operative management of intra-articular fractures include the presence of 4 mm or more of step off or gap (**Fig. 15.9**). Articular gap and step off is best visualized with two dimensional CT axial cuts (**Fig. 15.10**). Varying thresholds of 2–10 mm have been reported by different authors.

Isolated fractures of the acromion or coracoid process

Isolated fractures of the acromion or coracoid process are less common. While definitive indications for operative management remain to be established, our criteria include displacement of more than 10 mm in either process, double disruption of the superior shoulder complex, or symptomatic malunion/non-union. A supraspinatus outlet view is helpful to evaluate acromial depression as a potential cause of impingement syndrome, much like a type III 'hooked' acromion.

CONTRAINDICATIONS

Retrospective studies reporting outcomes of non-operatively treated fractures of the scapula are a testament to the shoulder's remarkable compensatory potential. The scapula can sufficiently compensate for degrees of displacement that would be deemed unacceptable in many other anatomic locations. Contraindications to surgery include extra-articular fractures that are displaced less than 10–15 mm and angulated less than 25°, because the outcomes of non-operative treatment for even moderately displaced fractures of the scapula are good. A shoulder sling, patient reassurance, and active elbow and wrist range of motion are encouraged for the first two weeks. Fractures of the scapula heal rapidly, due to the rich blood supply in the shoulder girdle. Active range of motion can be started by four weeks and maximized quickly. Resistive exercises are begun by eight weeks, and restrictions lifted, as symptoms allow, by three months.

TECHNIQUE

A variety of approaches are used for the open reduction and fixation of scapula fractures. Fracture location dictates which approach should be used. Available approaches are outlined below. The trend toward minimally invasive techniques is also observed in shoulder trauma, and the arthroscopic treatment of a glenoid fracture is included at the end of the section.

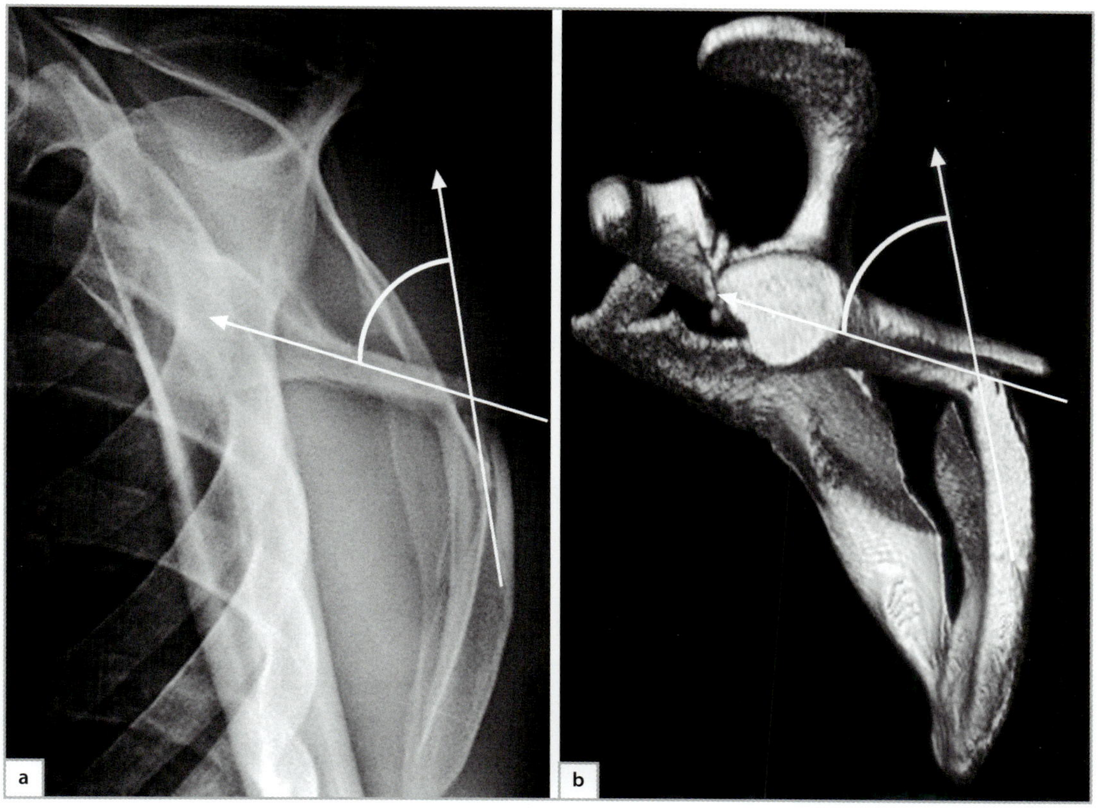

Figure 15.6 The determination of angular deformity on radiographs and on three-dimensional computerized tomography (3D CT). (a) Scapular 'Y' radiograph and (b) 3D CT rotated to 'Y' view demonstrating angular deformity. (From Anavian J, Conflitti JM, Khanna G, Guthrie ST, Cole PA. A reliable radiographic measurement technique for extra-articular scapular fractures. Clin Orthop Relat Res 2011;469:3371–3378, with permission.)

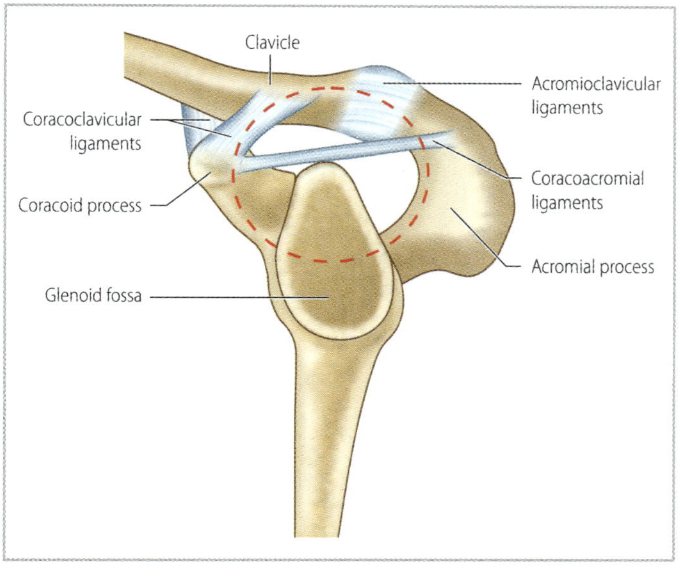

Figure 15.7 The superior shoulder suspensory complex. The complex is an osseoligamentous ring made up of the structures along the dotted line. Goss (1993) theorized that if two structures in the ring were disrupted, then a 'floating shoulder' lesion would be present, implying that there would be no osseous or ligamentous continuity between the axial skeleton and the forequarter. (Adapted from Goss TP. Double disruptions of the superior shoulder suspensory complex. J Orthop Trauma 1993;7:99–106.)

Posterior approaches

A posterior approach is utilized in the majority of extra-articular fractures. In addition, many glenoid fractures are best approached posteriorly, including all type IV and V fractures and many type III fractures (modified Ideberg classification).

The patient is positioned in the lateral decubitus position, 'flopping' slightly forward (**Fig. 15.11**). Bumps should be positioned on an arm-board to support the affected extremity. BoneFoam arm positioners are very helpful for this setup. The entire forequarter should be prepped and draped. This allows for manipulation, and is helpful for fracture reduction as well as manipulation after fixation. The preparation extends to the vertebral midline and inferior latissimus fold. The bony landmarks that guide incision should then be observed. The posterolateral acromion is palpated, and followed medially to the base of the spine of the scapula, and then caudad along the vertebral border. If there is difficulty identifying landmarks, the surgeon can retract or 'shuck' the shoulder while palpating the medial scapula. This maneuver will make the vertebral border more prominent

A Judet posterior incision is planned along these landmarks, 1 cm caudal to the acromion spine, and 1 cm lateral to the vertebral border, an adjustment which places the scar for better plate coverage, and allows for lateral retraction of a slightly less voluminous flap (**Fig. 15.12**).

The incision is taken down onto the bony ridge of the acromial spine, and splits the interval between the trapezius and deltoid insertions. The incision is curved distally at an acute angle just under 90° around the superomedial angle and down the vertebral border. The incision must be generous enough to allow for easy flap retraction if the surgeon wishes to use an extensile method mobilizing the infraspinatus. The fascial incision along the acromial spine and medial border should provide a cuff of tissue, which is sutured back to its bony origin at the end of the procedure.

Based on preoperative planning, the surgeon's decision making at this juncture depends on the desire for limited or complete exposure to the posterior scapula. Limited exposure, by developing intermuscular windows (Obremskey and Lyman 2004), is generally favored because it reduces trauma to the surrounding soft tissue, and helps protect the suprascapular and axillary nerves. This technique can be used to access fractures requiring reduction and fixation at the lateral border, acromial spine, and vertebral border.

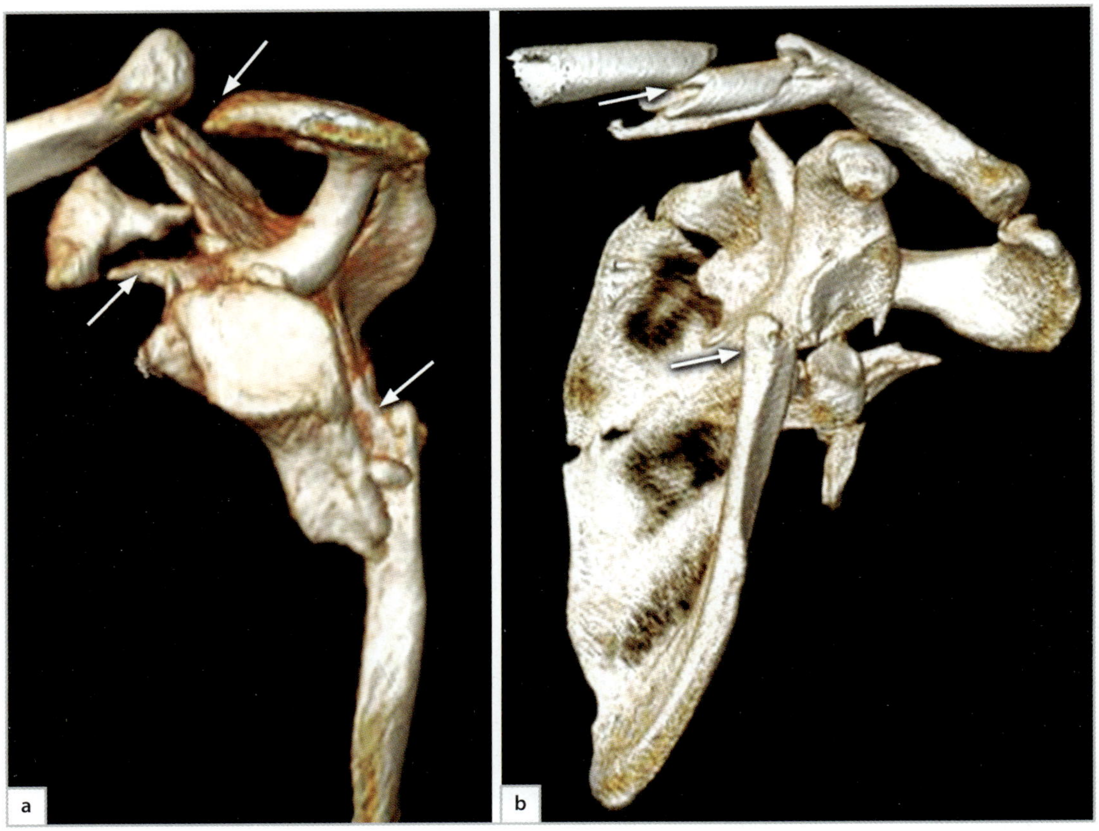

Figure 15.8 Disruption of the superior shoulder suspensory complex. (a) A triple disruption. The arrows highlight the disruption of the acromioclavicular joint, scapula neck, and coracoid. (b) A double disruption of the superior shoulder suspensory complex in a different patient. The arrows point to disruption caused by fracture of the scapular neck and clavicle.

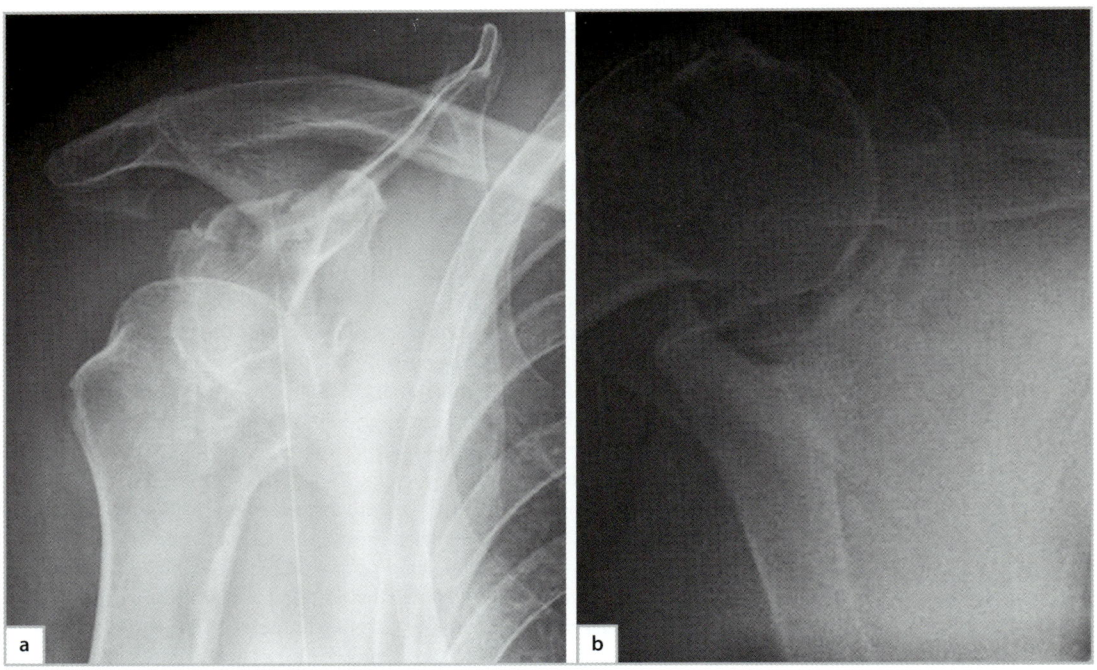

Figure 15.9 Radiographs showing a comminuted intra-articular fracture. (a) Anteroposterior and (b) axillary views. Fractures can often be visualized on radiographs. However, computerized tomography with multiplane reformatting is necessary for measurement of the displacement and operative planning.

Posterior Judet with limited exposure (modified Judet)

The Judet faciocutaneous flap is elevated laterally. Three intermuscular windows can then be utilized, depending on the fracture pattern (**Figs 15.12, 15.13**). Since almost all fractures of the scapula that require surgery have displacement on the lateral border, the most important window is between the infraspinatus and teres minor. This window gives access to the lateral border, the scapula, neck, and posterior glenoid. The glenohumeral joint can also be accessed for intra-articular fractures. It is imperative that the correct interval is used, to avoid injury to neurovascular structures located in the quadrangular space, which is more lateral and caudal to the desired interval. Once the appropriate interval is developed, the lateral border can be accessed for

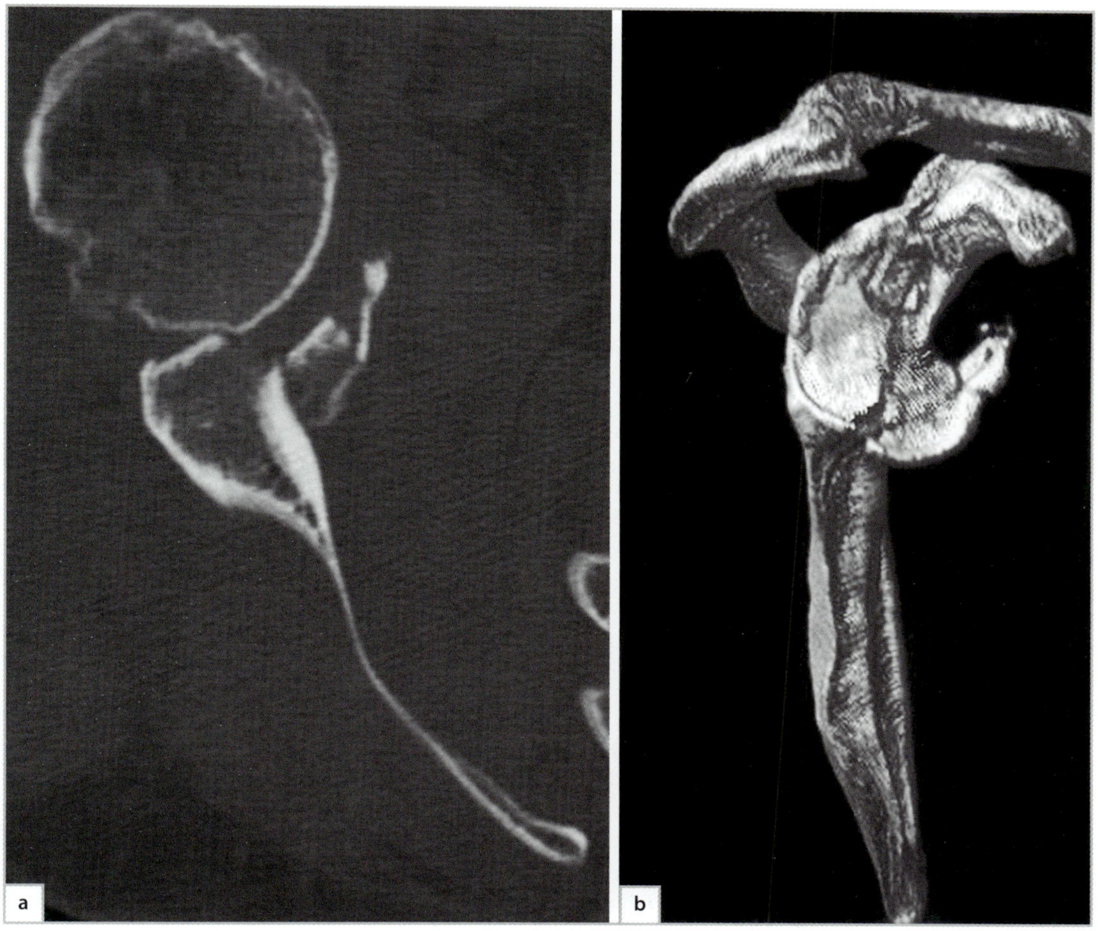

Figure 15.10 Computerized tomography images of a comminuted intra-articular fracture. This is the same fracture as in Fig. 15.9. The axial scan (a) and three-dimensional reconstruction (b) illustrate the benefits of this imaging modality.

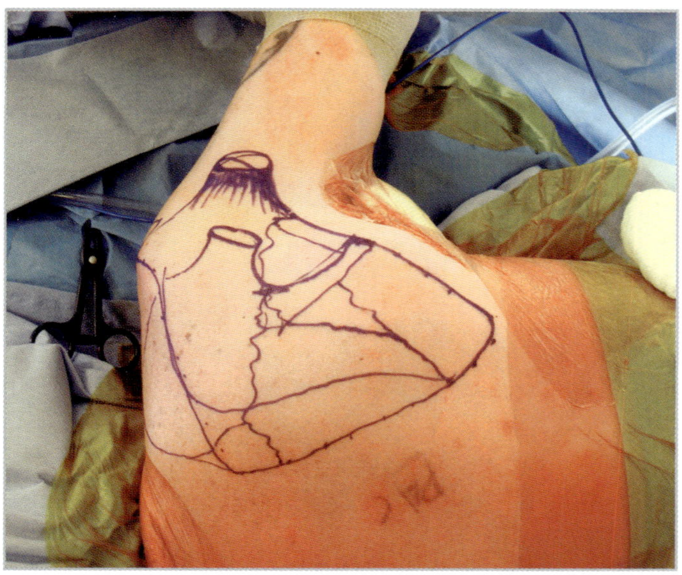

Figure 15.11 Position of the patient for a posterior approach to the scapula. Soft positioning wedges (BoneFoam, Excel Medical Solutions Inc., Plymouth, MN) allow for a supportive working surface, while protecting the downside arm. The patient's body, positioned on a beanbag, should be allowed to fall forward. The entire arm should be prepped to allow for manipulation and motion of the glenohumeral joint during the procedure.

reduction and plate placement. If needed, a transverse capsulotomy can be made, and the humeral head can be retracted for inspection of the articular surface. This maneuver is helpful to ensure restoration of the articular surface. During this arthrotomy, care must be taken to incise just distal to the labrum, an interval which can be appreciated with an 18-gauge needle.

The window to access the spine of the scapula is developed between the trapezius and the deltoid. The dissection is carried out subperiosteally, off the inferior margin of the spine, to uncover the rotator cuff muscles. The deltoid can be dissected off the muscular origin of the infraspinatus, and tagged through its fascial cuff for reattachment to osseous tunnels later or elevated with a retractor. The latter is more work of retraction during surgery, but spares taking down the deltoid and requiring its reattachment and healing.

At the vertebral border of the scapula, the intermuscular plane is between the infraspinatus and the rhomboids. We routinely use this exposure, as it is helpful to provide additional fixation at the medial spine, to render maximum stability.

While limited exposure is preferred, it is technically challenging to control all the fragments in highly comminuted scapula fractures. In addition, it is challenging to mobilize and reduce fractures treated after a delay, as fractures of the scapula rapidly form callus and contractures, which can be difficult to overcome. A general consideration for this approach could be fractures that are less than 10 days and have less than four exit points around the ring of the scapula perimeter. However, surgeon experience and skill will often dictate the operation, with open (versus less invasive) approaches being favored with less familiarity.

Extensile posterior approach/exposure

Alternatively, an extensile approach can be executed for entire posterior scapula exposure by elevating all musculature off the infraspinatus fossa with an elevator (**Fig. 15.12b**). This muscular flap can be elevated laterally as far as the lateral border, and allows exposure to the glenoid neck. The extensile approach exposes the entire posterior surface of the scapular body; however, the entire subscapularis muscular sleeve on the anterior surface of the scapula is preserved, maintaining blood supply to the scapular body. In this context, the extensile approach is biologically respectful, as supported by an extraordinarily low reported rate of non-union (just a single case report). It is most helpful to utilize an extensile approach by elevating the deltoid, infraspinatus, and teres minor in a single flap. As mentioned above, the extensile exposure grants the surgeon adequate control of the fracture at multiple points to effect the reduction and mobilize the fracture by breaking up intervening callus (**Fig. 15.14a**). It will not allow for exposure of the glenoid, due to the large flap; the surgeon should not try to retract this flap for joint exposure, because it will cause excessive retraction of the suprascapular neurovascular bundle. For adequate intra-articular exposure, an intermuscular dissection is necessary over the posterior glenohumeral joint.

Minimally invasive posterior approach

The use of small incisions distant from the fracture site to introduce implants and apply fixation is now a commonly accepted strategy in the management of fractures of the long bones, and we have recently applied this concept to fixation of the scapula. This approach allows for direct reduction of the fracture at its margins, without violating soft-tissue attachments along the majority of the fracture across the scapular body (Gauger and Cole 2011).

Straight skin incisions approximately 6 cm long are made at each fracture end (**Fig. 15.15**). Windows are then developed based on fracture pattern. For lateral border and posterior glenoid access, dissection is taken down to the inferior deltoid fascia, and the interval between the infraspinatus and teres minor is exposed by retracting the deltoid cephalad. The fascia overlying these rotator cuff muscles are then divided in line with their muscle fibers, and blunt dissection is used down to the lateral border, and the fracture site and glenoid neck is exposed.

Most fractures that exit the medial border are close to the base of the spine. The medial window is developed by dissecting down to the fascia and then periosteum, along the base of the spine and inferiorly on the vertebral border. A subperiosteal dissection is then performed to elevate the infraspinatus to the degree necessary to visualize the fracture and its reduction.

Straight posterior approach

A direct posterior approach can be used in the case of an isolated posterior glenoid fracture or an intra-articular glenoid fracture with a true glenoid neck fracture extending to the spinoglenoid notch. This exposure allows for the pathology to be determined, and for the desired reduction and fixation accomplished solely through the interval between the teres minor and the infraspinatus.

Straight posterior approach with infraspinatus tenotomy

Occasionally, in patients with substantial articular comminution, greater exposure of the joint can be gained with an infraspinatus tenotomy, where 1 cm of cuff insertion is left at the greater tuberosity

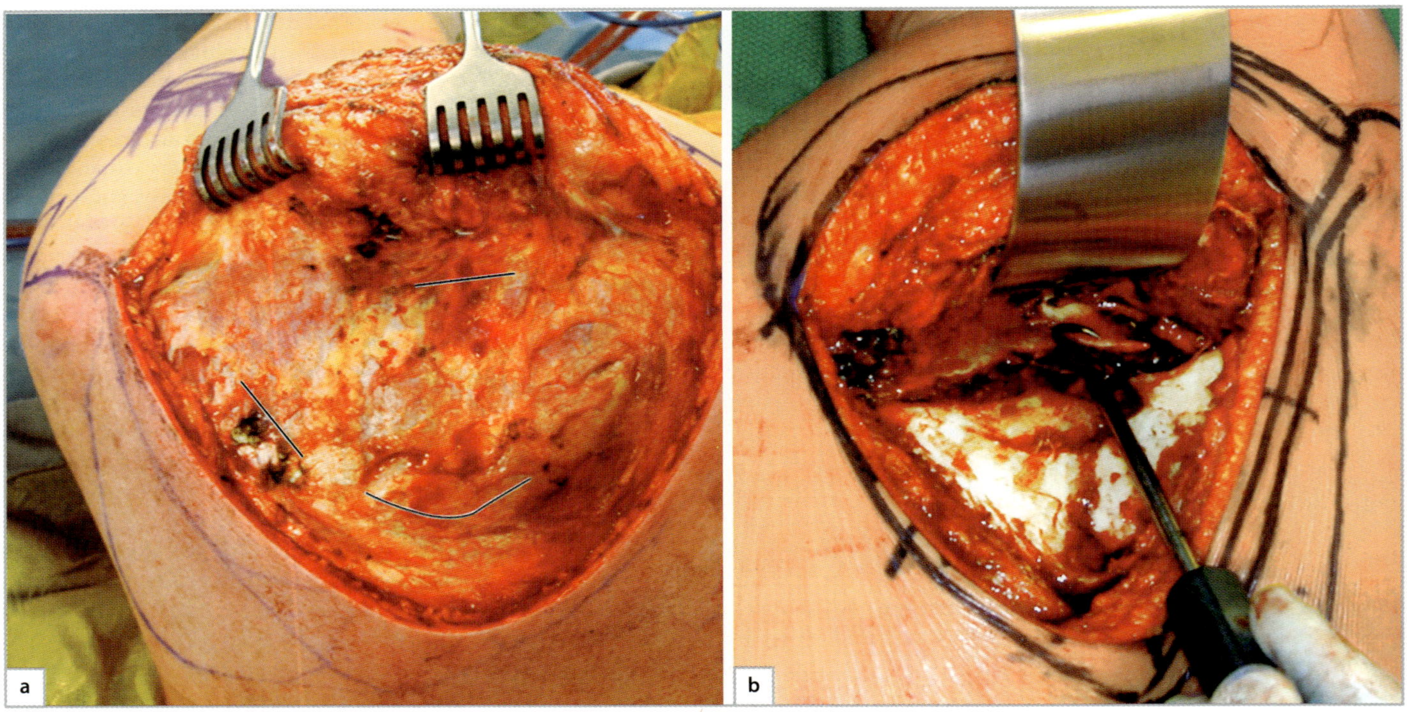

Figure 15.12 A Judet incision, the main posterior approach utilized for scapula fractures. The incision is planned along these landmarks: 1 cm caudal to the acromion spine, and 1 cm lateral to the vertebral border. (a) A Judet incision with subcutaneous flap elevated laterally. Intermuscular windows can then be developed to access bony anatomy. The white lines are the approximate location of window development. Alternatively, the surgeon can further dissect the Judet incision for the extensile exposure. (b) Infraspinatus, teres minor, and deltoid elevated laterally.

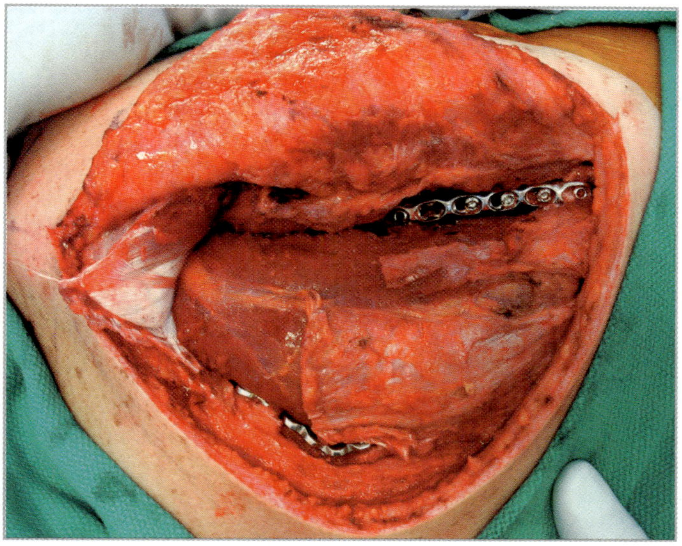

Figure 15.13 Management of a fracture via lateral and superomedial intermuscular windows.

for repair. This allows the slender musculotendinous portion of the infraspinatus to be retracted off the superior glenoid region, for better access to the glenohumeral joint. It is repaired with two heavy braided number 2 sutures at closure, and active external rotation against resistance should be protected for six weeks postoperatively.

Fracture reduction

To assist fracture reduction, a surgeon should have on hand at least two small pointed bone reduction clamps and two 4 mm Schanz pins with a small external fixator set, as well as a pair of small T-handle chucks. Often a 2.7 mm dynamic compression plate straddling a fracture of the lateral border can be helpful for reduction (as well as definitive fixation) since it is applied straight, without the need for contouring of this border. Pointed bone tenaculums can be applied at the periphery wherever there is a fracture exit point with displacement. The standard tenaculum frequently does not suit the pattern well, due to interference with the flap, so a Schanz pin in the proximal and distal segments can be secured in proper orientation, with a small external fixator bar and clamps to line up the lateral border for subsequent plating. If the reduction is still not stable, a provisional 2.0 mm plate and screws slightly more medial can be used to hold the lateral border appropriately aligned before a larger dynamic compression plate is placed. Further, a clamp can be placed at the medial extent of the fracture at the scapula spine or vertebral border to help offload stresses on the lateral border while maintaining reduction.

Fracture fixation

It is the senior author's experience that 2.7 mm plates are of adequate strength and seem to be the best suited for the scapula borders. This is based on a personal series of over 180 fractures without evidence of plate failure. The strategy of re-establishing the peripheral bony rim by fixation of all borders may have contributed to this absence of implant failure (**Fig. 15.14b**). The advantages of the 2.7 mm plates are their low profile, ease of contouring, and a greater number of screws per centimeter than with a 3.5 mm plate. Dynamic compression plates are preferred on the lateral border, where stresses are greatest, since they are stronger than reconstruction plates. Reconstruction plates are used for the spine and medial border of the scapula, as they are much easier to contour around the junction of the base of the spine and the vertebral border. Two pediatric Kocher clamps placed in adjacent holes are useful for bending and contouring these plates. Use of locking plates and screws gives better screw-hold, and allows for much shorter plates.

Before wound closure, it is important to ensure that all extrinsic adhesions and stiffness are eliminated, especially where there has been an extended delay to surgery. This is one reason why the entire extremity is prepped – for manipulation at the end of the procedure. The surgeon should proceed with closure over a self-suction drain under the flap, using a braided number 2 non-absorbable suture through several drill holes at the scapular spine and vertebral border, to ensure that the rotator cuff cannot avulse postoperatively. The rest of the musculofascial closure can be repaired with a number 1 resorbable braided suture. We prefer an absorbable subcuticular stitch for the skin to mitigate scar formation. However, in this region, scar formation can be excessive due to the high elastic multidirectional skin stretch, which should be anticipated during the early phase rehabilitation.

Treatment via an anterior approach

The patient is placed in a beach-chair position with an arm-board attached to support the extremity. A small towel roll is placed under the ipsilateral shoulder, to help thrust it forward. It is helpful to position an x-ray plate behind the shoulder during the setup so that an intraoperative film can be taken.

An incision is made from the palpable coracoid to a point just lateral to the axillary fold. This incision is taken down the deltopectoral interval, to where the cephalic vein is identified. If more exposure is desired, the incision can be extended distally on the humerus to the deltoid insertion, and proximally above the coracoid. The cephalic vein is then retracted laterally with the deltoid, and preserved throughout the procedure. The deltopectoral interval is dissected down to expose and release the clavipectoral fascia. The coracobrachialis and subscapularis tendons are now exposed. Superior and inferior retractors are placed, and the surgery can proceed either by releasing the subscapularis tendon, or by performing a coracoid osteotomy.

The subscapularis is released 1 cm from its insertion onto the humerus, which will leave a cuff of tendon attached to the tuberosity for repair at closure. Often the subscapularis seems indistinct from the joint capsule, due to capsular insertion or adhesion of its fibers. The humerus can be rotated to appreciate the subscapularis tendon's insertion onto the lesser tuberosity. It is helpful to discriminate and individually identify these two layers for an accurate closure, but, occasionally, it may be necessary to repair the two jointly. At the inferior margin of the tendon are vessels running transversely, which should be ligated. Below these vessels, the axillary nerve is at risk, and there is no reason to extend the dissection this far inferior. Stay sutures should be placed on each side of the subscapularis muscle, to identify it for closure, as well as to prevent medial displacement of the muscle. The joint capsule is now appreciated and can be cut and tagged longitudinally just off the palpable glenoid rim. A capsulotomy is mandatory if there is comminution and the surgeon needs to work on either side of the capsule. Alternatively, the surgeon can work through the fracture to wash out the joint and obtain an indirect articular reduction by working extra-articularly with the fragment. Releasing the subscapularis tendon is ideal for small rim lesions and non-comminuted anterior fragments that were determined in preoperative planning not to require a buttress plate for stable fixa-

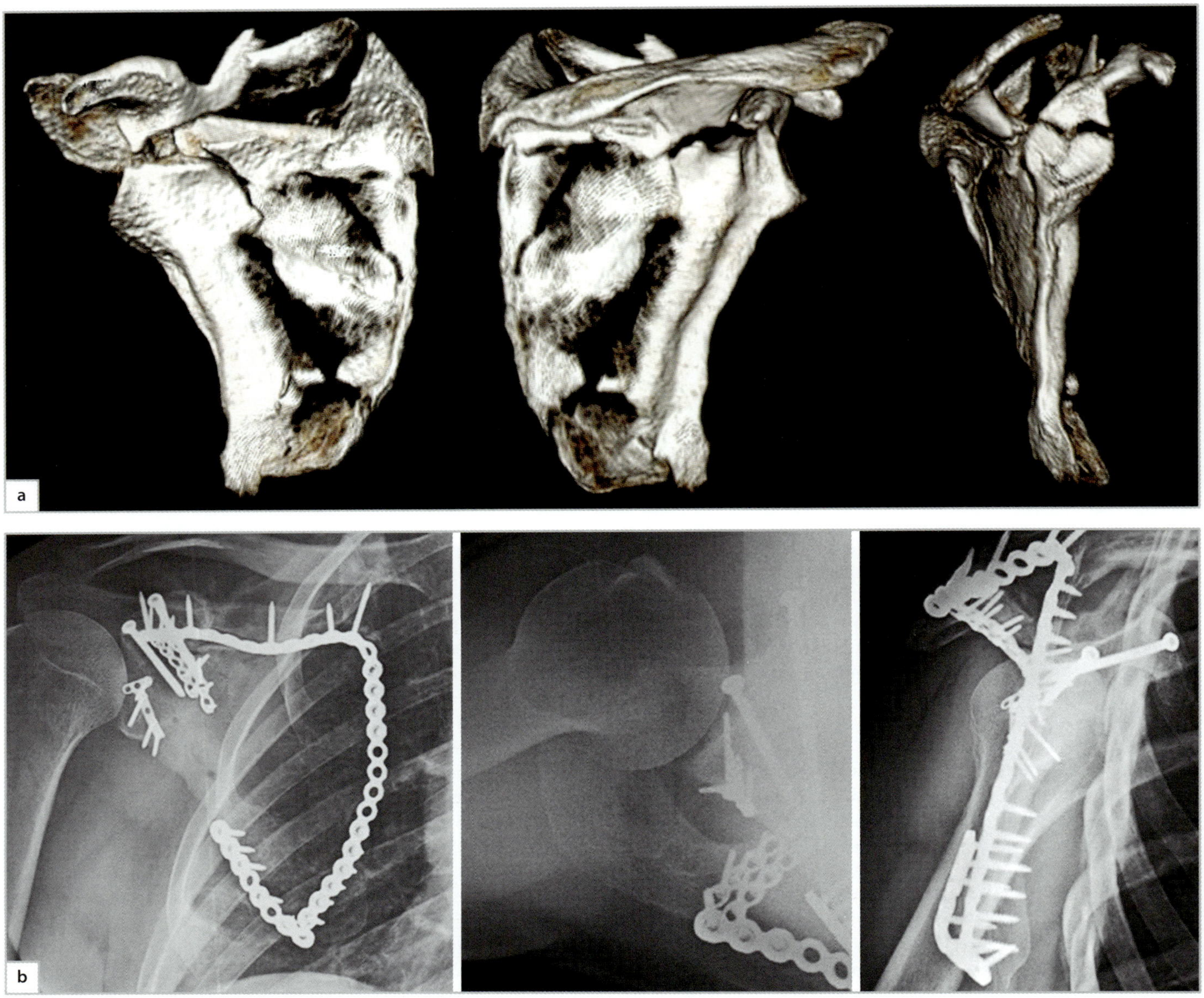

Figure 15.14 Extensile approach for the reduction and fixation of a fracture of the scapula. (a) Preoperative three-dimensional computerized tomography reconstruction of a scapula with six fracture exit points around the perimeter. The extensile approach is often necessary for reduction and fixation of highly comminuted fractures such as these. (b) Postoperative radiographs of the same fracture. Extensive plating was utilized for stable fixation of the bony perimeter.

tion. In some cases it may be difficult to obtain adequate exposure after releasing the subscapularis tendon. This is most often due to the presence of a large fracture of the anterior glenoid rim that extends medially along the neck, or anterior comminution requiring a buttress plate that extends medially. The surgeon may elect to perform a coracoid osteotomy to facilitate greater exposure.

The coracoid osteotomy begins by predrilling the coracoid with a 2.5 mm drill bit, and its surface can be scored with an osteotome or micro-oscillating saw. The osteotomy should be completed with an osteotome; however, care should be taken to create some degree of irregularity to the surfaces, as this will facilitate 'keying in' for anatomic repair at the end of the articular work. Once released, the conjoined tendon and coracoid may be reflected distally and medially. Excellent exposure of the anterior glenoid and scapular neck should now be appreciated. It is important to note that the musculocutaneous nerve penetrates the coracobrachialis approximately 5 cm from the tip of the coracoid. Care should be taken when reflecting the conjoined tendon distally so as to protect the musculocutaneous nerve from traction injury. Upon repair, the proximal cortex should be overdrilled with a 3.5 mm bit to lag the coracoid with a 3.5 mm cortical screw.

A dental pick or shoulder hook can assist in reduction of the anterior glenoid. Kirschner wires are helpful for provisional fixation. Fluoroscopy should not be needed, as direct inspection of the joint is possible, although the thickness of the articular cartilage and labral tissue must be taken into consideration. Depending on the size of the fragment, or the degree of comminution, implant (screw) choices may range in size from 2.0 mm to 3.5 mm. Most frequently, a 2.0 mm minibuttress plate is appropriate on the anteroinferior edge, particularly if there is any comminution.

Closure of the capsule and subscapularis may be executed with number 2 braided suture, the subcutaneous tissue approximated with

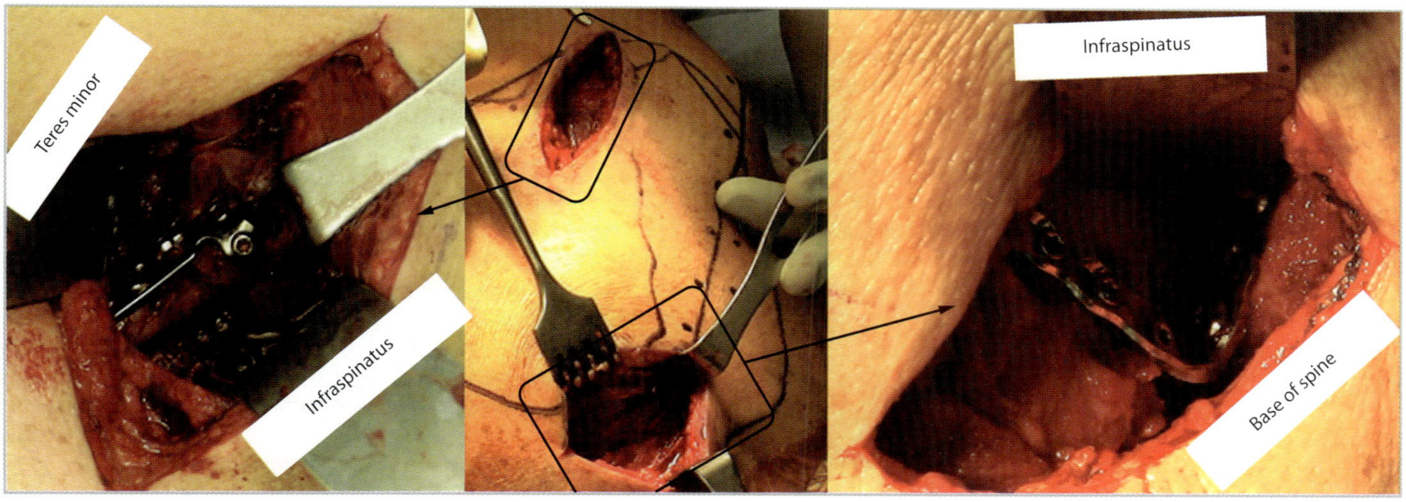

Figure 15.15 Intraoperative photographs showing minimally invasive limited incisions, deeper exposure, and clamp and plate application. The division between the deltoid and infraspinatus muscles can be seen. Once this important interval has been identified and developed, retractors can be placed to expose the lateral scapular border.

2-0 absorbable braided suture, and the skin closed with a monofilament, subcuticular, absorbable suture.

Arthroscopy (for intra-articular fractures of the glenoid)

As in other areas of surgery, the trend toward developing minimally invasive techniques is also observed in shoulder trauma. Cameron (1998) first reported an all-arthroscopic treatment of a glenoid fracture. The benefits of arthroscopic treatment are that the surgeon has a direct view of the articular surface, as well as the ability to assess the integrity of labrum and joint capsule, and it potentially minimizes the complications of open reduction and fixation. The literature suggests these methods are best reserved for fractures managed within two weeks of injury, and for relatively non-comminuted rim and fossa lesions that involve less than 30% of the articular surface. Both screws and suture anchors have been reported as methods of fixation. Fragment size and the presence of comminution dictate fixation choice. Suture anchors may be better suited for smaller fragments, as screws have the potential to split the fragment or penetrate the articular cartilage. Recently, Millett and Braun (2009) described a suture bridge technique as a means to give two-point fixation, to gain compression of fragments as well as to improve rotational stability.

Pearls and pitfalls

The first opportunity to diagnose a fracture of the scapula is with the initial trauma chest films. They are often missed with this imaging, due to the surrounding bone and soft tissue. The clinician should have a higher degree of suspicion for a fracture of the scapula when other proximal forequarter fractures are present. Dedicated shoulder radiographs should be ordered to rule out a fracture of the scapula if there is any pickup on the trauma chest film.

Fractures managed non-operatively should be closely followed radiographically to ensure fracture union and to monitor stability. Double disruptions of the SSSC as well as transverse extra-articular fractures that extend from the inferior glenoid neck to just inferior to the base of the spine may have a propensity to displace progressively into an operative category of displacement (Anavian, et al. 20010).

Certain fractures of the scapula are associated with injury of the suprascapular nerve, especially fractures of the scapula neck that extend into the spinoglenoid notch. The clinician should suspect nerve insult in this pattern when the fracture is displaced. Isometric testing of the infraspinatus helps the clinician to assess the integrity of this nerve without causing excess discomfort to the patient. Electromyography (EMG) will be inconclusive too soon after injury, but should be ordered after two or three weeks if there is suspicion of nerve damage. Intraoperatively, care should be taken during dissection, and the nerve should be liberated from the fracture before reduction is performed. Repair should be performed in the event that a lacerated nerve is identified. Often the crushed nerve can only be reattached to the anterior surface of the infraspinatus, approximating other branches.

It is the senior author's experience that surgery within the first 10 days is ideal. The callus is still immature and easy to take down, which allows the surgeon to utilize less invasive exposures to restore anatomy. Unfortunately, this is often not the case. Patients with abrasions in the surgical field are treated in a delayed fashion, to allow re-epithelialization. Additionally, associated injuries are very common, and higher-priority injuries will need to be stabilized. In addition, as mentioned above, fractures of the scapula are often missed, which will naturally delay treatment. Delayed surgery is technically more challenging for the surgeon, but we have previously reported that excellent outcomes can nevertheless be achieved in the majority of such patients (Herrera et al. 2009). In addition, we have also reported a case series showing that revision surgery for symptomatic malunions results in improved subjective and objective outcomes (Cole et al. 2011).

REHABILITATION

The goal of an orthopaedic trauma surgeon while fixing a fracture is to render it stable. Stable fixation is a construct that withstands physiologic passive motion. The adult shoulder has a propensity to get stiff quickly, and every effort must be directed at maintaining the full range of motion. At the end of every case, full passive range-of-motion exercises should be instituted immediately. The goal in the first four weeks postoperatively is to regain and maintain motion. A stable fixed fracture can soon feel quite comfortable, and the patient will be inclined to use it. The patient must understand that no lifting or weight bearing should be done for four weeks. However, ipsilateral elbow, wrist, and hand exercises, including with weights (around 2 kg, lifted with a supported elbow), are encouraged. These exercises will help to prevent any muscular atrophy in the arm, and help reduce edema.

Assistive devices such as pulleys, push-pull sticks in the opposite extremity, and supine assisted motion are necessary. Narcotic pain medications are useful during early rehabilitation, as they will help the patient to withstand greater ranges of motion. A regional anesthetic block with an indwelling interscalene catheter for the first 48–72 hours postoperatively is an excellent adjunctive method to promote early gains in confidence.

Postoperative orders

- Sling for comfort.
- Discontinue drain when discharge is less than 15 cc/8 hour shift.
- 24 hours of antibiotic perioperative coverage.
- Full-shoulder passive and active range of motion.
- Initiate strengthening at four weeks postoperatively, beginning with 2 kg (3–5 lb) weights.
- Advance strength program aggressively at eight weeks postoperatively.
- Remove all restrictions at 12 weeks postoperatively.

Patients who are still reluctant to progress their passive range of motion after six weeks should be taken for a manipulation under anesthesia, since most patients have almost full active range of motion by this time. Specific at-risk patients include those with injury to the head or brachial plexus (who may be totally dependent upon others for their therapy), as well as those with complex associated ipsilateral injuries and those with a halo vest for spine fractures. We prefer injecting 10 cc of an intra-articular solution of local anesthetic and steroid to mitigate reformation of intra-articular adhesions.

REFERENCES

Ada JR, Miller ME. Scapular fractures: analysis of 113 cases. Clin Orthop Relat Res 1991;269:174–180.

Anavian J, Wijdicks CA, Schroder LK, et al. Surgery for scapula process fractures. Acta Orthop 2009;3:344–350.

Anavian J, Khanna G, Plocher EK, et al. Progressive displacement of scapula fractures. J Trauma 2010;69:156–161.

Anavian J, Conflitti JM, Khanna G, et al. A reliable radiographic measurement technique for extra-articular scapular fractures. Clin Orthop Relat Res 2011;469:3371–3378.

Armitage BM, Wijdicks CA, Tarkin IS, et al. Mapping of scapular fractures with three-dimensional computed tomography. J Bone Joint Surg Am 2009;91:2222–2228.

Cameron SE. Arthroscopic reduction and internal fixation of an anterior glenoid fracture. Arthroscopy 1998;7:743–746.

Chadwick EK, van Noort A, van der Helm FC. Biomechanical analysis of scapular neck malunion – a simulation study. Clin Biomech (Bristol, Avon) 2004;9:906–912.

Cole PA, Talbot M, Schroder LK, Anavian J. Extra-articular malunions of the scapula: a comparison of functional outcome before and after reconstruction. J Orthop Trauma 2011;25:649–656.

Edwards SG, Whittle AP, Wood GW 2nd. Nonoperative treatment of ipsilateral fractures of the scapula and clavicle. J Bone Joint Surg Am 2000;6:774–780.

Gauger EM, Cole PA. Surgical technique: a minimally invasive approach to scapula neck and body fractures. Clin Orthop Relat Res 2011;469:3390–3399.

Goss TP. Double disruptions of the superior shoulder suspensory complex. J Orthop Trauma 1993;2:99–106.

Hardegger FH, Simpson LA, Weber BG. The operative treatment of scapular fractures. J Bone Joint Surg Br 1984;5:725–731.

Herrera DA, Anavian J, Tarkin IS, et al. Delayed operative management of fractures of the scapula. J Bone Joint Surg Br 2009;5:619–626.

Marsh JL, Slongo TF, Agel J, et al. Fracture and dislocation classification compendium – 2007: orthopaedic trauma association classification, database and outcomes committee. J Orthop Trauma 2007;10 Suppl:S1–133.

Mayo KA, Benirschke SK, Mast JW. Displaced fractures of the glenoid fossa. results of open reduction and internal fixation. Clin Orthop Relat Res 1998;347:122–130.

Millett PJ, Braun S. The 'bony Bankart bridge' procedure: a new arthroscopic technique for reduction and internal fixation of a bony Bankart lesion. Arthroscopy 2009;1:102–105.

Nordqvist A, Petersson C. Fracture of the body, neck, or spine of the scapula. A long-term follow-up study. Clin Orthop Relat Res 1992;283:139–144.

Obremskey WT, Lyman JR. A modified Judet approach to the scapula. J Orthop Trauma 2004;10:696–699.

Ogawa K, Naniwa T. Fractures of the acromion and the lateral scapular spine. J Shoulder Elbow Surg 1997;6:544–548.

Ogawa K, Yoshida A, Takahashi M, Ui M. Fractures of the coracoid process. J Bone Joint Surg Br 1997;1:17–19.

Ramos L, Mencia R, Alonso A, Ferrandez L. Conservative treatment of ipsilateral fractures of the scapula and clavicle. J Trauma 1997;2:239–242.

Romero J, Schai P, Imhoff AB. Scapular neck fracture – the influence of permanent malalignment of the glenoid neck on clinical outcome. Arch Orthop Trauma Surg 2001;6:313–316.

Chapter 16 Open reduction and internal fixation of fractures of the clavicle

Trevor R. Gaskill, Jared T. Lee, Robert E. Boykin,
Olivier A. J. van der Meijden, Peter J. Millett

INTRODUCTION

Clavicle fractures are common injuries and account for 2–5% of all adult fractures. Overall, the incidence is reported to be 29–64 per 100,000 in the adult population and these injuries appear to have a bimodal age distribution (Postacchini et al. 2002). Males aged under 30 years who are involved in sporting activities and patients over the age of 70 with osteoporotic bone appear to be two distinct groups at higher risk of fracturing the clavicle. More than two thirds of these injuries occur within the middle third of the clavicle, and these are more likely to be displaced than are fractures of the medial or lateral third. Lateral fractures account for approximately 25% of all clavicle fractures. Medial fractures are least common, comprising 2–3% of these injuries (Postacchini et al. 2002).

It has been suggested that non-surgical management of clavicle fractures uniformly results in union and satisfactory functional outcomes (Kashif Kahn et al. 2009) but in fact good outcomes are not universal. Recent evidence suggests that specific subsets of patients may be at high risk of non-union, shoulder dysfunction, or residual pain after non-surgical management (Nordqvist et al. 1997, Lazarides and Zafiropoulos 2006). In this subset of patients, acute surgical intervention may minimize suboptimal outcomes. Therefore, treatment of fractures of the clavicle should be individualized, based on fracture characteristics and patient expectations.

CLASSIFICATION

The first widely accepted classification system for fractures of the clavicle was described by Allman in 1967. It grouped fractures anatomically based on location and in descending order of incidence (Allman 1967). Therefore, fractures of the middle third of the clavicle are type I, as they are most common. Similarly, group II and type III fractures describe involvement of the lateral and medial thirds, respectively (**Fig. 16.1**).

The Allman classification was later modified by Neer, based on the recognition that the coracoclavicular (CC) ligaments were important to the stability of the medial fracture segment (Neer 1968). Therefore, fractures of the lateral third of the clavicle occurring distal to the CC ligaments were termed group I fractures. These injuries are typically stable, and are characterized by minimal fracture displacement because the CC ligaments function to maintain reduction of the medial fragment. By contrast, group II injuries are characterized by vertical displacement of the medial fracture fragment, implying discontinuity of the CC ligaments with the medial clavicle. These displaced fractures are subcategorized based on the integrity of the CC ligaments with the distal fracture fragment: group IIA fractures are defined by a fracture pattern that leaves both the conoid and trapezoid ligaments attached to the distal fracture segment, whereas a fracture occurring between the CC ligaments that results in the rupture of the more medial conoid ligament defines a group IIB injury. The displacement and vertical instability of the medial fracture fragment with these injuries results in a higher risk of non-union. group III fractures extend into the acromioclavicular (AC) joint, and are typically stable injuries, but may result in late traumatic arthrosis.

These early classification systems do not account for fracture pattern, displacement, or comminution, and are therefore less predictive of outcome. A more recent classification system was described by Robinson and is based on 1000 clavicle fractures occurring over a six-year period (Robinson 1998). This system classifies fractures of the clavicle according to their location, displacement, angulation, comminution, and intra-articular extension (**Fig. 16.2**). As in the earlier classification systems, fractures are initially described anatomically as occurring in the medial (type 1), middle (type 2), or lateral (type 3) third of the clavicle. Each is then subclassified based on fracture displacement. Subgroup A signifies displacement less than 100%, whereas those fractures more than 100% displaced are classified as subgroup B. These fractures are further subcategorized based on articular involvement (type 1 or 3) or degree of comminution (type 2). Despite the increased complexity of the classification system, it has prognostic value, as well as high interobserver and intraobserver reliability among orthopaedic trainees. Using this classification system, the authors report that both displacement and comminution were associated with a higher risk of delayed union or non-union (Robinson 2004).

INDICATIONS

Midshaft fractures

The primary goal of treatment is to achieve bony union and restore function to the shoulder girdle, thereby allowing patients to return to their preinjury activity level. Historically, displaced fractures were treated non-operatively, and studies reported a high level of patient satisfaction, and non-union rates of less than 1% (Rowe 1968). Thus, nearly all fractures of the middle third of the clavicle were initially treated non-operatively. These studies, however, did not take into account fracture severity, and included outcomes of clavicle fractures in children (who have the highest union rates). More recent evidence suggests that surgical fixation of some types of fracture results in a 16% reduction in the rate of non-union. Others have reported that restoration of clavicle length and alignment is associated with improved

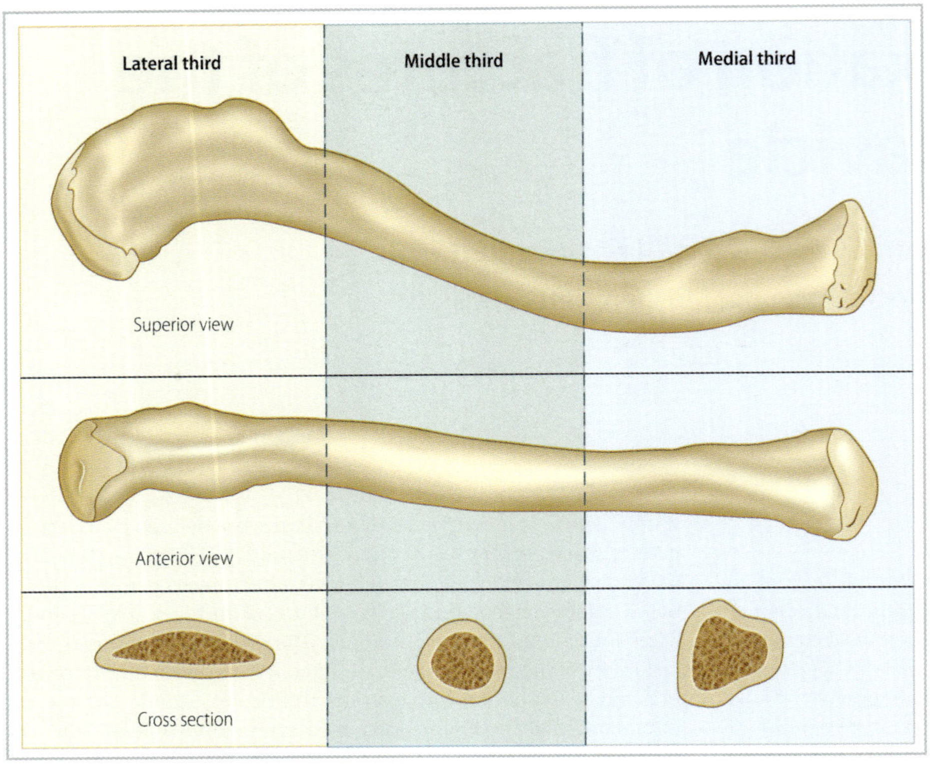

Figure 16.1 Anatomy and cross-sectional display of the clavicle. (Reprinted with permission from Craig EV. Fractures of the shoulder: Part II. Fractures of the clavicle. In: Rockwood CA, Green DP, Bucholz RW, eds. Rockwood and Green's Fractures in Adults, 3rd edition. Philadelphia, PA: JB Lippincott, 1991: vol 1, pp 928–990.)

functional outcomes (Kashif Kahn et al. 2009). Moreover, patient-based outcome scores indicate that many patients are dissatisfied with non-surgical management in certain circumstances. Therefore, it is now appreciated that all fractures of the clavicle do not behave identically, and that rates of non-union and symptomatic malunion in the adult population are likely higher than previously reported. It is also evident that advances in surgical technique and implants have resulted in less frequent operative complications. Others, however, continue to report high patient satisfaction with non-operative management (Zlowodski et al. 2005). The indications for surgical fixation of fractures of the midshaft of the clavicle therefore remain controversial.

It is generally agreed that non-displaced or minimally displaced fractures of the clavicle are best treated non-operatively. Sling immobilization has been reported to result in less discomfort, fewer complications including skin irritation, and similar clinical outcomes as compared to figure-of-eight bandaging (Andersen 1987). It appears that immobilization for between two and six weeks, tailored by patient discomfort, followed by structured shoulder rehabilitation, is successful for many patients. Contact sports should be avoided for a minimum of four months in these circumstances.

The treatment of displaced fractures is more controversial, although several absolute indications for acute surgical intervention do exist. These include skin tenting, open fractures, and the presence of neurovascular compromise. Fracture displacement or shortening greater than 2 cm, comminution, female gender, and advancing age have also been recently associated with less optimal outcomes, and may be considered relative indications for acute intervention (Nordqvist et al. 1997, Robinson et al. 2004, Nowak et al. 2005, Lazarides and Zafiropoulos 2006). Surgical intervention should also be considered in the context of polytrauma, and symptomatic non-union or malunion (Kashif Kahn et al. 2009).

Fractures of the lateral third of the clavicle

The indication for surgical fixation of fractures of the distal third of the clavicle is more clearly defined and is based on fracture stability. Neer type I and III injuries occur distal to the CC ligament insertion. This implies CC ligament continuity with the medial fracture fragment and, therefore, relative medial fragment stability. These injuries can typically be treated with immobilization, and commonly heal with minimal deformity. It is important to inform patients, however, that type III injuries may ultimately result in AC joint degeneration, and excision of the distal clavicle may be necessary if symptomatic. Neer type II injuries by definition are displaced, and imply vertical instability of the medial fragment. These injuries have been noted to exhibit a 30% risk of non-union if treated non-surgically (Oh et al. 2011). Therefore, surgical intervention is often recommended for this fracture pattern.

CONTRAINDICATIONS

There are several contraindications to surgical fixation of fractures of the clavicle. These include factors that place the patient at high risk for surgical complications related to wound healing, infection, anesthesia, or bony union. These complications should be considered in patients with active infection, irradiated tissues, or burns on the surgical site. Patients exhibiting decompensated medical conditions are also at higher risk of surgical complications, and these should be weighed against the potential benefits of surgical fixation. Elderly patients with low physical demands may also represent a relative contraindication to surgical treatment in the acute setting.

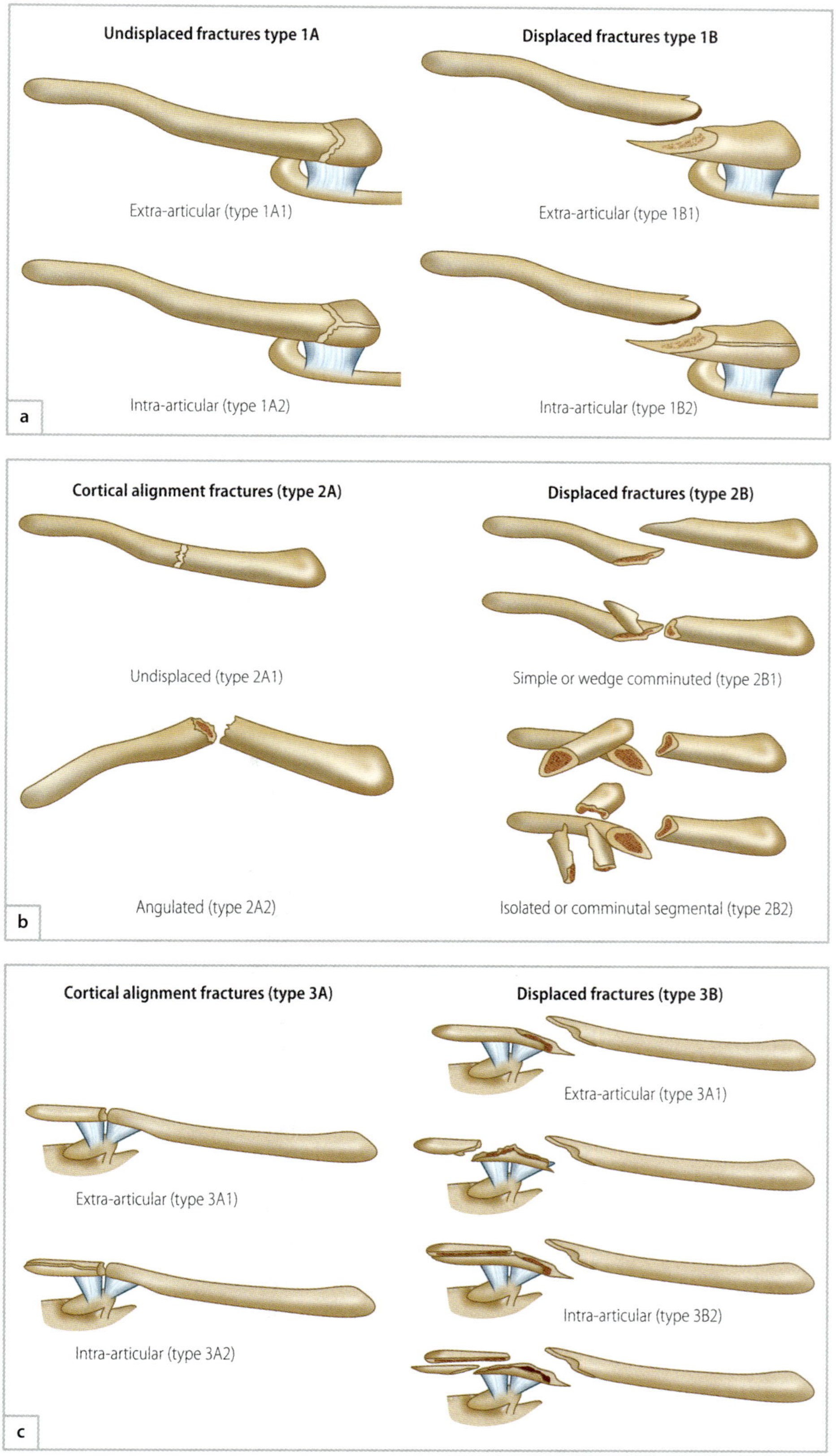

Figure 16.2 Edinburgh classification of clavicle fractures. (Reproduced with permission and copyright © of the British Editorial Society of Bone and Joint Surgery. Redrawn from Robinson CM. Fractures of the clavicle in the adult. Epidemiology and classification. J Bone Joint Surg Br 1998;80:476–484.)

TECHNIQUE

Midshaft fractures

Fractures of the midshaft of the clavicle are most commonly treated using plate or intramedullary pin fixation. Plates allow immediate rigid fixation. Plate fixation can be used to treat most fracture patterns, and allows for early mobilization. It has been shown to be biomechanically superior to other techniques, but may pose a greater risk to neurovascular structures; also, it can be more prominent than other types of fixation. Newer implants, precontoured to fit the clavicle anatomically, appear to reduce the need for hardware removal. Reconstruction-type plates are less favorable because they are biomechanically less rigid, and prone to deformation and failure at the fracture site.

Intramedullary fixation is also routinely used to treat these fractures. In contrast to plate fixation, this technique requires a smaller incision, which can be oriented within Langer's lines to produce a more cosmetic scar. It also requires less fracture stripping to accomplish, and is a load-sharing construct. However, because static locking options do not exist, intramedullary fixation provides less rotational and length stability than does plate fixation. Therefore, intramedullary pin fixation may be less beneficial in situations of severe comminution or segmental defects. It also requires hardware removal after bony union.

The complications with the two techniques are similar, although their incidence rates differ, and include infection, non-union, malunion, scar formation, refracture, and neurovascular injury. It has been recently reported that intramedullary pin fixation of high-risk fractures results in frequent early but temporary hardware prominence, and a non-union rate of 8.6% (Millett et al. 2011).

Plate fixation

Operative plating of the clavicle is complicated by its curved shape, which makes applying straight plates difficult. For this reason reconstruction plates have been traditionally been used for clavicle fixation, because they are easily contoured. These plates, however, provide less robust fixation, and frequently fatigue and fail at the fracture site. By contrast, limited-contact dynamic compression plates (LCDCP) provide more rigid fixation, but are more difficult to contour to the clavicle. For these reasons, anatomically contoured plates with locking-screw options have more recently been introduced, to provide rigid fixation while minimizing the need for anatomic contouring. These plates are frequently useful; however, they occasionally require manual contouring because the shape of the clavicle varies between patients.

Superior and anterior plate placement has been described for fractures of the clavicle. Superior plating may be accomplished with less stripping, and provides a broad surface for plate placement. This location, however, more commonly results in prominent and symptomatic hardware, and may pose a greater risk to neurovascular structures underlying the clavicle. By contrast, anterior placement may provide a less prominent hardware location, and greater protection of neurovascular structures. A larger amount of stripping is necessary for anterior placement, however, and the anterior surface of the clavicle tends to be narrower than the superior surface, which can complicate plate placement. On the basis of results from a simulated transverse fracture model, Iannotti et al. (2002) concluded that superiorly placed plates provide greater biomechanical rigidity than anteriorly placed plates. Others have suggested that anterior plating may be optimal if an inferior cortical defect is present. To date, no clinical studies have suggested that clinical outcome is correlated with the location of the plate.

Operative clavicle plating is performed under general anesthesia with or without a regional block. The patient is placed in the beach-chair position with a bump placed under the scapula, to assist with fracture reduction; this also makes the clavicle more prominent in the operative field. The head and endotracheal tube should be tilted away from the injured shoulder. In cases of considerable comminution, radiographic measurements of the uninjured clavicle can be used to help restore the injured side to appropriate length. The draped surgical field should include the base of the neck and sternum. The arm is typically prepped into the surgical field, to assist in reduction of the fracture. A C-arm should also be draped into the surgical field to facilitate intraoperative imaging.

The skin incision is centered over the fracture, parallel to the long axis of the clavicle (Millett and Heuer 2010). The length of incision should be consistent with the exposure necessary for fracture fixation. Typically, the incision overlies the clavicle, but it can also be placed slightly anterior, to maximize hardware coverage. The incision is carried through the subcutaneous tissue with care to preserve branches of the supraclavicular nerve as they cross over the clavicle subcutaneously. Injury to these branches may result in numbness below the clavicle, but typically has little long-term consequence. The platysma muscle is divided in line with its fibers, and the fracture hematoma is evacuated. Fracture fragments are then identified, and soft-tissue preventing reduction is removed. Care is taken to avoid stripping and devitalizing butterfly or comminuted segments. Reduction is achieved using reduction clamps and Kirschner wires (K-wires) as needed.

Once a satisfactory reduction is obtained, a plate is placed along the superior or anterior edge of the clavicle, and reduction forceps are used to reduce the plate to bone (**Fig. 16.3**). Simple oblique fracture patterns are often amenable to lag-screw placement, and small fragments can be cerclage sutured into place. If significant comminution is present, bridge plating using locking screws can often be performed. A minimum of three bicortical screws on each side of fracture should be used to ensure adequate fixation.

After screws are placed, the final reduction and screw length are confirmed under fluoroscopy prior to routine two-layer closure. Repair of the platysma and fascia over the clavicle helps prevent hardware irritation.

Intramedullary pin fixation

The patient is positioned, prepped, and draped in a manner similar to the plating technique described above. A large fluoroscopy C-arm unit is draped into the field perpendicular to the injured clavicle, and should allow visualization of the sternoclavicular and AC joints.

A skin incision 4–5 cm long is centered over the fracture, within Langer's lines, and perpendicular to the clavicle (Millett et al. 2010). Subcutaneous tissues are divided and the platysma is split in line with its fibers. Branches of the supraclavicular nerve are protected if encountered. Fracture fragments are identified, the fracture hematoma is evacuated, and large butterfly fragments are preserved with their soft-tissue attachments.

Once identified, the intramedullary portion of the medial fragment is tapped to accept the medial end of the appropriately sized clavicle pin (**Fig. 16.4**). Intraoperative imaging is used to ensure the sternoclavicular joint or anterior cortex of the clavicle is not breached while tapping occurs.

The lateral fragment is drilled to accept the lateral portion of the clavicle pin from medial to lateral. The posterolateral clavicle is perforated, and the selected intramedullary pin is passed in an antegrade fashion through the lateral bone fragment, and out through

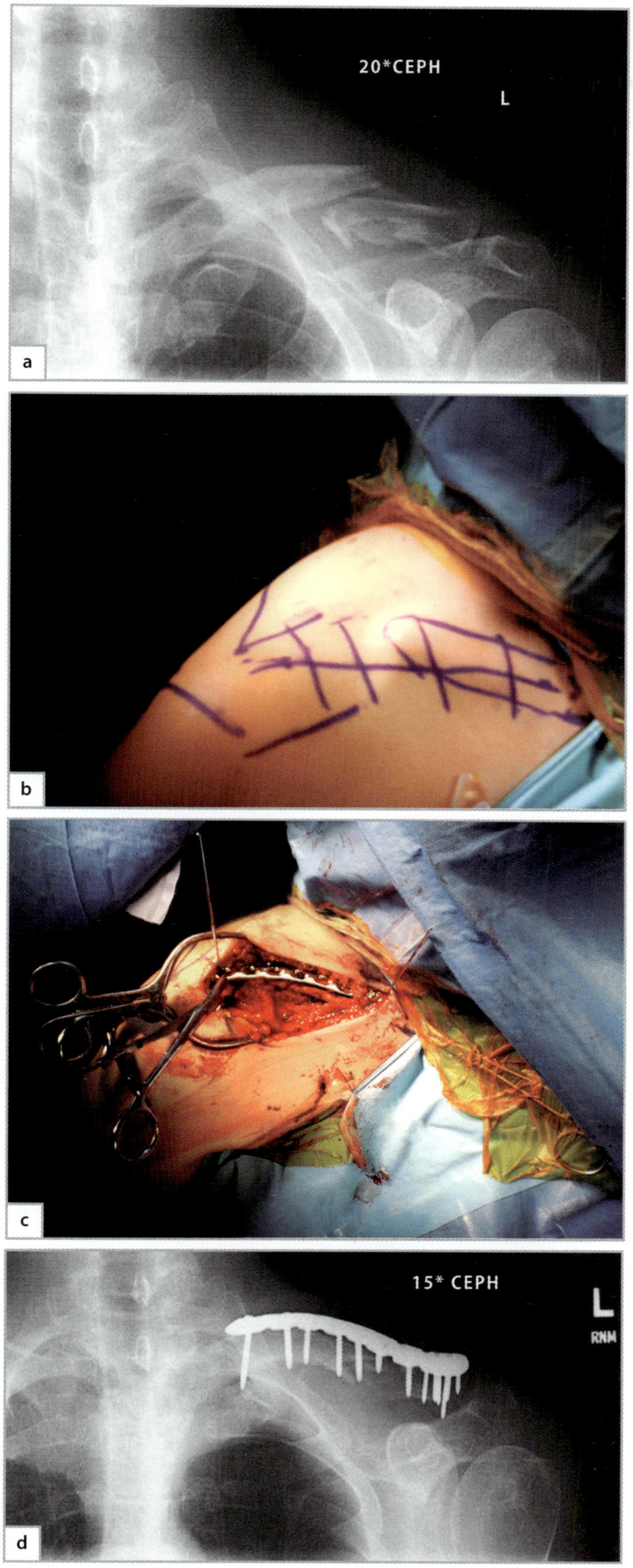

Figure 16.3 Plate fixation of a midshaft fracture of the left clavicle. (a) Preoperative anteroposterior image prior to superior plating. (b,c) Intraoperative images of superior plating. (d) Postoperative radiograph demonstrating completed superior plate fixation.

the posterolateral cortex of the clavicle. Once the pin is tenting the skin, a 1–2 cm incision is made to allow the pin to exit. In order to help minimize the prominence of the lateral locking nuts beneath the skin, the pin should exit the posterolateral clavicle as low as possible.

The drill is secured laterally to the clavicle pin exiting the posterolateral skin incision. It is further advanced until it is possible to place the blunt medial end of the intramedullary pin within the medial fracture fragment. The fracture is reduced, and the two hexagonal nuts are advanced and tightened together. The pin is then advanced further into the medial fragment by hand, using the lateral hexagonal nut wrench. Once the pin is in a satisfactory position, the medial hexagonal nut is advanced to the posterolateral clavicle cortex. When cortical apposition is present, this medial pin can be used to apply compression to the fracture site. The lateral hexagonal nut is then advanced and tightened to the medial nut, thereby 'locking' the construct and preventing migration of the pin.

The pin is cut flush with the lateral nut and a file is used to smooth sharp edges. This can be achieved more easily by backing the construct out of the wound using the medial wrench, cutting the pin flush, and advancing the pin back to its previous location.

Butterfly fragments are cerclaged into place using absorbable sutures prior to closure. Final fluoroscopic images are obtained and the wounds are closed in layers. The clavicle pin is removed on average of three months postoperatively, based on radiographic evidence of healing.

Fractures of the lateral third of the clavicle

Fractures of the lateral third of the clavicle should be treated based on their precise location and degree of displacement. Minimal displacement typically signifies intact periosteum and CC ligaments. These fractures are typically stable, and can be treated non-surgically. If the fracture is intra-articular, a late distal clavicle excision may be necessary if arthritic changes occur. When displacement is present, the risk of non-union without surgical intervention is high.

Many techniques have been popularized for the fixation of these fractures. Coracoclavicular stabilization, hook plating, K-wire, and intramedullary fixation have all been described as surgical options. To date, no single technique has emerged as superior, yet the use of several techniques have been limited by reported complications.

Migration and reported failure rates as high as 20% have led several authors to recommend that K-wire fixation is not used as a primary fixation technique. Coracoclavicular fixation techniques have also been popularized, but are limited by the location and extent of fracture comminution. Coracoclavicular screw fixation in particular has also been noted to limit shoulder girdle motion, and must be routinely removed. Alternatively, suture-type coracoclavicular fixation can be used to provide more dynamic fixation, and avoids the need for hardware removal. If the fragment of the distal clavicle is inadequate for screw placement, a hook plate may be indicated. Concerns regarding stiffness and arthritic progression necessitate routine plate removal after fracture healing. Dual plating of lateral clavicle fractures has also been recently described as a successful surgical technique, though long term follow up is not yet available (Kaipel 2010).

The hook-plate fixation technique

The patient is placed in the beach-chair position and the C-arm is draped into the field, similar to previous descriptions. The C-arm is positioned perpendicular to the clavicle and with a slight cephalic tilt. After standard prepping and draping of the patient, an incision is made parallel to the clavicle. This is typically made just anterior to the clavicle, to provide exposure of the distal clavicle, fracture site,

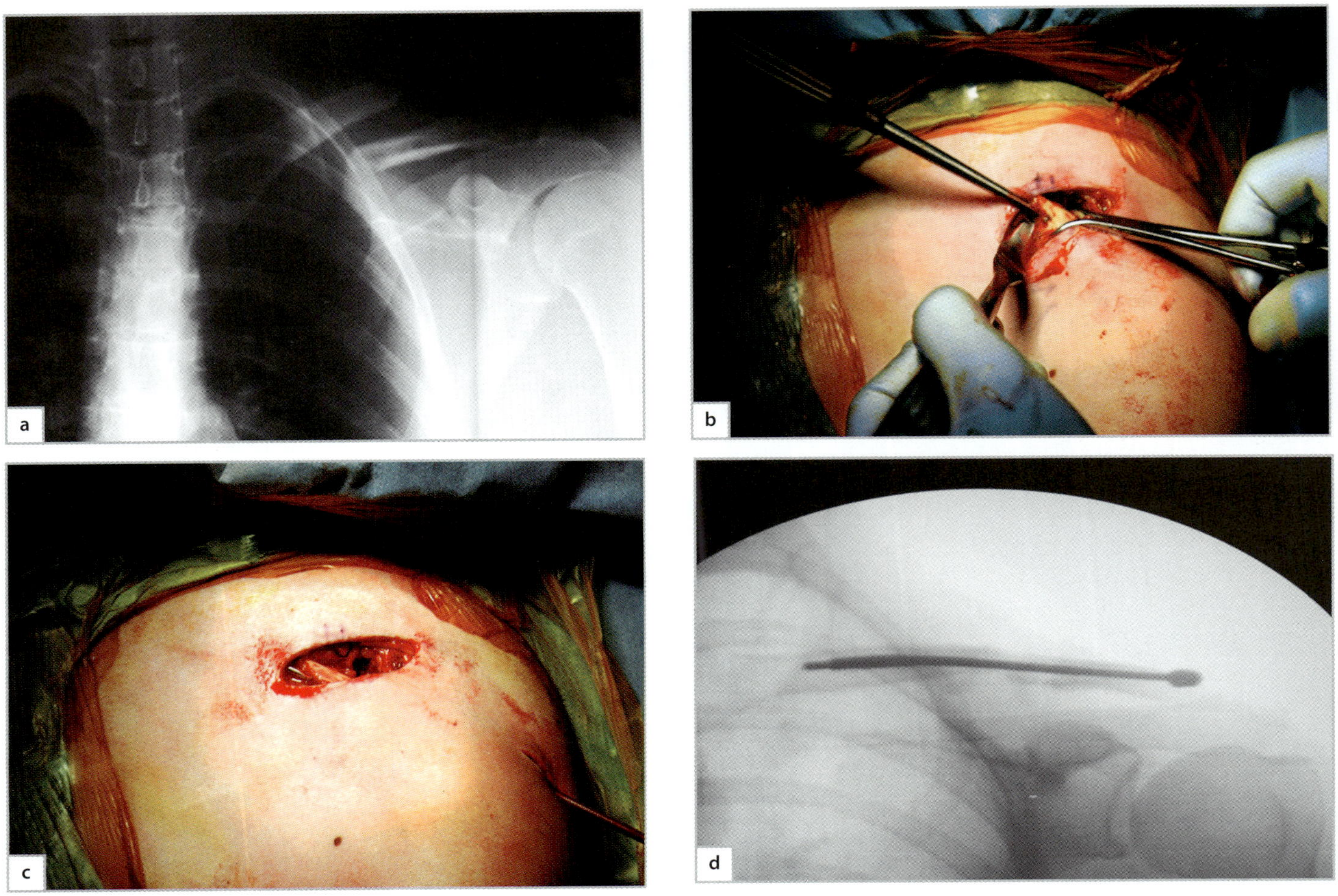

Figure 16.4 Intramedullary pin fixation of a midshaft fracture of the left clavicle. (a) Radiographic image prior to intramedullary fixation. Intraoperative images illustrating intramedullary tapping (b) and pin placement (c). (d) Postoperative radiograph demonstrating completed intramedullary pin fixation.

and AC joint, while maximizing soft-tissue coverage of the hardware. The subcutaneous tissues are sharply divided as one layer for later closure. The fracture and acromion are exposed, and any interposed soft-tissue removed.

Reduction is provisionally made using reduction forceps or K-wires. The soft tissue posterior to the AC joint is cleared, to allow placement of the hook under the acromion. An appropriately sized plate is placed along the superior aspect of the clavicle, with the hook contacting the undersurface of the acromion. An additional K-wire or reduction forceps is placed medially to hold the plate in place. Fluoroscopic imaging is used to confirm anatomic alignment of the clavicle and AC joint.

Screw holes are then sequentially filled, based on fracture orientation and comminution. A minimum of six to eight cortices should be used for fixation medial to the fracture site. The wound is irrigated and closed in layers.

The coracoclavicular fixation technique

The patient is placed in the beach-chair position with C-arm draped into the field in much the same fashion as described for fractures of the midshaft. One notable difference, however, is that the image intensifier is positioned from a posteromedial to anterolateral direction. This allows the coracoid to be radiographically visualized on end, as a 'cortical ring'.

A small incision overlying the fracture site is made within Langer's lines. The platysma is divided, and any soft tissue interposed between the fragments is removed. The fracture ends are reduced using reduction forceps or a 0.62 mm K-wire placed from lateral to medial through the acromion and into the fragment of the medial clavicle.

Through the same incision, if possible, the clavicle is drilled bicortically using an appropriately sized bit directly superior to the coracoid. A second bit is passed through this hole until it contacts the coracoid. This position is verified using fluoroscopy, and both cortices of the coracoid are drilled. Next, a button device is passed through both coracoid drill holes, and suture material is shuttled through the clavicle drill holes. Because the previously placed K-wire maintains clavicle reduction, it is now only necessary to place the second button over the sutures and tie them to secure the second button in place. After placing cerclage sutures to reapproximate larger fragments, the laterally placed K-wire can be removed. The soft tissues are closed in a routine two-layer fashion over the clavicle.

Using a similar surgical technique, it is possible to employ number of different coracoclavicular fixation types, based on surgeon experience and fracture characteristics. If screw fixation is selected, the screw should be removed 10–12 weeks after surgery.

Pearls and pitfalls

In the acute setting, a fractured clavicle may herald other injuries. Specifically, high-energy mechanisms should alert the clinician to be aware of other potential shoulder or chest injuries. Diastases of 1 cm or more may accompany a scapulothoracic dissociation injury.

Supraclavicular nerves can be injured while performing a surgical approach to the clavicle. There are typically two or three branches of the nerve, and these exhibit variable anatomy. The only reliable safe zones can be found in the medial 2.7 cm or lateral 1.9 cm of the clavicle (Nathe et al. 2011). Nerves should be protected if possible, but minimal long-term deficits are typically encountered if a branch is sacrificed for exposure.

Implants used for fixation of fractures of the clavicle can be prominent and irritating. Placing the incision along the anterior border of the clavicle prevents scar formation over a prominent area, and maximizes soft-tissue coverage of the implant. Additionally, a layered closure technique can help minimize symptoms produced by the hardware. To accomplish this, an effort should be made to elevate the deltotrapezial fascia as a single layer. This can then be imbricated over the clavicle, to decrease irritation, maximize wound healing, and reinforce the surgical repair.

REHABILITATION

Rehabilitation protocols are designed to protect the surgical repair while minimizing glenohumeral stiffness and muscular atrophy. The exact protocol should be individualized, based on the type and stability of the surgically repaired fracture.

For stable fractures, a sling is typically used for postoperative comfort 7–10 days after surgery. Full hand, wrist, and elbow motion is encouraged and, under supervision, full passive and active glenohumeral motion may begin immediately, as discomfort allows. Strengthening of the shoulder girdle can usually begin after four to six weeks. Return to full activity typically occurs six to eight weeks after surgical repair, but the precise timing should be based on clinical and radiographic evidence of fracture healing. Return to sport should be allowed after radiographic union, and full motion and strength are achieved no earlier than six weeks after surgery. For patients with intramedullary fixation, we recommend no shoulder motion above 90° of abduction until there is evidence of healing, as the intramedullary fixation does not provide as much rotational stability.

Fractures that demonstrate considerable comminution or poor bone quality should undergo a more conservative rehabilitation protocol. These patients are typically allowed to begin full passive range of motion in the supine position immediately, but active range of motion is delayed two to three weeks. The supine positioning helps support the shoulder throughout glenohumeral motion. The progression to active motion and strengthening is variable and should be based on clinical and radiographic findings. It is important to note, however, that the presence of callus formation will depend on the fixation technique and degree of fracture stability achieved.

If intramedullary fixation is used, the pin is removed once there are both clinical and radiographic signs of fracture healing, typically between 10 and 14 weeks after surgery. This is performed in an outpatient setting, using local anesthesia and sedation, with or without brief laryngeal mask anesthesia. With plate fixation, we remove the plate only if the hardware is producing symptoms. Radiographic union should be achieved prior to plate removal. It is our practice to avoid plate removal within 12 months, to allow fracture remodeling to occur.

Disclosure

The views expressed in this chapter are those of the authors and do not necessarily reflect the official policy or position of the Department of the Navy, Department of Defense, or the United States Government.

REFERENCES

Allman FL Jr. Fractures and ligamentous injuries of the clavicle and its articulation. J Bone Joint Surg Am 1967;49:774–784.

Andersen K, Jensen PO, Lauritzen J. Treatment of clavicular fractures. Figure-of-eight bandage versus a simple sling. Acta Orthop Scand 1987;58:71–4.

Iannotti MR, Crosby LA, Stafford P, et al. Effects of plate location and selection on the stability of midshaft clavicle osteotomies: a biomechanical study. J Shoulder Elbow Surg 2002;11:457–462.

Kaipel M, Majewski M, Regazzoni P. Double-plate fixation in lateral clavicle fractures - a new strategy. Journal Trauma 2010;69:896–900.

Kashif Kahn LA, Bradnock TJ, Scott C, Robinson CM. Fractures of the clavicle. J Bone Joint Surg Am 2009;91:447–460.

Lazarides S, Zafiropoulos G. Conservative treatment of fractures at the middle third of the clavicle: the relevance of shortening and clinical outcome. J Shoulder Elbow Surg 2006;15:191–194.

Millett P, Heuer H. Fixation of Midshaft Clavicle Fractures, Vumedi, June 2010 [video], http://www.vumedi.com/node/91627.

Millett P, Heuer H, Vaishnav S. Plate Fixation of Midshaft Clavicle Fractures, Vumedi, December 2010 [video], http://www.vumedi.com/node/106516?box=videos_related&link=1

Millett P, Hurst J, Horan M, Hawkins R. Complications of clavicle fractures treated with intramedullary fixation. J Shoulder Elbow Surg 2011;20:86–91.

Nathe T, Tseng S, Yoo B. The anatomy of the supraclavicular nerve during surgical approach to the clavicular shaft. Clin Orthop Relat Res 2011;469:890–894.

Neer CS 2nd. Fractures of the distal third of the clavicle. Clin Orthop Relat Res 1968;58:43–50.

Nordqvist A, Redlund-Johnel I, von Scheelel A, Petersson CJ. Shortening of clavicle after fracture: incidence and clinical significance, a 5-year follow-up of 85 patients. Acta Orthop Scand 1997;68:349–351.

Nowak J, Holgersson M, Larsson S. Sequelae from clavicular fractures are common. A prospective study of 222 patients. Acta Orthop 2005;76:496–502.

Oh JH, Kim SH, Lee JH, et al. Treatment of distal clavicle fracture: a systematic review of treatment modalities in 425 fractures. Arch Orthop Trauma Surg 2011;131:525–533.

Postacchini F, Gumina S, De Santis P, Albo F. Epidemiology of clavicle fractures. J Shoulder Elbow Surg 2002;11:452–456.

Robinson CM. Fractures of the clavicle in the adult. Epidemiology and classification. J Bone Joint Surg Br 1998;80:476–484.

Robinson CM, Court-Brown CM, McQueen MM, Wakefield AE. Estimating the risk of nonunion following nonoperative treatment of a clavicular fracture. J Bone Joint Surg Am 2004;86:1359–1365.

Rowe CR. An atlas of anatomy and treatment of midclavicular fractures. Clin Orthop Relat Res 1968;58:29–42.

Zlowodski M, Zelle BA, Cole PA, et al. Treatment of acute midshaft clavicle fractures: systematic review of 2144 fractures. J Orthop Trauma 2005;19:504–507.

Chapter 17 Operative treatment of injuries of the acromioclavicular joint

Knut Beitzel, Thomas J. S. Durant, Augustus D. Mazzocca

CLASSIFICATION

Classifications of dislocations of the acromioclavicular (AC) joint are based on the anatomy of the joint and its stabilizing soft-tissue structures. The AC joint is stabilized both by dynamic and static stabilizers. The dynamic stabilizers include the deltoid and trapezius muscles. The static stabilizers include the AC ligaments (superior, inferior, anterior, and posterior), the coracoclavicular (CC) ligaments (trapezoid and conoid), and the coracoacromial ligament. The AC joint capsule and the capsular ligaments are the primary restraints for anterior-to-posterior translation of the distal clavicle (Fukuda et al. 1986). The CC ligaments mainly contribute to vertical stability by preventing superior and inferior translation of the clavicle. This anatomic complex is made up of two structures: the trapezoid and the conoid ligaments. These two ligaments span the space between the coracoid and clavicle. The trapezoid is anterior and lateral to the conoid, and both the trapezoid and conoid are posterior to the pectoralis minor attachment on the coracoid (Bosworth 1949).

Fukuda et al. (1986) reported that with small displacements, the AC ligaments are the primary restrictors of posterior and superior translation of the clavicle. With larger displacements, the conoid ligament was found to be the primary restraint to superior translation, while the AC ligaments primarily restrict posterior translation (Fukuda et al. 1986). Debski et al. (2001), advancing on earlier research, recommended that the conoid and trapezoid ligaments should not be considered as one structure when surgical treatment is intended, and that capsular damage resulted in a shift of load to the CC ligaments.

Cadenat originally described a sequential injury mechanism based on the anatomy of the stabilizing structures, which Tossy later classified into three types. Rockwood (1984) expanded this classification to include types IV, V, and VI. In type I injuries, the AC ligaments are sprained, but the joint is intact, with no palpable displacement of the distal clavicle. Radiographically, there is no widening, separation, or deformity at the AC joint. The AC ligaments are torn in type II injuries, but the CC ligaments are intact. Type II injuries are characterized by moderate to severe pain at the AC joint, and a slightly superior position and increased horizontal mobility of the distal clavicle. In type III injuries, both the AC and CC ligaments are torn, but the deltoid and trapezial fascia are intact. Both plain and bilateral Zanca radiographs reveal that the distal clavicle is 100% displaced superiorly in relation to the acromion. A 'shrug test' can differentiate a type III injury from a type V injury: if the patient shrugs his or her shoulders and the joint reduces, then the deltotrapezial fascia is intact and a type V injury can be ruled out. In type IV injuries, the distal clavicle is displaced posteriorly into the trapezius muscle, and may tent the posterior skin; this usually causes pain. Examination of the seated patient from above will reveal that the distal clavicle is displaced posteriorly when compared with the uninjured shoulder. The posteriorly displaced clavicle is best appreciated on an axillary radiograph. Type V injuries represent a greater degree of soft-tissue damage, with the deltotrapezial fascia being stripped off the acromion and the clavicle. The distal end of the clavicle appears to be grossly displaced superiorly toward the neck. The scapula is translated anteriorly and inferiorly as it migrates around the thorax. On a bilateral Zanca view there is 100–300% increase in the CC interspace. Type VI injuries are inferior AC joint dislocations into a subacromial or subcoracoid position, and have been described only rarely in the literature; they mostly result from high-energy trauma. Associated injuries include fractures of the clavicle and upper rib, and injuries to the upper root of the brachial plexus. It is not uncommon for these patients to have transient paresthesias that subside after reduction.

The clinical examination should be performed with the patient in an upright position. Radiographic evaluation should include a bilateral Zanca view, which visualizes both AC joints on a single x-ray cassette while maintaining the same orientation of the x-ray beam. By visualizing both AC joints on the same cassette, the CC distance can be compared from side to side, pre- and postoperatively. An axillary view is particularly helpful in visualizing a type IV AC joint injury (posteriorly displaced distal clavicle).

INDICATIONS

The overall goal of treatment for AC joint injuries is pain-free shoulder movement with full range of motion and stability. Opinions vary regarding the optimal treatment (Tamaoki et al. 2010). The basis for this decision should be whether the treatment is meant to correct the anatomic deformity, functional impairment, or pain (Trainer et al. 2008). Type I and II lesions are generally treated conservatively, with a sling, ice, and a brief period of immobilization (typically three to seven days). However, no consensus exists regarding treatment for type III dislocations, although there is a trend toward initial non-operative management (Tamaoki et al. 2010). Some of these conservatively treated patients will have persistent pain and an inability to return to their sport or job, although subsequent surgical stabilization may allow them to so. It is important, however, to remember that, at two-year follow-up, non-operative versus operative treatment type III injuries results in no difference in joint strength. Also, in a prospective study of type III injuries conducted by Larsen and Hede, rates of persistent symptoms were similar between the operative (2/25, 8%) and non-operative (3/29, 10%) groups (Trainer et al. 2008). However, consideration of other factors, such as type of sport, timing of injury relative to athletic season, or the throwing demands in an uninjured dominant arm, may alter the procedure. In light of the controversy and lack of clear evidence supporting acute surgical management of type III AC separations, we recommend that all patients initially have three or four weeks of non-operative management (Trainer et al. 2008). If the patient is still in pain, intra-articular injection of local anesthetic may allow for immediate return to athletics. A patient with a type III AC separation qualifies for surgical reconstruction if symptoms persist after a course of non-operative management (Trainer et al. 2008).

Operative treatment is generally the accepted method for complete AC joint injuries (types IV, V, and VI) because of the significant morbidity associated with persistently dislocated joints and severe soft-tissue disruption.

CONTRAINDICATIONS

The common contraindications for any elective surgical procedure (unacceptable risks of anesthesia, risk of excessive intraoperative bleeding, increased risk of infection, etc.) may prohibit or delay surgical treatment for all types of AC joint dislocation. However, non-operative treatment is generally chosen as initial treatment for types I and II AC joint injuries. For type III injuries this decision is made on a case-by-case basis, but still with an emphasis on initial non-operative treatment. Such treatment is centered on a brief period of immobilization in a sling to reduce stress on the AC joint in lifting up the upper extremity. This is accompanied by ice and oral analgesic medication. The patient is encouraged to initiate range-of-motion activities within the first week of injury, to reduce pain and inflammation, in an effort to decrease associated morbidity. This is followed by strengthening exercises. Full rehabilitation should be achieved within 6–12 weeks.

TECHNIQUE

There is a wide range of procedures for the permanent reduction of AC joint dislocations, and none has been shown to be the 'gold standard' (Mazzocca et al. 2007, Geaney et al. 2010). Most techniques focus on reconstruction of the CC ligaments, as anatomic studies emphasize their biomechanical importance for vertical stability in repairs of the AC joint. Open and arthroscopically assisted procedures have been described. Of these surgical options, anatomic techniques emphasize the reconstruction of both the conoid and the trapezoid ligaments. However, improved horizontal stability may further be facilitated by a reconstruction of the CC ligaments early after injury, with an approach of clavicle and acromion, allowing subsequent healing of the torn ligaments by scar tissue. Alternatively, an additional reconstruction of the AC ligaments could be performed.

This chapter outlines the four principal surgical techniques. Such techniques are classified as open or arthroscopically assisted. For each, a non-anatomic and an anatomic technique are described. The modified non-anatomic technique described by Weaver and Dunn (1972) involves transfer of the coracoacromial ligament to the end of the distal clavicle to restore joint stability (**Fig. 17.1**). This approach, along with various technical modifications, is still widely utilized to reconstruct the CC ligaments, although it is not anatomic and in its biomechanical properties is considered to be inferior to other techniques (Mazzocca et al. 2007). The anatomic coracoclavicular reconstruction (ACCR) reconstructs the CC and AC ligaments for optimized restoration of biomechanical function (**Fig. 17.2**) (Carofino and Mazzocca 2010). As a non-anatomic, arthroscopically assisted technique, the single cortical button augmented with semitendinosus allograft enables CC ligament reconstruction in a one-step procedure with concurrent biologic augmentation (**Fig. 17.3**) (DeBerardino et al. 2010). The double cortical button technique is described according to the description of Walz et al. (2008) (**Fig. 17.4**). The basic idea of this technique is to place two cortical button pulley devices through the clavicle and coracoid into an anatomic position corresponding to both the conoid and the trapezoid ligament. Performed in an early stage after the initial injury, this approaches the clavicle and the acromion in a physiologic way to promote healing of the AC ligaments.

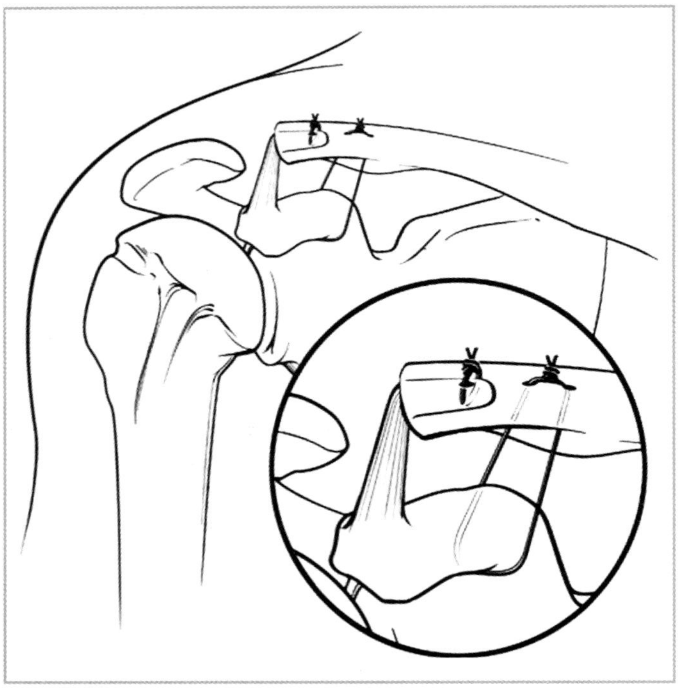

Figure 17.1 Modified Weaver–Dunn reconstruction of the acromioclavicular joint. (Reproduced with permission from Beitzel K, Obopilwe E, Chowaniec DM, et al. Biomechanical comparison of arthroscopic repairs for acromioclavicular joint instability: suture button systems without biological augmentation. Am J Sports Med 2011;39:2218–2225.)

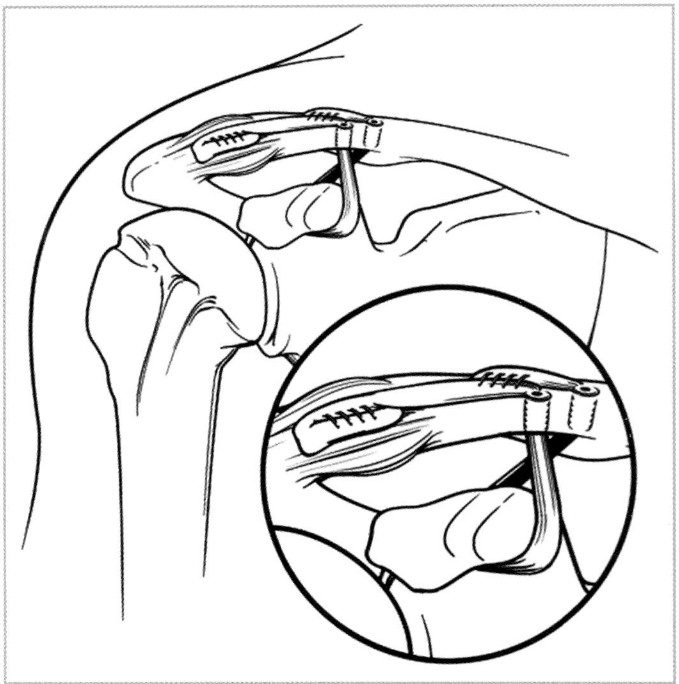

Figure 17.2 Anatomic coracoclavicular reconstruction (ACCR) of the acromioclavicular joint. (Reproduced with permission from Beitzel K, Obopilwe E, Chowaniec DM, et al. Biomechanical comparison of arthroscopic repairs for acromioclavicular joint instability: suture button systems without biological augmentation. Am J Sports Med 2011;39:2218–2225.)

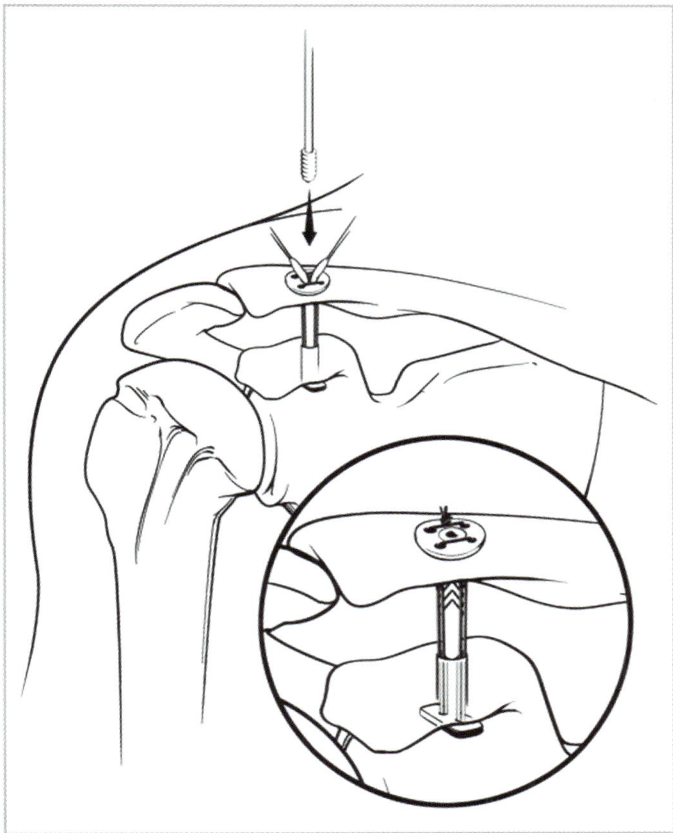

Figure 17.3 Suture button reconstruction with tendon augmentation. This is an arthroscopically assisted reconstruction of the acromioclavicular joint. (Reproduced with permission from Beitzel K, Obopilwe E, Chowaniec DM, et al. Biomechanical comparison of arthroscopic repairs for acromioclavicular joint instability: suture button systems without biological augmentation. Am J Sports Med 2011;39:2218–2225.)

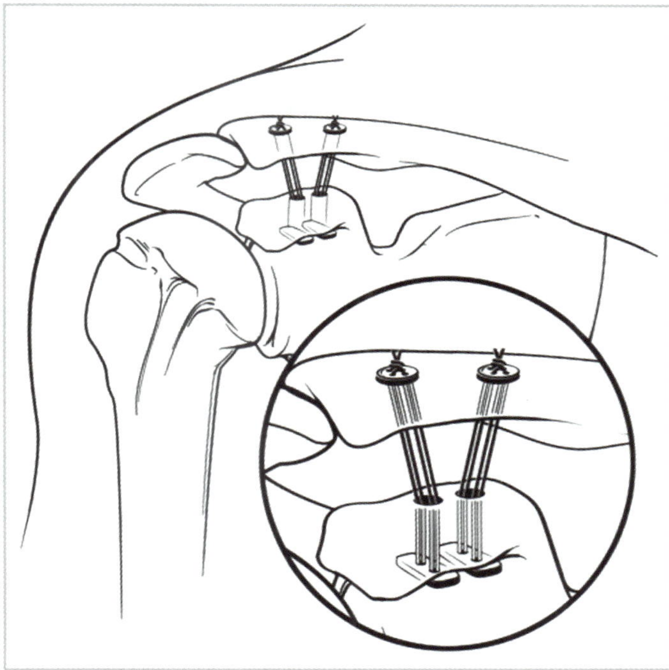

Figure 17.4 Anatomic suture button reconstruction technique. This uses two suture button pulley systems to reconstruct the conoid and the trapezoid ligament in an arthroscopically assisted procedure. (Reproduced with permission from Beitzel K, Obopilwe E, Chowaniec DM, et al. Biomechanical comparison of arthroscopic repairs for acromioclavicular joint instability: suture button systems without biological augmentation. Am J Sports Med 2011;39:2218–2225.)

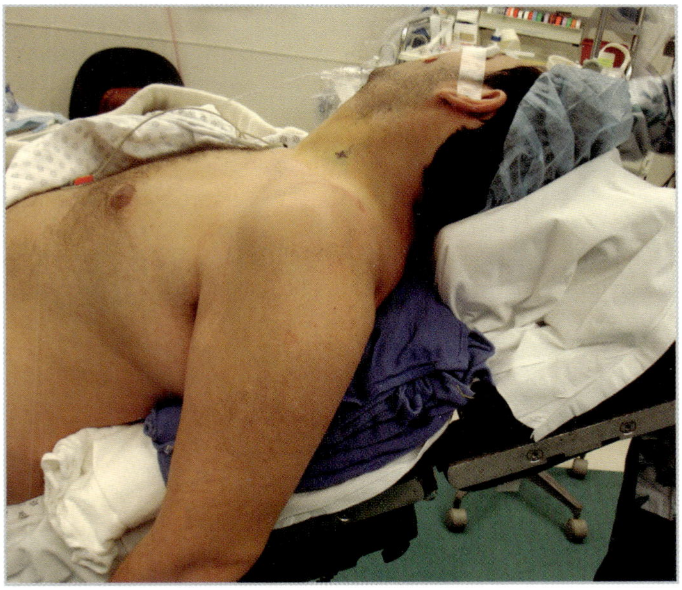

Figure 17.5 Preoperative positioning of the patient.

Open non-anatomic technique: modified Weaver–Dunn procedure

This technique represents an open procedure that does not restore the anatomy of the AC joint. It is included here because it is still widely used.

Setup

The patient is placed in a beach-chair position, with emphasis on good access to the clavicle for placement of the bone tunnels. Turning the patient's head slightly in the opposite direction, and making sure that the head can be repositioned intraoperatively, has been shown to be beneficial for this purpose. A small bump is placed at the medial border of the scapula to stabilize the AC joint for reduction. This also allows the shoulder to fall posterior, improving access to the coracoid. The sternoclavicular joint is included in the surgical field, and access to the posterior aspect of the clavicle should be possible (**Fig. 17.5**).

Surgical approach

While it is not essential, it is suggested that a glenohumeral and subacromial arthroscopic evaluation should be performed prior to the procedure, to address potential concomitant lesions. A small saber-type incision is made, starting slightly medial and posterior to the AC joint, and extending to just above the coracoid. A horizontal incision is made in the deltotrapezial fascia across the AC joint, and the coracoacromial ligament is prepared. It is then released, preserving its overall length, and a suture is placed into the end of a ligament with a whip stitch. The clavicle is excised by removing 2–3 mm from the medial edge of the acromion, and 7–8 mm from the lateral edge of the clavicle for a space of greater than 1 cm. The joint is exposed, and care is taken to maintain the strength of the periosteum and deltotrapezial fascia to allow a secure anatomic closure.

Clavicle preparation, reduction, and fixation

Two drill holes are made with a 1.6 mm drill 5 mm medial to the distal end of the clavicle. The sutures are placed through the end of the clavicle and tied over the holes. Reduction of the AC joint is maintained during this procedure by lifting up the scapulohumeral complex. For improved biomechanical function, the transfer of the coracoacromial ligament should be augmented. A cerclage suture can be guided around the coracoid and fixed on top of the clavicle. Finally, the deltotrapezoidal fascia as well as the skin is closed in layers, and the arm is placed in a sling postoperatively.

Open anatomic technique: anatomic coracoclavicular reconstruction (ACCR)

This technique restores the function of both the CC ligaments and the AC ligaments in an anatomic procedure with the use of semitendinosus auto- or allograft.

Setup

Patient setup is as described above.

Surgical approach

Operative treatment begins with a diagnostic glenohumeral and subacromial arthroscopy. This enables the surgeon to evaluate, and if necessary access, additional glenohumeral lesions. Such lesions have been shown to be commonly associated with AC joint dislocations, and should be carefully regarded (Tischer et al. 2009).

For the open part of the surgery, the skin incision begins at the posterior edge of the clavicle, approximately 3.5 cm medial to the AC joint, and extends inferiorly toward the coracoid. The deltotrapezial fascia is dissected, and generous skin flaps are raised above the fascia to improve visualization. The fascia is incised in line with the natural demarcation between the trapezius insertion onto the posterior aspect of the clavicle and the deltoid origin on the anterior clavicle. This incision extends medially beyond, to the conoid ligament insertion. Maintaining full-thickness flaps at this point is critical to obtaining a good closure. Additionally, tagging stitches are placed in the flaps at the medial extent of the exposure, to facilitate accurate reapproximation. The exposure is completed by freeing the clavicle and AC joint of soft tissues that are preventing joint reduction. Trial reduction is performed through elevation of the whole scapulohumeral complex. Routinely, visual inspection is necessary for control of adequate relocation. However, a mini C-arm should be kept available, and may be used for reassurance.

Tunnel placement

The conoid ligament tunnel should be placed in its anatomic insertion area 45 mm medial to the AC joint, at the posterior aspect of the clavicle. After placement of the guide pin, a cannulated reamer is used to create a 5 mm tunnel. Advancing the reamer under power and pulling it out after it has been disconnected prevents eccentric reaming. Finally, the tunnel is tapped. The trapezoid tunnel is placed at the anterior aspect of the clavicle, 30 mm lateral to the acromioclavicular joint, and prepared using the same technique. At this step, surgeons have to be aware of a possible 'blow-out' at the posterior or anterior cortex, and an insufficient distance between both tunnels to prevent fracture. A controlled placement of the guide wire is needed and helps to prevent such failure. If the clavicle is subluxated posteriorly, the tunnel should be placed more posterior (**Fig. 17.6**).

Graft preparation and passage

Different graft options exist, ranging from various allograft (e.g. semitendinosus or tibialis anterior graft) to autograft (semitendinosus tendon). We prefer to use a semitendinosus allograft, because it avoids donor site morbidity as well as the positioning and setup issues involved with harvesting the semitendinosus tendon. The graft is prepared as usual, and the ends are augmented with high-strength non-absorbable sutures in a 'bullet' technique (**Fig. 17.7**).

The graft is passed beneath the coracoid using either a clamp or a curved suture-passing device. To improve primary fixation strength of the graft, a high strength non-absorbable suture is added and passed simultaneously. After passing the graft and suture, limbs can be crossed before they are shuttled through the bone tunnels. The crossing of the limbs is more anatomical, however if the clavicle is posterior in relation to the acromion, we do not recommend crossing the limbs. After cyclically loading the graft to prevent any slack, it is arranged in a way that approximately 2 cm exit the conoid tunnel (**Fig. 17.8**). The remaining length of the graft exits the trapezoid tunnel. This will later reinforce the AC joint and create a reconstruction of the superior and anterior AC ligaments.

Reduction of displacement and graft fixation

The AC joint is then reduced by pushing up on the elbow to elevate the scapulohumeral complex. At this step, the possibility of posterior displacement has to be prevented. Prior to fixation, the quality of reduction is examined visually and fluoroscopically (with the mini C-arm). Anatomic reduction of the AC joint is critical. We recommend fixing the joint in a slightly over-reduced position (2–3 mm), to compensate for the loss of reduction that generally occurs in the postoperative period. While an assistant maintains the reduction, the graft limbs are secured with interference screws (5.5 × 8 mm PEEK). The graft exiting the posteromedial (conoid ligament) tunnels is secured first. It is placed in the anterior aspect of the tunnel, and tension is maintained on the graft during fixation. The other limb of the graft exiting the trapezoid

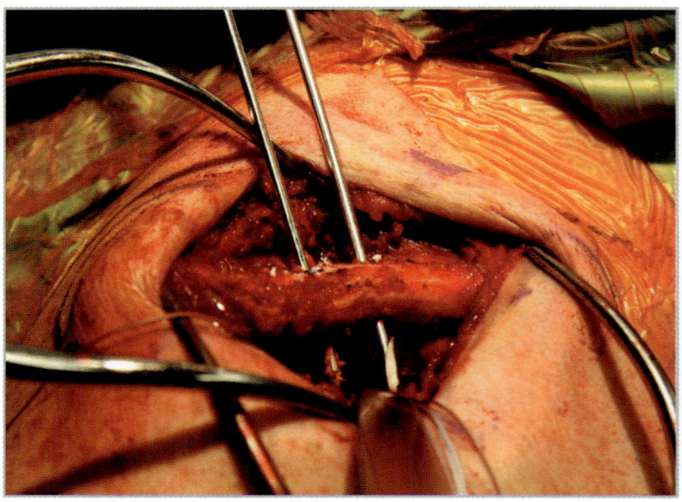

Figure 17.6 Anatomic coracoclavicular reconstruction of the acromioclavicular joint in an open procedure. Clavicle with Kirschner wires, and both tunnels in anatomic position.

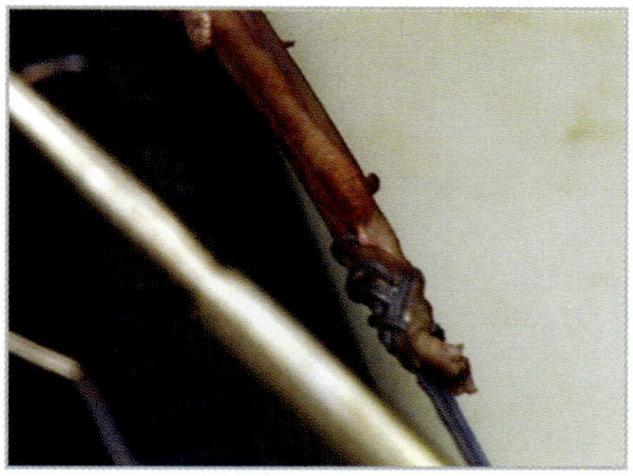

Figure 17.7 Prepared tendon graft with 'bulleted' ends.

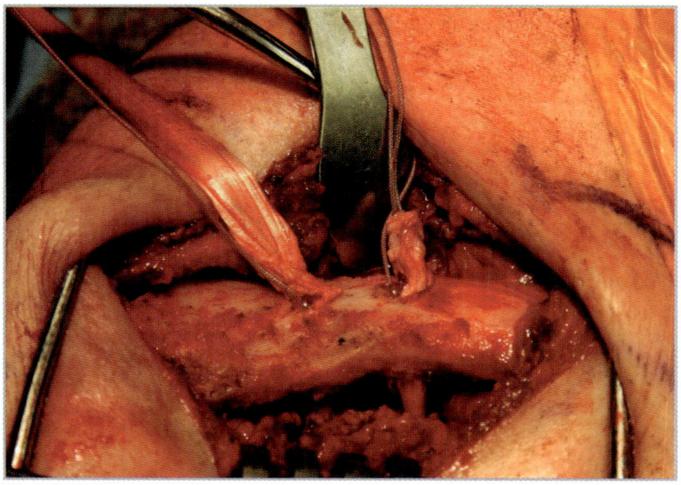

Figure 17.8 Graft passed through both clavicle tunnels. The medial limb is kept shorter and the lateral limb longer for later reconstruction of the acromioclavicular ligaments.

tunnel is again cyclically tensioned to remove any slack before being secured with a second interference screw. The non-absorbable suture is now tied on the superior aspect of the clavicle for additional security, after the suture has been passed through the cannulated portion of the screw. The shorter limb of graft exiting the conoid tunnel is sewn into the longer limb in order to reinforce this repair. High-strength non-absorbable suture is used to take the lateral limb (trapezoid) to the acromial side of the joint, where it is sutured into the most posterior tissue. The remaining graft is then taken posteriorly and sutured to the trapezial fascia, creating the posterior AC ligament (**Fig. 17.9**).

The deltotrapezial fascia is then closed with interrupted non-absorbable sutures. This is a critical step, and great care must be used to attach the deltoid to the anterosuperior aspect of the clavicle. Both attachments of the anterior deltoid fascia and the trapezius fascia are brought together with interrupted stitches. The knots are placed on the posterior side of the flap, to minimize skin irritation. Finally, the dermal layer is closed in the usual way.

Arthroscopically assisted, non-anatomic technique: single cortical button with semitendinosus augmentation

This technique combines a single cortical button pulley device with semitendinosus autograft or allograft. This technique only reconstructs the CC ligaments, and is not considered an anatomic reconstruction.

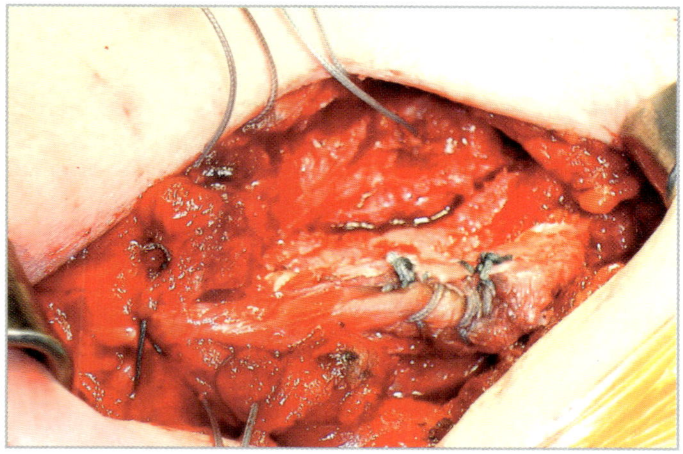

Figure 17.9 Lateral limb fixed posterosuperior at the acromioclavicular joint. This is used to reconstruct the acromioclavicular ligaments.

Setup

Patient setup is as described above.

Surgical approach

A standard 30°/40 mm arthroscope is used within the posterior portal. Additional working portals (straight lateral and anterolateral) are established for the coracoid preparation. A small skin incision (3–4 cm) is marked approximately 3.5 cm medial to the lateral edge of the clavicle, between the insertion of the conoid and trapezoid ligament. After routine glenohumeral arthroscopy, the anterior portal is placed lateral and under the CA ligament, with introduction of an 8.25 mm cannula. From this portal, working access to the base of the coracoid has to be ensured. If evident, any intra-articular pathology can be addressed at this time with standard arthroscopic techniques.

Tunnel placement

The rotator interval is cleared with a radiofrequency ablation device under arthroscopic view. Debridement is taken down to the level of the coracoid anteromedially, following the CA ligament. The coracoid undersurface is prepared circumferentially, to ensure visualization of the medial and lateral edge of the undersurface of the coracoid elbow, extending to the base. For this step, the arthroscope is placed in the anterolateral portal for improved visualization of the base of the coracoid. A vertical skin incision is made, 3 cm long, perpendicular to the clavicle and approximately 3.5 cm medial to the lateral border of the clavicle. The overlying fascia is incised, elevated to expose the entire anterior/posterior extent of the clavicle, and tagged for repair on closure. The AC joint is thoroughly reduced. Correct reduction is checked visually and radiographically. Maintaining an exact reduction throughout the following steps is essential.

A special drill guide (introduced through the anterior portal) is positioned close to the base, and medial to the midline of the coracoid, to direct the placement of the bone tunnel. On the clavicle, the guide is placed 3.5 cm medial from the lateral edge of the clavicle, along the midline, to prevent a cortical 'blow-out.' A Kirschner wire (K-wire) is placed to guide the 6 mm cannulated drill, which is done under arthroscopic visualization to ensure correct placement (**Fig. 17.10**). The K-wire remains in place until the final tunnel is drilled. Then the

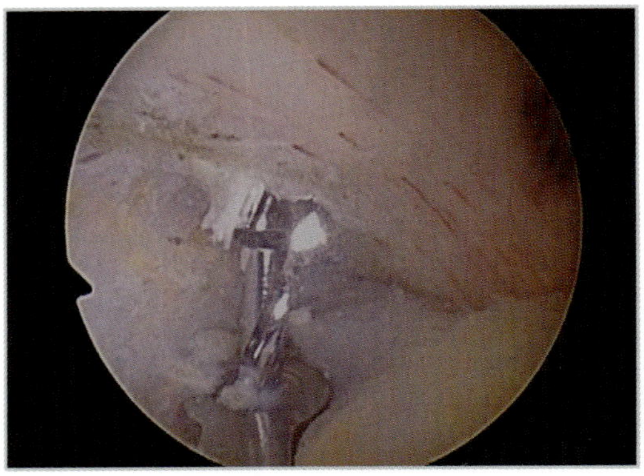

Figure 17.10 Arthroscopic view of the undersurface of the coracoid. The first tunnel is drilled with the help of an arthroscopic aiming instrument.

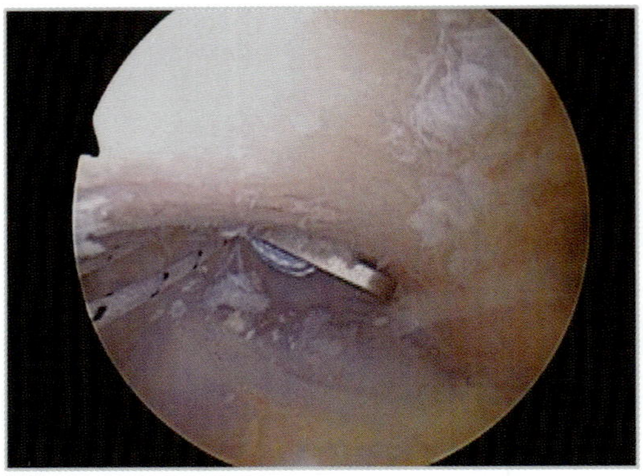

Figure 17.11 Arthroscopic view of the undersurface of the coracoid with the first flipped button of the suture pulley system.

drill bit is left in situ while the K-wires and the guiding instrument are removed. A passing suture is placed through the central cannel of the drill bit and, under arthroscopic visualization, pulled out through the anterior portal. At this point the drill bit may be removed with the suture lasso retained.

Graft preparation and passage

A soft-tissue allograft (semitendinosis or tibialis anterior) is commonly used as a looped graft for this reconstructive procedure. Its length should be approximately 12–15 cm, and the folded graft should pass through a 4.5–5.5 mm sizing block. The metal clavicle washer and coracoid button are joined by a continuous loop of high-strength, non-absorbable suture, providing fixation during the healing phase. The looped end of the graft is secured to a hole through a small keel in the coracoid button with another high-strength suture. The tails of the soft-tissue graft are secured with sutures, and passed up through the center of the clavicle washer.

Insertion and fixation of the cortical button device and graft

The cortical button device with the graft is connected to the loop of the passing suture, with the button in line with the suture to accommodate passage through the tunnels. Both are passed from superior, through the clavicle bone tunnel, followed by the coracoid bone tunnel, the shuttle suture being pulled through the anterolateral portal. It is imperative that the 'flip button' on the passing end of the device is not flipped until it can be completely visualized arthroscopically under the coracoid base and fully out of the coracoid tunnel. A suture retriever can be used as a hypomochlion to help pull the button of the pulley device through the bony tunnels and around the edge of the coracoid tunnel if needed. The device is 'armed' or flipped by pulling up on the suture still present superior to the entrance to the clavicle bone tunnel (**Fig. 17.11**). The passing suture is then removed from the button. After adequate reduction, the device is tightened by aid of the pulley system, and secured by alternating knots on top of the clavicle. A PEEK screw (5.5 mm diameter, 12 mm long) is then placed as an interference screw between the tensioned graft limbs for final fixation of the construct. The deltotrapezoidal fascia as well as the skin is closed in layers, and the arm is placed in a sling postoperatively.

Arthroscopically assisted anatomic technique: double bundle cortical suture button reconstruction

Both CC ligaments are reconstructed individually with a separate cortical button device. This reproduces their specific function, and enables a healing of the ruptured AC ligaments, if the technique is performed shortly after the injury.

Setup

Patient setup is as described above.

Surgical approach

The portal and surgical approaches are identical to those for a single cortical button with semitendinosus augmentation.

Tunnel placement

The rotator interval is cleared, and debridement is taken down to the level of the coracoid. The coracoid undersurface is prepared as described above, and the skin incision and clavicle preparation are the same. After preparation of clavicle and coracoid, the AC joint is reduced. Correct reduction should be maintained throughout the next steps.

The drill guide is positioned on the undersurface of the coracoid, at the elbow of the coracoid. On the clavicle, the guide is placed 4.5 cm medial from the lateral edge of the clavicle, along the midline or just slight posterior (at the insertion of the conoid ligament). Again a cortical 'blow-out' should be prevented. A K-wire is used to guide the 3.5 mm cannulated drill for the first tunnel. The drill bit is used to shuttle a passing suture through bone tunnels and pulled out through the anterior portal. Finally, the drill bit is removed. The second bone tunnel is completed with an identical series of steps. Its position is referenced from the first bone tunnel. At the coracoid it is critical that a bone bridge of at least 10 mm is preserved, to ensure lowest risk of fracture. The trapezoid tunnel position is typically around 2.5 cm medial from the lateral edge of clavicle, corresponding to the anatomic position of the trapezoid ligament. The sequence of K-wire placement, tunnel drilling, and passage of suture lasso is identical to the conoid tunnel.

Insertion and fixation of both cortical button devices

The cortical button device is connected to the loop of the passing suture, with the button in line with the suture to accommodate passage through the tunnels. Both are passed from superior, and the shuttle suture is pulled through the anterolateral portal. Pulling up on the superior suture blocks the cortical button beneath the coracoid, and the passing suture can be removed. The second cortical button device is inserted similarly. The end result has both buttons oriented mediolateral on the undersurface of the coracoid, allowing optimal bone purchase (**Fig. 17.12**). After adequate reduction, first the medial and then the lateral device is tightened by aid of the pulley system, and secured by alternating knots on top of the clavicle. The deltotrapezoidal fascia as well as the skin is closed in layers and the arm is placed in a sling postoperatively.

Pearls and pitfalls

The classification of AC joint injuries informs treatment decisions, and helps guide patient expectations and options. It emphasizes the various forms of AC injuries, and so helps to prevent improper recognition and hence improper treatment of an AC injury.

As concomitant injuries to the shoulder girdle are frequent, any successful AC joint surgery demands complete and accurate diagnosis of all pathology involved. Such additional injuries may be coracoid fractures, pectoralis major tendon tears, shoulder instability and dislocations, rotator cuff tears, or pulmonary contusions.

Surgeons should be aware of the importance of the superior and posterior AC ligaments, and should avoid sacrificing their competence in surgical procedures. If too much of the distal clavicle was excised, resulting in persistent instability despite reconstruction, the surgeon must ensure adequate anterior to posterior repair of the deltotrapezial fascia, with a resorbable suture in a 'pants over vest' fashion to regain sufficient stability.

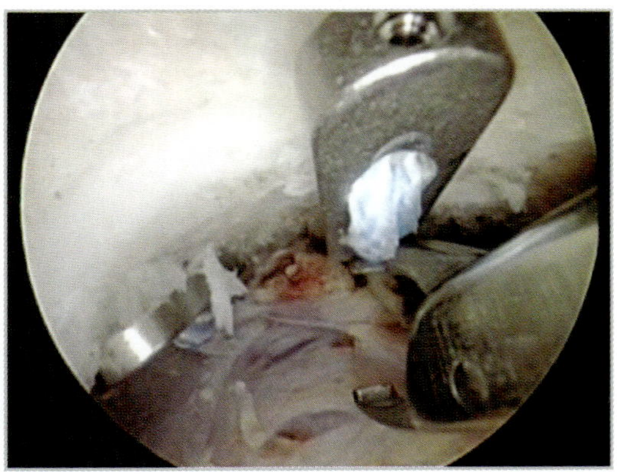

Figure 17.12 Arthroscopic view of the undersurface of the coracoid with both flipped buttons for the anatomic reconstruction of the acromioclavicular joint with two cortical buttons.

Understanding the anatomy of the CC ligaments reduces the potential for instability and, thus, continued pain. The insertion of the trapezoid ligament is, on average, 46.3±5 mm medial to the lateral edge of the clavicle, and the insertion of the conoid 21.4±4.2 mm.

When preparing the coracoid bone tunnel, an intraoperative coracoid fracture may result. This should be avoided by precise tunnel positioning. However, if it occurs, it can be fixed with a 3.5 mm screw or anchor device that was temporarily fixed with K-wire(s).

Inability to pass allograft or autograft under the coracoid process during anatomic CC ligament reconstruction can cause intraoperative frustration. Instrumentation such as a 90° clamp, or commercially available 90° suture-passers (akin to Hewson suture-passers) may be utilized to place passing sutures under the coracoid to transmit the graft.

Blowing out the posterior or anterior cortical rim of the clavicle when making drill holes or passing graft and/or sutures can be addressed by redrilling in another location. However, this may preclude reproduction of the anatomy.

REHABILITATION

Prior to surgery, patients are counseled in brace use and are taught a postoperative home program involving hand, wrist, and elbow exercises. Directly after surgery, the patient is placed in a platform brace for the first six to eight weeks. This provides support, and protects the surgical repair against the pull of gravity and excessive loads. The brace may be removed for grooming and supine range-of-motion exercises only. Guidelines for progression of activities following ACCR are based on the tissue-healing time frames on tendon healing in a bone tunnel.

Following removal of the brace, patients are referred to rehabilitation for active assistive range of motion in all planes. Motions that may increase stress on the AC joint, specifically internal rotation behind the back, cross-body adduction, and end-range forward elevation, are approached cautiously, and within the patient's pain threshold. The authors prefer to initiate range-of-motion exercises with limb-supported activities like the table or wall slide.

At 10 weeks postoperatively, patients typically present with near full restoration of range of motion, lacking only the ability to perform IR behind the back. Stretching exercises behind the back like towel internal rotation are allowed only if the patient can maintain scapular retraction while performing the exercise. At 12 weeks, if there is a pain-free range of motion, strengthening exercises are begun. All isotonic strength activities are withheld for 12 weeks because of concern about the ability of the surgical construct to tolerate a repetitively applied load. However, closed-chain scapular exercises and kinetic chain activities are allowed after eight weeks. From 12 to 18 weeks, exercise is progressed to include isotonic strength activities. Weight training may begin at three to five months postoperatively. Generally, it takes nine months to a year for patients to regain peak strength, particularly with pressing activities, or lifting from the floor (as in a dead lift).

REFERENCES

Bosworth BM. Complete acromioclavicular dislocation. N Engl J Med 1949;241:221–225.

Carofino BC, Mazzocca AD. The anatomic coracoclavicular ligament reconstruction: surgical technique and indications. J Shoulder Elbow Surg 2010;19 (2 Suppl):37–46.

DeBerardino TM, Pensak MJ, Ferreira J, Mazzocca AD. Arthroscopic stabilization of acromioclavicular joint dislocation using the AC graftrope system. J Shoulder Elbow Surg 2010;19 (2 Suppl):47–52.

Debski RE, Parsons IMt, Woo SL, Fu FH. Effect of capsular injury on acromioclavicular joint mechanics. J Bone Joint Surg Am 2001;83:1344–1351.

Fukuda K, Craig EV, An KN, et al. Biomechanical study of the ligamentous system of the acromioclavicular joint. J Bone Joint Surg Am 1986;68:434–440.

Geaney LE, Miller MD, Ticker JB, et al. Management of the failed AC joint reconstruction: causation and treatment. Sports Med Arthrosc 2010;18:167–172.

Mazzocca AD, Arciero RA, Bicos J. Evaluation and treatment of acromioclavicular joint injuries. Am J Sports Med 2007;35:316–329.

Rockwood. Injuries to the acromioclavicular joint: subluxations and dislocations about the shoulder. In: Rockwood CA Jr, ed. Fractures in Adults. Philadelphia, PA: JB Lippincott, 1984: 860–910.

Tamaoki MJ, Belloti JC, Lenza M, et al. Surgical versus conservative interventions for treating acromioclavicular dislocation of the shoulder in adults. Cochrane Database Syst Rev 2010;(8):CD007429.

Tischer T, Salzmann GM, El-Azab H, et al. Incidence of associated injuries with acute acromioclavicular joint dislocations types III through V. Am J Sports Med 2009;37:136–139.

Trainer G, Arciero RA, Mazzocca AD. Practical management of grade III acromioclavicular separations. Clin J Sport Med 2008;18:162–166.

Walz L, Salzmann GM, Fabbro T, et al. The anatomic reconstruction of acromioclavicular joint dislocations using 2 TightRope devices: a biomechanical study. Am J Sports Med 2008;36:2398–2406.

Weaver JK, Dunn HK. Treatment of acromioclavicular injuries, especially complete acromioclavicular separation. J Bone Joint Surg Am 1972;54:1187–1194.

Chapter 18 Elbow anatomy and surgical approaches

Andrew S. Neviaser, Bradford O. Parsons

INTRODUCTION

The elbow is formed by the articulations of the proximal ulna and radius with the distal humerus and with each other. It has evolved as a crucial link between the shoulder girdle and the distal extremity, allowing for positioning and orientation of the hand. The importance of the elbow to overall arm function is highlighted by the deficits incurred by elbow fusion. Whereas fusion of the wrist and shoulder are still done in some circumstances, fusion of the elbow is almost never indicated because there is no one suitable position that provides acceptable function. Furthermore, the elbow joint is among the least tolerant of traumatic injury: a single, simple dislocation can result in debilitating stiffness, heterotopic ossification, or recurrent instability. Although there have been several recent improvements in the treatment of elbow trauma, for example with precontoured locking-plate technology and advances in arthroscopic techniques, the surgeon must still respect the fickle soft-tissue envelope, proximity of neurovascular structures, and complex osseous anatomy in order to achieve optimal outcomes. This chapter focuses on the surgical landmarks that facilitate a safe approach and reconstruction of all parts of the elbow.

TOPICAL ANATOMY

The antecubital fossa is defined by the superficial contour of the biceps proximally, mobile wad laterally, and flexor–pronator mass medially. These structures form a triangular recess that may be further outlined by the subcutaneous cephalic and basilic veins. The visible flexion crease of the elbow lies roughly 1–2 cm proximal to the actual joint line when the arm is in extension (Morrey and Sanchez-Sotelo 2009). This is of particular importance when determining placement of a volar incision to access the joint or radial tuberosity. Posterolaterally, the borders of the olecranon, radial head, and lateral epicondyle define the so-called 'soft spot'. This point provides direct access to the joint for palpation of an effusion, aspiration, or insufflation prior to arthroscopy. Proximal to the lateral epicondyle, the lateral supracondylar ridge is the origin of the brachioradialis and extensor carpi radialis longus and is a palpable landmark for the lateral column approach. Medially, the epicondyle is quite prominent and forms the border of the cubital tunnel, which contains the ulnar nerve. Approaches to the medial elbow often require transposition of the ulnar nerve to facilitate exposure.

OSSEOUS ANATOMY

The cylindrical cortical tube of the humeral shaft flattens distally and transitions into divergent medial and lateral columns (**Fig. 18.1**). Centered between these is the spool-shaped trochlea, which lies distal to a narrow isthmus formed by the olecranon fossa posteriorly and coronoid fossa anteriorly. In approximately 6–10% of patients there is a bony defect within this space which has been termed a septal aperture. The triangle formed by the columns and trochlea is best appreciated when viewed posteriorly (Ring and Jupiter 2000). Reconstruction of the distal humerus after comminuted fracture requires that all sides of the triangle be adequately supported to achieve maximum stability.

The lateral column diverges from the humeral shaft at an angle of 20° and extends to the level of the distal trochlea. The capitellum forms its anterior surface and is spheroidal in shape. It is covered with hyaline cartilage that is approximately 2 mm thick. Proximal to the capitellum lies the radial fossa, which accepts the radial head as the elbow is flexed. Like the coronoid and olecranon fossae, encroachment into the radial fossa by screws or heterotopic bone can produce a physical block to

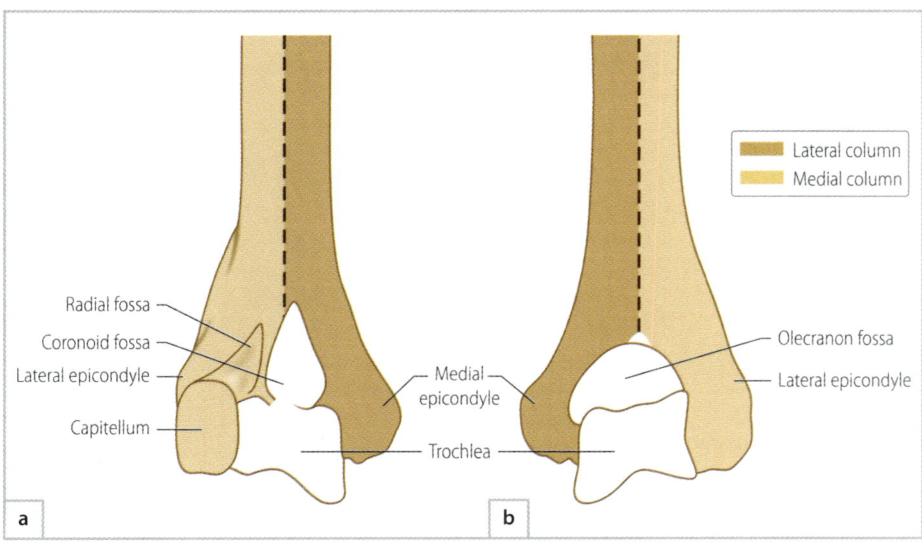

Figure 18.1 The distal humerus is formed by two columns and the trochlea. (a) Columns viewed from anterior. (b) Columns viewed from posterior. With permission from Browner BD, Jupiter JB, Trafton PG, Levine AM. Skeletal Trauma: Basic Science, Management, and Reconstruction, 3rd Edition (Vol. 2). Philadelphia, PA: Saunders/Elsevier, 2003.

motion. The posterior aspect of the lateral column is flat, devoid of cartilage, and amenable to plate placement.

The medial column subtends a more acute angle from the shaft (45°) and is smaller than the lateral column. It ends more proximally, terminating as the medial epicondyle at the level of the mid-trochlea. The proximal two thirds are cortical bone, whereas the distal one third is predominantly cancellous. Its size and make-up render it more susceptible to trauma than its lateral counterpart. The medial aspect of the triangular-shaped medial epicondyle provides a suitable location for a contoured plate, which can serve as buttress of the entire column. In 1–3% of individuals a bony medial supracondylar process is present 5–7 cm proximal to the medial epicondyle. A fibrous band which takes origin on this process and inserts on the medial epicondyle, termed the ligament of Struthers, may also be present. This anomaly has been associated with median nerve compression and fractures.

In contrast to the capitellum, which is considered part of the lateral column, the trochlea is centered between the two columns and forms the base of the distal humeral triangle. Its cartilaginous covering encompasses an arc of 300°. The medial portion is larger and projects more distally than the lateral. These two projections are separated by a groove which articulates with the guiding ridge of the greater sigmoid notch. The trochlear–capitellar articular axis is internally rotated 5–7° relative to the humeral epicondyles. It also has 6–8° of valgus tilt and 30° of anterior tilt relative to the humeral shaft.

The trochlea articulates with the proximal ulna, forming a ginglymus (hinged) joint. This articulation affords the elbow great stability. The greater sigmoid notch is highly congruent with the trochlea and forms an arc of 190°. When viewed in the sagittal plane, it is clear that the notch is more of an ellipse than a sphere. Anterior to the notch lies the coronoid, which functions as a bony buttress against anterior instability. The coronoid tip is devoid of soft-tissue insertions, and fractures of this should be considered hallmarks of an elbow dislocation. The anteromedial facet of the coronoid serves as an attachment site for the anterior band of the medial collateral ligament and also functions as a bony buttress to varus posteromedial instability. The lesser sigmoid notch articulates with the rim of the radial head. The olecranon is the most posterior structure in the elbow and lies subcutaneously, making it a frequent site of open fractures.

The radial head is an important secondary stabilizer of the elbow against valgus instability and also has a role in preventing posterolateral rotatory instability (Morrey et al. 1979, Schneeberger et al. 2004). It has a concave proximal surface that articulates with the capitellum. This entire surface is covered by articular cartilage, whereas only 280° of the rim is covered. The remaining uncovered portion of the rim is available for internal fixation of fractures of the radial head (**Fig. 18.2**). The radial neck lies distal to the head and is angled from the shaft a variable amount, but typically by about 15° (Bryce and Armstrong 2008). This angulation is in the opposite direction from the protuberance of the radial tuberosity, which lies more distally on the shaft.

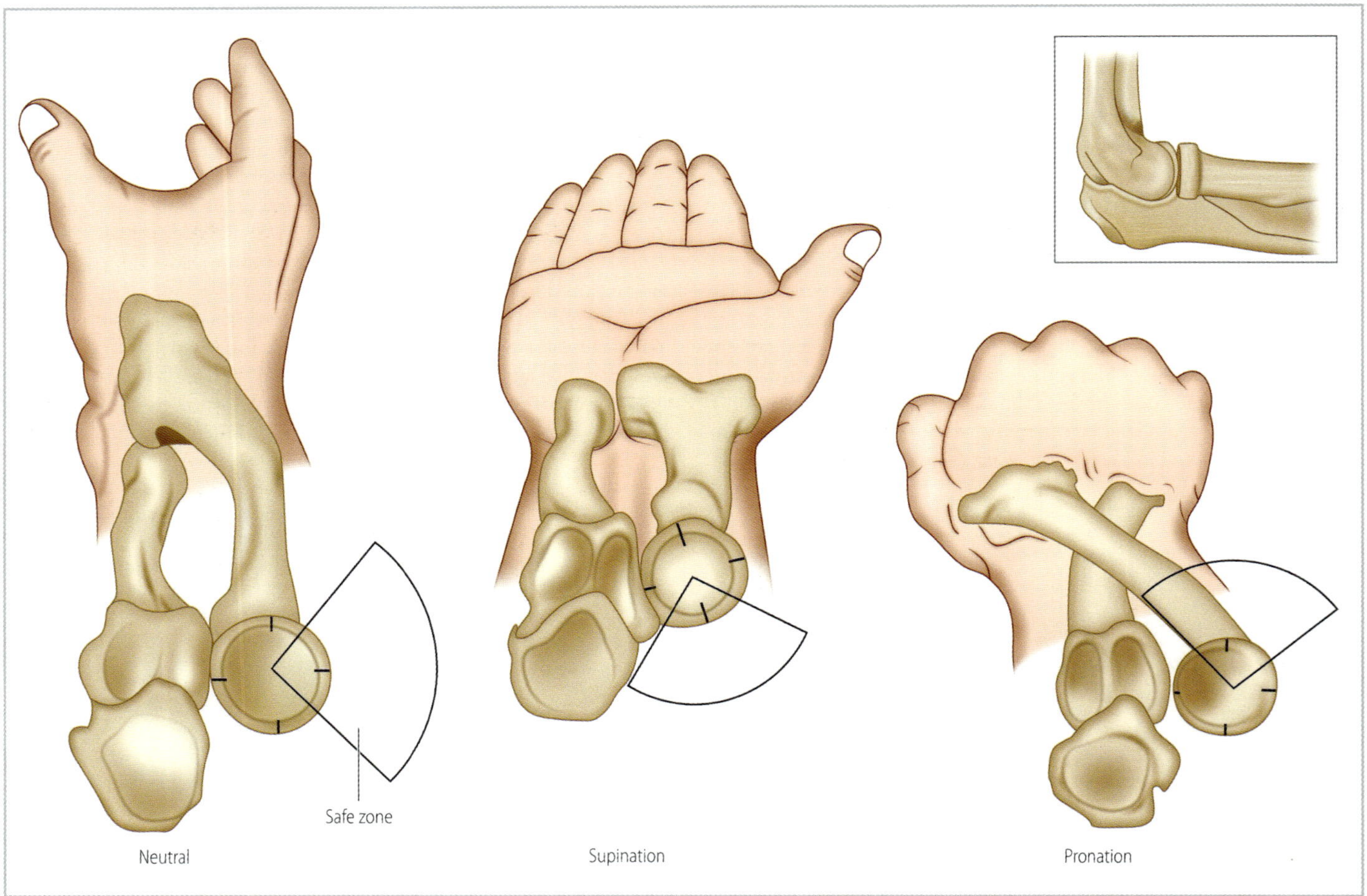

Figure 18.2 Two hundred and eighty degrees of the radial head articulate with the proximal ulna. Placing screws outside this zone (in the 'safe zone') is critical when internal fixation of the head is required. The 90° arc can be approximated by palpating the radial styloid and Lister's tubercle. © 1997 American Academy of Orthopaedic Surgeons. Redrawn from the Journal of the American Academy of Orthopaedic Surgeons 1997;5(1), 1–10, with permission.)

This is the site of insertion for the biceps tendon. Rotation of the forearm occurs through the radiocapitellar joint, and is independent of the flexion and extension which occur at the ulnotrochlear joint.

LIGAMENTOUS STRUCTURES

In addition to the inherent stability afforded by the ulnohumeral articulation, two ligamentous complexes, one on each side of the joint, contribute to elbow stability. The medial collateral ligament complex (**Fig. 18.3a**) consists of two or three parts – the anterior and posterior bundles are consistently present, whereas the transverse bundle is found only intermittently – and is the primary constraint against valgus torque. The anterior bundle is further subdivided into anterior and posterior bands, which tighten in a reciprocal fashion with flexion and extension of the elbow. The anterior band arises from the lateral two thirds of the anteroinferior epicondyle and inserts onto the sublime tubercle of the ulna. The posterior band of the anterior bundle runs from the posteromedial epicondyle to just proximal and posterior to the sublime tubercle. At flexion of 30°, 60°, and 90°, the anterior band is the primary restraint to valgus rotation (Callaway et al. 1997); the posterior band functions as a secondary restraint at these levels of flexion and is a co-primary restraint at 120°.

The posterior bundle of the medial collateral ligament complex acts as a secondary restraint to valgus rotation at 30° of flexion. The transverse bundle is inconsistently present and has little discernible function.

Because most activities of daily living are done with the arm somewhat abducted, the elbow is more frequently exposed to varus loads than to valgus loads. Thus injuries to the medial ligamentous complex are typically well tolerated. The exception to this is the throwing athlete, for whom valgus stability is extremely important.

The lateral collateral ligament complex consists of four parts, which are less distinct and more variable than those of the medial collateral ligament complex (**Fig. 18.3b**). The radial collateral ligament arises from the lateral epicondyle and blends into the annular ligament at its insertion. It originates near the axis of elbow rotation and remains taut throughout flexion and extension. The annular ligament is a distinct band of fibrous tissue encircling the proximal radius, taking origin from the anterior portion of the sigmoid notch and inserting onto the posterior portion. It maintains the radial head within the sigmoid notch of the ulna. The lateral ulnar collateral ligament provides stability to the ulnohumeral joint by resisting posterolateral rotator instability and is the main lateral stabilizer of the elbow. It has been suggested that the elliptical radial head acts in a cam-like fashion to tension the lateral ulnar collateral ligament resisting posterolateral rotatory instability. Disruption of this ligament has been proposed as the essential lesion in most complete elbow dislocations (O'Driscoll et al. 1992) (**Fig. 18.4**). This portion of the lateral complex originates on the lateral epicondyle, courses superficially over the annular ligament and the posterolateral radial head, to insert on the supinator crest of the ulna. The accessory lateral collateral ligament is the fourth component of the complex and functions to stabilize the annular ligament.

Traumatic injury to any single primary stabilizer may lead to elbow instability, and most injuries involve a spectrum of pathology. Understanding the pathoanatomy of instability is critical to the choice of treatment. The primary static stabilizers of the elbow include the ulnohumeral articulation, the medial collateral ligament, and the lateral ulnar collateral ligament. The secondary stabilizers include the radiocapitellar articulation, and the common flexor and extensor origins. The anterior capsule also functions as an anterior restraint, particularly in terminal extension. The muscles spanning the elbow act as dynamic stabilizers, including the brachialis, triceps, and anconeus. They impart a compressive force across the joint.

As our understanding of elbow pathology progresses and reconstruction techniques become more refined, surgical approaches are likely to become more specific. Several approaches to address specific pathology are presented in later chapters. The following sections describe approaches to the medial and lateral aspects of the elbow that can be used to address a wide range of pathology. Surgical options from a posterior approach are also discussed. The relevant neurovascular anatomy, which is densely concentrated in this region, is highlighted in relation to these approaches.

POSTERIOR APPROACH

Many different posterior approaches to the elbow have been described. They can be used for elbow arthroplasty, fractures of the distal humerus and olecranon, or ruptures of the triceps tendon. The elbow is tolerant of skin flaps, and a single posterior incision can be used to access both sides of the elbow joint simultaneously. Patient positioning can be either supine with the operative arm placed across the chest, or lateral decubitus with the arm in a position of forward flexion at the shoulder and the elbow resting on a post. Prone positioning is rarely used. The supine position is easiest for the anesthesiologist but requires more assistance to stabilize the arm. A longitudinal posterior incision is typically made. Care should be taken not to place the incision directly over the prominence of the olecranon. It can be curved laterally to avoid the boney prominence and the cubital tunnel on the medial side.

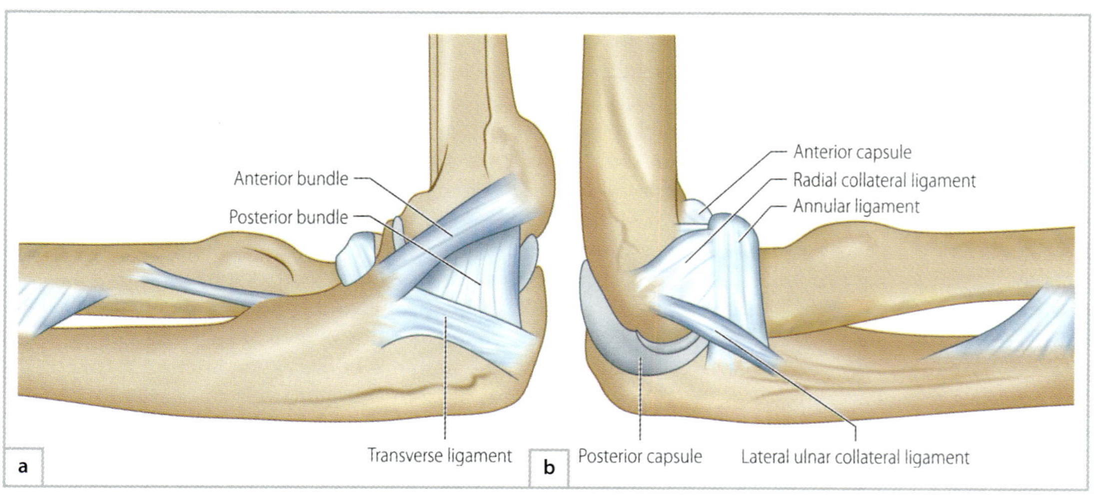

Figure 18.3 The main ligamentous stabilizers in the elbow. (a) The medial collateral ligament complex. (b) The lateral collateral ligament complex. © 2006 American Academy of Orthopaedic Surgeons. Redrawn from the Journal of the American Academy of Orthopaedic Surgeons 2006;14(5), 278–286, with permission.)

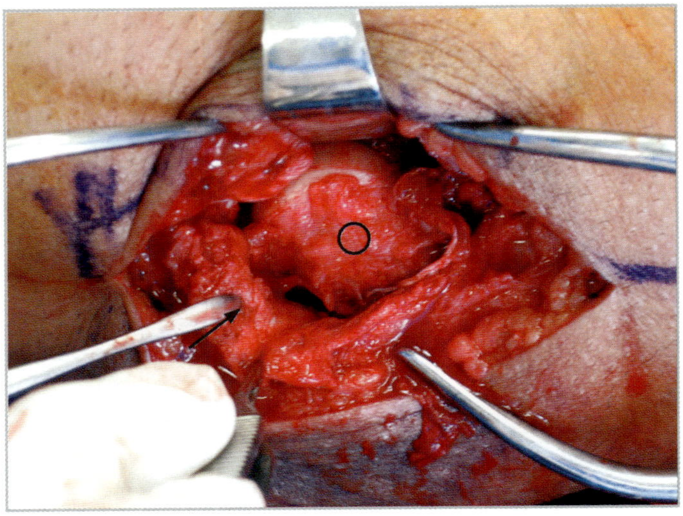

Figure 18.4 The essential lesion of an elbow dislocation. The lateral ulnar collateral ligament (arrow) has been torn from its humeral insertion. Repair of this lesion (circled) is critical to prevent recurrent stability.

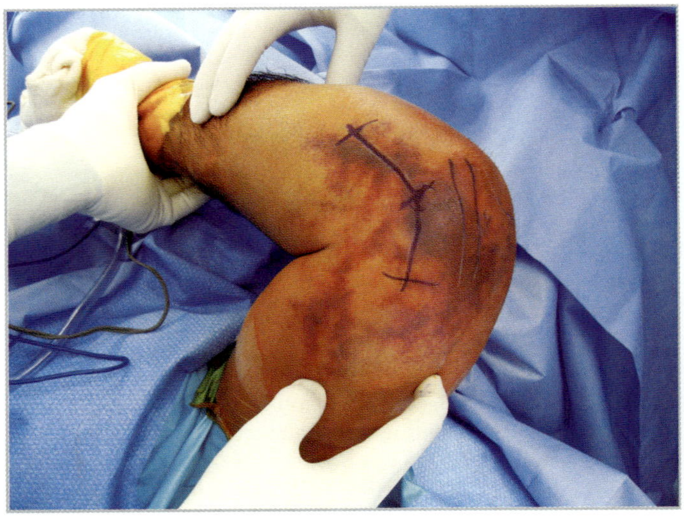

Figure 18.5 The medial incision lies posterior to the medial epicondyle and anterior to the course of the ulnar nerve (marked by the double lines).

Full-thickness flaps are raised as necessary. There are several ways to manage the extensor mechanism, the choice of which will be dictated by the exact pathology being addressed and surgeon preference. For most posterior approaches, the ulnar nerve can be found proximally between the medial intermuscular septum and the medial head of the triceps. It is freed distally beyond the elbow joint into the flexor–pronator mass to the level of the flexor carpi ulnaris. It is then transposed anteriorly.

A paratricipital approach has the advantage of leaving the triceps intact. The distal humerus is accessed through windows established on either side of the triceps tendon. This approach is useful for extra-articular and some intra-articular fractures of the distal humerus. Exposure of the joint is limited, however, and a fracture with severe comminution of the joint surface usually requires greater exposure. This can be achieved through an olecranon osteotomy, which allows complete visualization of the distal humerus but carries the morbidity of added hardware and the risk of non-union. The triceps-reflecting (i.e. Bryan–Morrey) approach preserves the extensor mechanism by releasing the triceps tendon, forearm fascia, and periosteum from the olecranon as one unit. This provides improved visualization of the joint surface, without the need for osteotomy.

MEDIAL APPROACH

This approach, described by Hotchkiss (see Green et al. 1999), can be used for contracture release or to address medial-sided coronoid fractures. The patient is placed in the supine position. A hand-table and sterile tourniquet are used. The entire humerus should be resting on the hand-table extension. The scapula is 'bumped' with two small towels. A longitudinal incision is placed posterior to the medial epicondyle, primarily for cosmetic reasons (**Fig. 18.5**). Dissection is through subcutaneous tissue to the level of fascia. It is in this plane that skin flaps are raised. Maintaining full-thickness flaps allows the medial antebrachial cutaneous nerve to be swept laterally within the superficial flap as dissection is carried laterally. When adequate visualization has been established, the ulnar nerve is identified adjacent to the intermuscular septum, as described above. In a revision setting, the nerve can be identified more proximally and dissection should proceed back toward the joint.

The medial intermuscular septum is identified and a triangular piece of its distal portion is excised. This exposes the medial column of the humerus. The anterior aspect of the medial column is then exposed distally to the level of the joint capsule. The median nerve lies approximately one finger's breadth anterior to the intermuscular septum and can be readily identified if necessary. A longitudinal split is made in the flexor–pronator mass, leaving an approximately 1.5 cm strip of flexor carpi ulnaris posteriorly. The brachialis, flexor carpi radialis, and pronator teres muscles are elevated anteriorly. In an open contracture release, the dissection is completed in the plane superficial to the joint capsule, which can later be excised. When excision of the capsule is not necessary, the capsule is incised and lifted anteriorly with the adjacent structures. A Bennett retractor can then be placed across the joint and the lateral compartment visualized. The median nerve, brachial artery, and vein lie superficial to the brachialis and are protected by it.

LATERAL APPROACH

Lateral approaches can be used to treat radial head and neck pathology, capitellum fractures, and elbow contractures. Compared with the traditional Kocher approach, which exploits the internervous plane between the anconeus (radial nerve innervation) and extensor carpi ulnaris (posterior interosseus nerve innervation), the more anterior lateral approach as described by Hotchkiss (1997) affords better visualization of the lateral joint and reduces the risk of iatrogenic injury to the lateral ulnar collateral ligament. Positioning of the patient is the same as for the medial approach. The length of the skin incision will depend on the need for exposure. The incision begins parallel and slightly posterior to the lateral epicondylar ridge and curves anteriorly as it extends distally over the radial head and neck (**Fig. 18.6**). Should extensive proximal exposure be needed (i.e. greater than 10 cm proximal to the epicondyle), the radial nerve should be identified at this level, lying between the brachialis and the brachioradialis. Full-thickness skin flaps are raised. Integral to this approach is identification of the supracondylar ridge and the posterior border of the extensor carpi radialis brevis. After finding the ridge, subperiosteal dissection proceeds distally to the epicondyle, but not posterior to it, especially distally. The capsule and tendinous insertions of the extensor muscles can be incised at the posterior border of the extensor carpi radialis brevis and elevated anteriorly. The joint is incised distally just anterior to the midline of the capitellum and radial head. Disruption of the lateral ulnar collateral ligament is avoided by not dissecting posterior to these boundaries. With more distal exposure, the common extensor

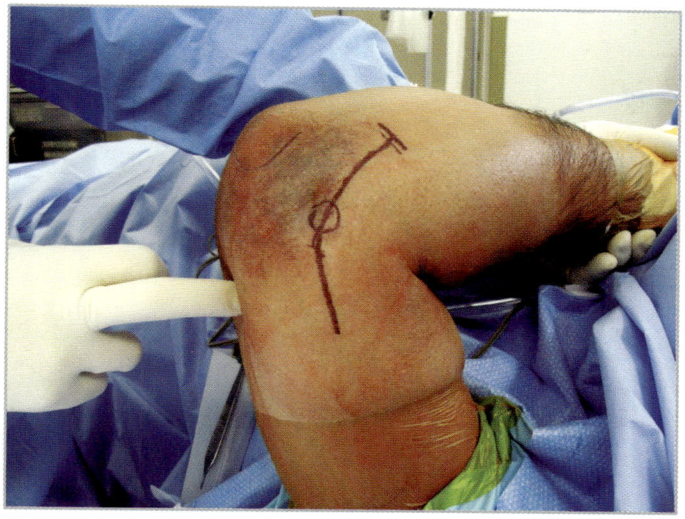

Figure 18.6 Incision for the lateral column approach. This is more anterior than the traditional Kocher incision.

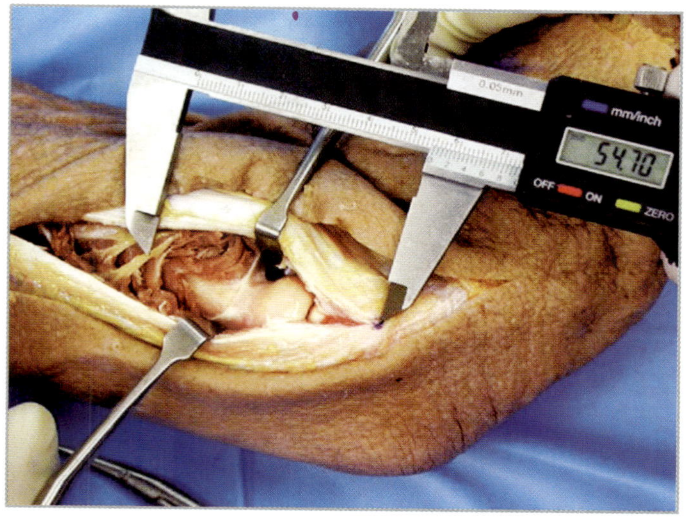

Figure 18.7 Dissection distal to the radial neck should be done with caution. The posterior interosseous nerve lies approximately 5 cm from the lateral epicondyle.

compartment is entered and the fibers of the supinator are identified by their oblique orientation. These should be teased anteriorly. The annular ligament can also be split and taken anteriorly, as needed, to expose the radial neck. This is completed with the arm in pronation, to increase the distance of the posterior interosseous nerve from the zone of dissection. It is an average of 48 mm from the radiocapitellar joint on the radial neck (Schimizzi et al. 2009) (**Fig. 18.7**).

CONCLUSION

The anatomy of the elbow is complex and densely concentrated. The described approaches allow a variety of elbow pathology to be addressed safely. Reconstruction after trauma should replicate the native anatomy when possible, and understanding of the intricacies of the elbow is vital to successful treatment.

REFERENCES

Bryce CD, Armstrong AD. Anatomy and biomechanics of the elbow. Orthop Clin North Am 2008;39:141–154.

Callaway GH, Field LD, Deng XH, et al. Biomechanical evaluation of the medial collateral ligament of the elbow. J Bone Joint Surg Am 1997;79:1223–1231.

Green DP, Hotchkiss RN, Pederson WC. Green's Operative Hand Surgery, 4th edn. New York: Churchill Livingstone, 1999.

Hotchkiss R. Displaced fractures of the radial head: internal fixation of excision? J Am Acad Orthop Surg 1997;5:1–10.

Morrey BF, Chao EY, Hui FC. Biomechanical study of the elbow following excision of the radial head. J Bone Joint Surg Am 1979;61:63–68.

Morrey BF, Sanchez-Sotelo J. The Elbow and Its Disorders, 4th edn. Philadelphia, PA: Saunders/Elsevier, 2009: 1211.

O'Driscoll SW, Morrey BF, Korinek S, An KN. Elbow subluxation and dislocation. A spectrum of instability. Clin Orthop Relat Res 1992;(280):186–197.

Ring D, Jupiter JB. Fractures of the distal humerus. Orthop Clin North Am 2000;31:103–113.

Schimizzi A, MacLennan A, Meier KM, et al. Defining a safe zone of dissection during the extensor digitorum communis splitting approach to the proximal radius and forearm: an anatomic study. J Hand Surg Am 2009;34:1252–1255.

Schneeberger AG, Sadowski MM, Jacob HA. Coronoid process and radial head as posterolateral rotatory stabilizers of the elbow. J Bone Joint Surg Am 2004;86:975–982.

Chapter 19 Arthroscopic treatment of fractures of the elbow

Michael R. Hausman

INTRODUCTION

Intra-articular fractures of the elbow rarely occur in isolation, and usually in conjunction with soft-tissue injury of the collateral ligaments and capsule. Adequate exposure to treat all components of the injury can involve extensive surgical approaches from multiple directions, thus compounding the effects of the injury. As with all surgery, exposure and visualization are the foundations of a successful procedure. The complex osteology of the elbow makes exposure challenging, and the problem is compounded by the need to spare critical ligaments to avoid complex instability problems that could exacerbate the effects of the injury.

Arthroscopy, while it may be challenging, offers several potential advantages, including access to multiple compartments with minimal trauma, as well as magnification, which can improve the precision of the procedure. Arthroscopic techniques can be applied to elbow trauma to improve exposure and visualization of the articular surface without an extensive approach, and to facilitate accurate reduction and fixation while minimizing surgical trauma. Given the challenges of elbow trauma and elbow arthroscopy individually, the combination may seem forbidding. However, immediately prior to the fracture, the elbow, in most patients, would have been normal, meaning a thin, pliable, non-contracted capsule, and normal joint volume. In addition, the fractured elbow comes pre-distended by fracture hematoma, making joint entry relatively easy. However, the surgeon must be able to irrigate or debride the hematoma and become oriented to the anatomy, despite distortion due to the fracture.

INDICATIONS

The indications for arthroscopic techniques in the management of intra-articular fractures of the elbow continue to evolve. Arthroscopy has proven useful in the management of fractures of the capitellum, coronoid, pediatric lateral condyle, and radial neck, as well as anterior coronal shear fractures, and has recently been used for unicondylar (AO type B), intra-articular fractures of the adult distal humerus (Hausman et al. 2007, Hausman et al. 2008). Other authors have reported arthroscopically assisted reduction and fixation of fractures of the radial head (Graveleau et al. 2006, Rolla et al. 2006, Michels et al. 2007). Basically, the technique is indicated when arthroscopy can help with the visualization of the articular surface to obtain an anatomic reduction of the joint surface.

CONTRAINDICATIONS

Contraindications are those applying to any elbow arthroscopic procedure. Submuscular transposition of the ulnar nerve is a contraindication, unless the entire procedure can be done without medial portals. Arthroscopy is also contraindicated if adequate visualization cannot be achieved or, simply, if the technique is not helpful and is not making the procedure either easier or better in terms of a more precise reduction. Prolonged and frustrating arthroscopy using high inflow pressures should be avoided. It is usually apparent within minutes whether arthroscopy will provide good visualization and be useful. If not, conversion to a standard open technique is advised.

TECHNIQUE

Elbow arthroscopy has been performed in the prone, lateral decubitus, and supine positions. Our preference is the supine position using a shoulder positioner to allow the patient's arm to be placed either across the chest or at the patient's side (**Fig. 19.1**). This confers several advantages, including: the ability to move the arm in space; easy access for fluoroscopy; elevation of the arm to minimize 'breakthrough bleeding'; and application of longitudinal traction to the elbow, which frequently assists with the reduction. The posterior compartment is accessed with the arm across the patient's chest, and the anterior compartment is accessed with the shoulder abducted 90° and the humerus parallel to the floor. A tourniquet is routinely used.

Timing of the intervention is important. Surgery during the acute period can be complicated by persistent, low-level bleeding from the fractured bone surfaces. This can require the use of elevated fluid inflow pressures and exacerbate swelling. A delay of one to two days, if possible, allows clot to form on the bone surfaces and there is much less bleeding, permitting the use of lower infusion pressures. Inflow pressures of approximately 25 mmHg are recommended to avoid swelling. Below 30–35 mmHg, working time is extended without distension of the elbow. Above 35 mmHg, working time is generally limited to 30–60 minutes, after which the elbow becomes severely swollen. As mentioned, entering a traumatized elbow joint and establishing a field of vision is generally easy with elbow fractures. The joint is pre-distended by the fracture hematoma, and the thin, compliant capsule is easily pierced with a safe, blunt trocar. Special trocars and cannulae (**Fig. 19.2**) without fenestrations should be used, to avoid extravasation of fluid into the subcutaneous layer. Other special instruments, such as 3.5 mm cannulated screws, a small Freer elevator with a hole drilled in the end, 28-gauge stainless steel wire, and a modified skin hook may be helpful in reducing, holding fragments, and passing sutures. In addition, a small drill guide, like an anterior cruciate ligament (ACL) guide or one used for drilling osteochondral lesions in the talus, may be helpful. Specific techniques for particular fractures are described below.

Pediatric fracture of the lateral condyle

Pediatric fractures of the lateral condyle were the first application of arthroscopic techniques to elbow trauma management attempted by the author. The rationale was to avoid the extensive dissection around the lateral condyle required to adequately visualize the articular

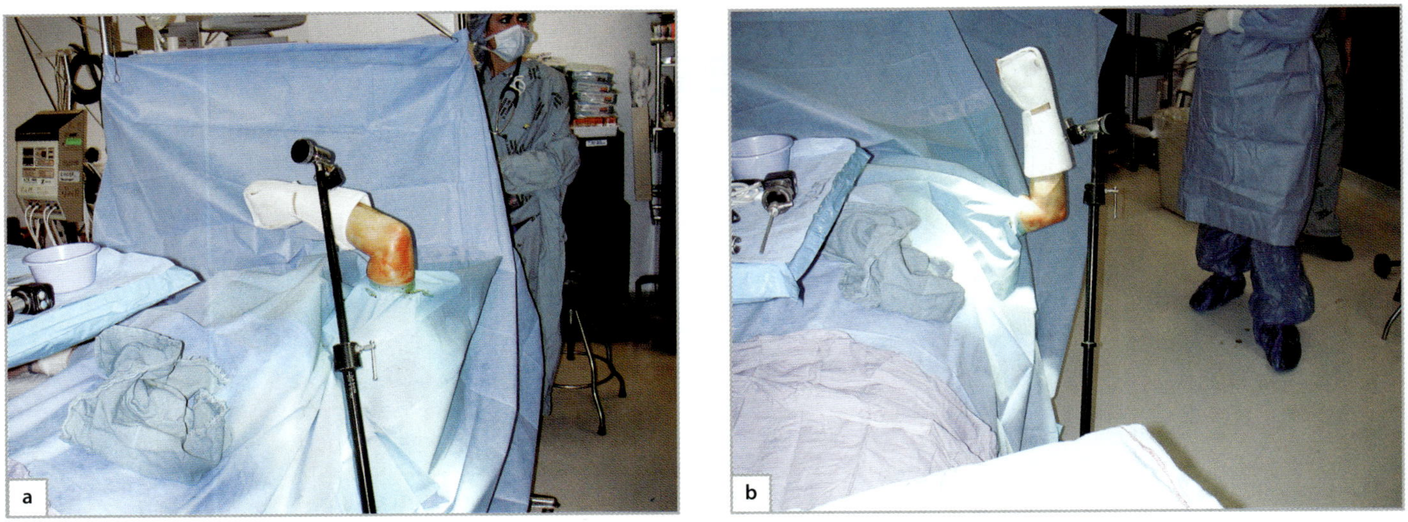

Fig. 19.1 Author's preferred position for elbow arthroscopy for fracture fixation, showing the use of the shoulder positioner. (a) Position that gives good access to the posterior compartment. (b) Position used to work in the anterior compartment. (All photographs in subsequent figures are shown in this orientation.)

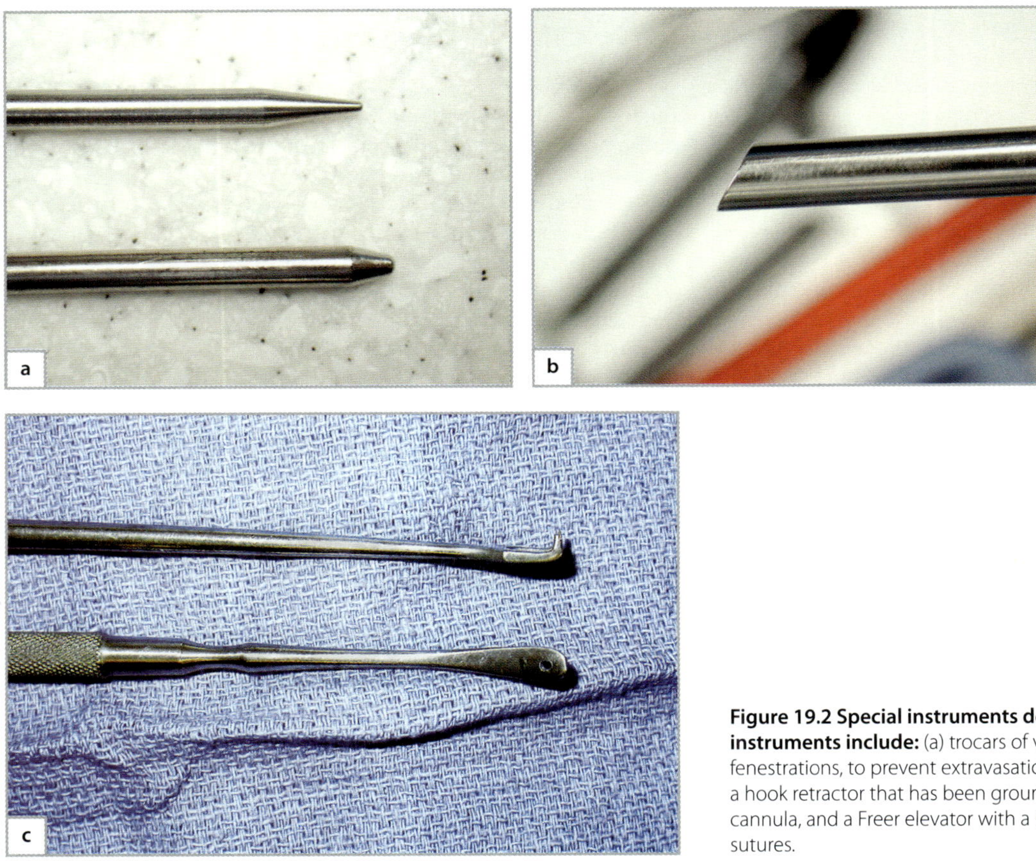

Figure 19.2 Special instruments designed for elbow arthroscopy. Such instruments include: (a) trocars of varying acuity; (b) cannulae without fenestrations, to prevent extravasation of fluid in the subcutaneous space; (c) a hook retractor that has been ground and modified to fit through a small cannula, and a Freer elevator with a hole drilled through the end for passing sutures.

surface and, thus, to protect the rather precarious blood supply and thereby minimize the risk of avascular necrosis.

After positioning the elbow as described above, a standard proximal anteromedial portal is created. Initially, hematoma in the joint obscures the view, but this can be evacuated and irrigated using the cannula. Once adequate visualization is achieved, the degree and direction of displacement can be seen. A 1.6 mm (0.062 inch) Kirschner wire (K-wire) or small-diameter Steinmann pin can be inserted percutaneously into the lateral condylar fragment. Alternatively, the arthroscope can be advanced to the trabecular bone of the secondary ossification center (**Fig. 19.3**) and the cannula placed in contact with the bone.

The arthroscope is then withdrawn and the K-wire is advanced through the cannula, into the fragment, and out through the skin. As the arthroscope is reinserted in the cannula, the K-wire is withdrawn out of the lateral aspect of the elbow, until just the tip of the pin is seen in the secondary ossification center. This technique ensures that the pin placement will be within the bone of the ossification center. Two or three such pins are placed under direct vision, and are used

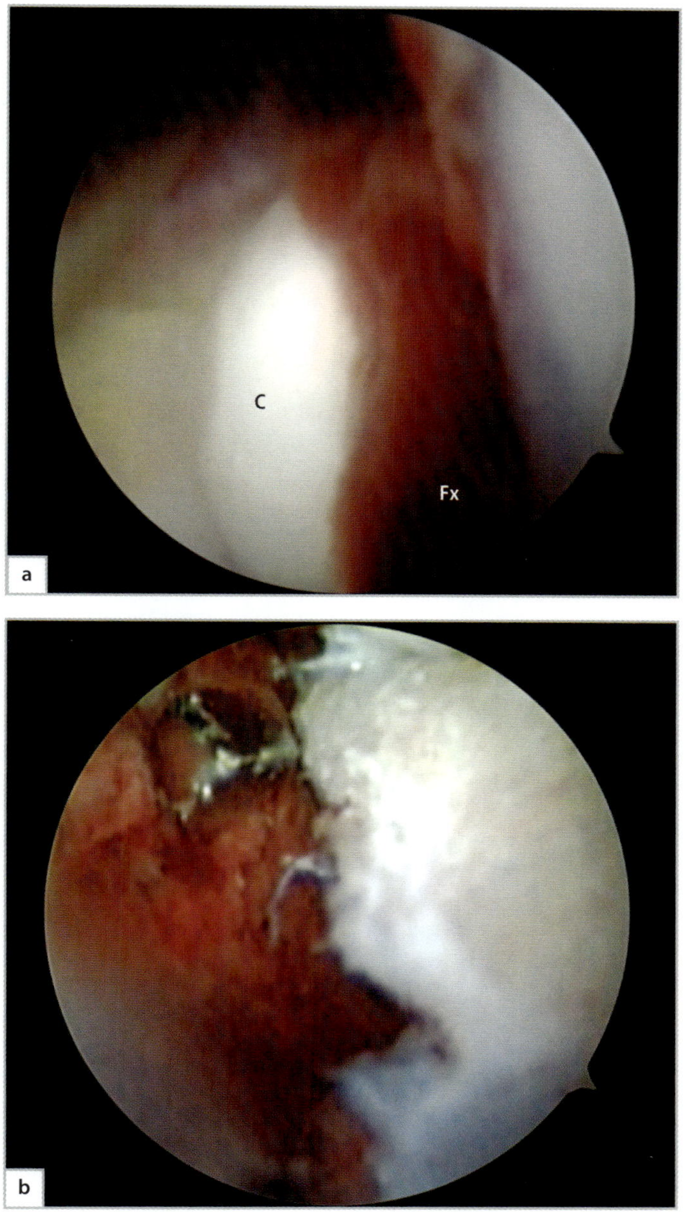

Figure 19.3 An arthroscopic view from the proximal anteromedial portal shows the displaced lateral condyle. (a) The cannula and scope are advanced up to the bone of the secondary ossification center, the arthroscope is withdrawn while holding the cannula in position, and a K-wire is advanced through the cannula into the bone. C = capitellum; fx = fracture line. (b) The wire is then withdrawn from the lateral aspect of the elbow until it is just piercing the surface of the bone.

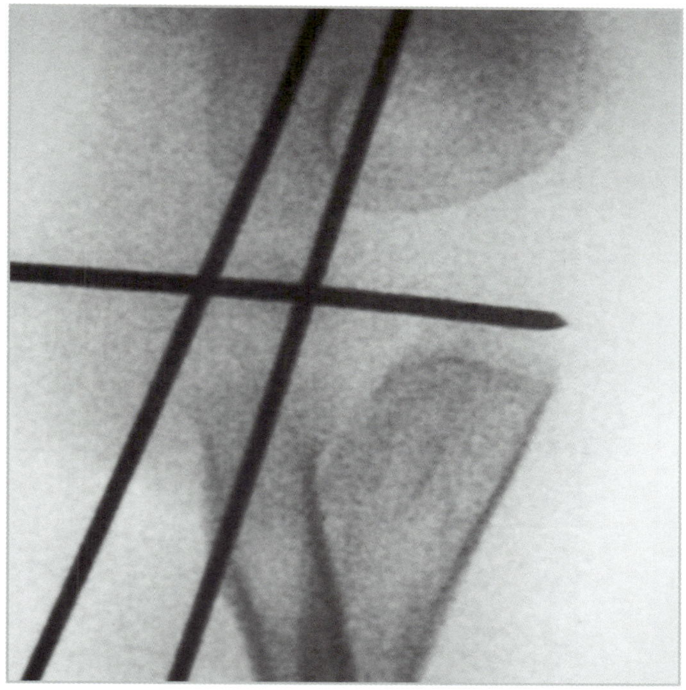

Figure 19.4 Position of the fixation pins to reduce a displaced lateral condyle. Note the use of a transcondylar pin to prevent rotation, in addition to the usual oblique pins.

as joysticks to reduce the fragment. The pins are then alternately advanced. The reduction is inspected both under direct visualization with the arthroscope and using fluoroscopy (**Fig. 19.4**). The pins are then trimmed and the elbow is put in a cast.

Fractures of the capitellum and anterior coronal shear fractures

Treatment of fractures of the capitellum and of anterior coronal shear fractures is similar to that for a pediatric fractures of the lateral condyle, except that examination of the posterior cortex of the distal humerus may be required. Once again, a proximal anteromedial portal is established, and the hematoma is evacuated from the joint. The fracture can frequently be reduced in elbow extension, but can then redisplace when the elbow is flexed. If so, a trocar is placed in the radiocapitellar joint to help the radial head 'ride over' the capitellum as the elbow is flexed (**Fig. 19.5**). A trocar placed in a proximal anterolateral portal is used to push and reduce the anterior coronal shear fragment, and is then interposed in the radiocapitellar joint to prevent displacement as the elbow is flexed. Once flexed more than 90°, the radial head will help to maintain the reduction. This trocar can be introduced either from the anteromedial portal or a proximal anterolateral portal can be made for it. The elbow is then flexed under fluoroscopic examination to ensure that the capitellar fragment is captured by the radial head and does not redisplace.

Once the initial reduction is performed, the elbow is kept in a flexed position to prevent loss of reduction. Ideally, the reduction should be assessed not only in the anterior aspect of the joint, but also at the distal humerus, where there can be comminuted fragments or plastic deformation of the posterior fragment of the distal humerus that prevents a perfect reduction. An arthroscopic approach through a trans-triceps or distal posterolateral portal, passing down the lateral gutter, will permit visualization of this area. A second, 'soft spot' posterior radiocapitellar portal is usually needed for a 3.5 mm shaver to remove debris in this area.

Once an accurate reduction is achieved and confirmed, 3.5 mm cannulated screws are inserted over the guide wires. The guide wires may be observed either from an anterior portal or from the lateral gutter, using a 70° scope, if necessary, to confirm the trajectory of the screws, assuring the proper length and position. The guide wires are advanced until just barely visible through the cartilage, and a screw 2–4 mm shorter than the measured length is selected. This process ensures that the longest possible screw is being used; the surgeon should avoid undersizing by judging the screw length in a sphere

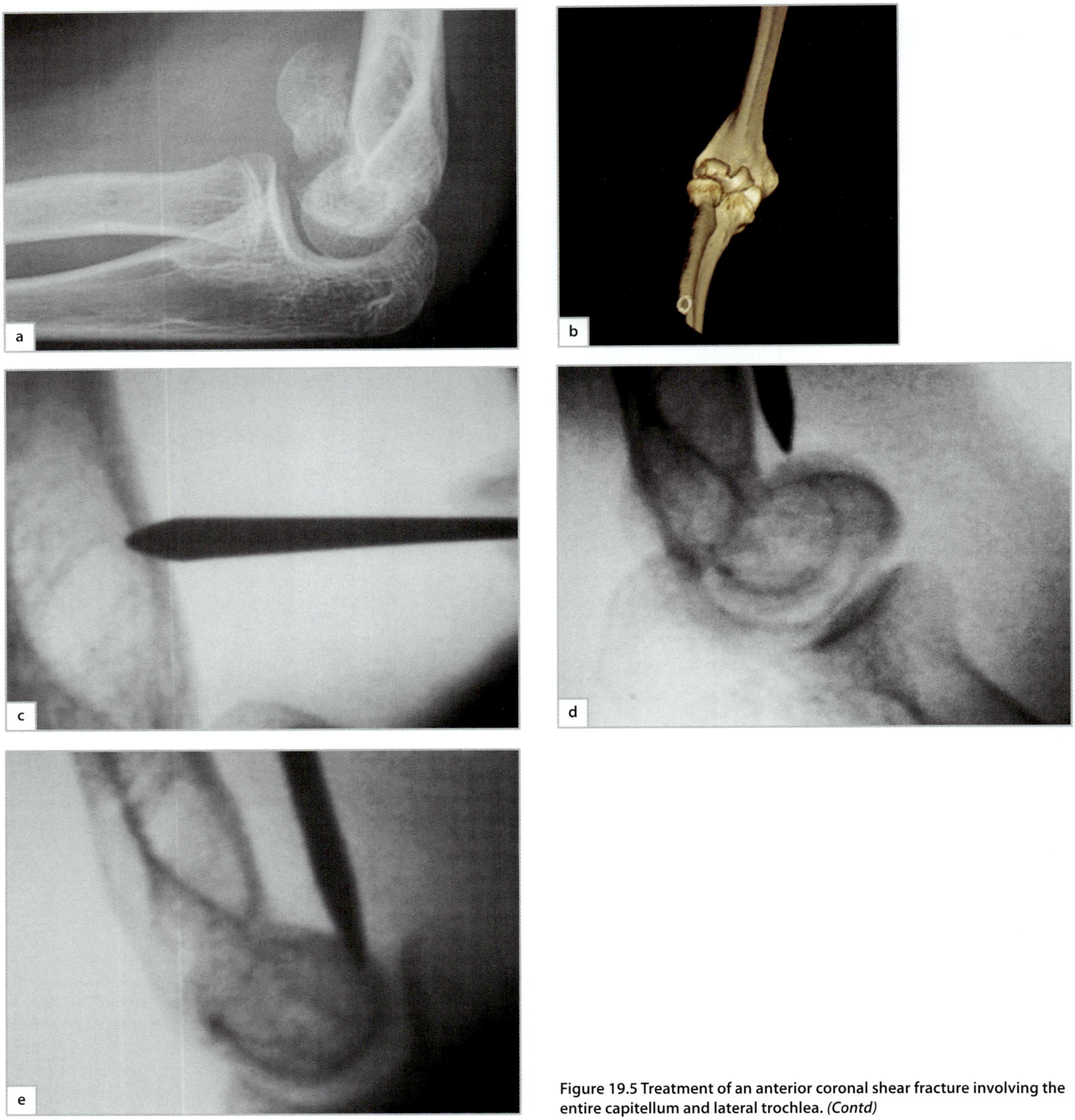

Figure 19.5 Treatment of an anterior coronal shear fracture involving the entire capitellum and lateral trochlea. ***(Contd)***

on a two-dimensional radiograph. A lateral-to-medial 2.7 or 3.5 mm transcondylar screw will substantially increase the strength of the fixation if necessary.

Unicondylar fractures (AO type B) of the distal humerus

Anatomically, one can think of a unicondylar intra-articular fracture of the distal humerus as an extension of a capitellar fracture or pediatric lateral condyle fracture. The critical principles of treatment are: accurate reduction of the articular surface; and reassociation of the distal articular surface to the shaft by means of a plate. The major challenge in such cases is adequate visualization of the articular surface, to ensure an anatomic reduction. Suggested approaches include the olecranon osteotomy, a triceps-on approach, or medial and lateral approaches. However it is done, a fairly large exposure and arthrotomy are needed solely to assess the articular reduction. Olecranon osteotomy affords excellent exposure. Other techniques,

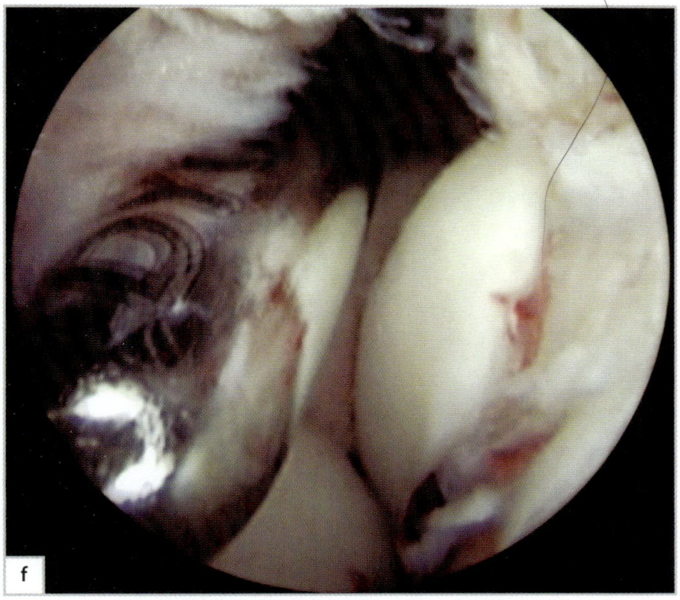

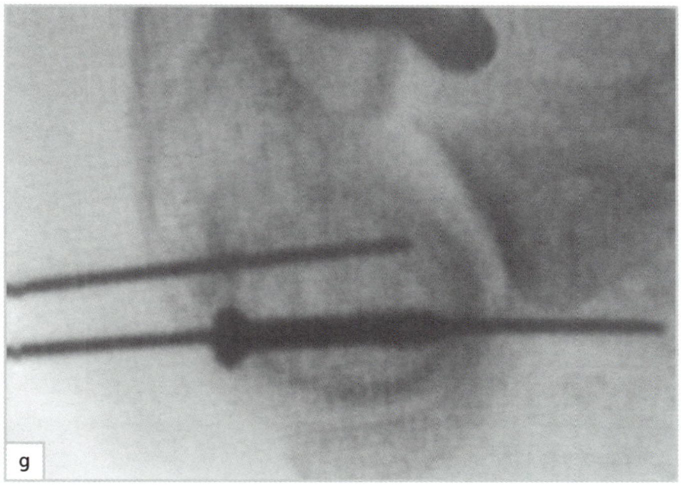

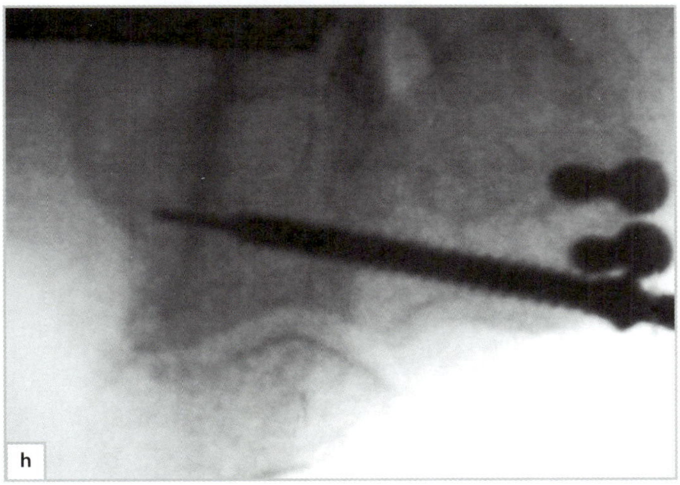

Figure 19.5 Treatment of an anterior coronal shear fracture involving the entire capitellum and lateral trochlea. (a) Radiograph and (b) computerized tomography scan of the fracture. (c) A 'high' anterolateral portal is created proximal to the fracture. (d,e,f) Extension frequently will reduce the fracture. In this case, a complete reduction does not occur with extension and a trocar is used to push the fragment into an anatomic reduction, which is confirmed with the arthroscopic view from the anterolateral portal. (g,h) Fixation is achieved with 3.5 mm cannulated screws, using the arthroscope to confirm optimal placement and length. Note the use of a 2.7 or 3.5 mm transcondylar screw to reinforce the fixation, permitting early use and therapy.

such as the triceps-on, compromise exposure unless extensive dissection and mobilization create some degree of instability to allow distraction of the elbow joint.

In this type of fracture, arthroscopy can provide the desired, excellent view of the articular surface for an anatomic articular reduction (**Fig. 19.6**) without the need for a more disruptive surgical approach. Visualization and assessment of the reduction are similar those for fractures of the lateral condyle and capitellum, described above. However, a thicker (1/8 inch or 3 mm) Steinmann pin will be required to manipulate the larger fragment with the attached muscle origins. Once the reduction has been evaluated both arthroscopically and radiographically, the fracture is temporarily fixed with transcondylar wires or pin - our preference is a stout, 3 mm (1/8 inch) Steinmann pin. Then, a medial or lateral mid-axial incision is made for application of the plate. However, only the skin and subcutaneous tissue need be incised, and no additional arthrotomy or musculotendinous dissection is required.

For a fracture of the medial column, the incision should be made prior to pin placement, because of the proximity of the ulnar nerve, which should be identified, retracted, if necessary, and protected as the pin is inserted. When reducing a fracture of the lateral column, care is needed not to advance the pin too far medially, to protect the ulnar nerve. On the medial side, the limited open surgical approach is performed, and the pin is inserted through the medial border of the trochlea. Arthroscopic and radiographic examination will then confirm that an anatomic reduction has been achieved.

A medial or lateral axial incision can then be made through the skin and subcutaneous tissues. The plate is applied over the K-wires or Steinmann pin in the correct position. The use of precontoured plates simplifies this task. The plate is then provisionally fixed, and a second distal transcondylar screw is placed. The initial pin can then be removed and replaced with a transcondylar screw through the plate, thus conforming with O'Driscoll's principles for fixation of fractures of the distal humerus. The remaining proximal and distal screws are then placed.

Coronoid fractures

Our understanding of the significance of coronoid fractures and the indications for repair are evolving. The traditional Reagan–Morrey classification has been modified in recognition that type I and type II coronoid fractures are frequently associated with ligament and soft-tissue injuries and significant instability. These modifications recognize the association of medial coronoid facet injuries (type II)

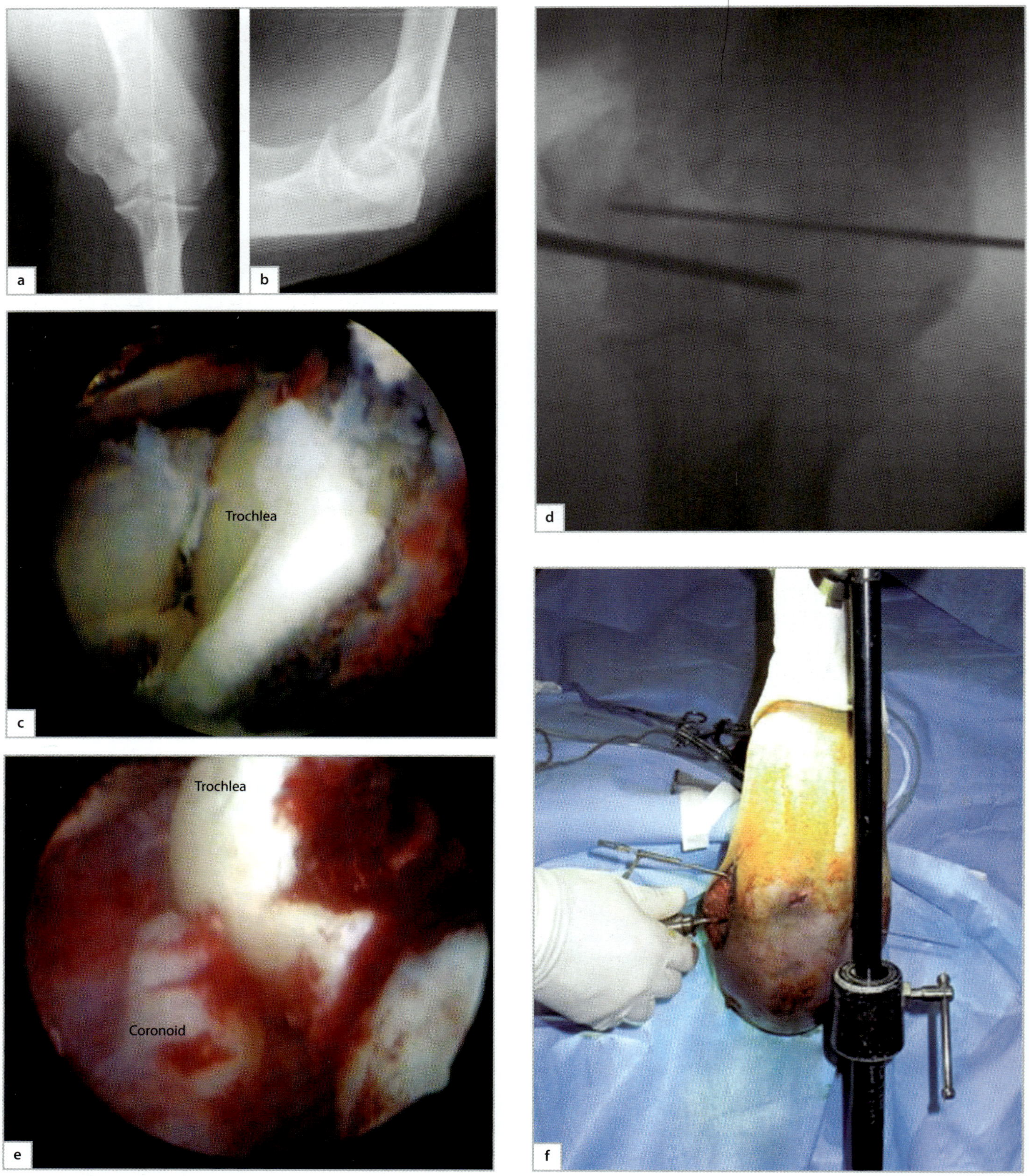

Figure 19.6 Treatment of a unicondylar, intra-articular fracture of the distal humerus. ***(Contd)***

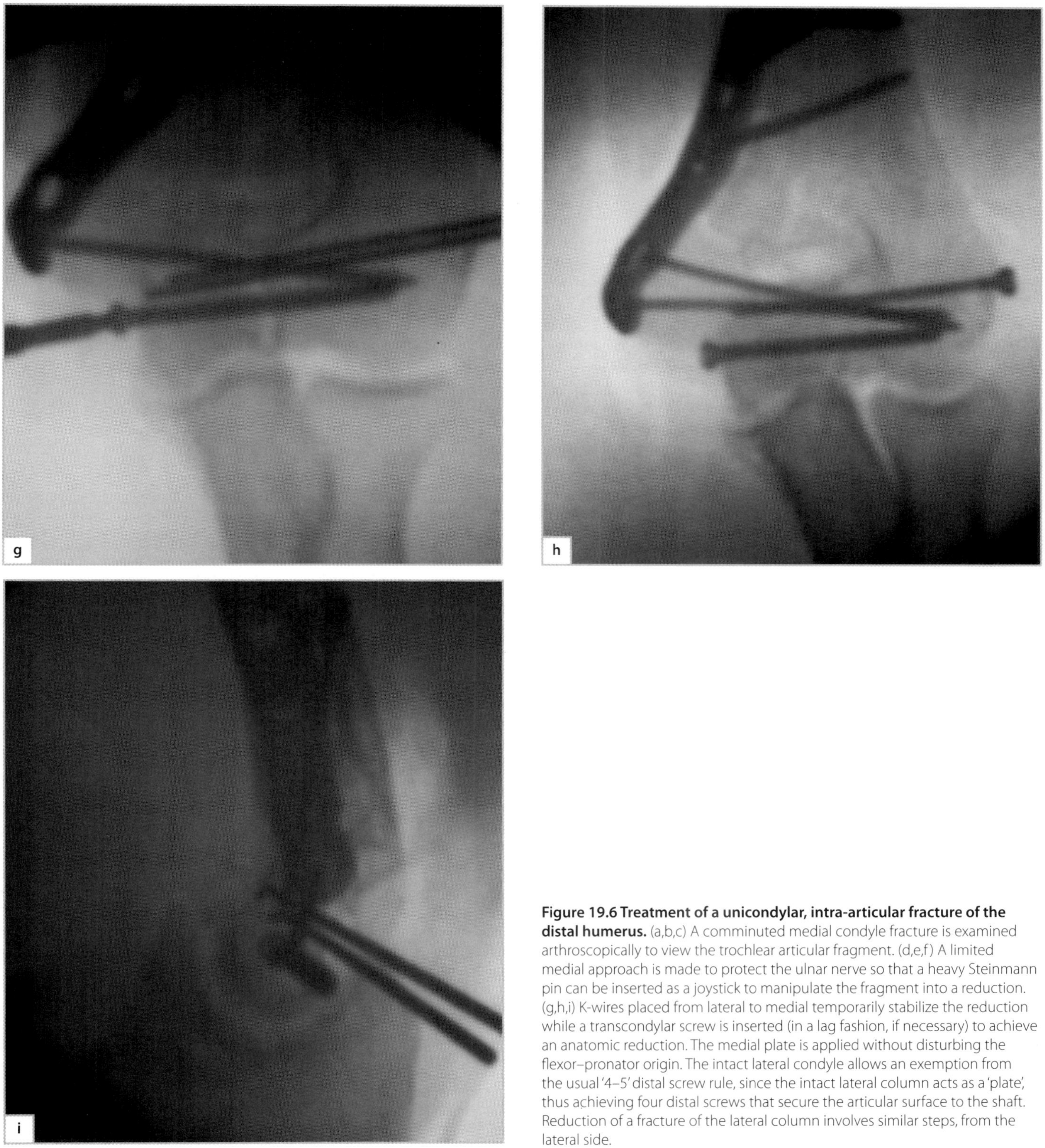

Figure 19.6 Treatment of a unicondylar, intra-articular fracture of the distal humerus. (a,b,c) A comminuted medial condyle fracture is examined arthroscopically to view the trochlear articular fragment. (d,e,f) A limited medial approach is made to protect the ulnar nerve so that a heavy Steinmann pin can be inserted as a joystick to manipulate the fragment into a reduction. (g,h,i) K-wires placed from lateral to medial temporarily stabilize the reduction while a transcondylar screw is inserted (in a lag fashion, if necessary) to achieve an anatomic reduction. The medial plate is applied without disturbing the flexor–pronator origin. The intact lateral condyle allows an exemption from the usual '4–5' distal screw rule, since the intact lateral column acts as a 'plate', thus achieving four distal screws that secure the articular surface to the shaft. Reduction of a fracture of the lateral column involves similar steps, from the lateral side.

with varus instability, and in turn Doornberg and Ring have shown this to be associated with posteromedial rotatory instability (Adams et al. 2007, Doornberg et al. 2007, Steinmann 2008, Adams et al. 2009). Similarly, transverse fractures of the coronoid tip and anterolateral coronoid facet (O'Driscoll type I) can be associated with medial collateral ligament rupture and posterolateral rotatory instability.

The exact indications for coronoid open reduction and internal fixation are not clear. Our current practice is to perform open reduction and internal fixation on fractures of the medial coronoid facet using a buttress plate, as an adequate buttressing effect cannot be achieved by arthroscopic techniques at present (Adams et al. 2009). Transverse fractures of the coronoid tip and anterolateral fractures can be treated by arthroscopic reduction and fixation (Hausman et al. 2008). Access to the coronoid from a lateral approach is relatively easy if the radial head is resected. If not, coronoid open reduction and internal fixation is possible but more difficult, requiring either proximal extension of the lateral approach or a substantial medial approach. Our preference is to perform arthroscopic reduction and fixation of the coronoid fragment if there is no fracture of the radial head, or if the radial head is to be preserved. This allows the coronoid fracture to be addressed, imparting additional stability to the elbow, with minimal additional surgical trauma.

Whether the fracture is treated arthroscopically or open, leaving the ulnar nerve in situ avoids trauma and additional scarring, and preserves the option of arthroscopic arthrolysis, should subsequent elbow release surgery be necessary. This principle applies to our treatment of all elbow fractures.

Once again, a shoulder positioner is used and anteromedial and anterolateral standard portals are established. Evacuation of hematoma will generally permit adequate visualization of the coronoid from the anterolateral portal. However, if there is significant synovitis, a debridement along the anterior capsule might be necessary to adequately visualize the fragment. Hematoma formed at the fracture site should be removed with a 3.5 mm shaver.

It should be remembered that when properly reduced, the coronoid fits intimately against the trochlea. A small modified skin hook introduced through a cannula in the anteromedial portal can be used to grab and reduce the coronoid fragment. A mini-fluoroscopy unit is used to locate the optimal site of entrance for cannulated screw guide wires through the posterior cortex of the proximal ulna, just distal to the coronoid process. Two or three wires are inserted to engage and fix the coronoid, ideally exiting just distal to the coronoid tip. The guide wires should angle slightly from distal posteriorly to proximal anteriorly, so that distally directed forces on the coronoid from the trochlea tend to compress, rather than distract, across the fracture site (**Fig. 19.7**).

A decision about the optimal fixation must now be made. If the fragment is of sufficient size to pass two partially threaded cannulated screws, this is the preferred fixation. It should be further reinforced with a cerclage loop of suture passed through the screws to achieve a mattress suture effect, which is like an umbrella embracing the tip of the fragment (**Fig. 19.7i**). Most fractures, however, will not accept two screws. Therefore, the screw is placed in the center across the largest dimension of the fragment. Confirmation of the correct position is done by arthroscopic and fluoroscopic examination. Once the correct position has been confirmed, the fragment is held into position with an elevator or modified skin hook while the cannulated drill is used. The guide wire may be grasped with an arthroscopic grasper both to hold the reduction and to prevent inadvertent extraction of the pin by the cannulated drill.

Next, a short-threaded cannulated screw is inserted. This screw should be slightly undersized so that there is 1 mm of bone between the cortex of the coronoid and the screw. This will avoid abrasion against the cerclage sutures.

The fixation is then reinforced by passage of cerclage sutures. If the coronoid fragment is an anterolateral fragment, a spinal needle is placed through the 'soft spot' at the proximal radioulnar joint, and a 28-gauge stainless-steel wire or other suture passer is passed through the spinal needle and extracted through the lateral portal, along with a cerclage suture that has been passed through the screw.

The wires are then used to pass a Kevlar-reinforced suture. An arthroscopic sliding knot can be used to tighten the cerclage suture. No adverse effects have been noted from an intra-articular suture of this type, although the knot present on the posterior border of the proximal ulna can be irritating. If this is the case, cutting the cerclage suture and removing the knot and the suture are easily performed once the fracture has healed.

If cerclage of the medial fragment is required, a small Freer elevator can be passed along the medial border of the proximal ulna. Extreme care must be taken to remain exactly on the bone and distal to the joint in order to be deep to the ulnar nerve. This requires very careful attention because of the proximity of the ulnar nerve. The modified Freer elevator is preloaded with a 28-gauge stainless-steel wire, which can be used to pass the cerclage suture exiting from the cannulated screw. Once again, an arthroscopic sliding knot is placed along the subcutaneous border of the ulna (**Fig. 19.7l**).

Arthroscopic fixation of the coronoid affords an excellent view of the reduction and fixation, a view that is probably even better than that achieved by an extensile open approach. However, careful attention to detail is required. The most difficult portion of the procedure can be visualization of the fragment due to hematoma and soft-tissue swelling, particularly if the anterior capsule is avulsed. A few extra minutes spent debriding this area can be very helpful, as can the use of retractors.

Osteochondritis dissecans

Osteochondritis dissecans carries a poorer prognosis in patients with closed growth plates and large, potentially unstable fragments. Preservation and healing of the osteochondral fragment will improve the outcome (Takahara et al. 2007, Takahara et al. 2008). However, the procedure is technically challenging and may require a very extensile and potentially destabilizing surgical approach. Several authors have described the advantages of arthroscopic visualization for drilling, picking, or debridement. The technique described here is for actual repair and internal fixation of loose, but not detached, osteochondral fragments.

The procedure is performed with the elbow over the patient's chest. The lesion is viewed from either a distal posterolateral portal with the arthroscope advanced down the lateral gutter, or from a 'soft spot' portal. Our preference is the posterior approach with a 3.5 mm shaver in the 'soft spot' posterior radiocapitellar portal. There is usually some degree of synovitis and reactive capsulitis in this zone, which must be debrided so that the fragment is easily seen. If the fragment is very proximal, which is unusual, a 70° arthroscope may be helpful.

A small stab incision is made over the posterior aspect of the lateral column and, using the image intensifier, the best entry point and trajectory are determined for passage of a guide wire (**Fig. 19.8c**). The osteochondral fragment is then directly observed with the arthroscope as the guide wire is advanced. Direct arthroscopic observation confirms that the guide wire is placed in the center of the lesion. A small elevator is placed through the 'soft spot' portal to stabilize the fragment and prevent it from detaching and becoming a loose body as the wire is advanced and, especially, during the drilling.

Next, with the fragment held in position, a cannulated drill is used to create a tunnel for the passage of sutures and bone graft. Multiple 0-PDS sutures are then placed to create an umbrella effect over the fragment, thus firmly securing it (**Fig. 19.8g,h**).

The cerclage sutures are then created by using guide wires and 18-gauge spinal needles to pass additional suture limbs medial and lateral and, if necessary, proximal and distal to the fragment (**Fig. 19.8i**). Once the sutures are passed and collected at the posterolateral incision, bone graft (our preference is for iliac crest graft harvested percutaneously with a special trephine needle) is packed again while observing the fragment to avoid displacement care. Care is taken to ensure that the drill crossed the non-union site into the subchondral

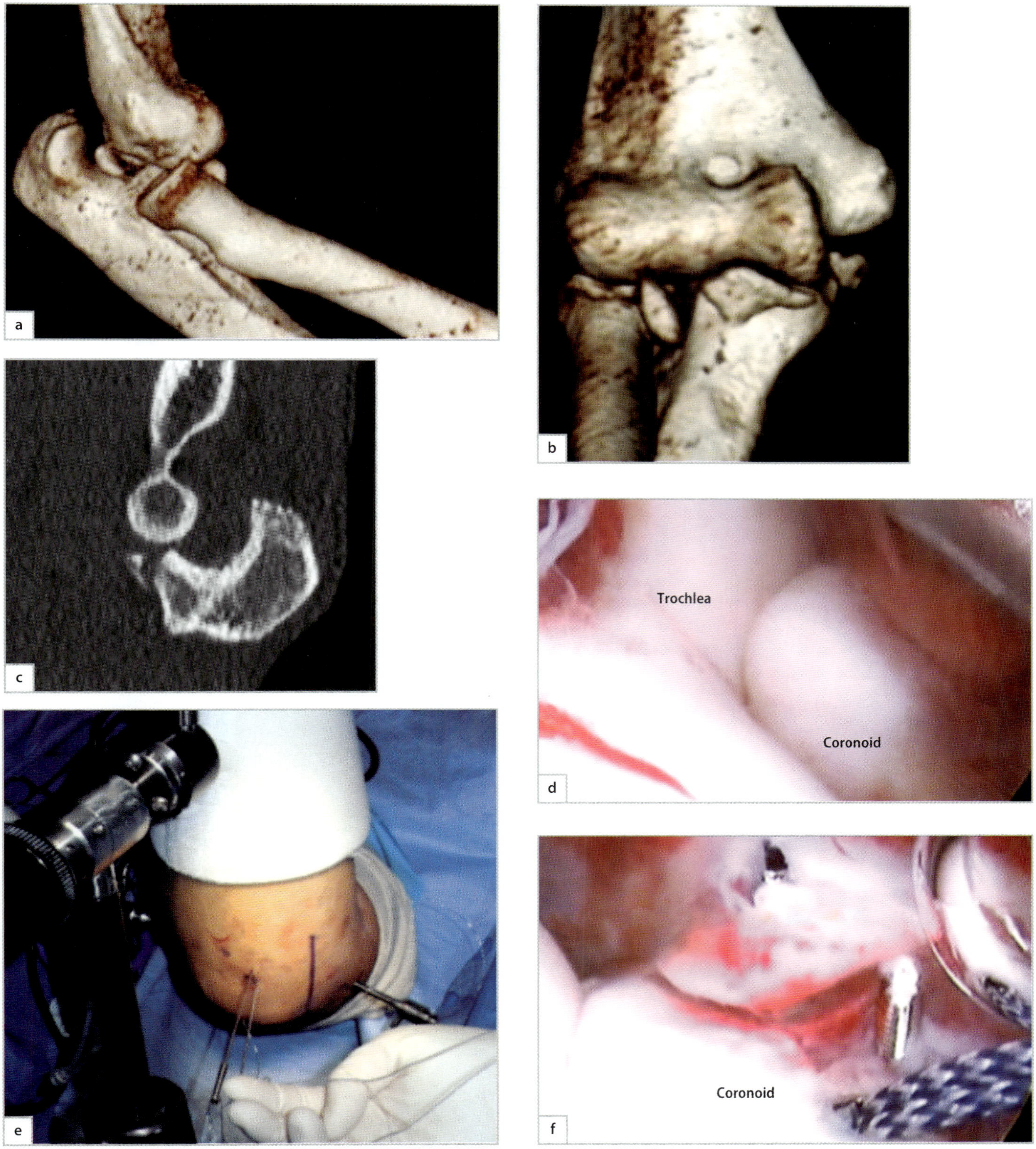

Figure 19.7. Treatment of a 'terrible triad' injury. (*Contd*)

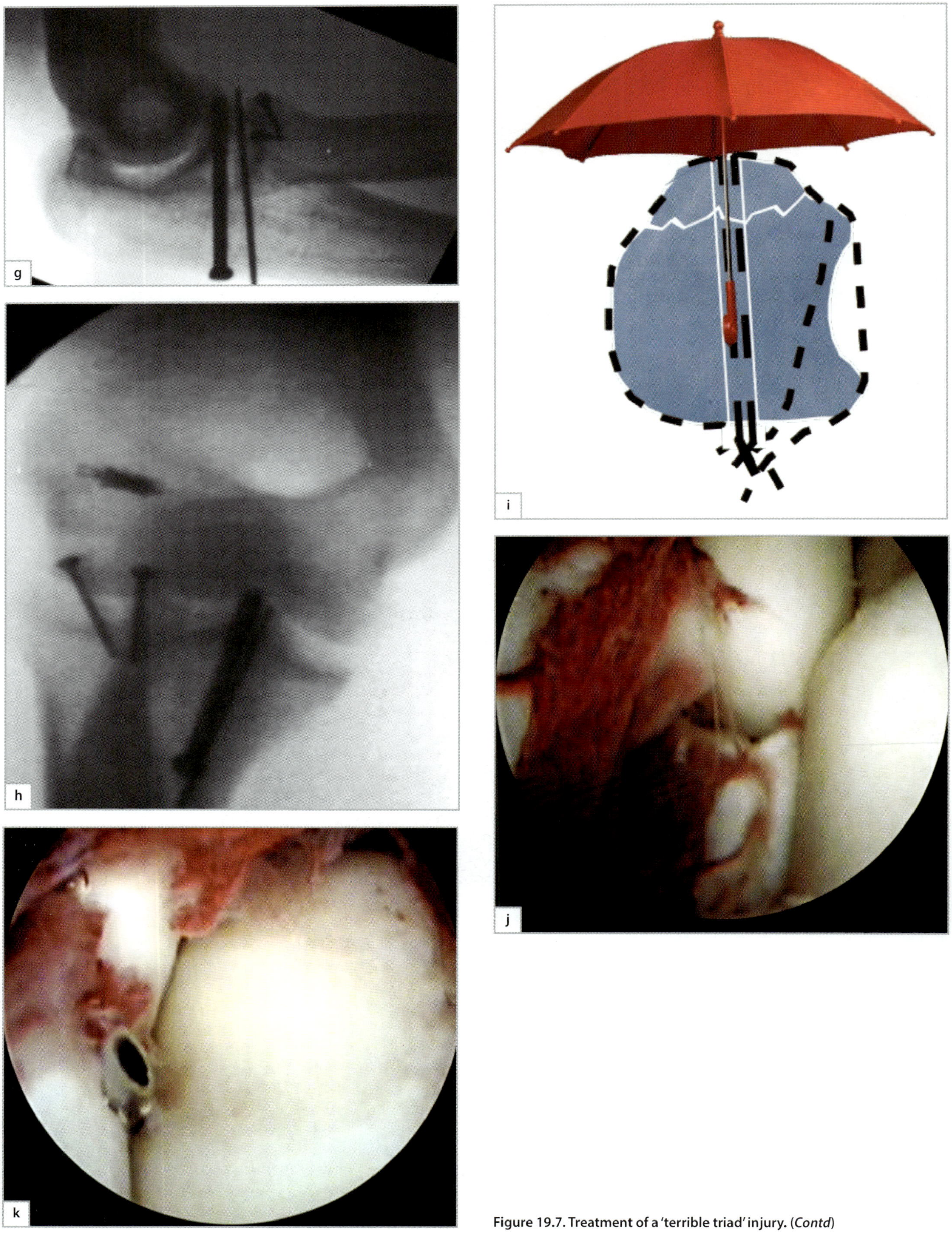

Figure 19.7. Treatment of a 'terrible triad' injury. (*Contd*)

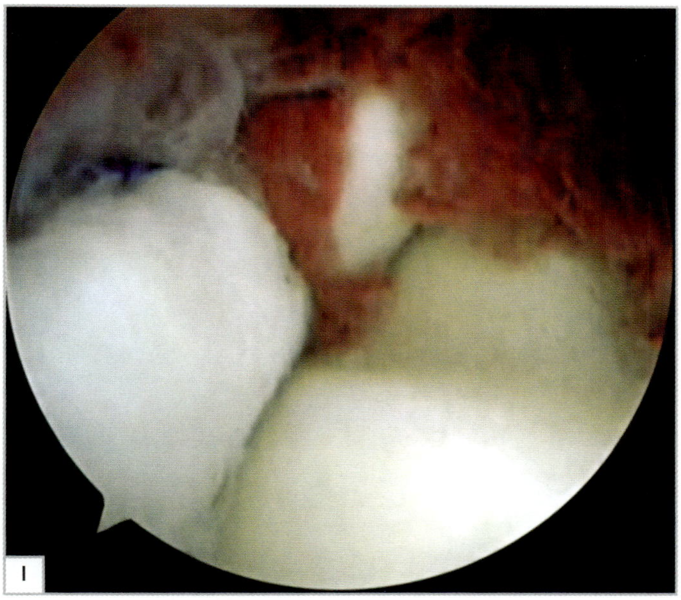

Figure 19.7. Treatment of a 'terrible triad' injury. (a-c) Preoperative CT scanning demonstrates a 'terrible triad' injury with an anterior marginal fracture of the radial head, characteristic of posterolateral instability, and an O'Driscoll Type I coronoid fracture. There is also anterior ulnohumeral instability, but the anteromedial facet of the coronid is intact, signifying that posteromedial rotatory instability will not be likely if the other injuries are fixed. The radial head will be preserved in this case, limiting access to the coronoid from the lateral approach, but the anterior ulnohumeral instability is an indication for ARIF of the coronoid. (d-h) The tip of the coronoid is reduced and, under arthroscopic visualization, a guide wire and cannulated screw are placed in the coronoid from the subcutaneous border of the proximal ulna. Fluoroscopy helps determine the approximate entrance point. A second, medial hole is drilled over another guide wire for passage of a circlage suture using a suture retriever or 28 gauge wire. A Kevlar reinforced suture is passed through the cannulated screw and through the second hole, then exiting to the posterior border of the ulna. The coronoid circlage suture is tied after ORIF of the radial head using an arthroscopic sliding knot. (i-l) The second case demonstrates the circlage suture passing through the proximal radioulnar joint to secure an anterolateral coronoid fragment. Note the vector of the suture's pull in a proximal direction, securing the fragment in a reduced position against the trochlea. As shown in the drawing of the umbrella, the goal is to circlage the coronoid fragment to anatomically reduce and firmly fix and compress the fragment. Circlage avoids the suture anchor effect of tying to a point which actually makes anatomic reduction impossible. If the fragment is large enough, the circlage suture can pass through two holes in the fragment. Otherwise, passing around the entire proximal humerus (deep to the ulnar nerve medially and through the joint laterally) may be required (i).

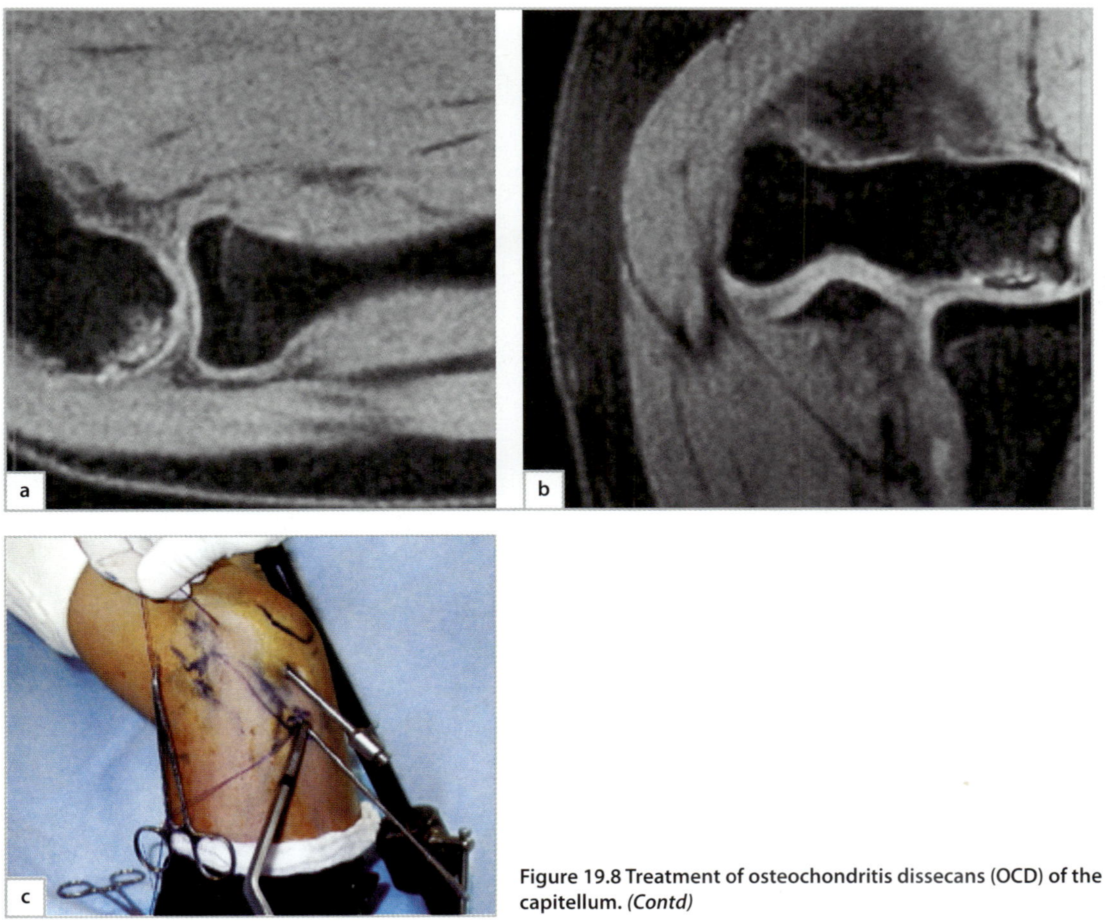

Figure 19.8 Treatment of osteochondritis dissecans (OCD) of the capitellum. ***(Contd)***

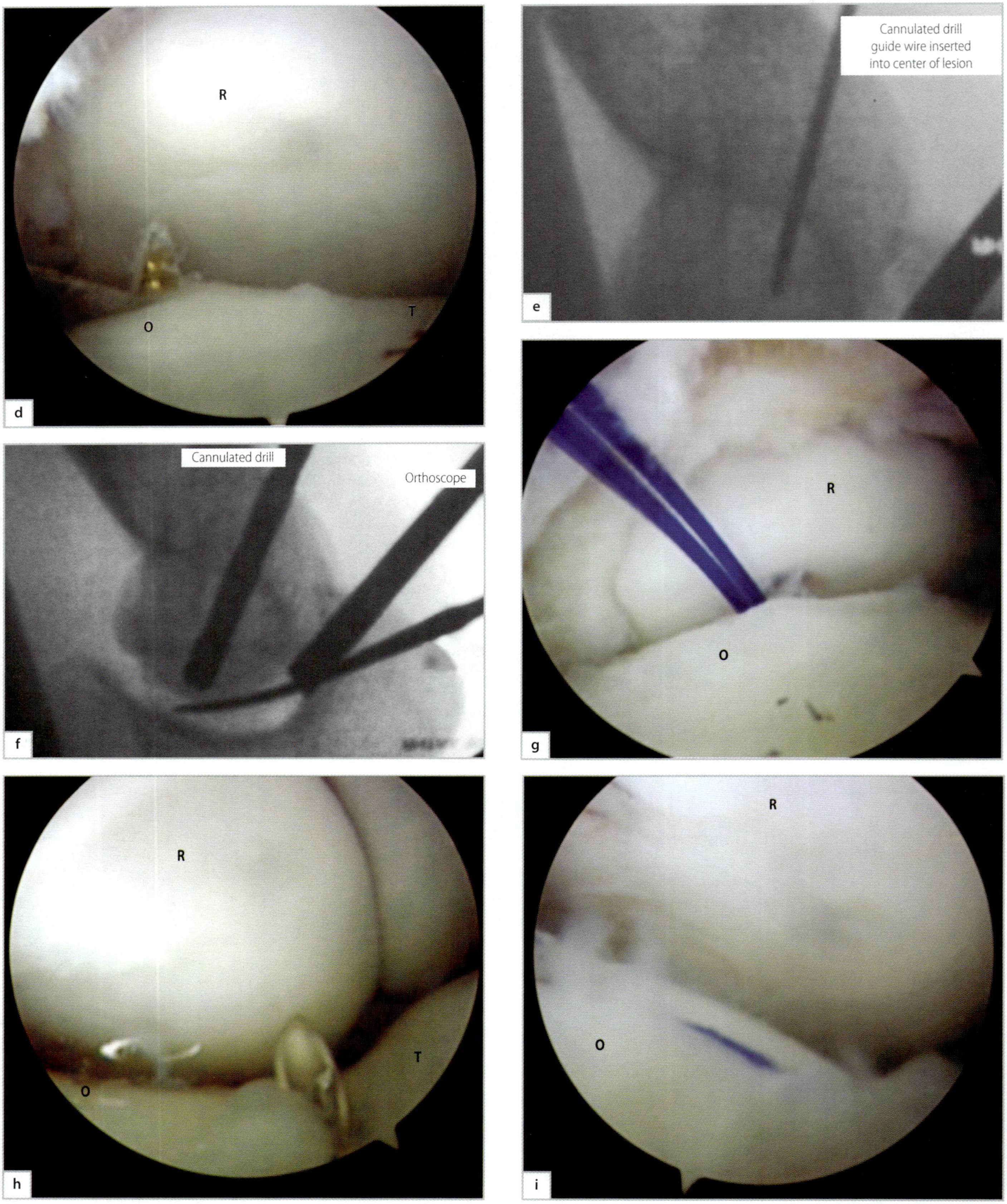

Figure 19.8 Treatment of osteochondritis dissecans (OCD) of the capitellum. ***(Contd)***

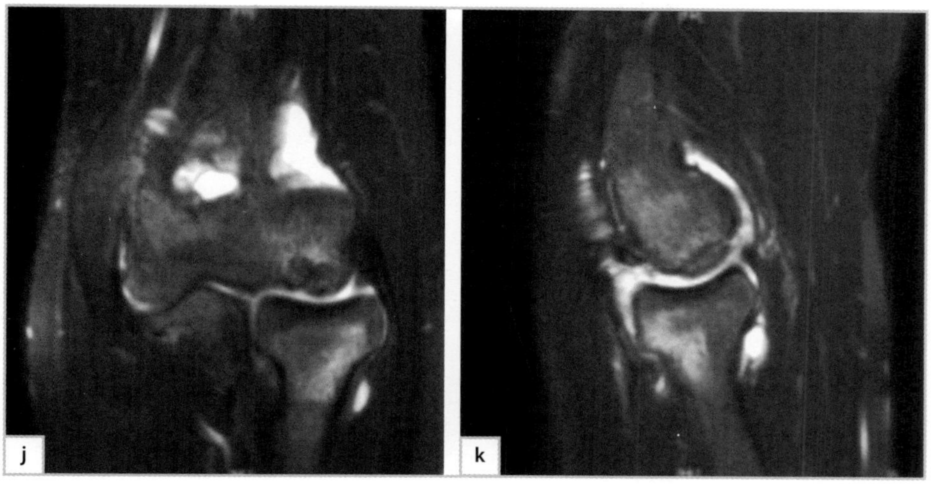

Figure 19.8 Treatment of osteochondritis dissecans (OCD) of the capitellum. (a,b) Magnetic resonance imaging demonstrates a large, loose but not displaced OCD lesion of the capitellum. (c,d,e) The lesion is visualized with the arthroscope in the distal posterolateral portal and a Freer elevator in the posterior radiocapitellar 'soft spot' portal stabilizes the fragment as a cannulated screw guide wire is passed into the center of the fragment. (f) The cannulated drill is then used to drill right up to the subchondral bone, while the elevator stabilizes the fragment to protect the cartilage. (g,h) 0-PDS sutures are then passed and another hole is drilled at the lateral trochlea to pass a suture-passing wire to create a mattress suture over the OCD fragment, similar to the coronoid technique. (i) The sutures are then tied posteriorly with sliding knots to stabilize the fragment and morsellized ICBG is packed, under radiographic control, across the fracture site and up to the subchondral bone. (j,k) Magnetic resonance scans at four months demonstrate healing and trabecular bridging of the subchondral fracture line. R = radial head; O = OCD lesion in capitellum; T = lateral trochlear ridge.

bone, and that the bone graft bridges the subcondral defect. The sutures are then tied using arthroscopic sliding knots and, as the sutures are tightened, compression of the articular cartilage beneath the suture is observed, demonstrating firm fixation of the fragment.

The elbow is kept in a cast until healing and bridging of the osteochondral fracture are demonstrated with magnetic resonance imaging (MRI). Despite the postoperative immobilization in a cast, none of our patients has required subsequent elbow release surgery, although this certainly might be necessary in some cases.

REHABILITATION

The rehabilitation protocol is dependent upon the type of fracture, and the stability of the fracture fixation and of the elbow. The guidance has evolved in recent years. Elbow motion was formerly the paramount concern, and early and aggressive rehabilitation was prioritized. Unfortunately, this could cause fixation failure and loss of critical bone stock and articular fragments, due to motion and avascular necrosis. Therefore, our current rehabilitation philosophy prioritizes healing over range of motion. As our facility and expertise with elbow contracture-release techniques has improved, we are now comfortable with elbow release surgery, by either arthroscopic or traditional open means, and recognize that certain injuries are best treated with two-stage reconstructive procedures, the first step being treatment of the fracture or dislocation, allowing for healing and contracture release as a second step. This is best summarized by the dictum 'we have a predictable solution for a stiff elbow, but we do not have a reliable solution for chronic instability or loss of bone stock and articular surface'.

For pediatric fractures of the lateral condyle, fixation is always somewhat tenuous with percutaneous pins. Such injuries are therefore immobilized in a long arm cast for four to six weeks, or until evidence of healing by periosteal bone apposition is seen radiographically. Any doubts about healing can be resolved with MRI. Once the fracture has healed, an aggressive rehabilitation protocol is begun. Most patients will regain full motion. However, long-term radiographic or MRI monitoring, looking for avascular necrosis of the lateral trochlea or a physeal bar at the lateral condyle, should be performed to prevent a fishtail deformity. Persistent loss of motion is treated with early arthroscopic release, and the physeal bar, if present, can also be resected arthroscopically. The surgeon should not be lulled into complacency by good short-term results and restoration of motion, as all pediatric elbow injuries should be followed long term for signs of growth disturbance, to prevent deformity and loss of function in adulthood.

Pediatric fractures of the radial neck are generally stable after reduction. This is particularly true if the periosteal hinge on one side of the fracture remains. Such injuries allow for more aggressive rehabilitation, with gentle exercise begun immediately after arthroscopic reduction. Sports activities are prohibited for approximately four weeks, after which time return to full function is permitted.

Intra-articular fractures of the lateral and medial condyle in adults can generally be securely stabilized by following the principles of fixation for fractures of the distal humerus, with all transcondylar screws passing through the plate that reassociates the distal articular spool with the humeral shaft. Such fractures are generally stable if these principles are followed, and rapid rehabilitation is then possible with early and aggressive range-of-motion exercises. However, if these fixation principles are not followed and fixation is done with inferior techniques, such as a single column screw or K-wires, early motion is likely to lead to loss of reduction or failure to heal, and should be avoided. Again, arthroscopy should not imply a lesser procedure or inferior fixation, but rather should be a technique for better visualizing the articular surface and the accuracy of the reduction. Standard, validated fixation principles should always be followed.

Fractures of the capitellum and anterior coronal shear fractures can generally be adequately stabilized to permit early range of motion by placing multiple screws and using arthroscopy to ensure correct placement of the screws of the appropriate length (**Fig. 19.9**). The lateral-to-medial transcondylar screw substantially improves the strength of fixation, if its use is appropriate. Such fractures can be treated with early and aggressive rehabilitation. However, if there is any concern about the strength of fixation, a two-stage procedure is an option if motion cannot be restored with therapy after healing has occurred. Loss of the capitellum due to avascular necrosis is to be avoided at all costs.

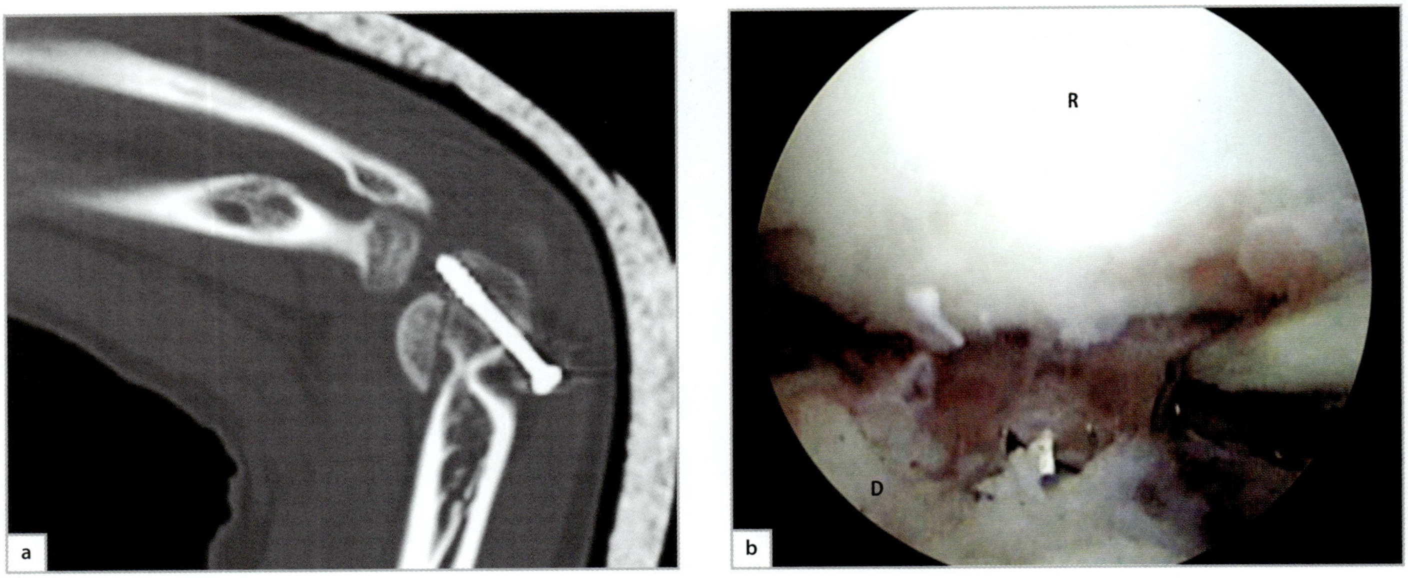

Figure 19.9 Loss of fixation after open reduction and internal fixation (ORIF) of a fracture of the capitellum. (a) A sagittal computerized tomography image demonstrates loss of fixation. (b) Arthroscopic examination confirms that the screw was too short, with barely one thread beyond the posterior fragment. Arthroscopic examination during revision ORIF allows use of the longest possible screw, for best fixation, without penetrating the articular surface. D = distal humerus; R = radial head.

REFERENCES

Adams JE, Merten SM, Steinmann SP. Arthroscopic-assisted treatment of coronoid fractures. Arthroscopy 2007;23:1060–1065.

Adams JE, Hoskin TL, Morrey BF, Steinmann SP. Management and outcome of 103 acute fractures of the coronoid process of the ulna. J Bone Joint Surg Br 2009;91:632–635.

Doornberg JN, de Jong IM, Lindenhovius AL, Ring D. The anteromedial facet of the coronoid process of the ulna. J Shoulder Elbow Surg 2007;16:667–670.

Graveleau N, Bauer T, Hardy P. [Arthroscopic treatment of acute elbow fractures.] [In French.] Chir Main. 2006;25 Suppl 1:S114–120.

Hausman MR, Qureshi S, Goldstein R, et al. Arthroscopically-assisted treatment of pediatric lateral humeral condyle fractures. J Pediatr Orthop 2007;27:739–742.

Hausman MR, Klug RA, Qureshi S, et al. Arthroscopically assisted coronoid fracture fixation: a preliminary report. Clin Orthop Relat Res 2008;466:3147–3152.

Michels F, Pouliart N, Handelberg F. Arthroscopic management of Mason type 2 radial head fractures. Knee Surg Sports Traumatol Arthrosc 2007;15:1244–1250.

Rolla PR, Surace MF, Bini A, Pilato G. Arthroscopic treatment of fractures of the radial head. Arthroscopy 2006;22:233.e1–233.e6.

Steinmann SP. Coronoid process fracture. J Am Acad Orthop Surg 2008;16:519–529.

Takahara M, Mura N, Sasaki J, et al. Classification, treatment, and outcome of osteochondritis dissecans of the humeral capitellum. J Bone Joint Surg Am 2007;89:1205–1214.

Takahara M, Mura N, Sasaki J, et al. Classification, treatment, and outcome of osteochondritis dissecans of the humeral capitellum. Surgical technique. J Bone Joint Surg Am 2008;90 Suppl 2 Pt 1:47–62.

Chapter 20 Management of radial head and neck fractures

Lauren H. Redler, Stephanie H. Hsu, William N. Levine

INTRODUCTION

Fractures of the head of the radius are the most common adult elbow fracture. They are frequently associated with elbow dislocations, concomitant fractures, and injury to the interosseous ligament, the medial collateral ligament (MCL) complex, and/or lateral collateral ligament (LCL) complex. Appropriate management is essential, as the radial head is critically important to elbow and forearm stability and motion. An improved understanding of the complexity of injury in fractures of the radial head and neck has improved our ability to devise a successful treatment plan based upon clinical examination, imaging, intraoperative findings, and advanced surgical techniques and implants.

The radial head, along with other bony and ligamentous restraints, allows for load transfer from the wrist to the elbow, provides stability against valgus instability, posterolateral rotatory instability, and translation, as well as proximal migration of the radius. The stabilizing role of the radial head becomes more obvious with concurrent injury to the interosseous membrane or the distal radioulnar joint (DRUJ), as in Essex-Lopresti injuries (**Figs 20.1, 20.2**).

Fractures of the radial head and neck often occur from a fall on an outstretched arm, with a valgus pronation force directing the proximal radius against the capitellum. They less commonly occur with a pure valgus injury or direct blow. Fractures of the radial head are identified in 5–10% of all elbow dislocations, and are often found in combination with coronoid fractures, 'terrible triad' injuries (Chapter 25), fractures of the ulna, and injuries of the interosseous ligament (Essex-Lopresti injuries), of the triangular fibrocartilage complex, and of the collateral ligament.

Recognizing the importance of associated injuries is paramount in determining the appropriate treatment. Clinical examination should focus on elbow stability, additional areas of tenderness, including the DRUJ, as well as an evaluation for a mechanical block to motion. Aspiration of the fracture hematoma and intra-articular injection of local anesthetic can assist in the identification of a mechanical block to motion.

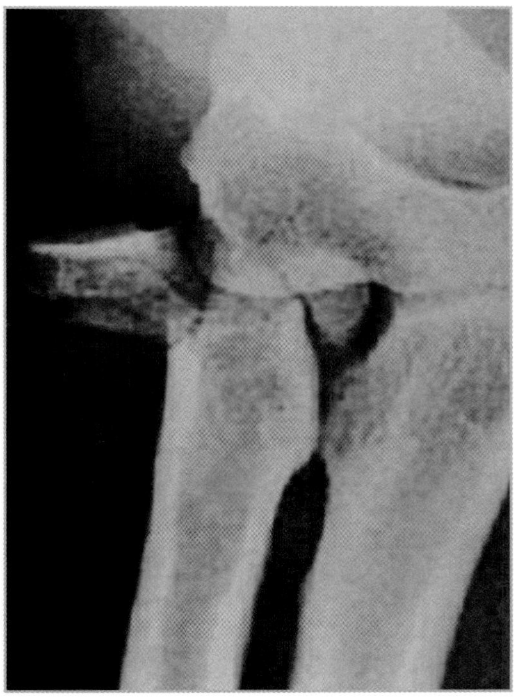

Figure 20.1 Essex-Lopresti injury. This 27-year-old man fell from 5 m and landed on his outstretched dominant right wrist. This anteroposterior radiograph of the elbow shows the comminuted, displaced fracture of the radial head and neck. (Figure courtesy of Columbia University Center for Shoulder, Elbow and Sports Medicine.)

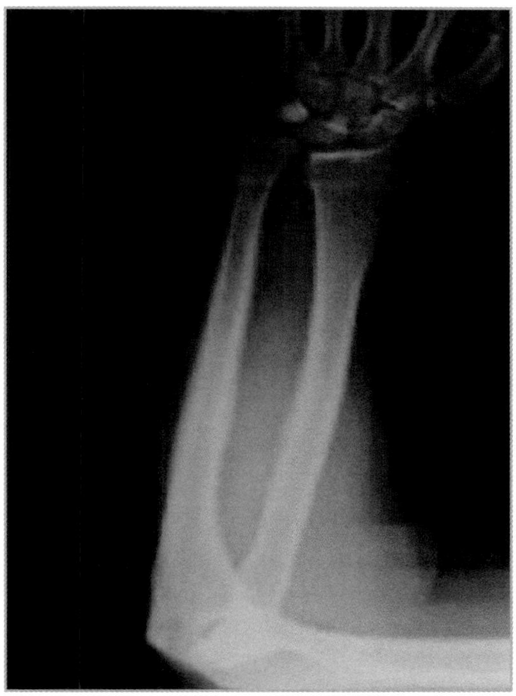

Figure 20.2 Essex-Lopresti injury. This anteroposterior radiograph of the wrist of the same patient as in Fig. 20.1 demonstrates significant proximal radial migration with dislocation of the distal radioulnar joint (DRUJ). (Figure courtesy of Columbia University Center for Shoulder, Elbow and Sports Medicine.)

Standard radiographic evaluation of the elbow should include an anterolateral (AP), lateral, and often oblique views focused upon the radiocapitellar joint. The Greenspan view, a modified lateral view with the beam angled 45° toward the radial head, or other modifications of radiocapitellar views, are used to avoid coronoid overlap and improve visualization of the radial head and capitellum. Elevation of the anterior and posterior fat pads due to hemarthrosis may be the only radiographic evidence of a non-displaced fracture of the radial head. Articular injury is often more severe than plain radiographs reveal (O›Driscoll and Jupiter 2003). Bilateral posteroanterior (PA) views of the wrist may be obtained to assess ulnar variance if there is concern about injury to the interosseous ligament or DRUJ. Computerized tomography (CT) scans and reconstructions are particularly helpful in delineating fragment number, size, displacement, comminution, depression of the articular surface, and bone quality; they can also provide important information for preoperative planning if open reduction and internal fixation (ORIF), or radial head arthroplasty is planned. Magnetic resonance imaging (MRI) may occasionally be used to provide additional information regarding injury to the collateral ligament and interosseous ligament, chondral injury, or non-ossified loose bodies.

CLASSIFICATION

There are several systems that classify fractures of the radial head (**Table 20.1**). That first developed by Mason in 1954 is based solely on radiographic findings and thus fails to take into account associated soft-tissue injury and does not help determine management (Mason 1954). A Mason type I fracture is non-displaced (**Figs 20.3, 20.4**). A type II injury is a minimally displaced partial fracture. A type III injury is a comminuted fracture of the radial head. Johnston's modification added a type IV, taking into account associated elbow dislocation (Johnston 1962). Morrey's modification allowed for quantification of the head involvement and included fractures of the radial neck (Broberg and Morrey 1987): a type I fracture involves the radial head or neck with <2 mm displacement; a type II fracture involves the radial head or neck with ≥2 mm displacement and involving ≥30% of the articular surface; a type III is a comminuted fracture of the radial head or neck; a type IV is any fracture of the radial head associated with an elbow dislocation.

Hotchkiss described a modified classification that involves assessment of associated injuries as well as the presence or absence of a mechanical block to motion to determine treatment (Hotchkiss 1997). Type I fractures are minimally displaced with no mechanical block to motion, ≤2 mm intra-articular displacement, or marginal lip fracture; they are generally treated non-operatively with early range of motion.

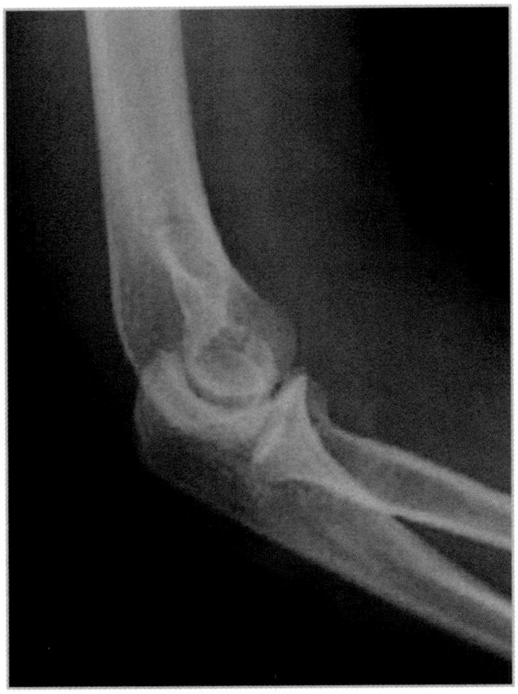

Figure 20.3 Mason type I fracture of the head of the radius. This lateral radiograph of a 52-year-old woman shows the fracture of the radial head with <2 mm displacement. (Figure courtesy of Columbia University Center for Shoulder, Elbow and Sports Medicine.)

Type II fractures have ≥2 mm displacement or neck angulation, often with a limitation to motion requiring surgical treatment. Type III fractures have severe comminution with or without a block to motion, and require open reduction and internal fixation (ORIF), or radial head arthroplasty.

INDICATIONS

Treatments for fractures of the radial head and neck include non-operative management, fragment excision, radial head excision, ORIF, and radial head arthroplasty. Characteristics of the fracture, in addition to clinical presentation, and the results of examination and imaging, dictate fracture management. Fragment number, size, displacement, comminution, impaction, bone quality, and associated ligamentous injuries or fractures are carefully considered. The principal goals of surgical treatment are to obtain stable fixation that restores anatomy and articular congruity, to allow for early range of motion.

Table 20.1 Mason classification of fractures of the head of the radius, as modified by Johnston, Morrey, and Hotchkiss

	Mason (1954)	Johnston (1962)	Morrey (1987)	Hotchkiss (1997)
Type I	Non-displaced		Head or neck fracture with <2 mm displacement	Minimally displaced, no mechanical block to motion, ≤2 mm intra-articular displacement, marginal lip fracture
Type II	Minimally displaced, partial head fracture		Head or neck fracture with ≥2 mm displacement and involving ≥30% of the articular surface	≥2 mm displacement, neck angulation, often with limitation to motion
Type III	Comminuted fracture of radial head		Comminuted head or neck fracture	Severe comminution with or without block to motion
Type IV		Radial head fracture with elbow dislocation	Radial head fracture with elbow dislocation	

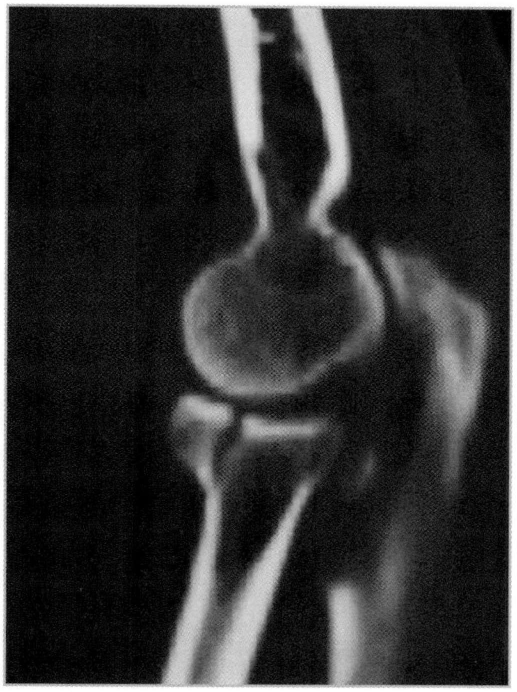

Figure 20.4 Mason type I fracture of the head of the radius. This computerized tomography scan of same patient as in Fig. 20.3 confirms there is no displacement of the radial head fragment. The patient had no mechanical block to motion. The fracture was treated non-operatively and went on to heal without any functional deficits. (Figure courtesy of Columbia University Center for Shoulder, Elbow and Sports Medicine.)

Table 20.2 Indications for open reduction and internal fixation

Less than a third of the articular surface is involved
Fracture displaced >2 mm, with a possible block to mechanical motion
2–3 mm articular depression
Ability to achieve stable fixation
High-demand patient
Fractures with associated ligamentous or soft-tissue injuries
Fractures distal to the annular ligament

Table 20.3 Indications for arthroplasty

Medial collateral ligament-deficient elbow
Comminuted fracture of the radial head with elbow or forearm instability (elbow dislocation or injury to the distal radioulnar joint)
When stable open reduction and internal fixation is not possible
Fractures involving over a third of the radial head
Radial head/neck non-union
Associated coronoid or olecranon fracture that is displaced or comminuted and unstable

Approximately 40–60% of radial head fractures are non-displaced or minimally displaced (Akesson et al. 2006). Usually, there is no mechanical block to motion or significant articular incongruity and, therefore, these stable fractures can be treated non-operatively with good functional outcomes and minimal loss of motion. Fractures involving less than one third of the articular surface with <2 mm displacement, or fractures in low-demand elderly patients, are at a low risk of further displacement (Beingessner et al. 2005). Multiple groups have reported good results in 85–95% of patients, with a sling for comfort and early active range of motion (Herbertsson et al. 2004, Akesson et al. 2006, Duckworth et al. 2011). Although rare, displaced fractures involving over 33% of the articular surface may occur, in which case cautious rehabilitation or operative fixation is required to prevent poor outcomes.

Operative treatment is indicated in patients with a mechanical block to motion, displaced articular fractures, more than three fragments, significant articular depression, associated fractures, or concurrent injury to the MCL, LCL, interosseous membrane, or DRUJ (**Tables 20.2, 20.3**). Plain radiographs may not reveal the primarily cartilaginous pieces; however, fragments from the radial head or capitellum may cause a mechanical block to motion and may be excised if not amenable to ORIF or arthroplasty. Fragment excision should not exceed 35% of the surface of the radial head or 25–33% of the capitellar surface area (Beingessner et al. 2005, Caputo et al. 2006). Excision is rarely recommended, due to the large number of complications, especially in the setting of concomitant soft-tissue injuries. These complications include premature arthritis, instability, altered biomechanics, pain, proximal migration of the radius, cubitus valgus, and decreased strength. Excision of the radial head should be considered only in isolated scenarios of comminution and displacement, in which there is no associated ligamentous or bony injuries. The reported outcomes of treating fractures of the radial head or neck with excision have been mixed. Herbertsson et al. (2004) reported fair or good results in a series of 61 fractures of the radial head, with Mason type IV fractures having the worst results, and showed no difference between primary or delayed excision. Antuña et al. (2010) reported satisfactory results for Mason type II or type III fractures at a mean of 25 years' follow-up in over 90% of 26 patients younger than 40 years of age treated with primary radial head excision. Iftimie et al. (2011) reported satisfactory functional results in 96% of patients with Mason type II, III, or IV fractures treated with primary excision at a mean follow-up of 17 years. However, 53% were lost to follow-up and 25% experienced proximal migration of the radius. Conversely, Ikeda et al. (2005) showed improved clinical outcomes for 13 consecutive patients with Mason type III fractures treated with ORIF versus 15 consecutive patients with Mason type III fractures treated with excision, including preserved range of motion, greater strength, and better function.

For comminuted fractures in young, active patients, ORIF can be attempted to achieve stable fixation. Successful and stable fracture fixation of the articular surface and restoration of the head to neck anatomy is possible with ORIF. King et al. (1991) reported 100% excellent results with ORIF for Mason type II fractures but only 33% excellent results for Mason type III fractures, suggesting that more comminuted fractures should be managed with alternative treatments, such as excision. Ikeda et al. (2003) reported excellent results for ORIF with Mason type III and IV fractures using low-profile precontoured mini-plates. However, this was a series of only 10 patients and 9 of the 10 required removal of hardware. Ring (2004) recommends ORIF for fractures of the radial head with three or fewer articular fragments, based on his series of 56 fractures of the radial head treated with ORIF. Thirteen of 14 Mason type III fractures with more than three fragments had unsatisfactory results, whereas 15 of 15 Mason type II fractures had satisfactory results.

Arthroplasty or ORIF restores the lateral column of the elbow, providing axial as well as varus–valgus stability, and so allowing healing of associated injuries. Radial head arthroplasty is essential in cases of fractures associated with MCL disruption or injury to the interosseous ligament or DRUJ, as it avoids the poor functional outcomes associated with excision (Mirzayan and Itamura 2004). In a consecutive series of 65 Mason type III fractures, Liu et al. (2010) reported that ORIF produced excellent or good results in 57% of patients, as compared with 73% for arthroplasty.

CONTRAINDICATIONS

Contraindications to the surgical management of fractures of the radial head or neck include infection, major soft-tissue injury, and medical instability.

Excision of the radial head is rarely undertaken, due to the high rates of postoperative complications, including proximal migration of the radius, wrist pain, decreased grip strength, valgus instability, early recurrent posterolateral rotatory instability, osteoarthritis, and cubitus valgus.

Contraindications to ORIF include older age, underlying osteoarthritis, and injury to the capitellum. ORIF for a highly comminuted fracture may result in unreliable fixation, non-union, and poor outcomes. In these situations, radial head arthroplasty is preferred.

In the setting of ligamentous injuries and instability, radial head arthroplasty may be preferable to marginal ORIF. Radial head arthroplasty should be considered carefully in the young patient and those without instability, as its long-term effects on the capitellar articulation and long-term implant survivability are still not fully known.

TECHNIQUE

Surgical approaches

Lateral approaches provide exposure and visualization of the radial head and neck. Depending on the location and extent of the fracture, a Kaplan or Kocher approach may be chosen, or one splitting the extensor digitorum communis (EDC).

The patient may be positioned in a supine position, with a roll under the ipsilateral side allowing slight rotation of the patient's torso so the operative arm can be draped across the chest. Alternatively, a hand-table may be used with the patient's shoulder abducted. A sterile tourniquet is used.

The Kaplan approach maintains exposure anterior to the LCL, to prevent iatrogenic injury to the lateral ulnar collateral ligament (LUCL) and resultant posterolateral instability. A skin incision is made from the lateral epicondyle distally 3–4 cm toward Lister's tubercle. The interval is between the EDC and the common origin of the extensor carpi radialis brevis (ECRB) and extensor carpi radialis longus (ECRL). The raphe is incised longitudinally and a Hohmann retractor may be used to elevate the anterior flap made in the capsule. Disruption of the LCL should be avoided. When using the Kaplan approach, the surgeon should be aware of the risk to the posterior interosseous nerve (PIN) anteriorly, and the need to elevate the remaining EDC origin to access the LCL if repair is necessary. An EDC-splitting approach also remains anterior to the LCL and is another option if the LCL is intact. These more anterior approaches also allow better access to anterolateral fracture fragments of the radial head.

The Kocher approach may be preferred if the LCL is known to be disrupted. A lateral incision over the radial head or a posteriorly based incision with full-thickness skin flaps may be used. The interval is between the anconeus (radial nerve) and extensor carpi ulnaris (PIN) and is best identified distally and extended proximally. The deep fascia is incised and muscles released from the ligamentous–capsular layer. A longitudinal or Z-type capsulotomy may be used at the annular ligament for repair or more distal exposure of the neck. The LCL should be carefully protected, or recognized if ruptured for later repair. An anterior flap is elevated from the epicondyle to expose the radiocapitellar joint, while the posterior flap is left intact to maintain stability. Pronation of the forearm allows for protection of the PIN. A cadaveric study by Diliberti et al. (2000) established a safe zone of ≥38 mm from the capitellum of the lateral aspect of the radius to the PIN with pronation. Flexion and extension did not affect the location of the PIN.

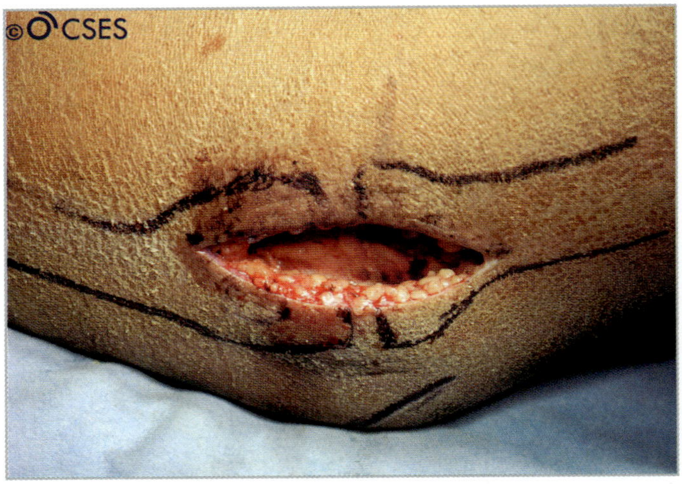

Figure 20.5 Lateral skin incision and lateral approach to an isolated fracture of the head of the radius. (Figure courtesy of Columbia University Center for Shoulder, Elbow and Sports Medicine.)

The Boyd approach is also an option for improved visualization and access to the radial head and neck for extended fractures or arthroplasty. With this exposure, the radioulnar, radiohumeral, and ulnohumeral articulations may be visualized. A posteriorly based incision is used with an approach to the radial head and neck by periosteally elevating the anconeus, annular ligament, and ulnar base of the LCL for exposure. Suture anchors are then used to repair the LCL complex back to the ulna, or crista supinatoris (Mirzayan and Itamura 2004).

A posterior approach may be used to access the medial elbow if the MCL needs to be repaired (Mirzayan and Itamura 2004). A midline posterior skin incision is made distal to the tip of the olecranon. Full-thickness fasciocutaneous flaps are raised to avoid injury to the cutaneous nerves. This allows access to both the medial and lateral sides, as well as fixation of a fracture of the proximal ulna (if present).

ORIF of the radial head

Open reduction and internal fixation has predictable results and good outcomes (Ring 2004) and is thus the preferred treatment for fractures of the radial head (**Fig. 20.6**). The articular surface should be reduced under direct visualization using a dental pick or bone tamp and confirmed with intraoperative fluoroscopy. Provisional fixation is achieved with small Kirschner wires (K-wires). Larger fragments may often be fixed to one another prior to fixation at the radial neck, to help restore anatomy. Hardware is then placed, with the goal of providing enough stability to allow postoperative functional mobilization. Choices of hardware include: mini-fragment screws (1.5 or 2.0 mm), self-compressing mini-screws, mini-condylar plates, variable-pitch headless screws, or precontoured radial head, neck, and T-plates. If a plate is used, it must be long enough for three screws distal to the fracture site but should not be placed distal to the bicipital tuberosity, due to risk of injury to the PIN.

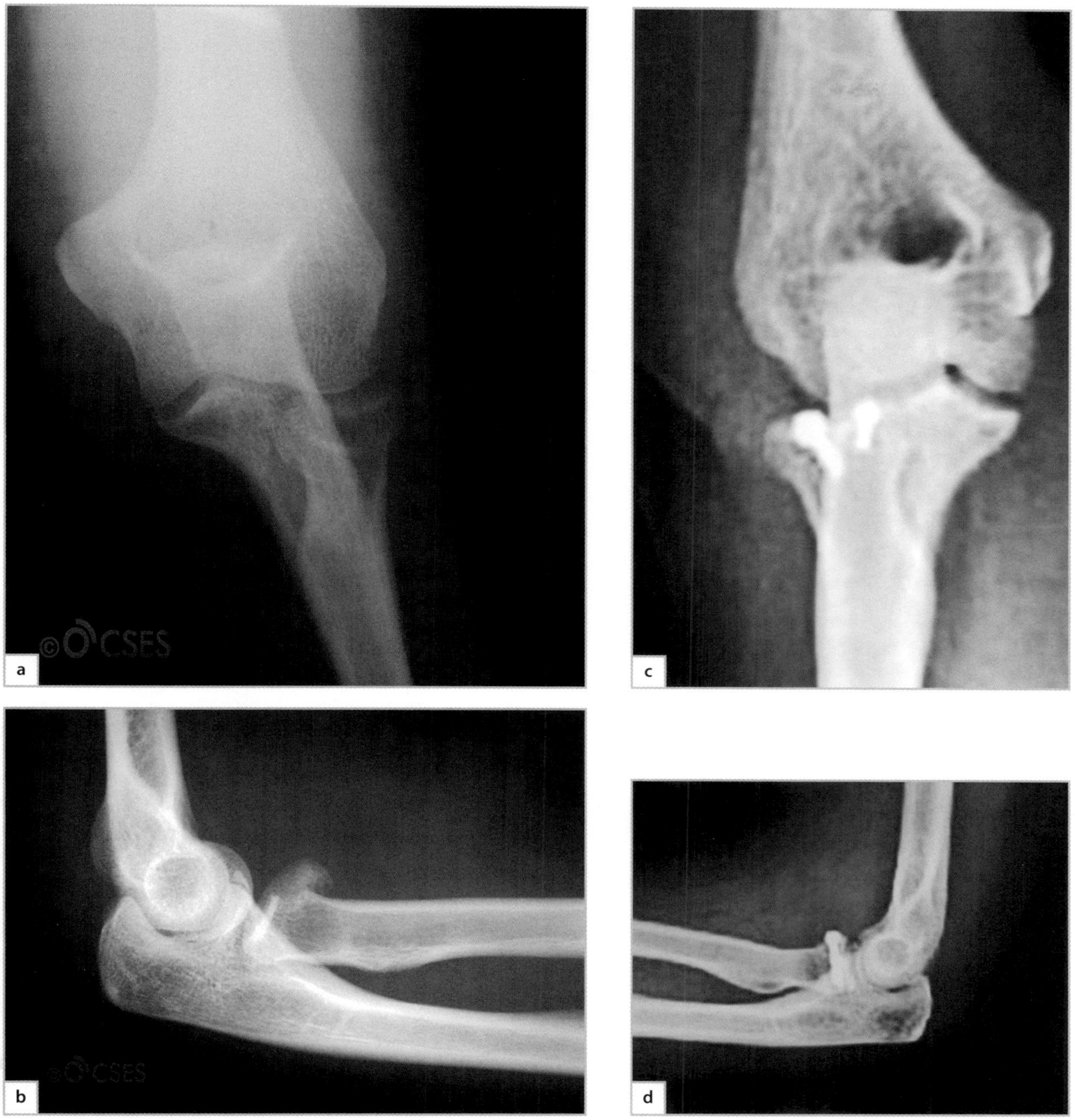

Figure 20.6 Treatment of a displaced fracture of the head of the radius. This 33-year-old right-handed man slipped and fell. (a) Preoperative anteroposterior radiograph. (b) Preoperative lateral radiograph. (c) Anteroposterior radiograph after open reduction and internal fixation (ORIF). (d) Posteroperative lateral radiograph. (Figures courtesy of Columbia University Center for Shoulder, Elbow and Sports Medicine.)

Several biomechanical studies have reported on various constructs used for internal fixation. One study comparing three locking plates with two non-locking plates and 2.0 mm crossed screws found equivalent or improved stability with each of the 2.0 mm locking plates compared with the bulkier 2.4 mm non-locking plates or the crossed screws (Burkhart et al. 2007). Another biomechanical study compared 3.0mm headless compression screws (Synthes, West Chester, PA) with standard 2.0mm cortical screws (Synthes, West Chester, PA) and found no significant difference in stability to axial and transverse loading (Burkhart et al. 2010b). Ertürer et al. (2010) compared ORIF with mini-screws (2.5 mm headless compression screws) to 2.0 mm K-wires and found equivalent outcomes both clinically and radiographically. There were no significant differences between the two groups with respect to time to union, range of motion, Morrey score, or time to return to work. Regardless of the implant chosen, stable anatomic fixation that allows early postoperative motion should be achieved.

ORIF of the radial neck

Open reduction and internal fixation of the radial neck (**Fig. 20.7**) is more technically challenging and has less predictable results than that of the radial head. Extending the lateral incision distally increases exposure of the neck. The muscle fibers of the common extensors are lifted anteriorly, which exposes the posterior margin of the supinator.

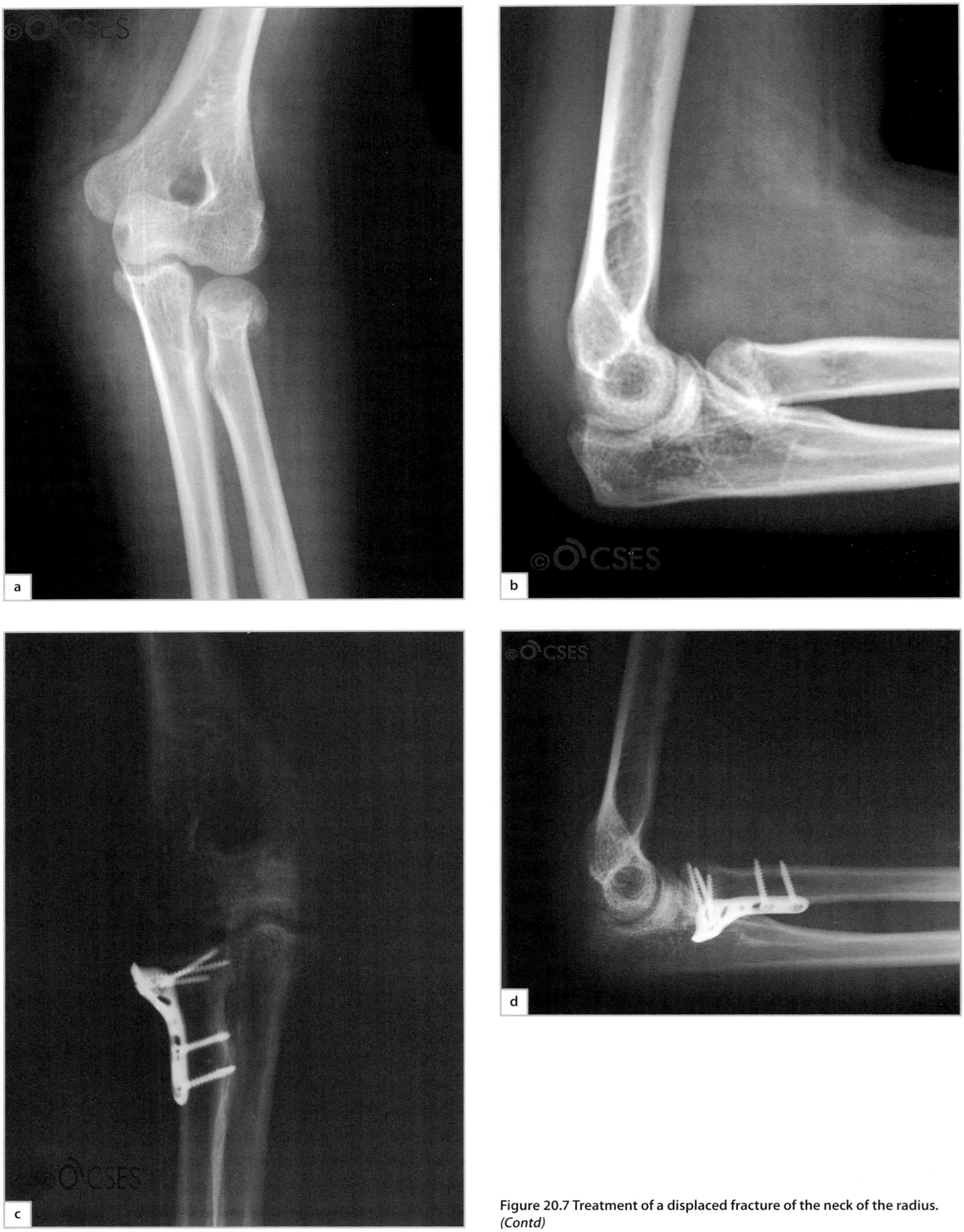

Figure 20.7 Treatment of a displaced fracture of the neck of the radius. *(Contd)*

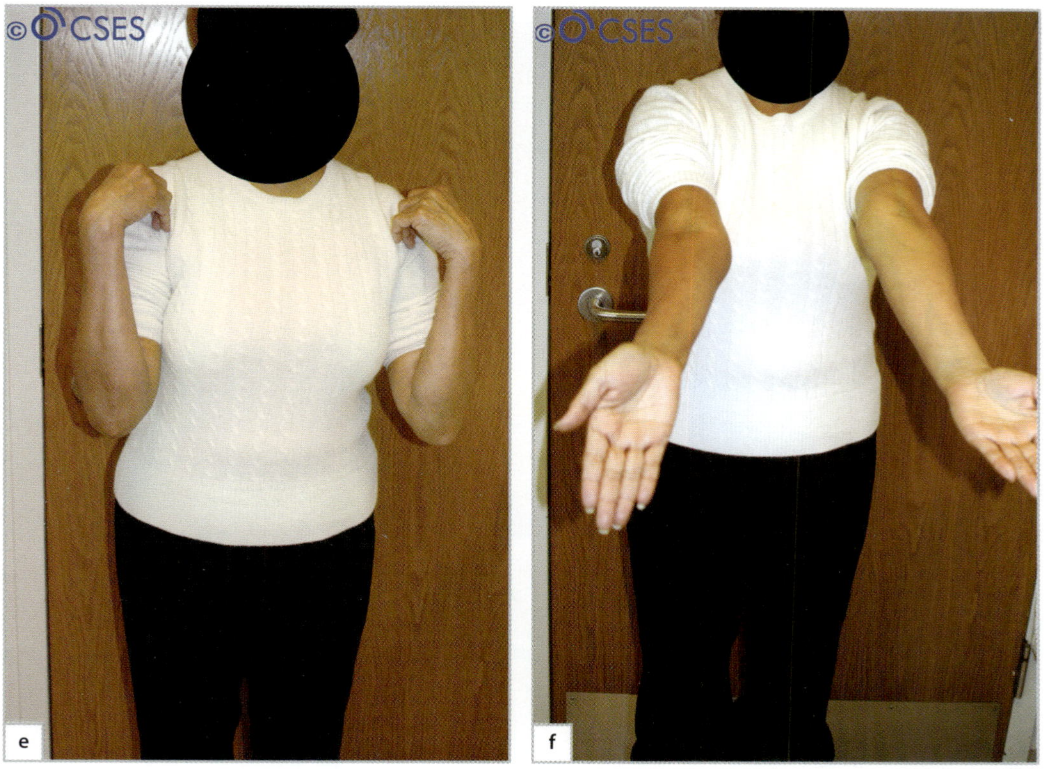

Figure 20.7 Treatment of a displaced fracture of the neck of the radius. This 52-year-old right-handed woman fell off a bicycle. (a) Preoperative anteroposterior radiograph. (b) Preoperative lateral radiograph. (c) Anteroposterior radiograph after open reduction and internal fixation (ORIF), with low-profile radial neck plate. (d) Posteroperative lateral radiograph. (e) Clinical picture showing bilateral elbow flexion three months postoperatively. (f) Clinical picture showing bilateral elbow extension three months postoperatively. (Figures courtesy of Columbia University Center for Shoulder, Elbow and Sports Medicine.)

The supinator is easily identifiable, as the fibers run at a 45° angle to the longitudinal fibers of the extensor compartment. This increases exposure for correct fracture reduction and plate placement.

Often these fractures require a mini-fragment T-plate as well as bone grafting to fill in any defects, which are usually in the area of the neck. If a large plate is needed, the PIN should be identified before distal exposure, to ensure protection. Instrumentation should be placed in the safe zone, a 90° arc of non-articular radial head encompassing the right angle formed by the radial styloid and Lister's tubercle, so as not to impinge on the proximal radioulnar joint (Caputo et al. 1998, O›Driscoll et al. 2003). The safe zone is anterolateral in the neutral position, and posterolateral with the forearm in supination. Assessment of the cartilage in the safe zone may also be useful, as it is most often thinner and less opaque. In a cadaveric study, Caputo et al. (1998) found that regardless of approach (anterior, lateral, posterolateral), internal fixation with a 2.7 mm mini-T-plate (Synthes, West Chester, PA) allowed full forearm rotation. Alternatively, Soyer et al. (1998) showed that a plate applied directly laterally on the radial head and neck with the arm in neutral position does not impinge on the proximal radioulnar joint.

Arthroplasty of the radial head

Arthroplasty of the radial head is the preferred treatment for acute comminuted fractures that cannot be stably reconstructed with ORIF **(Fig. 20.8)**. There are reports of non-union, fixation failure, and loss of forearm rotation when comminuted fractures have been treated with ORIF (Ring 2004, Ikeda et al. 2005). It is important to assess for an associated non-displaced fracture of the radial neck so that it may be prophylactically wired prior to arthroplasty, to prevent displacement during ulnar preparation and prosthesis insertion. The native head should be resected at the metaphyseal flare to preserve the attachment of the annular ligament. The maximum amount of radial neck should be preserved, to provide a stable rim for the prosthesis and also a measure of length.

One of the keys to successful arthroplasty of the radial head is optimal sizing of the implant (Ring 2004, Athwal et al. 2010). If the diameter is too large, it will load the margins of the sigmoid notch. If the diameter is too small, it will point load on the sigmoid notch. An incorrect diameter of the prosthesis will also have abnormal loading on the capitellum. Overstuffing can lead to lateral-sided elbow pain, limited elbow flexion, capitellar erosions, or implant dislocations, whereas understuffing will prevent proper loading of the capitellum and lead to persistent instability. The correct size of prosthesis should be chosen by comparing the excised fragments of the radial head to the trial implants. Measuring the height of the fractured head from the fracture surface with the least amount of radial neck will prevent overlengthening of the radius (Athwal et al. 2010). If detached or torn, repair of the LCL complex is essential to restore elbow stability after radial head arthroplasty.

The elbow should be ranged throughout the full range of motion once the prosthesis is implanted to ensure joint congruity and the absence of impingement. The ulnohumeral joint should be directly visualized to assess for any gapping, as this is the most sensitive intraoperative test for overlengthening (Frank et al. 2009). Full assessment of elbow stability should be performed with stress testing at 30° flexion with a pronated forearm to check the integrity of the ulnar collateral ligament. It is intact if there is less than 2 mm radiocapitellar opening; axial loading of the radius is then used to assess any disruption of the interosseous membrane if there is more than 2 mm of proximal displacement.

Good results have been shown with metallic radial head implants but no data exist showing better outcomes with modular or bipolar implants compared with monoblock prostheses. Burkhart et al. (2010a) reported an 8.8-year follow-up on 17 fractures of the radial head treated with arthroplasty using the Judet (Tornier, Edina, MN) bipolar

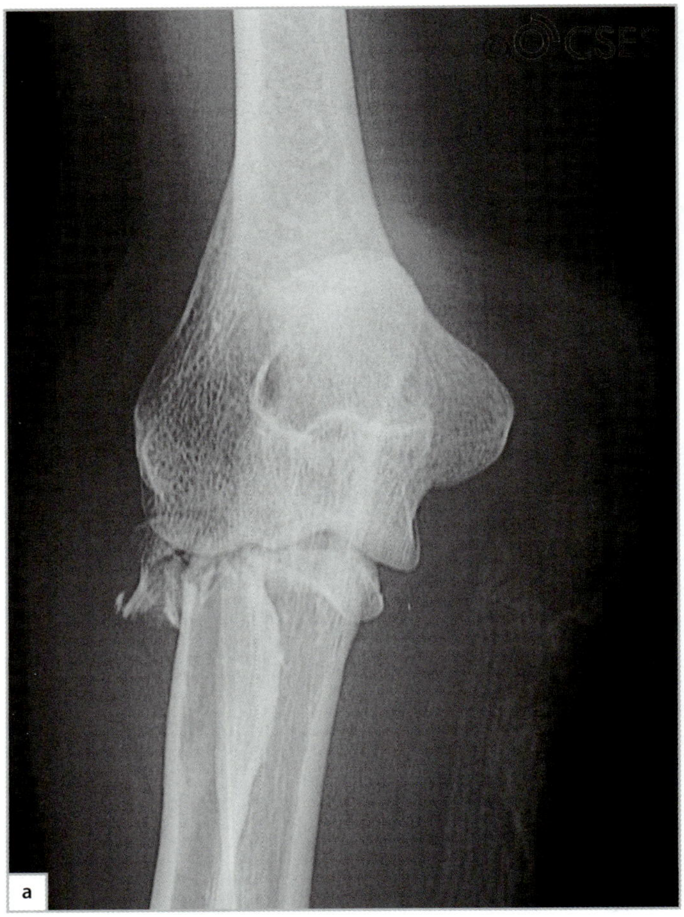

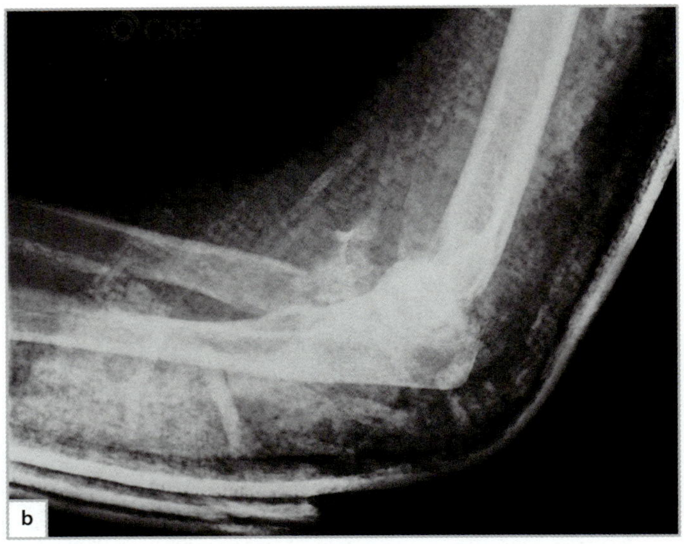

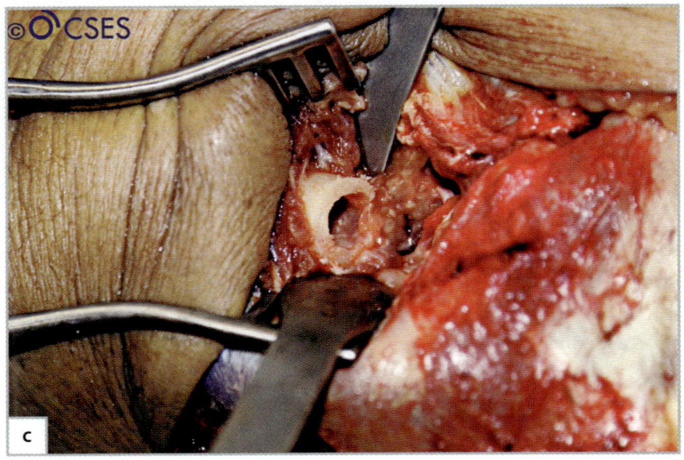

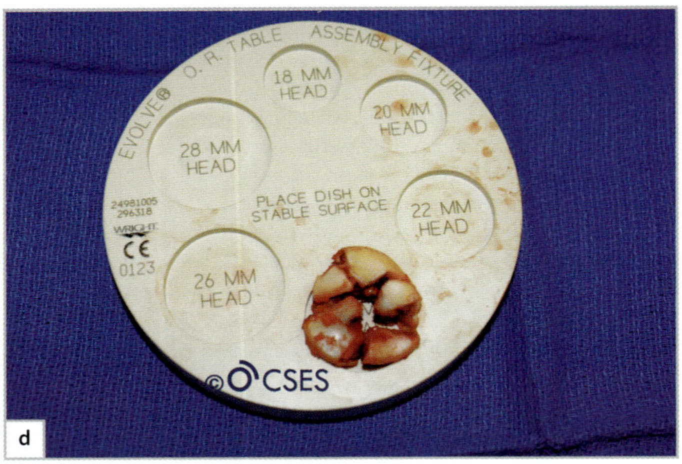

Figure 20.8 Arthroplasty for a comminuted displaced fracture of the head of the radius.

prosthesis: the results were excellent in six cases, good in 10, and fair in one, according to the Mayo Elbow Performance Score. Short-term complications included two dislocations, degenerative changes of the capitellum in eight cases, and ulnohumeral arthrosis in 12 cases. An important limitation of this series is that the authors did not separate out Monteggia-like lesions, Essex-Lopresti lesions, or 'terrible triad' injuries. Bain et al. (2005) reported on 16 patients with Mason type III fractures treated with titanium prostheses and found good to excellent results in 80% at 2.8-year follow-up. Compared with metallic implants, silicone implants have increased rates of reactive synovitis, inflammatory arthritis, and fractures of the silastic implants. Complications of arthroplasty of the radial head include persistent pain, restricted range of motion due to impingement, aseptic loosening, capitellar osteopenia, infection, nerve damage, heterotopic ossification, and synostosis formation. Heterotopic ossification is the most common complication reported in ORIF but it can also occur after arthroplasty; however, it rarely requires excision, except in patients with significant limitation to the motion of their arm.

Pearls and pitfalls

Recognition of the difficulties in the operative treatment of fractures of the radial head is important for successful outcomes and to avoid complications.

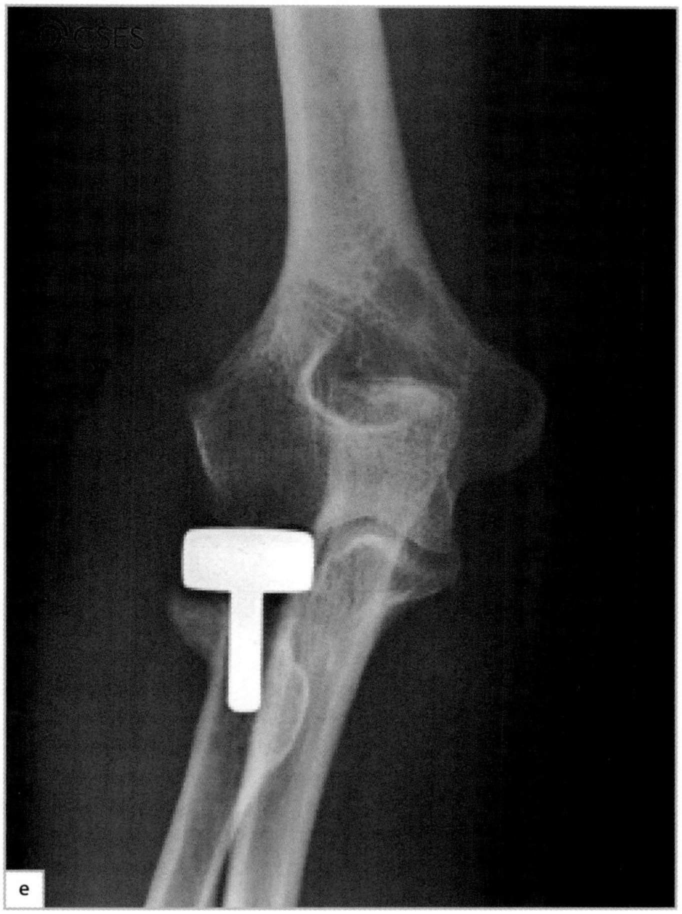
e

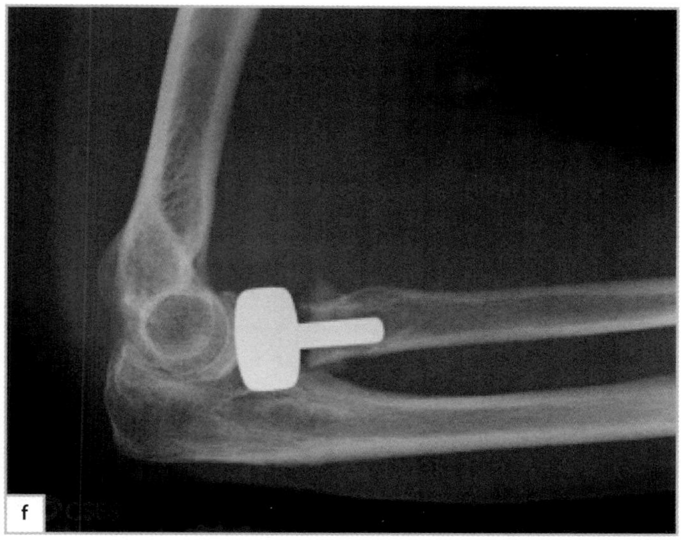
f

Figure 20.8 Arthroplasty for a comminuted displaced fracture of the head of the radius. This 48-year-old man fell onto his outstretched hand. (a) Preoperative anteroposterior radiograph. (b) Preoperative lateral radiograph showing posterior splint. (c) Intraoperative photograph demonstrating radial neck cut in preparation for radial head replacement. (d) Fragments assembled on sizer block on back table (Wright-Medical, Evolve). (e) Postoperative anteroposterior radiograph. (f) Postoperative lateral radiograph. (Figures courtesy of Columbia University Center for Shoulder, Elbow and Sports Medicine.)

Careful preservation of the LCL complex during lateral approaches to the elbow is essential to maintaining overall stability.

Protection of the PIN is aided by forearm pronation during a lateral approach, and its proximity should be acknowledged when accessing the radial neck.

Understanding the concave anatomy of the radial head helps to avoid intra-articular penetration of hardware.

Impacted articular fragments should be elevated to restore joint congruity. The defect may be filled with bone graft from the lateral epicondyle or olecranon.

The safe zone for hardware placement is an approximately 90° arc between the radial styloid and Lister's tubercle. The cartilage of the radial head in this area is thinner and less opaque.

The surgeon should attempt to maintain the length of the radial neck during arthroplasty, to provide a stable rim for the implant, to maintain annular ligament attachments, and to provide an anatomic marker of native anatomy.

Overstuffing of a radial head arthroplasty can lead to many complications.

It is important to check intraoperatively for full range of motion, as well as elbow and interosseous stability.

REHABILITATION

Rehabilitation focuses on the balance between concern for recurrent instability and the need for early mobilization to prevent stiffness. Non-operative treatment with early mobilization is the treatment of choice for stable fractures involving less than a third of the articular surface and most fractures in elderly, low-demand individuals. Active individuals with fractures involving more than a third of the articular surface benefit from a few days of sling support and then protected functional activities for 7–10 days. If the LCL is also repaired, supination should be limited for the first four to six weeks after surgery. If the MCL is repaired, a functional brace is added for stability, with a gentle increase in range of motion. Due to the known loss of full extension, some authors advise the use of an extension splint, worn at night, for 10–12 weeks.

REFERENCES

Akesson T, Herbertsson P, Josefsson PO, et al. Primary nonoperative treatment of moderately displaced two-part fractures of the radial head. J Bone Joint Surg Am 2006;88:1909–1914.

Antuña SA, Sánchez-Márquez JM, Barco R. Long-term results of radial head resection following isolated radial head fractures in patients younger than forty years old. J Bone Joint Surg Am 2010;92:558–566.

Athwal GS, Frank SG, Grewal R, et al. Determination of correct implant size in radial head arthroplasty to avoid overlengthening: surgical technique. J Bone Joint Surg Am 2010;92 Suppl 1 Pt 2:250–257.

Bain GI, Ashwood N, Baird R, Unni R. Management of Mason type-III radial head fractures with a titanium prosthesis, ligament repair, and early mobilization. Surgical technique. J Bone Joint Surg Am 2005;87 Suppl 1(Pt 1):136–147.

Beingessner DM, Dunning CE, Gordon KD, et al. The effect of radial head fracture size on elbow kinematics and stability. J Orthop Res 2005;23:210–217.
Broberg MA, Morrey BF. Results of treatment of fracture-dislocations of the elbow. Clin Orthop Relat Res 1987;(216):109–119.
Burkhart KJ, Mueller LP, Krezdorn D, et al. Stability of radial head and neck fractures: a biomechanical study of six fixation constructs with consideration of three locking plates. J Hand Surg Am 2007;2:1569–1575.
Burkhart KJ, Mattyasovszky SG, Runkel M, et al. Mid- to long-term results after bipolar radial head arthroplasty. J Shoulder Elbow Surg 2010a;19:965–972.
Burkhart KJ, Nowak TE, Appelmann P, et al. Screw fixation of radial head fractures: compression screw versus lag screw – a biomechanical comparison. Injury 2010b;41:963–967.
Caputo AE, Mazzocca AD, Santoro VM. The nonarticulating portion of the radial head: anatomic and clinical correlations for internal fixation. J Hand Surg Am 1998;23:1082–1090.
Caputo AE, Burton KJ, Cohen MS, King GJ. Articular cartilage injuries of the capitellum interposed in radial head fractures: a report of ten cases. J Shoulder Elbow Surg 2006;15:716–720.
Diliberti T, Botte MJ, Abrams RA. Anatomical considerations regarding the posterior interosseous nerve during posterolateral approaches to the proximal part of the radius. J Bone Joint Surg Am 2000;82:809–813.
Duckworth AD, Watson BS, Will EM. Radial head and neck fractures: functional results and predictors of outcome. J Trauma 2011;71:643–648.
Ertürer E, Seçkin F, Akman S, et al. The results of open reduction and screw or K-wire fixation for isolated type II radial head fractures. Acta Orthop Traumatol Turc 2010;44: 20–26.
Frank SG, Grewal R, Johnson J, et al. Determination of correct implant size in radial head arthroplasty to avoid overlengthening. J Bone Joint Surg Am 2009;91:1738–1746.
Herbertsson P, Josefsson PO, Hasserius R, et al. Uncomplicated Mason type-II and III fractures of the radial head and neck in adults. A long-term follow-up study. J Bone Joint Surg Am 2004;86:569–574.
Hotchkiss RN. Displaced fractures of the radial head: internal fixation or excision? J Am Acad Orthop Surg 1997;5:1–10.
Iftimie PP, Calmet Garcia J, de Loyola Garcia Forcada I, et al. Resection arthroplasty for radial head fractures: long-term follow-up. J Shoulder Elbow Surg 2011;20:45–50.
Ikeda M, Yamashina Y, Kamimoto M, Oka Y. Open reduction and internal fixation of comminuted fractures of the radial head using low-profile mini-plates. J Bone Joint Surg Br 2003;85:1040–1044.
Ikeda M, Sugiyama K, Kang C, et al. Comminuted fractures of the radial head. Comparison of resection and internal fixation. J Bone Joint Surg Am 2005;87:76–84.
Johnston GW. A follow-up of one hundred cases of fracture of the head of the radius with a review of the literature. Ulster Med J 1962;31:51–56.
King GJ, Evans DC, Kellam JF. Open reduction and internal fixation of radial head fractures. J Orthop Trauma 1991;5:21–28.
Liu B, Lin Z, Cao L, Kang Y. [Effectiveness comparison between open reduction combined with internal fixation and artificial radial head replacement in treating Mason type-III comminuted fractures of radial head]. [Article in Chinese.] Zhongguo Xiu Fu Chong Jian Wai Ke Za Zhi 2010;24:900–903.
Mason ML. Some observations on fractures of the head of the radius with a review of one hundred cases. Br J Surg 1954;42:123–132.
Mirzayan R, Itamura JM. Shoulder and Elbow Trauma. New York: Thieme, 2004.
O'Driscoll SW, Jupiter JB, Cohen MS, et al. Difficult elbow fractures: pearls and pitfalls. Instr Course Lect 2003;52:113–134.
Ring D. Open reduction and internal fixation of fractures of the radial head. Hand Clin 2004;20:415–427.
Soyer AD, Nowotarski PJ, Kelso TB, Mighell MA. Optimal position for plate fixation of complex fractures of the proximal radius: a cadaver study. J Orthop Trauma 1998;12:291–293.

Chapter 21 Fractures of the capitellum

Shahryar Ahmadi, Scott P. Steinmann

CLASSIFICATION

Capitellum is a Latin word meaning 'little head.' It is part of the lateral distal articular aspect of the humerus that articulates with the radial head. Its articular surface is over the anterior and inferior aspect of the bone.

Isolated fractures of the capitellum account for 0.5–1% of all elbow fractures. The fracture line typically runs in the coronal plane. There is a female predominance, which is thought to represent either biomechanical vulnerability – to which increased valgus carrying angle and hyperextensibility of the elbow are contributory factors – or metabolic susceptibility (osteoporosis) (Grantham et al. 1981). These fractures typically occur via a shear mechanism after a fall on an outstretched hand with the elbow extended. The force is transmitted through the radius, fracturing the capitellum (Grantham et al. 1981, McKee et al. 1996, Clough et al. 2001).

Bryan and Morrey classified this fracture into three types and McKee et al. (1996) added a fourth (**Fig. 21.1**). Type I (the Hahn–Steinthal fracture) involves articular cartilage and the underlying osseous portion of the capitellum. Type II (the Kocher–Lorenz fracture) involves the articular cartilage with a thin layer of underlying subchondral bone. Type III fractures are defined by severe comminution of the articular surface. Finally, type IV fractures include a coronal shear fracture of the capitellum and part of the trochlea. A coronal shear fracture involving the capitellum and a major portion of the trochlea was initially described by Mouchet in 1898 and Kocher in 1904 as well as by Lindem in 1922, but the significance of this type of fracture was not described until 1996 by McKee et al. (see also Stamatis and Paxinos 2003). The type I fracture is the most common and type III the least (Stamatis and Paxinos 2003). The fracture fragment typically displaces proximally toward the radial fossa (Ma et al. 1984, McKee et al. 1996).

The lateral view is diagnostic. The fracture will appear as a semicircular shadow of the capitellum seen in the radial fossa in varying degrees of rotation (Alvarez et al. 1975). Often the exact pattern of the fracture cannot be defined in plain radiographs. Computerized tomography (CT) with three-dimensional reconstructions to aid the preoperative assessment of the fracture and operative decision making is recommended in most of these injuries. These scans are especially useful to identify posterior or medial extension of the fracture and this can influence the surgical approach (anterolateral approach, extended Kocher approach with reflection of the lateral collateral ligament and olecranon osteotomy) (Ring et al. 2003). A lateral radiograph may show a double-arc sign in a type IV fracture. The double-arc sign represents the subchondral arc of bone of the capitellum and the lateral trochlear ridge (McKee et al. 1996). The fragment is usually in mild internal rotation. The double-arc sign may not be clear if rotation is increased, since the subchondral bone of the trochlear ridge is projected in an oblique and not a lateral plane (Stamatis and Paxinos 2003).

INDICATIONS

Indications for surgery include displaced fractures of the capitellum, fractures which extend into the trochlea, and open fractures. Treatment options include closed reduction, fragment excision, and open reduction with or without internal fixation. When open reduction and internal fixation are performed, techniques include the use of partially threaded cancellous lag screws, cannulated screws, Kirschner wires (K-wires), bioabsorbable pins or screws, headless screws, and small plates. **Table 21.1** summarizes the results reported in the literature with different approaches to the four types of fracture.

Type I fractures

Splint and observation

Alvarez et al. (1975) reported on seven patients who were treated by splinting and observation. All of these patients had poor results.

Excision

Good results have been reported with excision and early mobilization of the displaced capitellar fragment, although others have reported

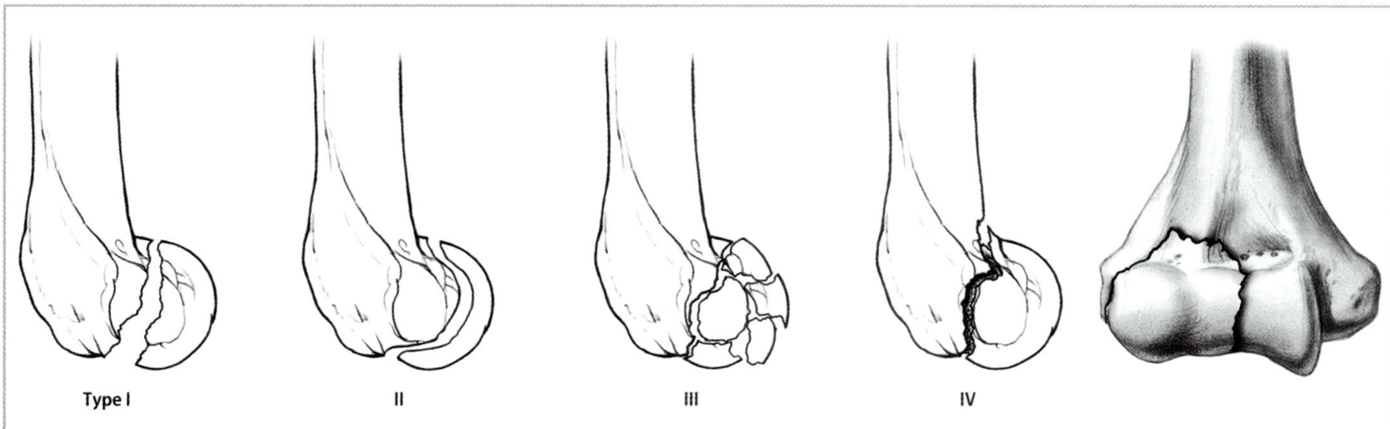

Figure 21.1 Capitellum fracture classification. By permission of Mayo Foundation for Medical Education and Research.

Table 21.1 Summary of case series using different approaches to the four types of fracture of the capitellum

	Fracture type										
	I	II	III	IV	Male/ female	Age	Dominant arm	Treatment	Range of motion	Follow-up	Result
Grantham et al. (1981)	19/29	2/29	8/29	*	24/5	16–92	2/3	ORIF 4, CR 5, excision 20	Average restriction of motion for early excision 20°, for late excision70°, for ORIF 25°, for CR 20°	1–15 years	E 1, G 8, F 4, P 4
Ring et al. (2003)	Different classification	–	–	–	2/19	50 (20–74)	9/21	ORIF	Average arc of ulnohumeral motion 96° (range 55–144°)	40 months	E 4, G 12, F 5
Imatani et al. (2001)	0	0	0	6/6	1/5	47 (38–66)	3/6	ORIF	Arc of motion 105–140°	40.3 (24–54) months	E 1, G 4, F 1
McKee et al. (1996)	0	0	0	6/6	1/5	38 (10–63)	4/6	ORIF	141°	22 (18–26) months	E 3, G 3
Hirvensalo et al. (1993)	6	0	0	2	0/8	40 (17–68)		ORIF	Only 4 patients had 5–15° restriction of extension	1 year	G 8
Poynton et al. (1998)	12	0	0	0	2/10	18 (12–40)		CR and K-wire 6, CR and Herbert screw 6	11 patients with an average 5° (range 4–8°) extension lag	35 (6–65) months	S 11
Fowles and Kassab (1974)	5	0	0	1	2/4	14–51		Open excision	Extension lag from 0° to 45°, elbow flexion from 90° to 150°	12–42 months	G 3, P 3
Ma et al. (1984)	9	0	0	0	3/6	15–74		Percutaneous probe reduction	Limitation of elbow motion: 3 patients 0°, 2 patients 10°, 1 patient 15°, 1 patient 30°	19–80 months	E 3, G 4, reduction failure 2
Alvarez et al. (1975)	14	0	0	0	1/9**	49 (26–65)**		Excision 10, CR 3, open reduction and K-wire fixation 1	15–140° **	20 (8–108) months	S for excision, P for CR and fixation
Clough et al. (2001)	4	0	0	0	0/4	51 (22–83)		ORIF with plate	Extension lag 6° (0–15°), restriction of full flexion 10° (0–20°)	30 (20–51) months	S 4
Stamatis and Paxinos (2003)	0	0	0	5	0/5	27–53		ORIF	4 patients with full ROM, 1 patient with 10° extension lag	39–50 months	E 5
Mosheiff et al. (1991)	5	0	0	0	1/4	20–70		ORIF	45–130°	9–18 months	S 5

ORIF = open reduction and internal fixation, CR = closed reduction, P = poor, F = fair, G = good, E = excellent, S = satisfactory.
*12 patients with some and 5 patients with significant trochlear involvement.
** Excision group.

less favorable results because of pain, loss of motion, and resultant late instability, particularly if the fracture initially was associated with medial joint instability (Fowles and Kassab 1974, Alvarez et al. 1975, Ma et al. 1984, Clough et al. 2001).

A cadaveric study showed that the removal of the capitellum instead of the radial head did not lead to elbow instability if the medial collateral structures were intact, but this is the case in only 50% of capitellar fractures (Hardy et al. 2002).

Alvarez et al. (1975) reported on 84 patients treated by excision of the capitellar fragment. Sixty-six patients had good to excellent results. The other 18 had poor results, which in 12 patients were attributed to delay (from one to six months) in excision of the fragments. The reasons for other poor results included incomplete excision of fragments, valgus deformity, and exuberant new bone formation at the capitellar bed. Alvarez et al. reported just two patients with valgus deformity and instability in the excision group. They felt that, compared with radial head excision, isolated capitellar excision did not lead to residual instability.

Mancini et al. (1989) reported on 39 resections of the capitellum with an average follow-up of 12 years. The result was excellent or good in 59% of the cases and fair or poor in 41%. Grantham et al. (1981) reported poor or fair results after excision of the capitellar fragment. They reported better results with early excision (under three weeks in this series) and poor results with delayed excision. It is possible that some of the instability following excision was due to poorer fixation options compared with modern techniques, where cannulated screws, headless screws, and bioabsorbable screws have improved the clinical results (Hardy et al. 2002).

The advantages of excision include the simplicity of the procedure, the short period of immobilization, and the elimination of complications associated with other treatment modalities (Mosheiff et al. 1991). The disadvantages of excision include risk of capsular adhesions and restricted range of motion, instability, and osteoarthritis (Mosheiff et al. 1991). In spite of all of these concerns, for the older patient with less functional demand or poor bone stock, excision is a practical method of management (McKee et al. 1996).

Closed reduction

Because of the lack of soft-tissue attachments on the fragment, anatomic closed reduction is difficult to achieve, partly because the fragment can easily slip position, and the elbow has to be immobilized at 90° for at least three weeks before active mobilization can be started (Clough et al. 2001). Christopher and Bushnell (1935) reported good results, with full range of motion and no pain at follow-up, in two cases with type I capitellar fractures treated by closed reduction.

Open reduction

Alvarez et al. (1975) reported on 41 patients treated by open reduction with or without internal fixation. Twenty-one had good to excellent results. The complications included avascular necrosis, redisplacement, valgus or varus deformity, malunion, and pain.

Ma et al. (1984) performed percutaneous probe reduction with Steinmann pins to treat nine patients with type I fracture, and reported favorable late results.

Poynton et al. (1998) compared K-wire fixation with Herbert screw fixation. They had one pin-tract infection in the K-wire group, with a poor result. Patients in the Herbert screw group returned to their previous activities at 5.5 weeks while the K-wire group did not do so until 9 weeks. In addition to pin-tract infection, the risks of K-wire fixation include penetration of the articular surface of the capitellum; furthermore, there is the need for subsequent K-wire removal, as well as for supplementary cast immobilization (Clough et al. 2001). Open reduction and fixation with bioabsorbable polyglycolide pins has been reported in an attempt to eliminate the problem of pin-tract infection and K-wire removal. However, this technique does not offer compression at the fracture site, and sterile synovitis has been a reported complication. Böstman reported this as a causative factor of subsequent joint arthritis (Böstman 1998). Clough et al. (2001) reported excellent results with open reduction and fixation using a maxillofacial Y-shaped plate for the treatment of type I fractures of the capitellum.

Arthroscopy

Arthroscopy permits better evaluation of the fracture and associated lesions. It can be used for more precise articular fracture reduction without significant soft-tissue dissection. Hardy et al. (2002) reported good results with arthroscopic reduction.

Type II and III fractures

The treatment of choice for the very small or comminuted capitellar fragment, with or without trochlear involvement, is usually resection. At present there is not enough evidence to support primary prosthetic replacement (Mosheiff et al. 1991). Feldman (1997) reported two cases of arthroscopic excision of type II fractures of the capitellum with satisfactory results. Fowles and Kassab (1974) reported on three immediate and three delayed excisions of type II fractures. They reported good results in the first group and poor results in the second. The follow-up was from 12 to 42 months.

Type IV fractures

The significance of the type IV fracture is the potential instability of the elbow joint because of involvement of the lateral trochlear ridge and the difficulty in accurately visualizing and reducing the medial extent of the fracture. Failure to reduce this fracture anatomically may adversely affect the intrinsic stability and range of motion of the elbow joint (Stamatis and Paxinos 2003).

The results of non-operative treatment of type IV fractures of the capitellum with closed reduction and immobilization in a cast are unpredictable, leading many investigators to recommend operative reduction (McKee et al. 1996).

CONTRAINDICATIONS

Excision may give good results, particularly in older patients. However, it should be avoided in young and active patients with type I or IV fractures. Reduction without fixation requires longer immobilization and has a high failure rate (Hardy et al. 2002).

TECHNIQUE

In a cadaveric study, Elkowitz et al. (2002) compared the fixation stability achieved with 4 mm partially threaded cancellous lag screws inserted in the anteroposterior (AP) direction, screws inserted in the posteroanterior (PA) direction, and headless compression screws. The headless screws provided more stable fixation of the fractures of the capitellum than the 4 mm partially threaded cancellous lag screws. When they tested the cancellous lag screws, insertion in the PA direction provided more stable fixation than insertion in the AP direction. Also, the PA screws have the clinical benefit of not violating the articular surface (as can happen with the countersinking process). When screws are countersunk, the stronger subchondral bone of the fragment is unavailable for purchase, but the subchondral bone of the fragment can be captured with PA screws. Also in this study, screw insertion in the AP direction increased the risk of fragment splitting (Elkowits et al. 2002).

Closed reduction

The elbow is placed in full supination and 90° flexion. Closed reduction is performed by placing traction on the elbow while posteriorly directed pressure is applied to the capitellar fragment. The elbow has then to be immobilized at 90° for at least three weeks. Obtaining and maintaining the reduction is very difficult because of the lack of soft-tissue attachments on the fragment (Clough et al. 2001).

Open reduction and internal fixation

A direct lateral or lateral Kocher approach can be used for optimal exposure of the articular surface and the posterior aspect of the condyle (**Fig. 21.2**). The surgeon will not be able to subluxate the joint posterolaterally or visualize and reduce the trochlear extension of a type IV fracture with this method unless the humeral origin of the lateral collateral ligament is reflected.

A pneumatic tourniquet is applied on the proximal arm. An 8 cm lateral skin incision is centered over the lateral humeral epicondyle. Through a lateral approach, the origin of the extensor carpi radialis longus is partially detached and the common extensor tendon is completely detached. The operative exposure can be extended proximally, along the lateral humeral ridge between the biceps and the triceps. In the Kocher approach, the exposure also can be extended distally, between the anconeus and the extensor carpi ulnaris. The posterior interosseous nerve can be protected by keeping the forearm pronated. The lateral collateral ligament should be preserved in most cases. In some type IV fractures, however, it is necessary to reflect the lateral collateral ligament from the humerus to gain enough access for reduction and fixation. A suture is placed in the ligament to facilitate its accurate reattachment. The elbow joint is opened longitudinally anterior to the lateral condyle. By elevating the anterior portion of the elbow capsule, retractors can be placed over the medial column of the distal end of the humerus, and the entire anterior articular surface of the distal end of the humerus can be visualized. The triceps is partially elevated to expose the posterior aspect of the lateral condyle.

The fracture is then reduced and provisionally fixed with K-wires. Definitive fixation is achieved by screws (partially threaded 4 mm cancellous screws, short threaded 3.5 mm cannulated screws, or headless screws), which are inserted from either the anterior or the posterior surfaces. Alternatively, a small plate can be used if the fracture line exits more posteriorly into the lateral condyle. The internal fixation and position of the screws can be checked by using fluoroscopic intensification. The lateral collateral ligament is repaired back to the humerus through drill holes in the lateral epicondyle, or with suture anchors.

Imatani et al. (2001) reported on an anterolateral approach to fix six type IV fractures (**Fig. 21.3**). They claimed better exposure was obtained for these fractures, without the need for olecranon osteotomy or reflection of the humeral origin of lateral collateral ligament. A curved incision is made over the anterolateral elbow and the interval between the brachioradialis and biceps is entered. The radial nerve is identified between the brachialis and brachioradialis. The brachioradialis and radial nerve are retracted laterally and the biceps is retracted medially. A longitudinal incision is made in the anterior capsule to expose the capitellum. The elbow is flexed for better exposure. K-wires are used for provisional fixation and two or three Herbert screws, placed from anterior to posterior, are used for definitive fixation. Imatani et al. (2001) reported no complications.

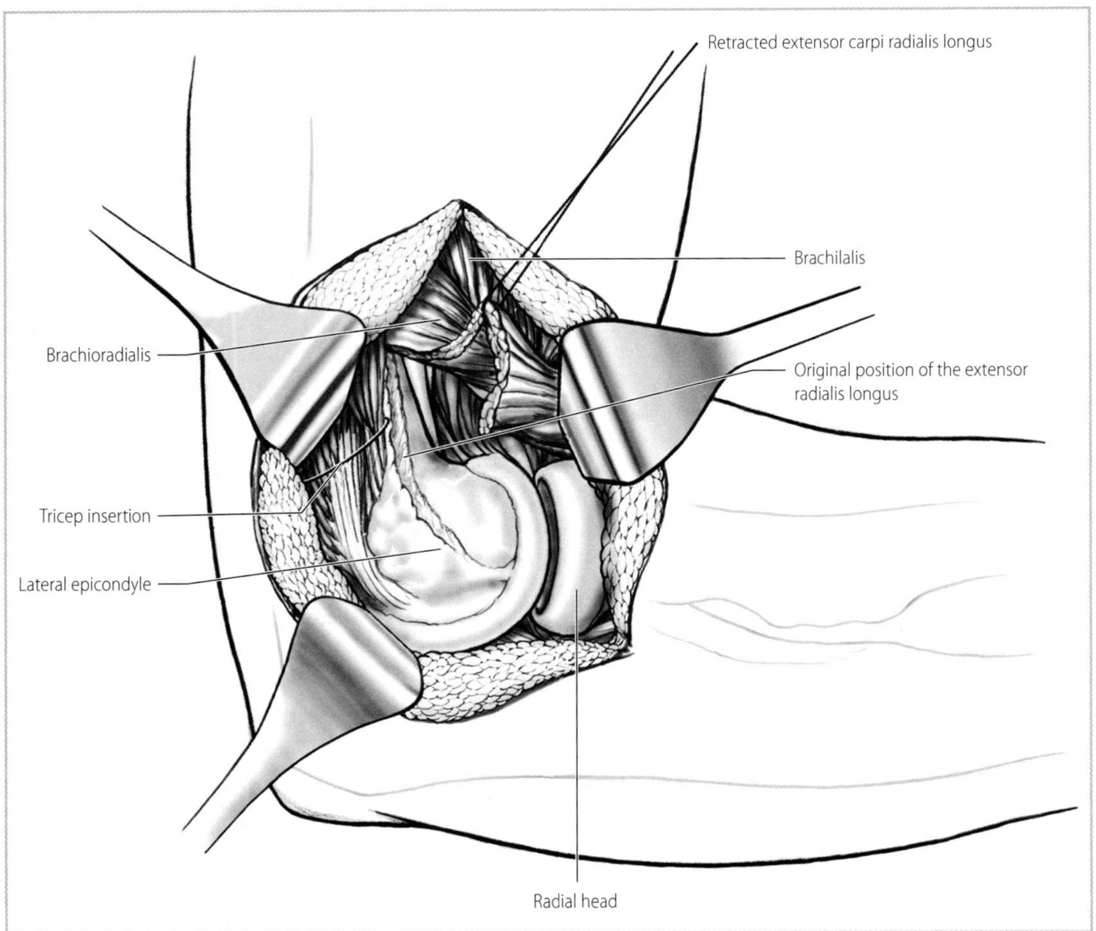

Figure 21.2 Lateral approach to the distal humerus. By permission of Mayo Foundation for Medical Education and Research. All rights reserved.

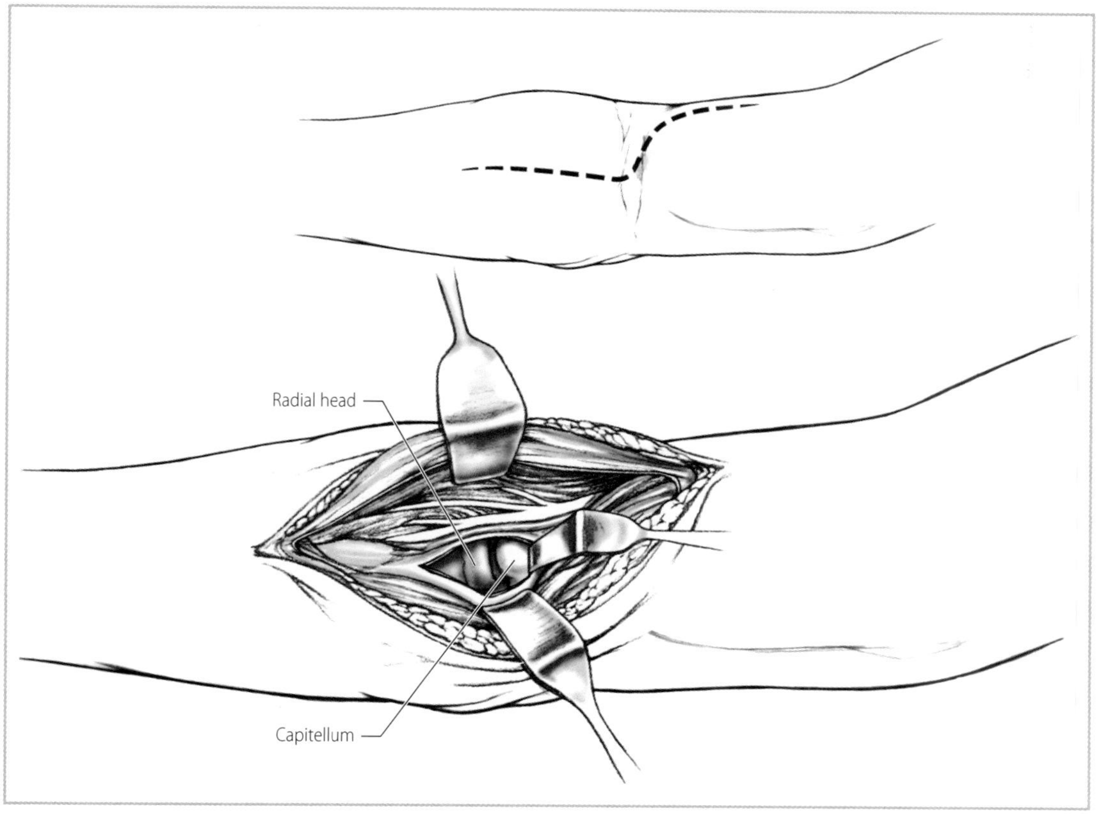

Figure 21.3 Anterolateral approach to the elbow. By permission of Mayo Foundation for Medical Education and Research. All rights reserved.

Open excision

This can be done through a limited lateral approach, as described above.

Arthroscopic excision or reduction

The advantage of elbow arthroscopy is less soft-tissue dissection and damage compared with an open approach. Elbow arthroscopy can be used for fragment reduction and fixation or excision. The patient should be placed in the lateral decubitus position with the arm on a bolster. A tourniquet is placed on the proximal arm. A proximal anteromedial portal is used for viewing. An anterolateral portal is used to remove the fragment. Anterolateral and proximal anterolateral portals are used for reduction (**Fig. 21.4**).

First, the joint is irrigated and evacuated of clots. The fracture site is prepared with a shaver. The fragment is reduced carefully by using a grasper introduced through the anterolateral portal. To obtain reduction, it may be necessary to apply traction to the axis of the forearm with the elbow flexed at 30°. The fracture can be definitively fixed with a cannulated screw. The head of the screw is buried in the articular cartilage (Hardy et al. 2002).

For type II fractures, after the fragment is impacted into anatomic position, with the elbow splinted at 90°, the radial head alone can help to maintain the reduction without screw fixation.

Pearls and pitfalls

Surgeons should be aware of the potential complexity of these fractures and should be prepared to reflect the lateral collateral ligament if more exposure is needed.

Complications include elbow stiffness, damage to the lateral collateral ligament, ulnar nerve neuropathy, articular damage, prominent hardware, loss of fixation, and avascular necrosis of the capitellum.

Despite separation of the fracture fragments from the underlying metaphyseal bone and soft-tissue attachments, osteonecrosis of these fragments is rare (Ma et al. 1984, McKee et al. 1996, Poynton et al. 1998, Clough et al. 2001, Imatani et al. 2001).

Stamatis and Paxinos (2003) reported a case of osteonecrosis that caused collapse of the capitellar portion of the fragment. The patient regained full range of motion and remained asymptomatic, with no signs of valgus instability of the elbow. This finding has also been noted in other studies (Ring et al. 2003).

Ring et al. (2003) reported on profound ulnar neuropathy in two patients within a few months of surgery. The fracture was treated through an extended lateral approach without exposure or manipulation of the nerve. They developed ulnar neuropathy with pain and progressive loss of elbow motion. Early recognition and subcutaneous transposition led to rapid resolution of the symptoms and recovery of elbow function in both patients.

REHABILITATION

Biomechanical testing has shown that the greatest amount of force transmitted from the radial head to the capitellum occurs between 0°and 30° of elbow flexion. Therefore, the elbow should be immobilized in 90° of flexion (Morrey et al. 1988).

Fragment excision

Immobilization should be brief (about two weeks) and then range of motion should be initiated (Alvarez et al. 1975).

Closed reduction

Because of the lack of soft-tissue attachments on the fragment, the elbow has to be immobilized at 90° for at least three weeks (Clough et al. 2001).

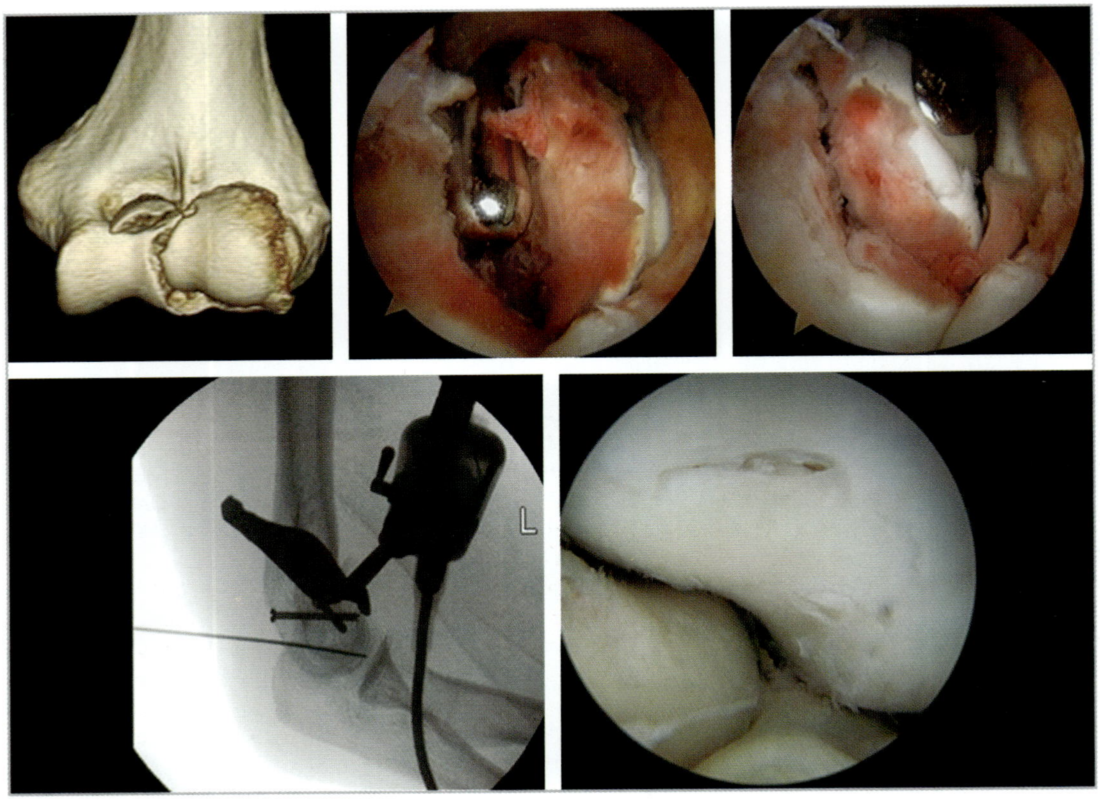

Figure 21.4 Arthroscopic reduction and fixation of a fracture of the capitellum

Open reduction and fixation

The choice of postoperative treatment should be selective and individualized according to the patient's age, the character of the bone, the type of fracture, the surgical approach (especially whether the lateral collateral ligament has been detached or not), and the fixation technique.

The security of the fixation should be assessed intraoperatively. The elbow can be immobilized for two weeks in 90° of flexion if secure fixation with screws has been achieved. The elbow should be immobilized for six weeks, on the other hand, if K-wires have been used for fixation (Poynton et al. 1998).

Supination should be restricted for the first four postoperative weeks, to eliminate the risk of residual instability if the lateral collateral ligament has been reflected during the surgical approach (Stamatis and Paxinos 2003).

Dynamic elbow splinting can be used in patients who find it difficult to regain elbow mobility with active assisted exercises. Splinting can be started at an average of six weeks (range 4–12 weeks) after surgery. Arthroscopic or open release is an option for patients who do not respond to dynamic splinting (Ring et al. 2003).

REFERENCES

Alvarez E, Patel MR, Nimberg G, Pearlman HS. Fracture of the capitulum humeri. J Bone Joint Surg Am 1975;57:1093–1096.

Böstman OM. Osteoarthritis of the ankle after foreign-body reaction to absorbable pins and screws: a three- to nine-year follow-up study. J Bone Joint Surg Br 1998;80:333–338.

Christopher F, Bushnell LF. Conservative treatment of fracture of the capitellum. J Bone Joint Surg Am 1935;17:489–492.

Clough TM, Jago ER, Sidhu DPS, Markovic L. Fractures of the capitellum: a new method of fixation using a maxillofacial plate. Clin Orthop Relat Res 2001;384:232–236.

Elkowitz SJ, Polatsch DB, Egol KA, et al. Capitellum fractures: a biomechanical evaluation of three fixation methods. J Orthop Trauma 2002;16:503–506.

Feldman MD. Arthroscopic excision of type II capitellar fractures. Arthroscopy 1997;13:743–748.

Fowles JV, Kassab MT. Fracture of the capitulum humeri, treatment by excision. J Bone Joint Surg Am 1974;56:794–798.

Grantham SA, Norris TR, Bush DC. Isolated fracture of the humeral capitellum. Clin Orthop Relat Res 1981;181:262–269.

Hardy P, Menguy F, Guillot S. Arthroscopic treatment of capitellum fracture of the humerus. Arthroscopy 2002;18:422–426.

Hirvensalo E, Bostman O, Partio E, et al. Fracture of the humeral capitellurn fixed with absorbable polyglycolide pins: 1-year follow-up of 8 adults. Acta Orthop Scand 1993;64:85–86.

Imatani J, Morito Y, Hashizume H, Inoue H. Internal fixation for coronal shear fracture of the distal end of the humerus by the anterolateral approach. J Shoulder Elbow Surg 2001;6:554–556.

Ma YZ, Zheng CB, Zhou TL, Yeh YC. Percutaneous probe reduction of frontal fracture of the humeral capitellum. Clin Orthop Relat Res 1984;183:17–21.

Mancini GB, Fiacca C, Picuti G. Resection of the radial capitellum: long-term results. Ital J Orthop Traumatol 1989;15:295–302.

McKee MD, Jupiter JB, Bamberger HB. Coronal shear fractures of the distal end of the humerus. J Bone Joint Surg Am 1996;78:49–54.

Morrey BF, An KN, Stormont TJ. Force transmission through the radial head. J Bone Joint Surg Am 1988;70:250–256.

Mosheiff R, Liebergall M, Elyashuv O, et al. Surgical treatment of fractures of the capitellum in adults: a modified technique. J Orthop Trauma 1991;5:297–300.

Poynton AR, Kelly IP, O'Rourke SK. Fracture of the capitellum: a comparison of two fixation methods. Injury 1998;29:341–343.

Ring D, Jupiter JB, Gulotta L. Articular fractures of the distal part of the humerus. J Bone Joint Surg Am 2003;85:232–238.

Stamatis E, Paxinos O. The treatment and functional outcome of type IV coronal shear fractures of the distal humerus: a retrospective review of five cases. J Orthop Trauma 2003;17:279–284.

Chapter 22 Fractures of the coronoid process

Thomas S. Obermeyer, Guido Marra

INTRODUCTION

The coronoid process of the ulna is one of the key stabilizers of the ulnohumeral joint and is vulnerable to injury with elbow dislocation. The recent observation that certain types of coronoid fracture are strongly associated with specific patterns of elbow instability has improved the ability to diagnose and treat these fractures. Surgical indications for coronoid fractures are dependent upon fracture location and size, associated osseous and ligamentous injuries, and congruency of the ulnohumeral joint. Adequate evaluation of these fractures often requires advanced imaging, including computerized tomography (CT), and fluoroscopic evaluation.

CLASSIFICATION

Regan and Morrey (1989) first classified coronoid fractures into three types based on the size of the coronoid fragment seen on a lateral radiograph. Type I fractures involve only the tip, type II involve <50% of the height of the coronoid process, and type III >50% (**Fig. 22.1**). A modifier was added to indicate the presence (type B) or absence (type A) of an elbow dislocation. This initial classification had prognostic implications, as larger fractures were associated with worse outcomes, although the majority of the fractures in the initial description were treated non-operatively (Regan and Morrey 1989). Recent outcomes data have confirmed the poorer prognosis associated with the operative management of higher Regan and Morrey types, despite trends toward treating these fractures with operative fixation (Adams et al. 2009). Although the Regan and Morrey classification system predates CT and does not provide information about the mechanism of injury or obliquity of the fracture (O'Driscoll et al. 2003), due to its simplicity and prognostic utility it remains a useful classification in the management of coronoid fractures.

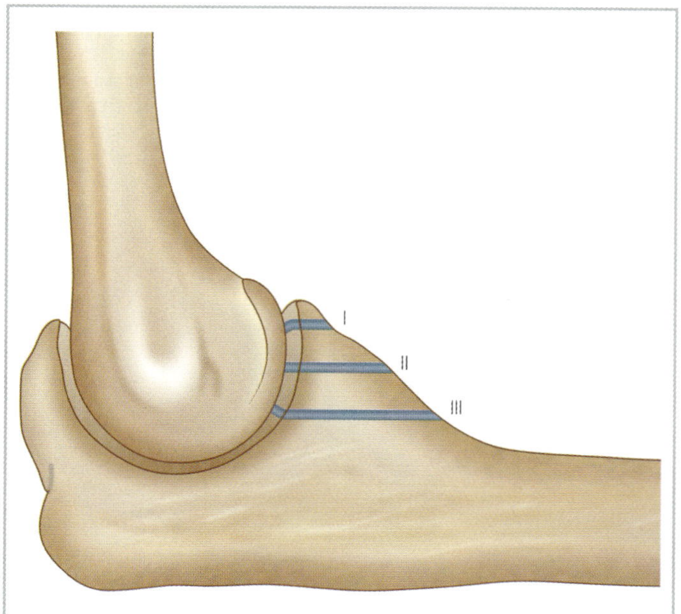

Figure 22.1 The Regan and Morrey classification, based on the size of the coronoid fracture on the lateral radiograph.

Since Regan and Morrey's classification, the availability of CT has improved the delineation of coronoid fracture morphology. In 2003, O'Driscoll et al. proposed a new classification system (**Fig. 22.2**) that more accurately describes the pathoanatomic features of coronoid fractures (O'Driscoll et al. 2003). This classification also comprises three main types: type I is a transverse fracture of the tip of the coronoid process, type II is a fracture of the anteromedial facet, and type III is a fracture of the base of the coronoid. These three types can be further subdivided based on the severity of coronoid involvement (**Table 22.1**). While not validated in clinical studies, this classification accounts for the mechanism of injury and provides information about the associated osseous and soft-tissue injuries (**Table 22.1**), and so serves as a useful guide in management.

In the O'Driscoll classification, type I fractures of the coronoid process involve the tip but do not extend medially into the sublime tubercle or distally into the coronoid body. They are transverse in orientation and usually include the insertion of the anterior capsule (Ring 2006). Type I fractures are commonly seen in association with 'terrible triad' injuries, and are on average 39% of the total coronoid height (Doornberg and Ring 2006a). These fractures occur as a result of a shearing mechanism as the coronoid is driven against the distal humerus during an elbow dislocation (O'Driscoll et al. 2003). Type I fractures are further classified into two subtypes, based on size of the fractured coronoid tip: subtype 1 fractures involve a flake of coronoid (≤2 mm) and subtype II fractures involve more than 2 mm of the coronoid tip.

Type II fractures involve the anteromedial aspect, and are associated with a varus/posteromedial mechanism of injury. Radiographically, they can appear as an isolated osseous injury with an intact radial head. Anteromedial coronoid fractures are associated with disruption to the lateral collateral ligament (LCL), which produces elbow instability and post-traumatic arthritis if not recognized and treated appropriately. Ulnar neuritis can occur secondary to edema and scar formation surrounding a torn posterior band of the medial collateral ligament (MCL) (O›Driscoll et al. 2003). Anteromedial subtype 1 fractures are located between the tip of the coronoid and the sublime tubercle, with the fracture line exiting medially at the cortex in the anterior half of the sublime tubercle, within the substance of the anterior bundle of the MCL. Laterally, the fracture line exits just medial to the tip of the coronoid. The fragmentation can extend to involve the tip (subtype 2), or the entire sublime tubercle (the insertion site of the anterior bundle of the MCL) (subtype 3).

Basal coronoid fractures (type III) involve the body of the coronoid, indicated by the fracture involving at least 50% of the height of the coronoid. These fractures are often associated with a less severe soft-tissue

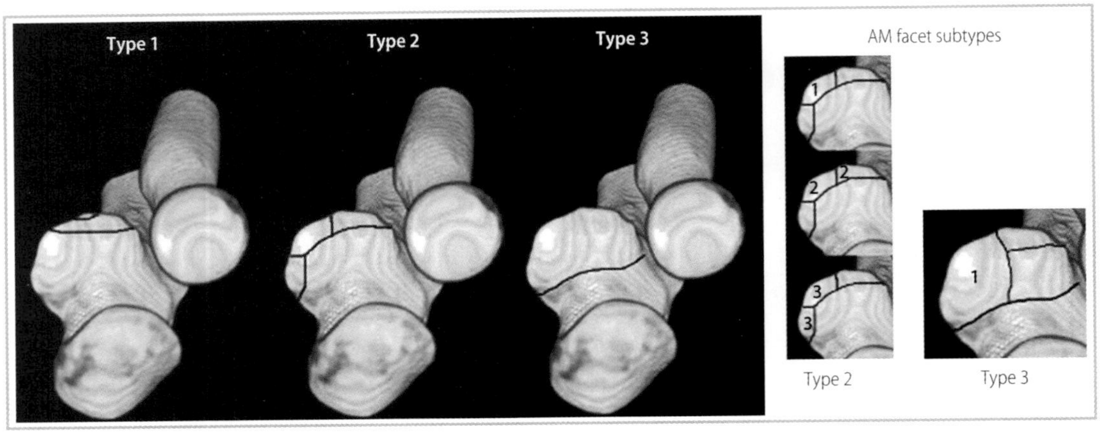

Figure 22.2 The O'Driscoll classification of coronoid fractures. Type I is a transverse fracture of the tip, type II is a fracture of the anteromedial facet, and type III is a fracture of the base.

Table 22.1 The O'Driscoll classification system

Type	Location	Mechanism	Associated injuries	Subtype	Description
I	Tip	Valgus posterolateral rotation with axial load	Radial head fracture ('terrible triad'), LCL avulsion from lateral epicondyle, with or without aMCL disruption	1	Flake involving ≤ 2 mm of coronoid height
				2	Fragment >2 mm of coronoid height
II	Anteromedial	Varus posteromedial rotation with axial load	Intact radial head, LCL avulsion from lateral epicondyle, pMCL disruption	1	Anteromedial rim
				2	Anteromedial rim and tip
				3	Anteromedial rim and sublime tubercle, with or without involvement of tip
III	Basal	Varus posteromedial rotation with axial load (subtype 1) or direct blow to olecranon (subtype 2)	Less soft-tissue injury, radial head fracture (subtype 1), olecranon fracture (subtype 2)	1	Coronoid body or base
				2	Transolecranon basal coronoid fracture

This system (O'Driscoll et al. 2003) provides information about the mechanism of injury and associated bony and soft-tissue injuries.
LCL = lateral collateral ligament, aMCL = anterior medial collateral ligament, pMCL = posterior medial collateral ligament.

injury compared with tip and anteromedial fractures, and thus good outcomes can be achieved with stable fracture fixation (O'Driscoll et al. 2003). The distinction between basal subtype 1 and subtype 2 fractures is that basal subtype 2 fractures involve the olecranon. A basal subtype 1 fracture is fragmented and usually involves the sublime tubercle and extends into the proximal radioulnar articulation. These fractures are commonly associated with fracture of the radial head as well. A basal subtype 2 fracture involves the body of the coronoid as well as the olecranon in a transolecranon fracture dislocation mechanism. Basal subtype 2 fractures frequently have a single large coronoid fragment.

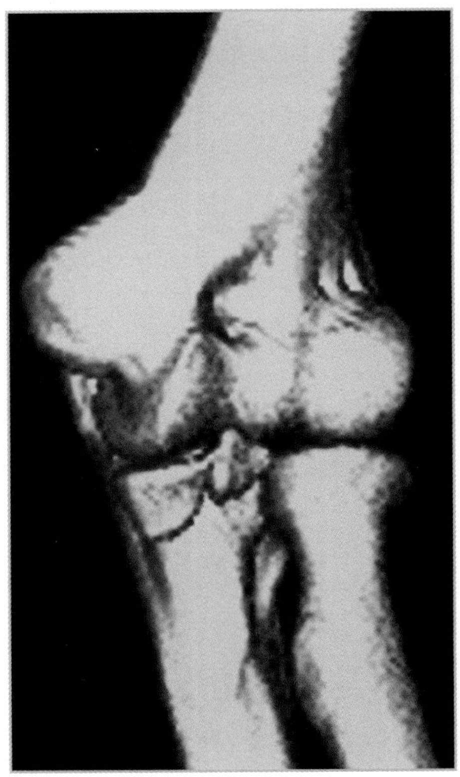

Figure 22.3 Three-dimensional computerized tomography can be helpful in allowing the surgeon to understand the fracture fragments and plan treatment. (Image courtesy of David Ring, MD, PhD.)

INDICATIONS

The two primary indications for coronoid fracture repair are valgus posterolateral rotatory instability and varus posteromedial rotatory instability (Doornberg and Ring 2006b, Pugh et al. 2004) (**Table 22.1**). The indication for coronoid fixation is based on the presence of associated injuries (**Table 22.1**), coronoid fracture morphology as determined by imaging, and elbow stability. Coronoid fracture morphology is best assessed by CT; when available, three-dimensional reconstructions may improve the characterization of fracture fragments (Lindenhovius et al. 2009) (**Fig. 22.3**). A large coronoid fracture associated with ulnohumeral subluxation on radiographs presents a clear indication for operative repair. In more subtle cases, elbow stability may be assessed by fluoroscopic examination in the operating room with the patient under anesthesia (**Fig. 22.4**). Varus and valgus

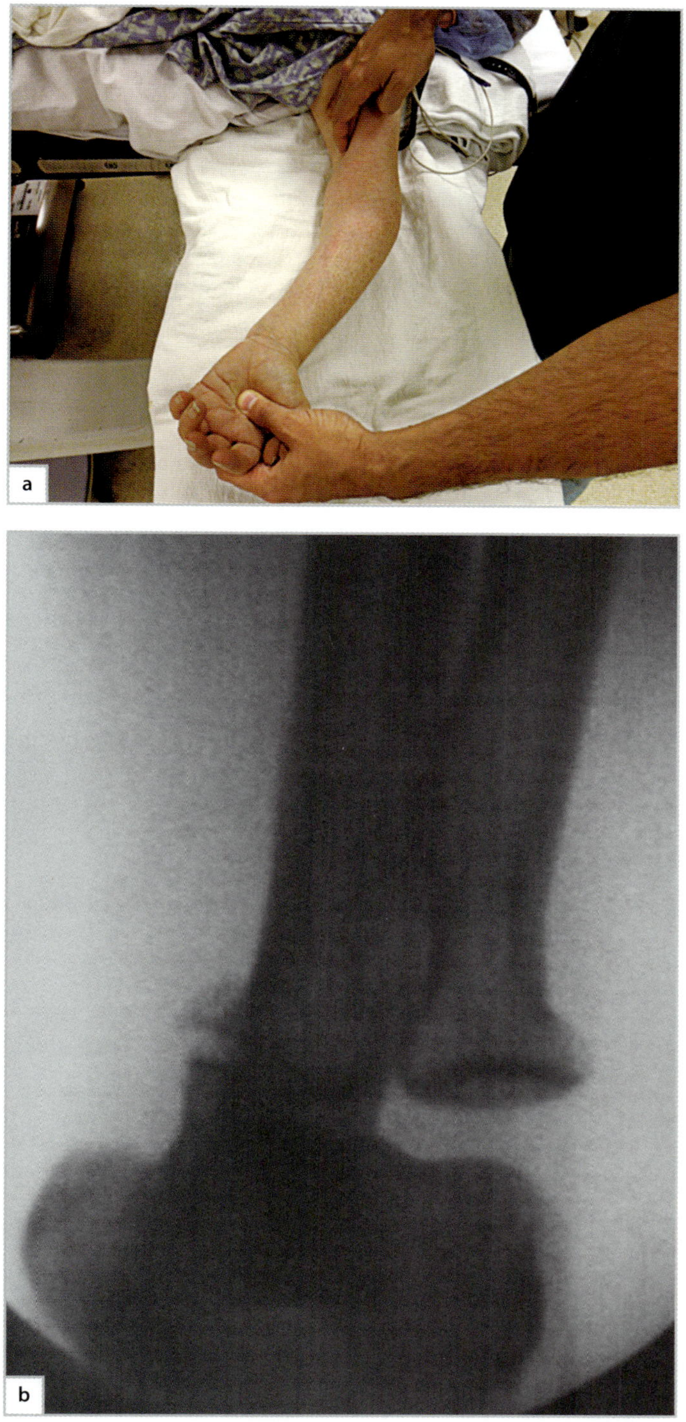

Figure 22.4 Assessment of elbow stability. (a) Intraoperative fluoroscopic examination provides useful information about elbow stability. (b) In this case, instability is observed with gapping of the radiocapitellar articulation. (Image courtesy of David Ring, MD, PhD.)

stress is applied by varying flexion angles with the forearm in supination and pronation. Any evidence of subluxation of the ulnohumeral joint dictates the need for surgical repair.

An exact set of indications about the size and shape of coronoid fractures that require repair to regain elbow stability is lacking, due in part to the infrequency of these fractures and in part to the large number of associated injuries. With small transverse fractures in the setting of the 'terrible triad', there is disagreement as to how the coronoid should be managed. Some authors feel that although these fractures are small, repairing them may contribute to elbow stability and thus improve outcomes (Pugh et al. 2004), while others feel these small fractures should be managed non-operatively (Adams et al. 2009). For the rare type I coronoid fracture that is too small for repair and represents a free loose body in the joint, simple excision is satisfactory. Despite the relatively new recognition and understanding of anteromedial fractures (O'Driscoll et al. 2003, Sanchez-Sotelo et al. 2005), the available clinical data suggest secure fixation affords good outcomes (Doornberg and Ring 2006b). Long-term follow-up studies will be required to determine the effect of coronoid fixation on the prevention of post-traumatic arthritis.

Biomechanical studies provide insight about the importance of the ligamentous injuries associated with coronoid fractures, but do not provide definitive surgical indications regarding coronoid fracture size (Closkey et al. 2000, Schneeberger et al. 2004, Hull et al. 2005, Beingessner et al. 2007, Pollock et al. 2009a, Pollock et al. 2009b). Closkey et al. (2000) demonstrated that transverse resection of 50% or more of the coronoid process will result in increased axial displacement of the ulnohumeral joint. This study was limited by not examining the stabilizing effects of the medial and lateral ligamentous structures, and by not investigating the effects of oblique coronoid resection. Hull et al. (2005) examined the role of the coronoid process in osteoarticular elbow stability and showed that after a 50% transverse resection of the coronoid process, the load-resisting varus displacement of the elbow decreased. As with the study by Closkey et al. (2000), this study did not evaluate the stabilizing effects of the medial and lateral ligaments. Schneeberger et al. (2004) reported that with resection of the radial head and 30% of the coronoid process, posterolateral rotatory laxity was induced. Additionally, this study also showed that radial head replacement alone is not sufficient to stabilize a ligamentously intact elbow when 50% or more of the coronoid is resected. Taken together, these studies suggest that large transverse fractures (30–50%) will generate elbow instability, and should be fixed.

A recent biomechanical study (Pollock et al. 2009a) provided the first data about how the size of anteromedial coronoid fractures affects elbow kinematics, particularly in varus stress. With varus stress after repair of the lateral collateral ligament, 5 mm anteromedial subtype 1 fractures and 2.5 mm anteromedial subtype 2 fractures demonstrated increased internal rotation of the ulna when compared with intact elbows. Anteromedial subtype 3 fractures demonstrated severe valgus instability, due to involvement of the sublime tubercle (ulnar attachment of the MCL) in addition to varus instability, even with LCL repair. These in vitro data suggest that with large anteromedial coronoid fractures (approximately 5 mm), fixation should be considered, to restore elbow stability.

CONTRAINDICATIONS

For small transverse coronoid fractures (i.e. <30%), biomechanical studies suggest ulnohumeral stability may be achieved by ignoring the coronoid fracture and focusing the plan on restoring the radial head and repairing the collateral ligaments (Schneeberger et al. 2004, Hull et al. 2005, Beingessner et al. 2007). A cadaveric study demonstrated no improvement in elbow kinematics with suture repair of a small (10%) transverse coronoid fracture (Beingessner et al. 2007). In this study, MCL deficiency was shown to play a much more important role in elbow instability than a small coronoid fracture. Thus, in vitro studies suggest that small transverse coronoid fractures may be left alone in the setting of posterolateral elbow instability with a fracture of the radial head. Clinical studies are needed to substantiate this treatment algorithm in patients.

With isolated non-displaced coronoid fractures, non-operative treatment is possible if physical examination demonstrates a stable elbow. Fluoroscopic examination with the patient under anesthesia should be performed if there is any question as to elbow stability. In posteromedial instability with a small subtype 1 anteromedial coronoid fracture and deficient LCL (with an intact MCL), in vitro data suggest that normal elbow kinematics can be achieved in the vertical (dependent) position (Pollock et al. 2009a). Patients with this combination of injury may be managed non-operatively if strict rehabilitation protocols with avoidance of varus stress are followed to allow healing of the LCL. These in vitro data also suggest that when secure fixation is not possible due to comminution, initial stability can be achieved with isolated repair of the LCL, and a postoperative rehabilitation protocol consisting of active (rather than passive) motion of the elbow with the forearm maintained in supination (Armstrong et al. 2000). In these cases, the integrity of the MCL must be confirmed prior to the initiation of treatment, and the patient should be followed closely with weekly clinical and radiographic examination to assure congruency of the ulnohumeral joint.

TECHNIQUES

Medial approach

A single midline posterior longitudinal incision is preferred in most cases of posteromedial instability, as it avoids sensory cutaneous nerves and permits elevation of medial and lateral skin flaps (Dowdy et al. 1995). It allows access to the medial and lateral aspects of the elbow, and access to all potential injury patterns through a single incision. The single posterior incision is easiest to perform with the patient supine and the arm across the chest (**Fig. 22.5**). A sterile tourniquet can be used to maximize the tissue included in the sterile field. Alternatively, two separate incisions can be made medially and laterally, centered over the epicondyles.

When a single posterior midline incision is used, the medial flap is developed and the ulnar nerve is identified and released. It is protected for the remainder of the procedure. The ulnar nerve can be carefully retracted with a vessel loop (**Fig. 22.6**) or can be placed in an anterior subcutaneous pocket (Ring 2006).

The medial approach develops the natural split in the flexor carpi ulnaris (FCU) distally to expose the ulnar nerve. In most elbows, the first few branches of the ulnar nerve are posterior articular branches that can be sacrificed if necessary to facilitate anterior transposition (Ring and Doornberg 2007). The flexor-pronator musculature is elevated off the coronoid fragment, exposing the anterior band of the MCL and the sublime tubercle. Dissecting the flexor-pronator musculature in a distal-to-proximal direction allows a clear distinction to be made between the distal musculature and the ligamentous tissue of the MCL (**Fig. 22.7**), which can tend to blend together (Steinmann 2008).

Smaller, more anterior fractures can be approached by the medial over-the-top technique described by Hotchkiss and Kasparyan (2000), which splits the flexor-pronator mass in half, and takes down a portion of its origin from the humerus and anterior capsule. The anterior half of the flexor-pronator mass, along with the brachialis muscle, is reflected anteriorly from the anterior part of the humerus and elbow capsule (Hotchkiss and Kasparyan 2000). Recent data suggest that

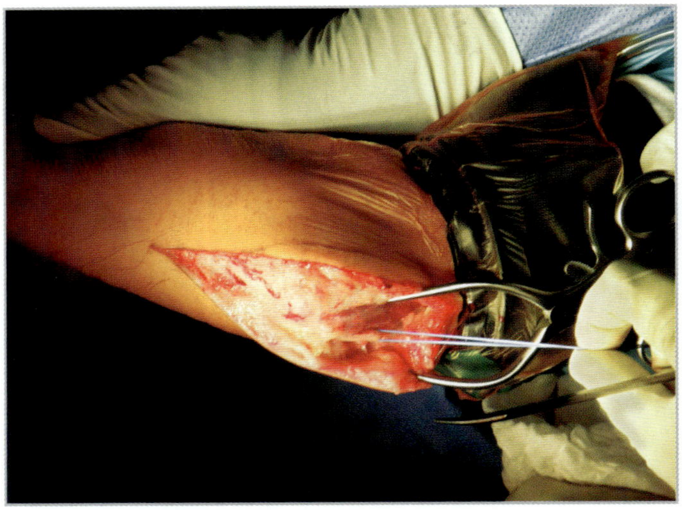

Figure 22.6 The ulnar nerve is identified and released in situ and tagged with a vessel loop to facilitate retraction.

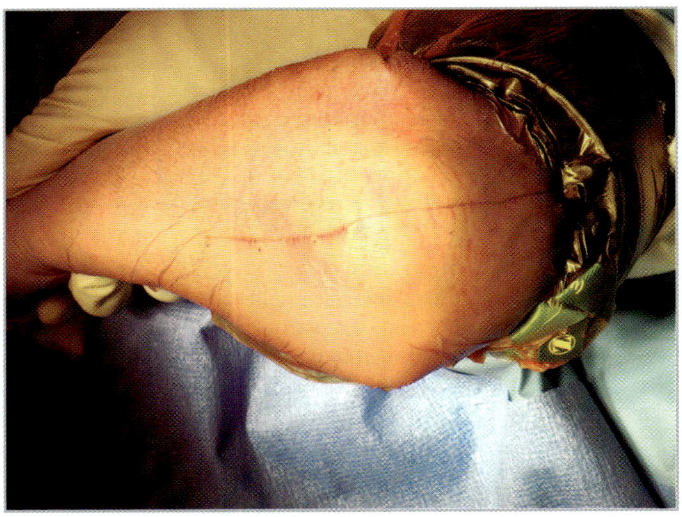

Figure 22.5 The line of a single midline posterior elbow incision. The incision is curved around the tip of the olecranon and permits access to medial and lateral sides via elevation of skin flaps. The arm is placed across the chest with a sterile tourniquet.

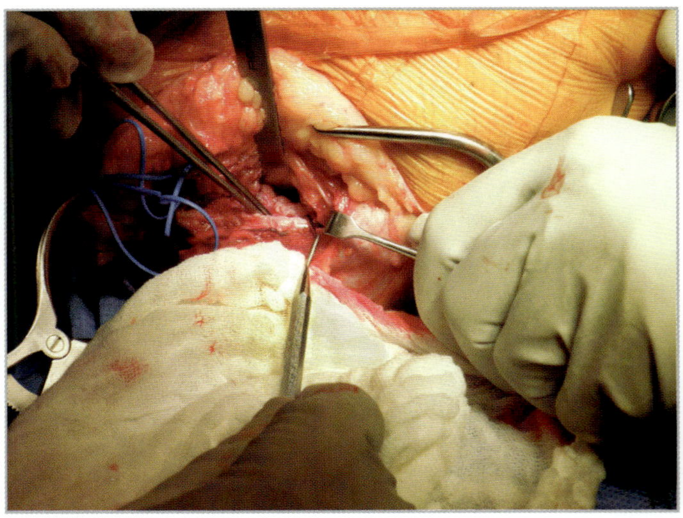

Figure 22.7 Medial coronoid exposure. The flexor carpi ulnaris is split and the flexor–pronator musculture is elevated. The pickups in the figure are tensioning the medial collateral ligament and the dental pick is pointing at the coronoid fracture.

this medial approach provides one third the osseous exposure as the FCU-splitting technique, and does not provide predictable exposure of the sublime tubercle/anterior bundle of the MCL (Krueger et al. 2011), which may be necessary in selected cases. In the case of very large fractures extending into the base, or when associated with an olecranon fracture, the entire flexor–pronator mass can be elevated, as described by Taylor and Scham (1969).

Once the coronoid is exposed, the fracture is reduced and provisionally stabilized with a large pointed reduction forceps or a Kirschner wire (K-wire). Definitive fixation is achieved with a small plate or screws. Specially designed coronoid plates are available which function as a buttress against posterior translation of the ulna on the humerus and provide fixation for the common, shearing-type anteromedial coronoid fragments. Other options for plate fixation include a locking T-plate or a small contoured 3.5 mm reconstruction plate.

With larger fractures, an anterior cruciate ligament (ACL) drill guide can facilitate placement of partially threaded cannulated screws, which are placed from the posterior aspect of the ulna. The ACL drill guide increases the accuracy of placement of the guide wire, allowing the surgeon to avoid intra-articular penetration and to achieve fixation in the region of the coronoid with the best bone quality. Two screws are generally needed for adequate fixation (**Fig. 22.8**). If the coronoid fragment is not large enough to accommodate two screws, fixation of a single screw should be supplemented with suture through the anterior capsule to protect the fixation (as in transverse fractures, discussed below, under 'Lateral approach') or with a contoured buttress plate (with anteromedial fractures). The presence of the large flexor–pronator musculature reflected anteriorly can make it difficult to place screws from anteriorly, and biomechanical studies suggest anterior-to-posterior screws provide inferior fixation when compared with screws placed in a posterior-to-anterior direction (Moon et al. 2009). Small threaded K-wires can sometimes be placed anteriorly and cut flush to the fracture fragment.

Very small coronoid fragments can be secured by suture (**Fig. 22.9**). Suture passed through drill holes placed through the dorsal ulna into the coronoid fracture bed secures the fracture fragments via anterior capsular attachments. Two drill holes are created laterally and medially. Sutures are passed through these holes using a suture-passing device, or a Keith needle with a loop is passed dorsal to palmar into the coronoid bed and the loop is delivered into the wound bed (Ring and Doornberg 2007). After suturing the coronoid fragment and passing each end of the suture through its corresponding drill hole, the ends of the suture are then tensioned over the dorsal aspect of the ulna and tied.

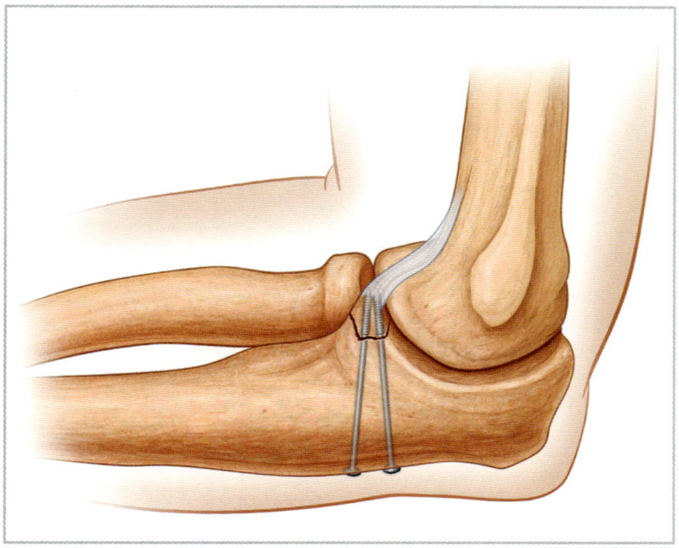

Figure 22.8 Two screws placed posterior to anterior can provide adequate fixation. An anterior cruciate ligament (ACL) drill guide can facilitate their placement.

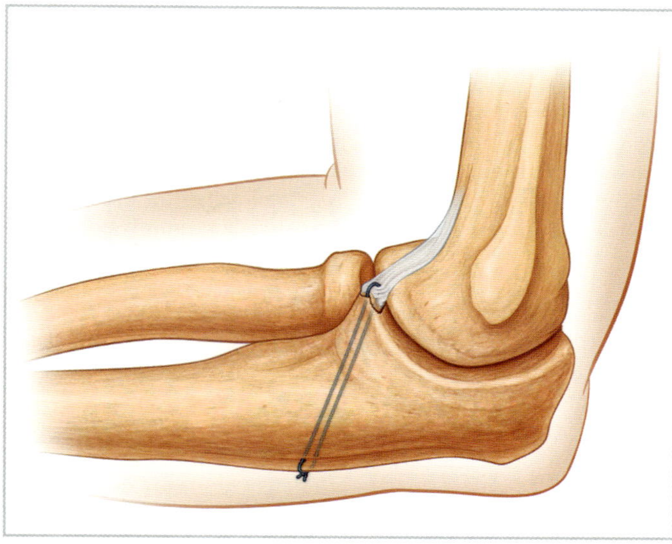

Figure 22.9 Anterior capsular fixation with suture to secure the coronoid fragments.

Once the coronoid is securely fixed, the LCL is then repaired. The lateral skin flap is raised, and tearing of the lateral common extensor mechanism is noted in many cases, which provides easy exposure to the LCL complex. If there is no tearing of the common extensor tendon, a Kocher approach may be developed, which facilitates the identification and repair of the LCL. The LCL and common extensor tendon can be repaired as one layer, to provide enough tissue for a robust repair, which is secured with no. 2 braided suture to the lateral epicondyle via drill holes or with suture anchors. A strong repair of the LCL is critical, as it protects the coronoid fixation during postoperative rehabilitation and ensures elbow stability against varus stress of the elbow.

Lateral approach

The lateral approach to the coronoid is performed in the setting of posterolateral rotatory instability, which frequently presents as an elbow dislocation with a small transverse fracture of the coronoid and a fracture of the radial head (Pugh et al. 2004). The lateral approach to the coronoid can again be made through a midline posterior incision or a direct lateral approach can be centered over the lateral epicondyle and extended distally in line with a point approximately 7–10 cm distal to the tip of the olecranon. With the 'terrible triad' injury pattern, there will often be a traumatic rent in the common extensor tendon. This defect facilitates exposure of the LCL and radial head. When no defect is appreciated in the extensor musculature, the Kocher interval is developed between the extensor carpi ulnaris and the anconeus.

With exposure of the fractured radial head, the radial head is either fixed or excised. Excision of the radial head and posterolateral subluxation of the elbow facilitate clear visualization of the coronoid. If the coronoid fracture is very small and devoid of capsular attachments, it can simply be excised. Large fractures should be treated with screw fixation in posterior-to-anterior fashion using the ACL drill guide

(**Fig. 22.10**) or with suture fixation via capsular attachments (**Fig. 22.9**). Screw fixation of large coronoid fractures is performed with a large pointed reduction forceps to hold the fracture reduced while an ACL drill guide is used to pass a guide wire from the posterior ulna to the coronoid fragment, just off the articular surface of the coronoid. The ACL drill guide facilitates accurate placement of the guide wire into a coronoid fracture fragment with a relatively small visible surface area. A partially threaded cannulated screw is then advanced over the guide wire and the fracture is compressed. A second screw may be placed in the same manner if the size of the coronoid fragment will accommodate a second screw. Suture fixation is performed by lassoing the coronoid fracture and anterior capsule with braided suture passed through drill holes in the posterior ulna. These drill holes are again accurately placed with the use of an ACL drill guide. The lasso suture is then tied to the posterior ulna after replacement of the radial head is complete, since replacement requires subluxation of the ulna.

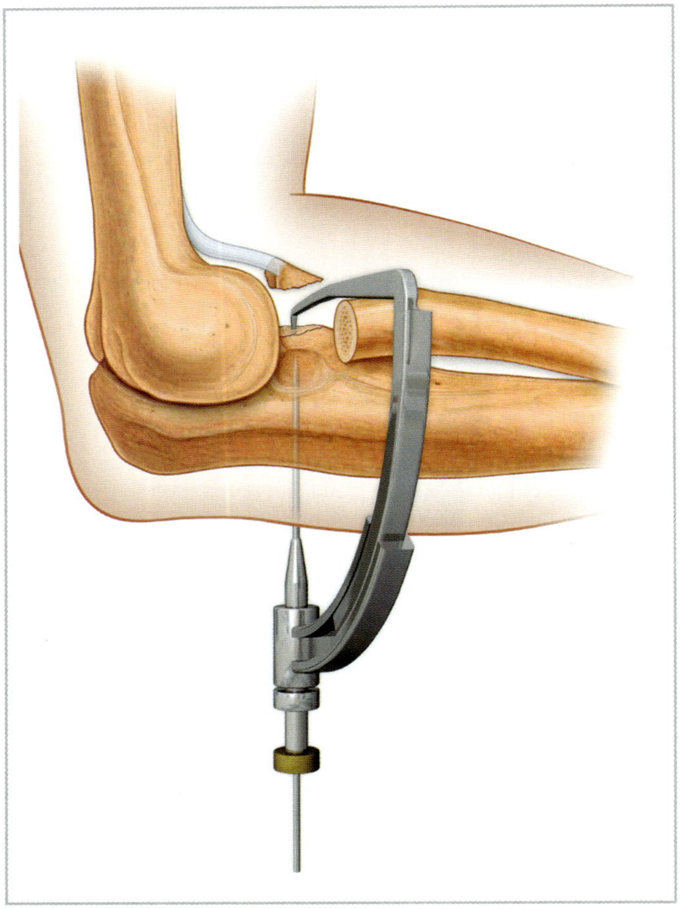

Figure 22.10 Use of the anterior cruciate ligament (ACL) drill guide for placement of a guide wire in the fixation of large coronoid fractures associated with posterolateral rotatory instability.

Pearls and pitfalls

The largest pitfall in treating isolated coronoid fractures is failure to recognize the severity of the soft-tissue injury. Many small isolated fractures can be more problematic than larger ones, and their significance should not be underestimated (Sanchez-Sotelo et al. 2005, Ring and Doornberg 2007). In cases of posteromedial instability, incongruent ulnohumeral motion can lead to rapid arthrosis. When this instability pattern is identified, a strong LCL repair must accompany coronoid fixation, to protect the elbow against varus stress.

Another pitfall is excising a coronoid fragment that has been mistaken as a fragment of the radial head (O'Driscoll et al. 2003). Any bone fragment in the coronoid fossa on radiographs should be assumed to derive from the coronoid itself, and not from the radial head. A CT scan with three-dimensional reconstruction can assist in clarifying the origin of fracture fragments should there be any question as to their identity. Finally, hinged external fixation (Chapter 26) should be considered for highly comminuted fractures treated with tenuous fixation, for complex injuries with persistent instability postoperatively, and for delayed treatment (two weeks or more after injury) of complex fractures.

REHABILITATION

Patients are instructed to avoid varus stress of the elbow for one month postoperatively. Gravitational varus stress is probably the major culprit in causing late displacement of the coronoid (O'Driscoll et al. 2003), and patients should be counseled thoroughly on avoiding such stress. Active assisted elbow exercises are initiated within one week of repair, when the postoperative splint is removed. Resistance exercises are started six weeks postoperatively.

Heterotopic ossification is a potential complication from any surgery around the elbow. Radiation or non-steroidal anti-inflammatory drugs may be used as prophylaxis.

REFERENCES

Adams JE, Hoskin TL, Morrey BF, Steinmann SP. Management and outcome of 103 acute fractures of the coronoid process of the ulna. J Bone Joint Surg Br 2009;91:632–635.

Armstrong AD, Dunning CE, Faber KJ, et al. Rehabilitation of the medial collateral ligament-deficient elbow: an in vitro biomechanical study. J Hand Surg Am 2000;25:1051–1057.

Beingessner DM, Stacpoole RA, Dunning CE, et al. The effect of suture fixation of type I coronoid fractures on the kinematics and stability of the elbow with and without medial collateral ligament repair. J Shoulder Elbow Surg 2007;16:213–217.

Closkey RF, Goode JR, Kirschenbaum D, Cody RP. The role of the coronoid process in elbow stability. A biomechanical analysis of axial loading. J Bone Joint Surg Am 2000;82:1749–1753.

Doornberg JN, Ring D. Coronoid fracture patterns. J Hand Surg 2006a;31:45–52.

Doornberg JN, Ring D. Fracture of the anteromedial facet of the coronoid process. J Bone Joint Surg 2006b;88:2216–2224.

Dowdy PA, Bain GI, King GJ, Patterson SD. The midline posterior elbow incision. An anatomical appraisal. J Bone Joint Surg Br 1995;77:696–699.

Hotchkiss RN, Kasparyan NG. The medial 'over the top' approach to the elbow. Techniques in Orthopaedics 2000;15:105–112.

Hull JR, Owen JR, Fern SE, et al. Role of the coronoid process in varus osteoarticular stability of the elbow. J Shoulder Elbow Surg 2005;14:441–446.

Krueger CA, Kirby JM, Hsu JR, et al. Medial elbow exposure: FCU-split versus over-the-top. Poster presentation, American Academy of Orthopaedic Surgeons Annual Meeting 2011: 304.

Lindenhovius A, Karanicolas PJ, Bhandari M, et al. Interobserver reliability of coronoid fracture classification: two-dimensional versus three-dimensional computed tomography. J Hand Surg 2009;34:1640–1646.

Moon JG, Zobitz ME, An KN, O'Driscoll SW. Optimal screw orientation for fixation of coronoid fractures. J Orthop Trauma 2009;23:277–280.

O'Driscoll SW, Jupiter JB, Cohen MS, et al. Difficult elbow fractures: pearls and pitfalls. Instr Course Lect 2003;52:113–134.

Pollock JW, Brownhill J, Ferreira L, et al. The effect of anteromedial facet fractures of the coronoid and lateral collateral ligament injury on elbow stability and kinematics. J Bone Joint Surg 2009;91:1448–1458.
Pollock JW, Pichora J, Brownhill J, et al. The influence of type II coronoid fractures, collateral ligament injuries, and surgical repair on the kinematics and stability of the elbow: an in vitro biomechanical study. J Shoulder Elbow Surg 2009;18:408–417.
Pugh DM, Wild LM, Schemitsch EH, et al. Standard surgical protocol to treat elbow dislocations with radial head and coronoid fractures. J Bone Joint Surg 2004;86:1122–1130.
Regan W, Morrey B. Fractures of the coronoid process of the ulna. J Bone Joint Surg 1989;71:1348–1354.
Ring D, Doornberg J. Fracture of the anteromedial facet of the coronoid process: surgical technique. J Bone Joint Surg 2007;89 (Suppl 2, Part 2):267–283.
Ring D. Fractures of the coronoid process of the ulna. J Hand Surg 2006;31:1679–1689.
Sanchez-Sotelo J, O'Driscoll SW, Morrey BF. Medial oblique compression fracture of the coronoid process of the ulna. J Shoulder Elbow Surg 2005;14:60–64.
Schneeberger A, Sadowski M, Jacob H. Coronoid process and radial head as posterolateral rotatory stabilizers of the elbow. J Bone Joint Surg 2004;86:975–982.
Steinmann S. Coronoid process fracture. J Am Acad Orthop Surg 2008;16:519–529.
Taylor TK, Scham S. A posteromedial approach to the proximal end of the ulna for the internal fixation of olecranon fractures. J Trauma 1969;9:594–602.

Chapter 23 Fractures of the olecranon

Daniel G. Schwartz, Bradley R. Merk, Sara L. Edwards

CLASSIFICATION

Colton (1973) first classified fractures of the olecranon, and that system has provided the basis for what is used today. The fracture is first classified as non-displaced (type I) or displaced (type II). A non-displaced fracture is displaced less than 2 mm, has an intact extensor mechanism, and is stable in up to 90° of flexion. Displaced fractures are divided according to their anatomic patterns: avulsion, oblique, transverse, oblique with comminution, comminuted, and fracture dislocation.

Also commonly used is Schatzker's (1987) system, which takes into consideration the fracture's biomechanical pattern. The six categories from this classification are the following: transverse, transverse impacted, oblique, comminuted, oblique distal, and fracture dislocation. The comminuted and oblique distal types are less stable patterns, and require the use of a plate and screw construct.

A system with a useful treatment algorithm is the Mayo classification, which is our preferred one. Type I fractures are minimally displaced (up to 2 mm) and further classified into subtype A (no comminution) and subtype B (comminution). Type I fractures may be treated non-operatively. In contrast, type II fractures are displaced over 2 mm. Type IIA (displaced, non-comminuted) can be treated with a tension-band construct, whereas IIB fractures (displaced and comminuted) (**Fig. 23.1**) may be treated with open reduction and internal fixation with a plate. Type III fractures demonstrate instability of the ulnohumeral joint and require a secondary operative intervention (Morrey 1995).

INDICATIONS

As described by the classification systems, indications for surgery include displacement greater than 2 mm, a disrupted extensor mechanism, and increased displacement with flexion. Additionally, complex elbow trauma (a concomitant fracture of the coronoid process or radial head) or a floating elbow are clear indications for surgery. Surgical objectives are to restore the extensor mechanism, reconstruct the articular surface, and allow for early range of motion. If this cannot be accomplished, then non-operative management should be attempted.

Most displaced, non-comminuted, stable fractures (Mayo type IIA) can be treated with an intramedullary screw or Kirschner wire (K-wire) and tension-band fixation, or a combination of such techniques.

For displaced, comminuted and unstable fractures (Mayo type IIB), our treatment preference is a contoured plate fixed with both an interfragmentary screw and plate construct as well as an intramedullary screw.

CONTRAINDICATIONS

Inability to obtain a stable construct that would allow early range of motion is a contraindication to surgical management of a fracture of the olecranon. There are few other absolute contraindications; however, a minimally or non-displaced fracture that is stable in flexion, with an intact extensor mechanism, is an indication for a trial of non-operative management, after appropriate discussion of the risks and benefits with the patient. If comminution is too severe, an external fixator or distraction device could be applied to provide stability and early range of motion. In an elderly patient with severe comminution and instability, a primary total elbow arthroplasty is sometimes performed.

Small avulsion fractures of the triceps with an intact extensor mechanism do not require surgery. Avulsion fractures that are less than 50% of the olecranon in elderly and osteoporotic patients can often be excised and treated as a triceps tendon rupture, with advancement of the tendon and repair through bone tunnels.

TECHNIQUE

The patient is placed in the supine position with a large bolster placed beneath the ipsilateral shoulder. Perioperative antibiotics are administered prior to incision. The bed is placed in an oblique or 90° position from the anesthesia staff to provide maximum room for fluoroscopic equipment. Care is taken to prepare the entire arm and shoulder to the neck to ensure room for a sterile tourniquet. Once the patient is draped, the tourniquet is placed as proximal as possible on the upper arm, so that it will not be in the field. A padded Mayo stand or chest bolster can be used across the bed to help support the arm. Tilting the bed to the contralateral side can also help keep the arm abducted throughout the procedure.

Type IIA: displaced stable fractures

Our preferred technique for a stable, displaced fracture of the olecranon (**Fig. 23.2**) is a tension-band construct applied using K-wires. A midline skin incision is made from the distal humerus, extending in a curvilinear fashion on the radial side of the olecranon, and returning to the midline to extend down the proximal ulna (**Fig. 23.3**). The subcutaneous fascia is incised, exposing the bone both proximal and distal to the fracture site. The proximal fragment can be reflected to evacuate hematoma and any debris that may lie in the joint. The surgeon should be aware of the location of the ulnar nerve throughout the procedure, but we do not routinely dissect or transpose it when operating on a stable fracture.

A 2 mm drill bit is used to place a transverse tunnel in the ulna distal to the fracture, equidistant from the fracture line to the tip of the olecranon, and an 18-gauge wire is passed through the bone tunnel.

Provisional reduction is obtained using a pointed reduction clamp or towel clip. Making a small pilot hole on the distal ulna with a K-wire, equidistant from the fracture line, is helpful to keep the reduction device from slipping. Accurate reduction should be assessed visually as well as fluoroscopically from the dorsal, lateral, and medial surface. Both sides of the joint should be examined to ensure that rotational alignment is adequate.

Two 1.6 mm K-wires are inserted from the dorsal surface of the proximal fragment to the anterior surface of the distal fragment, crossing the fracture line perpendicularly in the anterior–posterior plane and engaging the far cortex on the volar side of the ulna. Care is taken to ensure that the two wires are parallel to one another and not inadvertently crossing into the joint.

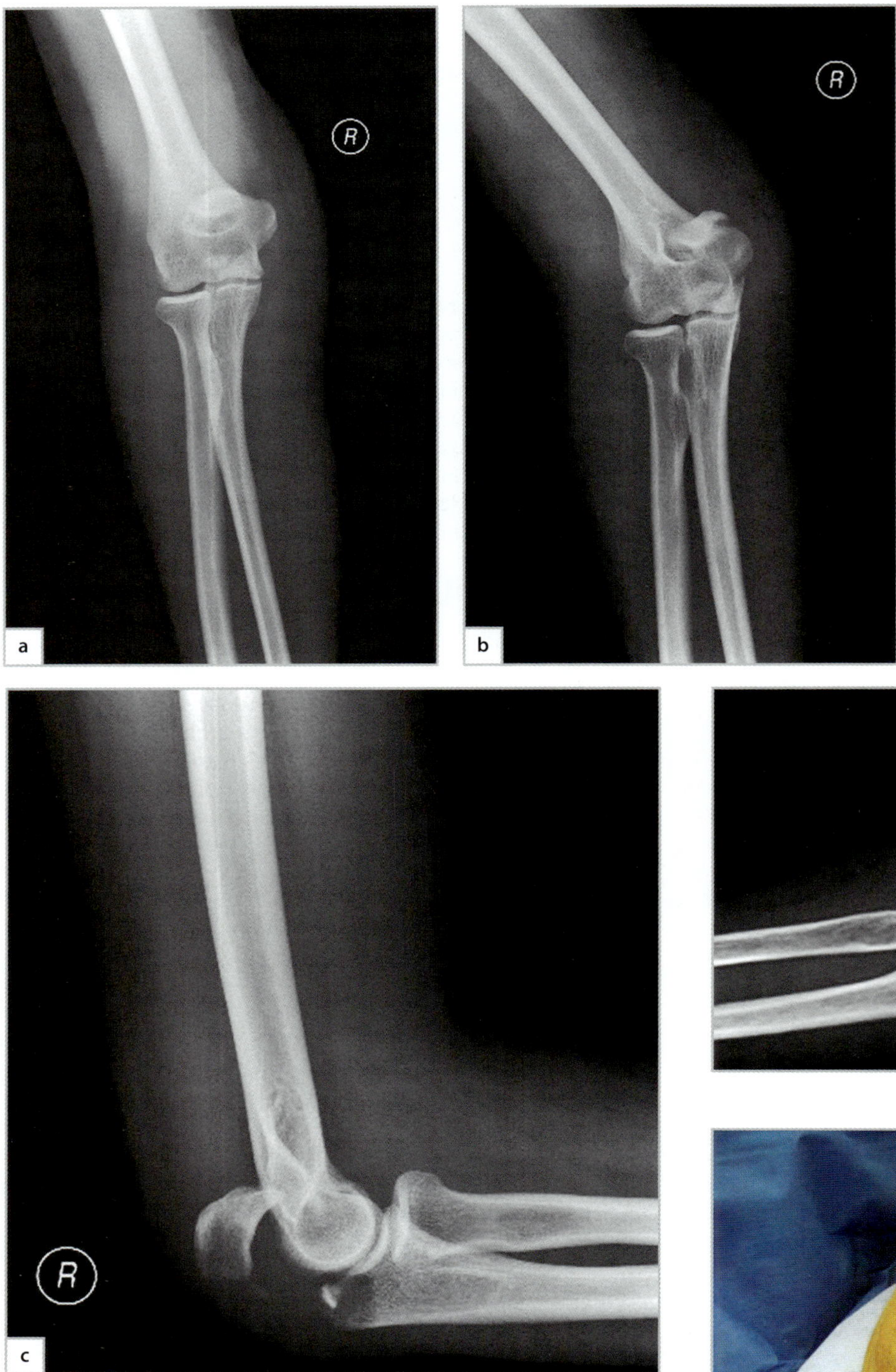

Figure 23.1 Radiographs of a comminuted displaced fracture of the olecranon. (a) Anteroposterior, (b) oblique, (c) lateral.

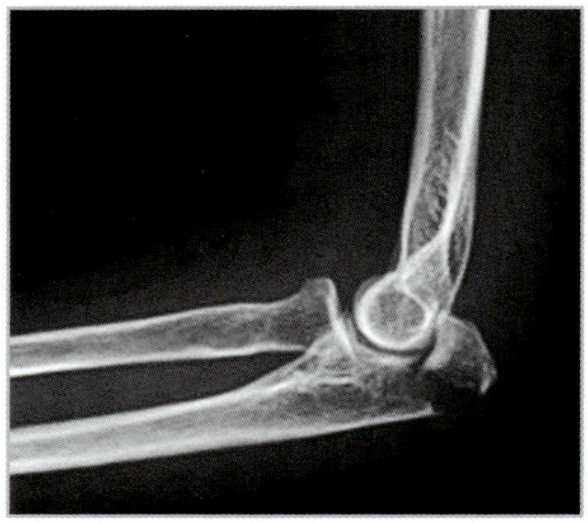

Figure 23.2 Stable, displaced fracture of the olecranon.

A 16-gauge angiocatheter is used to penetrate just proximal to the wires, deep to the triceps insertion. The central core of the angiocatheter is removed and the remaining end of the 18-gauge wire is passed from medial to lateral so that it is deep to the triceps and deep to the two K-wires. Once the figure-of-eight wire has been passed, two heavy needle-drivers are placed on both sides of the wire construct (**Fig. 23.4**). Using a twisting motion, the wires are tightened at the same time to symmetrically compress the fracture. Alternatively, one loop can be tightened.

Using heavy wire-cutters, the wires are clipped, leaving approximately 3 mm of wire exposed. The sharp end is curved down using a bone tap and placed into the soft tissue to minimize irritation.

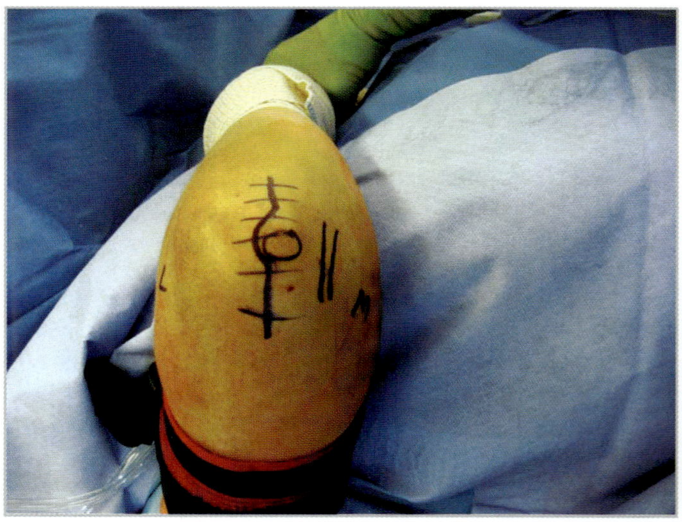

Figure 23.3 Curvilinear incision with notations to delineate the medial and lateral side of the elbow, as well as the ulnar nerve. Note that the incision is curved away from the ulnar nerve at the tip of the olecranon.

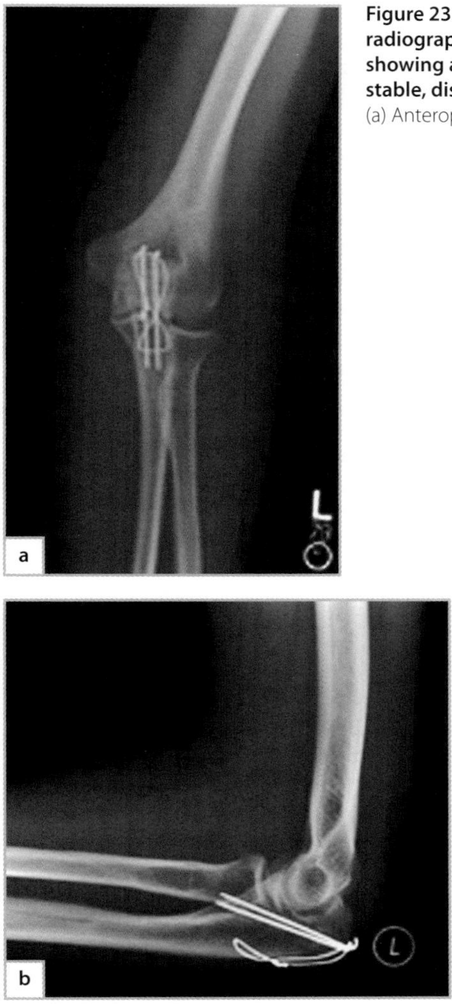

Figure 23.4 Postoperative radiographs of the elbow showing a tension band to treat a stable, displaced fracture. (a) Anteroposterior, (b) lateral.

The K-wires are bent using a needle-driver and heavy suction tip for leverage. The hooked piece of wire is turned 180° and gently tapped into the triceps insertion, advancing the wire several millimeters through the far cortex.

The elbow is taken through a range of motion to ensure fracture stability. Final images should ensure appropriate positioning of the hardware and fracture reduction. The wound is thoroughly irrigated with sterile saline and the incision is closed using 3-0 absorbable sutures on the subcutaneous layer and interrupted nylon sutures on the skin. Care should be taken in handling the skin, as wound breakdown can occur in this area.

After a sterile dressing is applied, the arm is splinted with a well padded splint in 90° of flexion and a neutral rotation.

Type IIB: displaced comminuted fractures

The patient positioning and exposure are as described above. Once the fracture is exposed, care is taken not to devascularize the multiple small pieces. It is important in this fracture type to look carefully at the small pieces and identify any substantial fragments that have articular cartilage, as they often will rotate from the trauma. Thorough irrigation of the joint is performed to clear any small pieces of debris and bone. Gentle manipulation and elevation of any articular fragments are performed using a Freer instrument or dental pick. Provisional reduction is obtained with extension of the arm and can be secured using small K-wires.

A precontoured plate is then chosen to span the fracture. Using fluoroscopic guidance, the screws are sequentially placed, beginning with an ulnar shaft screw, followed by proximal screws. With significant proximal comminution, the screws may be placed in a divergent pattern and locked to provide additional stability. The most proximal hole of the plate, which curves around the tip of the olecranon, can be used to place one long 'home run' intramedullary screw. Care should be taken not to compress this screw to the distal fragment if there is significant comminution. The rest of the screws can be filled in using a standard interfragmentary lag technique, with care taken not to penetrate the joint. When there is significant comminution around the joint, placing a long screw into the coronoid process will help provide stability. Bone graft or cancellous chips can be placed into the defect to help support the underlying articular surface. When placing the more distal shaft screws, care should be taken not to plunge with the drill, to avoid iatrogenic nerve damage.

After imaging confirms adequate reduction and placement of screws (**Fig. 23.5**), the incision can be closed using the technique described above. A posterior mold splint is placed with the arm in a neutral position.

Pearls and pitfalls

- Careful assessment of the fracture preoperatively is required. While the fracture may appear to be a simple transverse type, further investigation can demonstrate comminution. We have a precontoured plating system available for any olecranon fracture, in case it appears unstable upon direct visualization.
- Patients should be counseled preoperatively about the risk of painful hardware, regardless of technique, due to the subcutaneous location of the implants. The risk that the hardware will later need to be removed is high.
- To minimize pain from hardware with the tension-band technique, the two larger K-wires are embedded into the triceps insertion. Double loops in the tension band may improve compression across the fracture site, but a single loop may minimize pain.
- For the tension-band technique, it is important to verify that the parallel K-wires are just through the anterior cortex on the distal ulna, to prevent back-out.
- Following fixation with either technique, varus and valgus stability should be tested. With any gross instability, primary repair of the lateral collateral ligament or ulnar collateral ligament should be performed.
- More complex fracture patterns may be more easily treated using a lateral decubitus or prone position to aid in fracture reduction.
- The surgeon should be mindful of impaction of the ulnohumeral joint. If marginal impaction is present, this is reduced first, followed by reduction of the primary fracture fragments. It is important to identify and address any intra-articular debris at the fracture site prior to fixation.
- A small pointed reduction tool can be placed on the proximal fragment in order to make fine adjustments to rotation and translation. A medium-sized pointed reduction clamp can be placed from the small pilot hole on the ulna diaphysis to the olecranon tip. Extension can aid in reduction as well.

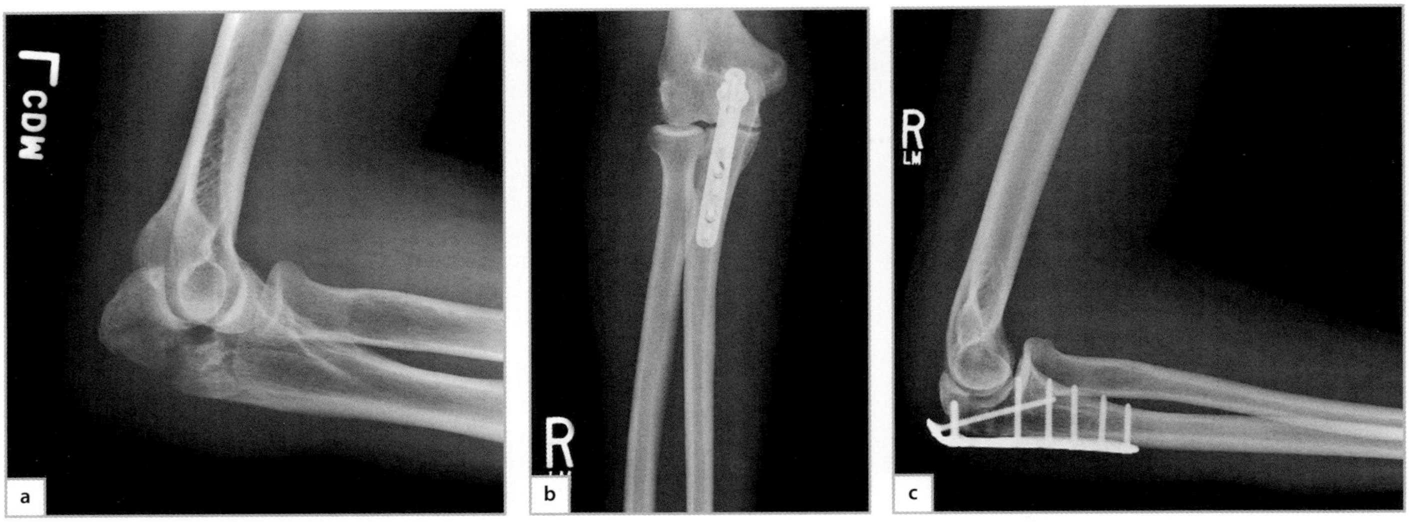

Figure 23.5 Radiographs showing open reduction and internal fixation of a comminuted, unstable olecranon fracture. (a) Pre-operative view, (b) anteroposterior postoperative view and (c) lateral postoperative view.

REHABILITATION

The splint is removed after 5–10 days. We then allow the patient to begin passive assisted range of motion of the elbow and to wear a sling (only for protection). The sutures are removed and replaced with steri-strips two weeks after surgery. At six weeks, active range of motion with formal physiotherapy is implemented. The patient may begin to lift light weights (less than 2.5 kg) with the arm at this time. The authors feel that allowing this early range of motion is instrumental in preventing significant postoperative stiffness; with the rigid fixation techniques described above, mechanical failure is unusual. If concomitant ligament repair was performed, the patient should be protected with a hinged elbow brace after the splint has been removed. Static progressive splinting or dynamic splinting can be considered if the range of motion remains 80–90% of normal at six weeks.

REFERENCES

Colton CL. Fractures of the olecranon in adults: classification and management. Injury 1973;5:121–129.

Morrey BF. Current concepts in the treatment of fractures of the radial head, the olecranon, and the coronoid. J Bone Joint Surg Am 1995;77:316–327.

Schatzker J. Olecranon fractures. In: Schatzker J, Tile M, eds. The Rational Basis of Operative Fracture Care. New York: Springer-Verlag, 1987: 89–95.

Chapter 24

Open reduction and internal fixation of fractures of the distal humerus

Michael S. Ferrell, Douglass E. Stull and Patrick M. Connor

INTRODUCTION

Fractures of the distal humerus remain one of the most challenging problems in orthopaedics, due to the difficulties involved in the surgical approach, the complexity of the normal bone morphology, and the absolute necessity of stable fixation to allow for early motion to restore elbow function. These fractures are often further complicated by osteoporotic bone, metaphyseal bone loss, and severe comminution. This chapter focuses on the management of these technically demanding fractures.

CLASSIFICATION

The AO/OTA classification system (of the Arbeitsgemeinschaft für Osteosynthesefragen/Orthopaedic Trauma Association) is commonly used for fractures of the distal humerus (Muller et al. 1990). It divides fractures into types A, B, and C. Type A fractures are extra-articular metaphyseal, transcondylar and apophyseal. Type B fractures are partial articular and include the coronal shear fractures. Type C fractures are articular fractures. Each type has three subclassifications, numbered 1–3, with the fracture being more comminuted or severe as the number increases (**Fig. 24.1**). Two other classification schemes bear discussion, that of Jupiter and Mehne (1992) and the combined scheme of Davies and Stanley (2006). Jupiter and Mehne divide the fractures into six types (**Fig. 24.2**): high T, low T, Y, H, medial lambda, and lateral lambda. Their system is based on intraoperative findings and is designed to inform the choice of surgical approach. The combined system of Davies and Stanley is the most recent (**Fig. 24.3**), and combines the systems of the AO/OTA, Jupiter and Mehne, and Riseborough and Radin (1969). Davies and Stanley report high reliability and reproducibility with their system.

To properly classify any severe fracture of the distal humerus, adequate and consistent imaging studies are necessary. Standard orthogonal views of the elbow are recommended, and traction views may be of assistance in classifying the fracture. Computerized tomography (CT), with both standard two-dimensional and three-dimensional reconstruction, has assisted the surgeon dramatically in defining the degree of comminution, the column involvement, and the amount of articular displacement. For articular fractures, CT is highly recommended, as it will assist in determining the best type of treatment, the surgical approach, and the type and location of implants to be used (**Fig. 24.4**).

INDICATIONS

It is now generally accepted that the long-term functional results are improved after surgical intervention for fractures of the distal humerus. In an analysis performed by Nauth et al. (2011) on pooled data from two studies that compared functional outcomes between operatively and non-operatively treated patients (Zagorski et al. 1986, Srinivasan et al. 2005), those treated non-operatively were almost three times more likely to have an unacceptable result. Further, Robinson et al. (2003) compared results of 273 operatively treated patients with those of 47 non-operatively treated patients and showed that the non-operative group was almost six times more likely to have a non-union and four times more likely to have a delayed union.

The goal of internal fixation is anatomic reduction of the ulnohumeral and radiocapitellar articulation, as this will allow range-of-motion rehabilitation to begin early. Therefore, any displaced fracture of the distal humerus in an adult is a candidate for open reduction and internal fixation if there is adequate soft-tissue coverage, adequate bone stock to provide stable fixation for early range of motion, and a viable arm in a patient who can medically tolerate surgery.

CONTRAINDICATIONS

Contraindications to open reduction and internal fixation of fractures of the distal humerus are considered from the patient perspective, the soft-tissue perspective, and the bone perspective. Patients with a profound preoperative paralysis of the affected arm and those who are demented should be considered poor candidates. Any medical condition that elevates the risks associated with general anesthesia should, of course, be strongly considered a contraindication. An adequate soft-tissue envelope to allow implant coverage and closure is necessary. Massive soft-tissue defects are best treated initially with external fixation. Soft-tissue coverage procedures and definitive fixation can be done later. Lastly, the fractured bone, which is often highly comminuted, must be of adequate density to provide for stable purchase of implants. Elderly patients, who comprise a large proportion of these cases, with highly comminuted fractures may be better served with arthroplasty (Frankle et al. 2003). Supracondylar bone loss is not necessarily a contraindication to open reduction and internal fixation but should alert the surgeon to the possibility of the need for structural bone grafting.

TECHNIQUE

The operation begins with surgical positioning of the patient. This procedure can be performed with the patient supine, prone, or in the lateral decubitus position with the operative arm draped across a well padded bolster. We prefer the last, for several reasons. The lateral decubitus is certainly easier from an anesthesia perspective. It orients the operative site so the posterior aspect of the elbow is easily accessible, and obviates the need to have an assistant hold the extremity.

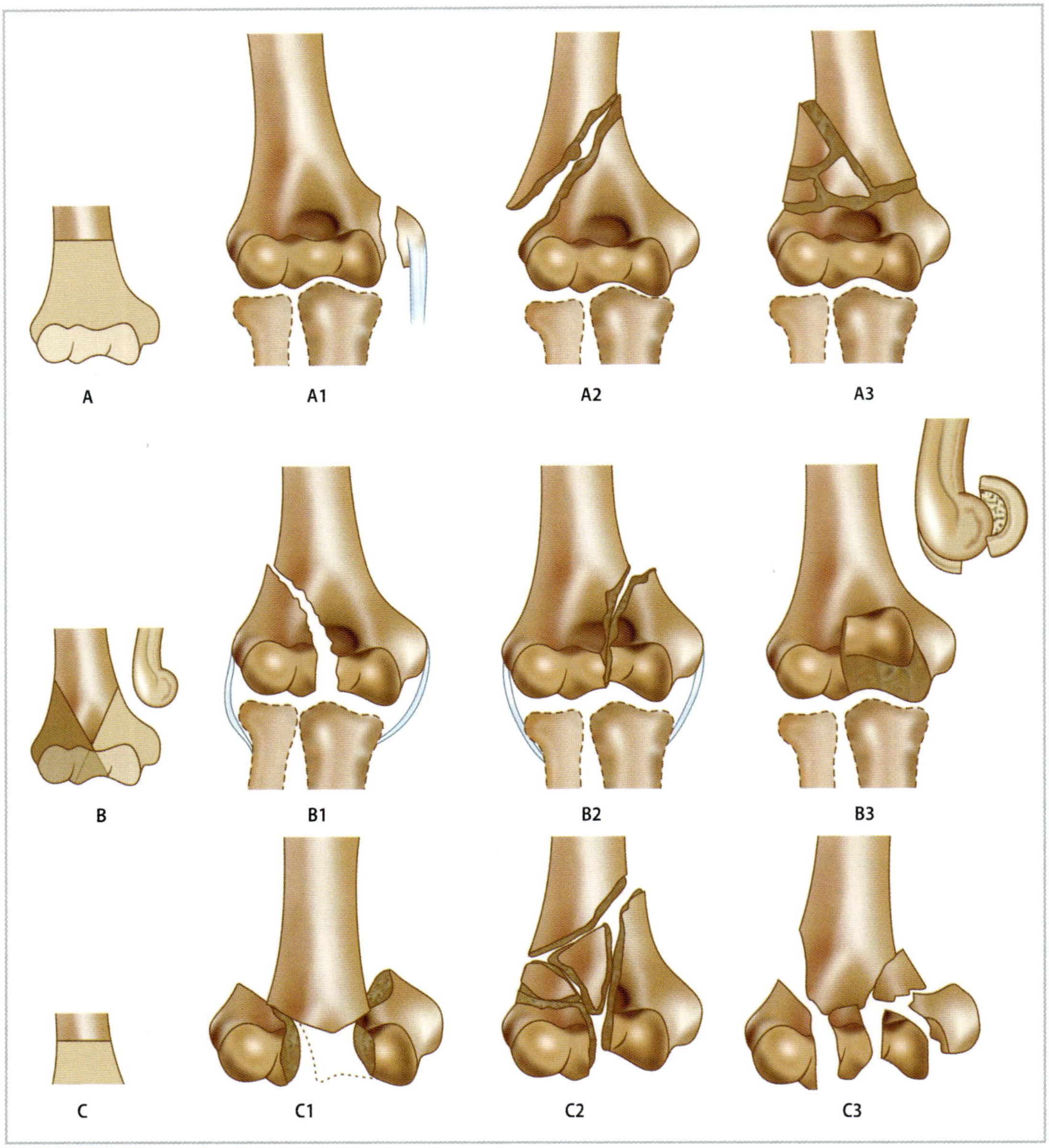

Figure 24.1 AO/OTA classification system (of the Arbeitsgemeinschaft für Osteosynthesefragen/ Orthopaedic Trauma Association) for fractures of the distal humerus.

The elbow is easily flexed and extended in this position. The surgical scrub assistant is positioned across the patient to avoid having to turn from the operative field, which allows the first surgical assistant to be on the same side of the table as the surgeon. When needed, the fluoroscopy unit can be brought in obliquely on the same side as the surgeon. A sterile tourniquet is used to provide hemostasis, especially during the dissection of the ulnar nerve.

The preferred surgical incision is a straight longitudinal incision 1–2 cm lateral to the tip of the olecranon. This location avoids the bony prominence of the olecranon and the medial side of the elbow, both of which are common resting positions for the elbow in daily life. This incision can be extended proximally and distally as needed. The dissection is taken down to the level of the fascia of the triceps.

The first step in the procedure is to dissect medially and identify the ulnar nerve. It is the surgeon›s choice whether to perform an anterior transposition of the ulnar nerve, and the decision to do so routinely is somewhat controversial. Although Chen et al. (2010) found a nearly fourfold higher incidence of postoperative ulnar neuritis in cases where the ulnar nerve was transposed (33%) versus left in situ (9%), there are multiple reasons to move the nerve, some of which were not addressed in the Chen study. The most obvious reason is to move the nerve out of harm›s way, to a protected position, at the initial stages of the procedure. A medial plate is best placed either at the level of medial epicondyle or distal to the medial epicondyle, both of which will potentially violate the cubital tunnel and cause iatrogenic injury to the ulnar nerve. Perhaps the most important issue regarding transposing the nerve to an anterior position concerns the most common complication following this surgery: postoperative stiffness. If the patient develops stiffness in the perioperative period, an examination and manipulation of the elbow under anesthesia can help restore the range of motion if performed in the first four to six weeks postoperatively. However, if the patient has stiffness in flexion and the ulnar nerve has not been transferred to an anterior position, then a manipulation of the elbow into further flexion will stretch a nerve that is scarred in the cubital tunnel, potentially causing an ulnar nerve palsy. Transposing the ulnar nerve mitigates this risk.

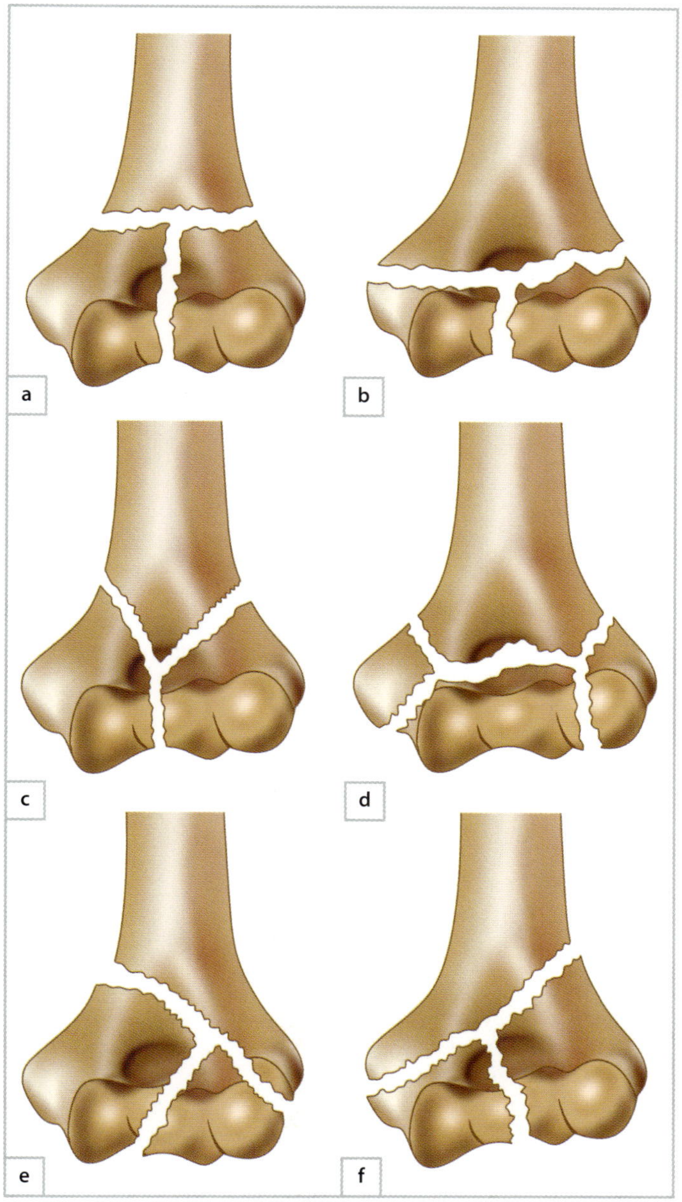

Figure 24.2 Jupiter and Mehne classification of distal humerus fractures. (a) High T, (b) low T, (c) Y, (d) H, (e) medial lambda, (f) lateral lambda.

Risks to the ulnar nerve during the transposition can be minimized by diligent handling, avoiding excessive surgical retraction, completely releasing the nerve, and dissecting an adequate flap to eliminate any postoperative subluxation at the end of the case. Further, Black et al. (2000), in their two-year follow-up of ulnar nerve transpositions (with good or excellent results in 91% of cases), found that the function of the ulnar nerve was more closely related to the preoperative intrinsic nerve pathology than to surgical technique. It is therefore possible that preoperative, postinjury nerve function in the Chen study played a role in the incidence of postoperative neuritis, irrespective of the decision to transpose the nerve.

Several approaches to the management of the triceps have been described in the literature: a triceps-sparing; triceps-reflecting; triceps-reflecting anconeus pedicle (Bryan–Morrey approach) (Morrey 2000); triceps-splitting; and transolecranon via an osteotomy. The fracture pattern and surgeon preference will usually dictate the appropriate technique. However, if there is significant articular comminution or if there is an anterior coronal shear fracture of the trochlea or capitellum, an olecranon osteotomy is necessary. Coles et al. (2006) found no olecranon non-unions in 67 patients who had received an osteotomy for the treatment of a fracture of the distal humerus, half of which were open fractures, over their six-year experience. These osteotomies were repaired by either plate stabilization, or with an intramedullary screw with supplemental wiring of the dorsal ulna.

The preference of the senior author is to perform a triceps-sparing approach except when the fracture dictates that an osteotomy should be performed, as noted above. This is begun by elevating the medial and lateral triceps off the intermuscular septum and sweeping the triceps off the humerus with a periosteal elevator. The posterior capsule is then excised to provide direct visualization of the fracture. The lateral side of the distal humerus is accessed without disturbing the anconeus. A large Penrose drain or Ray-Tec sponge can then be placed around the triceps to retract the triceps medially and laterally, depending on the angle needed. It is important not to release the medial or lateral flexors off the anterior distal humerus. Regardless of the fixation chosen, it is important to minimize soft-tissue stripping, especially the anterior soft tissues, from the distal humerus, to minimize the potential development of heterotopic ossification.

Once the fracture has been exposed and debrided, restoration of the articular surface should precede addressing the columns if a triceps-sparing approach is used. The exception to this general rule occurs when the integrity of the columns is necessary to appreciate the landmarks necessary to reduce the articular fragments. Otherwise, by not re-establishing the continuity of the columns initially, the arm is shortened, which decreases tension on the triceps and other soft tissues, allowing a much easier exposure of the articular surface than if the humerus is at its normal length. Of course, this is not an issue when an olecranon osteotomy is performed. Provisional fixation of the articular surface with Kirschner wires (K-wires) is performed if there is comminution of the articular surface. In cases of severe comminution, definitive fixation of very small articular fragments can be performed with threaded K-wires in the subchondral bone. The threaded K-wires can be cut flush with the bone and left in situ. Once the articular surfaces are provisionally fixed, the distal portion can be provisionally fixed to the columns, which are then anatomically reduced to the humeral shaft.

Plate placement follows provisional fixation. There has been a long-standing lack of consensus regarding optimal plate orientation on the distal humerus. The biomechanical data presented by Stoffel et al. (2008) showed statistically greater stability of the parallel double-locking plating system as regards compression, external rotation, and a greater ability to resist axial plastic deformation when compared with perpendicular constructs. These plates are now available precontoured to fit the distal humerus, which greatly facilitates anatomic reduction and minimizes hardware prominence. Following provisional fixation of the plates proximally, the articular surface is fixed with interdigitating screws through each plate, which, in effect, create a fixed-angle device and link the columns together 'by closing the arch', as described by O'Driscoll (2009). The fragments can be compressed prior to screw placement using a clamp to obviate the need for lag screws to achieve fragment compression. The plates are then fixed to the proximal humeral diaphysis under the maximum achievable compression, via the proximal slotted holes in each plate (**Fig. 24.5**).

At this point, it is important to critically evaluate hardware placement, the stability of definitive fixation, and elbow range of motion under fluoroscopy. The reduction should be anatomic or as close as possible given the degree of comminution and bone loss, and of

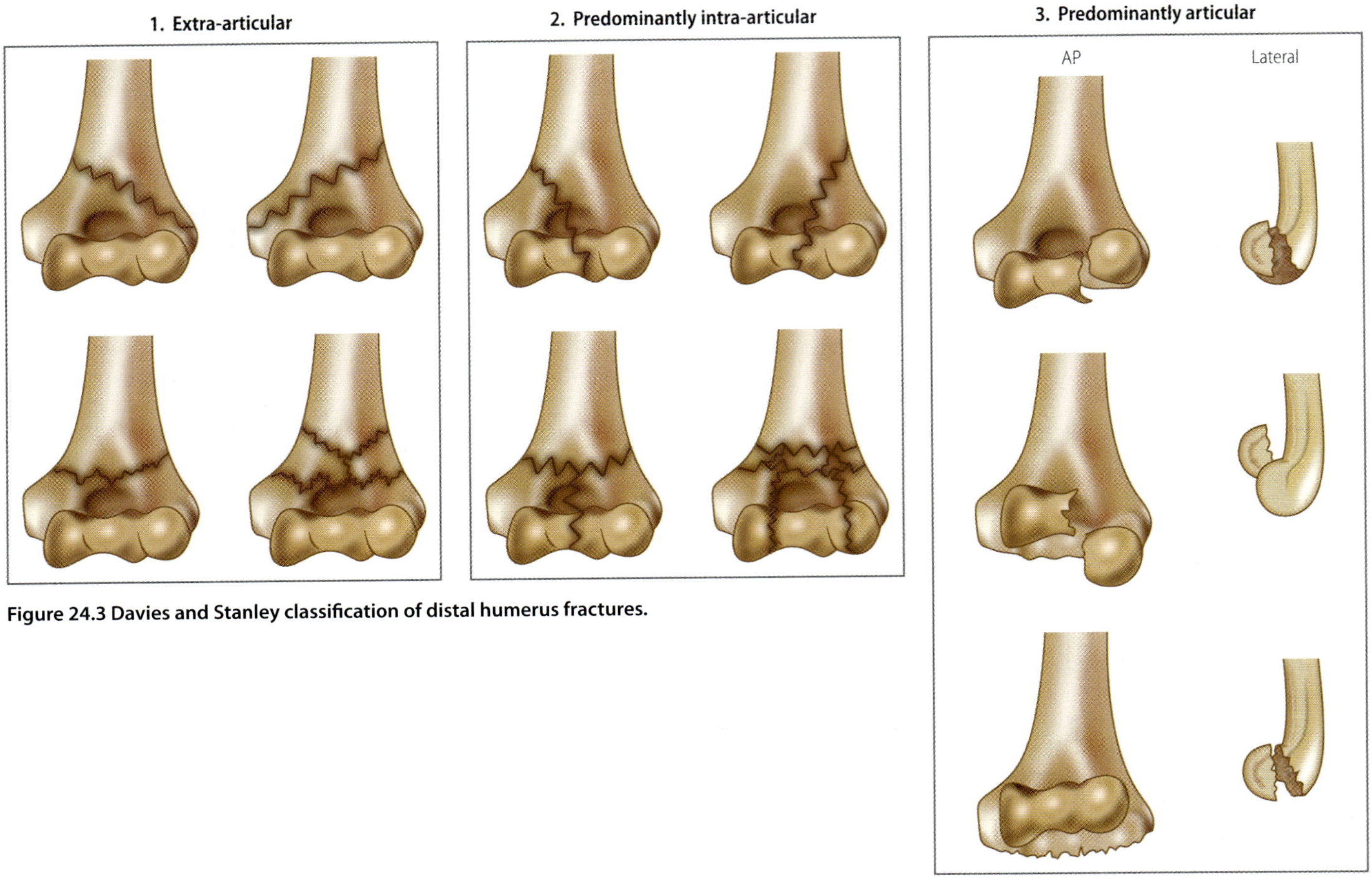

Figure 24.3 Davies and Stanley classification of distal humerus fractures.

sufficient stability to allow immediate, unrestricted motion. There should be no intra-articular hardware, including in the coronoid fossa anteriorly and the olecranon fossa posteriorly, which will allow unencumbered flexion and extension.

The wound is then closed over a medium Hemovac drain. A volar splint is used to hold the elbow in full extension for a brief period (12–36 hours) to minimize postoperative swelling. Thereafter, full and unrestricted range of motion is initiated. The use of continuous passive motion, physiotherapy, patient-initiated self-assisted range of motion, and static splints have all been successfully used. How they are integrated into the postoperative regimen is based on surgeon preference and experience. Dynamic splints and 'aggressive' therapy should be avoided.

Pearls and pitfalls

Obtaining accurate preoperative radiographs is critical to all aspects of preoperative planning, not only of the surgical approach but also the type of fixation used. Sometimes traction radiographs (anteroposterior and lateral) can be helpful; CT scans with two-dimensional and/or three-dimensional reconstructions are ubiquitously obtained. The CT scan should be performed in the coronal and sagittal planes of the distal humerus, with the elbow splinted at 90° of flexion. It is not unusual for CT scans to be obtained in oblique planes, but these make interpretation of the axial cuts as well as the reconstructions more difficult.

Surgery should be performed as soon as all the preoperative planning can be done, although complex fractures of the distal humerus should not be operated upon in the middle of the night, or with staff or assistants who are unfamiliar with the implants, technique or procedure. Grade I open fractures can be addressed the next day, after appropriate preoperative planning has been done and when the appropriate staff are available.

Care is taken throughout the procedure not to dissect around anterior to the distal humerus; an anterior capsular release is typically not necessary. This anterior dissection is discouraged because it is felt that this may increase the risk of heterotopic ossification. Copious irrigation and lowering the tourniquet to establish hemostasis may also help minimize the risk of heterotopic ossification.

When performing the triceps-sparing approach, visualization can be improved by removing a small portion of the olecranon tip, by either excising with a rongeur or an osteotome, to help facilitate exposure of the posterior articular surface with some degree of flexion. Again, the triceps-sparing approach can be used for nearly all fractures. However, those with substantial anterior comminution or an anterior coronal shear fracture require an olecranon osteotomy (**Fig. 24.6**).

If an olecranon osteotomy is used, our preference is to perform a distal chevron osteotomy, completed using an osteotome. This produces interdigitating bone that aids in reduction. The ideal fixation construct for the osteotomy uses a precontoured olecranon plate, which is preliminarily placed in order to predrill the proximal olecranon intramedullary screw prior to the osteotomy. Compression across the osteotomy is performed through the plate, using standard AO techniques. We prefer this pre-contoured compression plating technique over the historic technique which utilizes smooth K-wires or a long compression screw with tension band wire or sutures (**Fig. 24.7**).

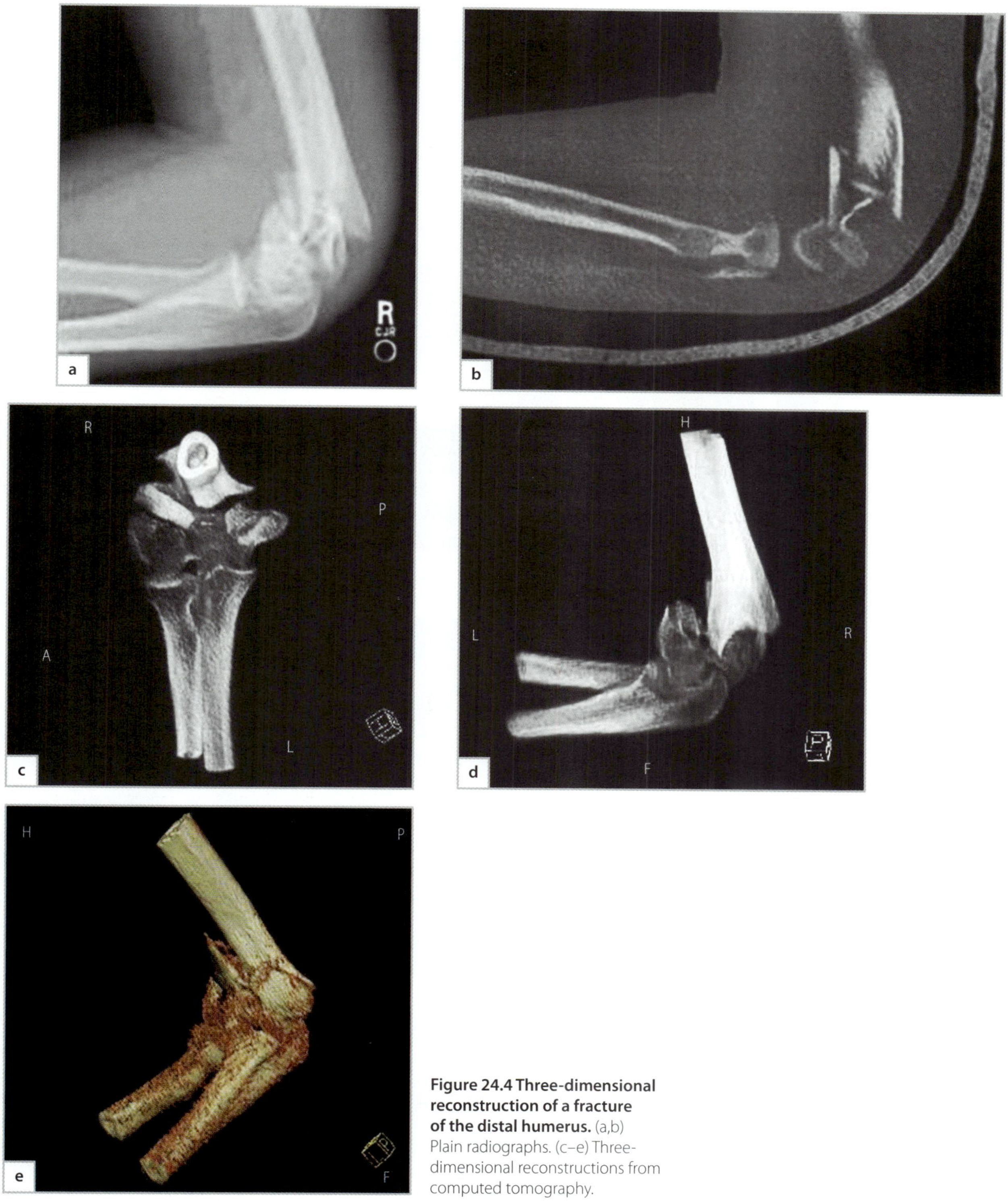

Figure 24.4 Three-dimensional reconstruction of a fracture of the distal humerus. (a,b) Plain radiographs. (c–e) Three-dimensional reconstructions from computed tomography.

The lateral humeral plate should extend distally as far as possible without releasing the lateral collateral ligament complex. The medial plate typically extends around the medial epicondyle but not necessarily into the cubital tunnel and down the medial trochlea. It is unusual for the fracture pattern to require use of a precontoured plate that extends this far distally.

It is preferable for the medial and lateral plates not to end at the same level proximally. Staggering the plates reduces the risk of a stress riser in the distal third of the humeral diaphysis compared with both plates ending at the same location. Stair-stepping the plates proximally is preferable.

At the conclusion of the procedure, taking the arm through a rather vigorous range of motion and rotation is suggested to test the stability of the construct. A stable construct minimizes concern for hardware failure and allows unencumbered rehabilitation, which will facilitate normal or near-normal range of motion postoperatively. If there are concerns regarding the stability of the fixation, it is better to know

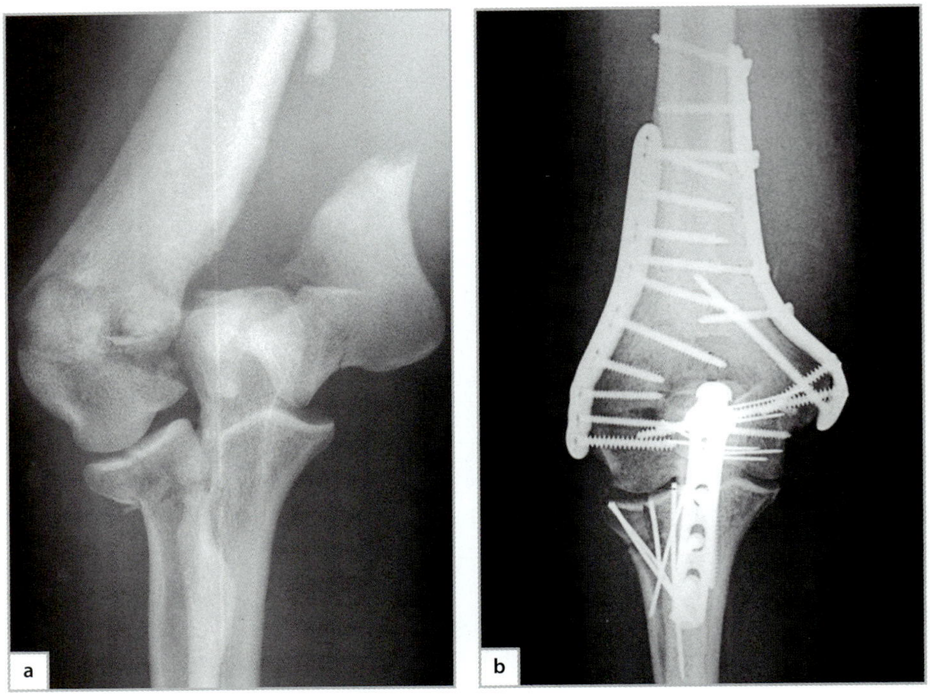

Figure 24.5 Parallel plating of a fracture. (a) Preoperative and (b) postoperative views.

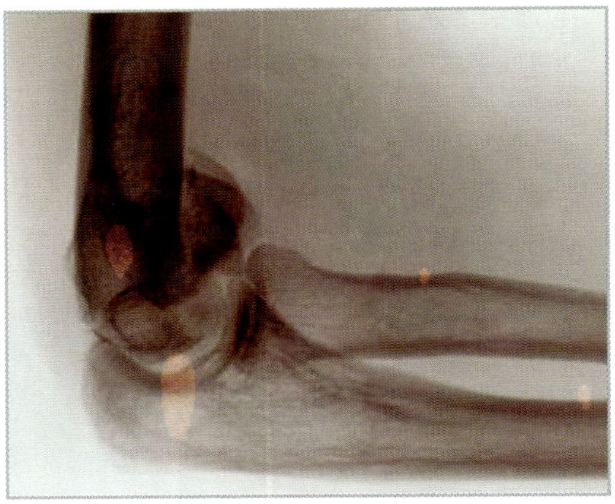

Figure 24.6 Coronal shear fracture of the distal humerus.

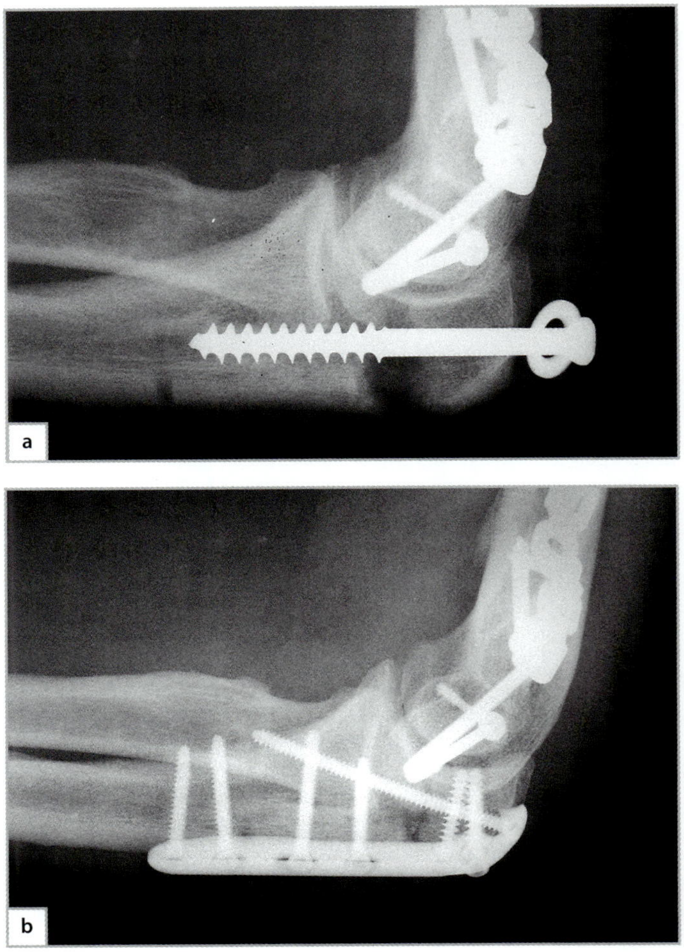

Figure 24.7 Olecranon osteotomy. Comparison of fixation techniques: (a) compression screw with tension band suture, and (b) pre contoured compression plating.

intraoperatively and address these as needed, rather than have postoperative fixation failure, which would require reoperation.

REHABILITATION

The goal of rehabilitating the elbow after open reduction and internal fixation of a complex fracture of the distal humerus is to provide a functional range of motion while allowing bony union of the entire fracture pattern. As noted, the most common complication after this surgery is arthrofibrosis, in particular loss of terminal extension. Preventing this complication begins at the time of surgery, with stable fixation that allows full unencumbered extension of the elbow, followed by postoperative splinting of the limb in full extension for 12–36 hours. While some surgeons elect to use continuous passive motion immediately postoperatively, our preference is to splint the elbow in full extension to minimize swelling and anterior hematoma formation. Active and active assisted range of motion of the elbow is then instituted, often by using static splints to help the patient progressively improve range of motion. Dynamic splints, which do not allow a period of stress relaxation for the periarticular soft tissues and which often aggravate periarticular inflammation, are not used in our practice. The patient is taught self-assisted exercises, consisting of long static stretches at the extremes of flexion and extension.

Pain management is important, as patients need to be able to tolerate range of motion and the demands of physiotherapy. Active hand, wrist, and shoulder motion should be incorporated into the rehabilitation program. Strength will return predictably if anatomic alignment is restored, fractures have healed, and full range of motion is achieved. Progressive resistance exercises can begin when there is radiographic evidence of bony union.

There is a belief that certain severe fracture patterns and/or co-morbid conditions (e.g. traumatic brain injury) increase the risk of symptomatic heterotopic ossification (**Fig. 24.8**). Prophylaxis with a single dose of soft-tissue radiation can be considered. If radiation treatment (XRT) is to be implemented, care should be taken to focus on the anterior soft tissues and to shield both the fracture fixation and the olecranon osteotomy repair, to avoid increasing the chance of non-union (Hamid et al. 2010). Orders for postoperative XRT must explicitly indicate the area of treatment, to avoid radiation exposure to the distal humerus and olecranon.

Additional pharmacological strategies (e.g. botulinum toxin) to prevent the development of stiffness are currently being investigated and may hold promise. Other complications include recalcitrant stiffness, non-union, ulnar neuropathy, implant failure, infection, osteotomy non-union, and symptomatic implants requiring reoperation for hardware removal.

Postoperatively, it is important clinically to follow these patients very closely, some on a weekly basis. Frequently, the staples or sutures are left in place for two or three weeks. The incision is on the tensile side of the elbow and prone to dehiscence with premature staple or suture removal. If a patient demonstrates an obvious lack of progression of range of motion by four weeks, an examination and gentle manipulation under anesthesia are appropriate. The gentle manipulation is intended to work through evolving capsular, periarticular, and intra-articular contractures. An aggressive manipulation under anesthesia should not be performed after six to eight weeks postoperatively, as iatrogenic fracture of the olecranon may result from the combination of strong, thick scarring and osteopenic bone (**Fig. 24.9**).

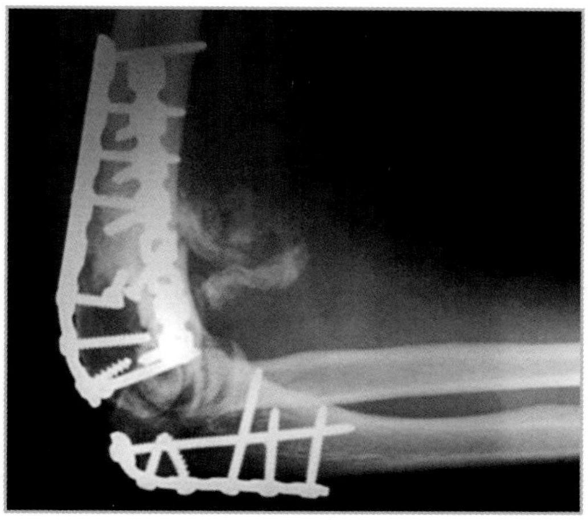

Figure 24.8 Anterior heterotopic ossification.

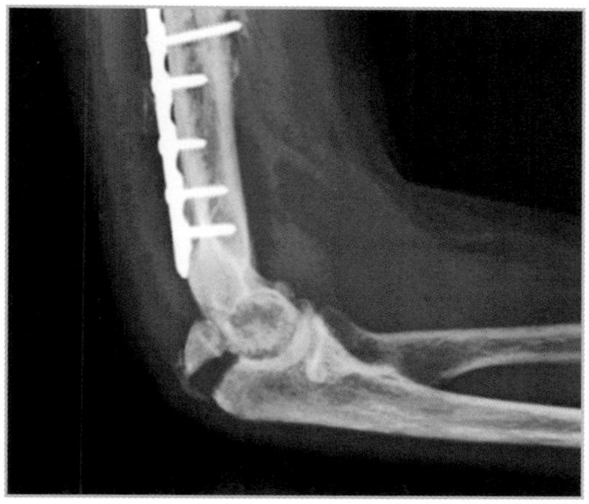

Figure 24.9 Iatrogenic olecranon fracture following aggressive manipulation.

REFERENCES

Black BT, Barron OA, Townsend PF, et al. Stabilized subcutaneous ulnar nerve transposition with immediate range of motion: long-term follow-up. J Bone Joint Surg Am 2000;82:1544–1551.

Chen RC, Harris DJ, Leduc S, et al. Is ulnar nerve transposition beneficial during open reduction internal fixation of distal humerus fractures? J Orthop Trauma 2010;24:391–394.

Coles CP, Barei DP, Nork SE, et al. The olecranon osteotomy: a six-year experience in the treatment of intraarticular fractures of the distal humerus. J Orthop Trauma 2006;20:164–171.

Davies M, Stanley D. A clinically applicable fracture classification for distal humerus fractures. J Shoulder Elbow Surg 2006;15:602–608.

Frankle MA, Herscovici D Jr, Di Pasquale TG, et al. A comparison of open reduction and internal fixation versus total elbow arthroplasty for displaced intra-articular distal humerus fractures in women older than age 65. J Orthop Trauma 2003;17:473–480.

Hamid N, Ashraf N, Bosse MJ, et al. Radiation therapy for heterotopic ossification prophylaxis acutely after elbow trauma: a prospective randomized study. J Bone Joint Surg Am 2010; 92:2032–2038.

Jupiter JB, Mehne DK. Fractures of the distal humerus. Orthopedics 1992;15:825–833.

Morrey BF. The Elbow and Its Disorders. Philadelphia, PA: WB Saunders, 2000: 150–154.

Muller ME, Nazarian S, Koch P, Schatker J. The Comprehensive Classification of Fractures of the Long Bones. Berlin: Springer-Verlag, 1990.

Nauth A, McKee MD, Risevski B, et al. Distal humeral fractures in adults. J Bone Joint Surg Am 2011;93:686–700.

O'Driscoll SW. Parallel plate fixation of bicolumn distal humeral fractures. Instr Course Lect 2009;58:521–528.

Riseborough EJ, Radin EL. Intercondylar T fractures of the humerus in the adult. A comparison of operative and non-operative treatment in twenty-nine cases. J Bone Joint Surg Am 1969;51:130–141.

Robinson CM, Hill RM, Jacobs N, et al. Adult distal humeral metaphyseal fractures: epidemiology and results of treatment. J Orthop Trauma 2003;17:38–47.

Srinivasan K, Agarwal M, Matthews SJ, Giannoudis PV. Fractures of the distal humerus in the elderly: is internal fixation the treatment of choice? Clin Orthop Relat Res 2005;434:222–230.

Stoffel K, Cunneen S, Morgan R, et al. Comparative stability of perpendicular versus parallel plating systems in osteoporotic comminuted distal humerus fractures. J Orthop Res 2008;26:778–784.

Zagorski JB, Jennings JJ, Burkhalter WE, Uribe JW. Comminuted intraarticular fractures of the distal humeral condyles. Surgical vs nonsurgical treatment. Clin Orthop Relat Res 1986;202:197–204.

Chapter 25 Management of 'terrible triad' injuries

Ash K. Moaveni, George S. Athwal

INTRODUCTION

Hotchkiss (1996) originally coined the term 'terrible triad' injury of the elbow due to the historically poor outcomes. The triad of injuries refers to a combination of an elbow dislocation with fractures of the radial head and coronoid process. Recently, clinical and biomechanical studies have better defined surgical indications and protocols that have led to improved patient outcomes (Pugh et al. 2004). Despite this, complications are still frequent and include stiffness, residual instability, and post-traumatic arthritis (Ring et al. 2002).

This chapter focuses on the surgical management of these complex elbow injuries. A systematic approach to the management of terrible triad injuries is provided, with an emphasis on understanding the pathoanatomy.

CLASSIFICATION

The individual components of the terrible triad can be classified to aid in the surgical management of this injury.

Fractures of the radial head

Several classification systems exist for fractures of the radial head. Broberg and Morrey (1987) modified Mason's original classification of radial head fractures. Their classification is based on preoperative imaging. A type I radial head fracture is minimally displaced, typically described as less than 2–3 mm. Type II fractures are displaced >2–3 mm and involve >30% of the radial head. Type III fractures are comminuted. This classification, when used for terrible triad injuries, is primarily descriptive.

Fractures of the coronoid process

Two classification schemes describe the fracture patterns seen in injuries to the coronoid process. The Regan and Morrey (1989) classification is based on the height of the coronoid fragment on a lateral radiograph of the elbow. Type I fractures involve the tip of the coronoid process and typically measure less than 10% of the coronoid height. They are believed to be shear fractures, where the coronoid tip is fractured off by the trochlea as the radius and ulna dislocate posteriorly. Type II fractures are fragments 10–50% of the coronoid height, and type III are greater than 50%. This classification is frequently used for coronoid fractures that occur in terrible triad injuries and is the authors' preferred system.

The second classification system, described by O'Driscoll et al. (2003), is based on the size and location of the fracture fragments. This classification recognizes that not all coronoid fractures occur in the coronal plane, and describes the complex patterns of injury that may occur. The injury patterns described are coronoid tip fractures, anteromedial coronoid facet fractures, and basal fractures. The category of injury is best determined by clinical observation and computerized tomography (CT).

Injury to the lateral collateral ligament

McKee et al. (2003) described the pattern of lateral soft-tissue injury in a clinical series with elbow dislocations. Six injury patterns to the lateral collateral ligament (LCL) were described: proximal avulsion of the LCL; bony avulsion of the lateral epicondyle; mid-substance rupture of the LCL; ulnar detachment of the LCL; ulnar bony avulsion of the LCL (cristae supinatoris fracture); and a combination of patterns. In this series of elbow dislocations, LCL disruption was seen in all elbows. The LCL injury pattern was of proximal avulsion in more than half the patients. In addition to the LCL injury, two thirds of elbows had a concomitant rupture of the common extensor origin.

INDICATIONS

Following closed reduction of a complex elbow dislocation, the elbow joint often remains unstable and incongruent. Prolonged immobilization may be required, resulting in long-term stiffness. As such, most terrible triad injuries of the elbow are best managed with surgical stabilization.

A systematic approach helps to address the critical components of this injury (**Fig. 25.1**) (Mathew et al. 2009). This includes fixation or replacement of the radial head, fixation of the coronoid fragment, and repair of the LCL. Once this has been done, the elbow is intraoperatively assessed for stability, preferably with fluoroscopy, to determine whether repair of the medial collateral ligament (MCL) is required, and whether an external fixator is required (see Chapter 26), although it rarely is.

The goals of treatment for the fracture of the radial head are to have a stable construct, to allow the radial head to function as an elbow stabilizer and to allow early mobilization. Most fractures of the radial head in terrible triad injuries are Broberg and Morrey type II or III. Type I fractures are rare and most can be fixed. Fragment excision for these fractures is, in general, contraindicated. However, if fragment excision is to be considered, the fragment should be <25% of the head, non-articular with the proximal radioulnar joint, and the remainder of the radial head should provide adequate stability.

Radial head excision in the setting of complex elbow instability is contraindicated (Beingessner et al. 2004). The radial head is an important secondary stabilizer. First, it resists valgus load when the MCL is injured. Second, it acts as a buttress to posterior instability with a deficient coronoid. Third, it tensions the repaired LCL to resist varus and posterolateral rotatory instability. Clinical studies have reported persistent instability and early post-traumatic arthritis following resection of the radial head in complex elbow dislocations (Ring et al. 2002).

Treatment options for type II and type III fractures of the radial head include open reduction and internal fixation, and arthroplasty. On occasion, an associated fracture of the radial neck will require stabilization.

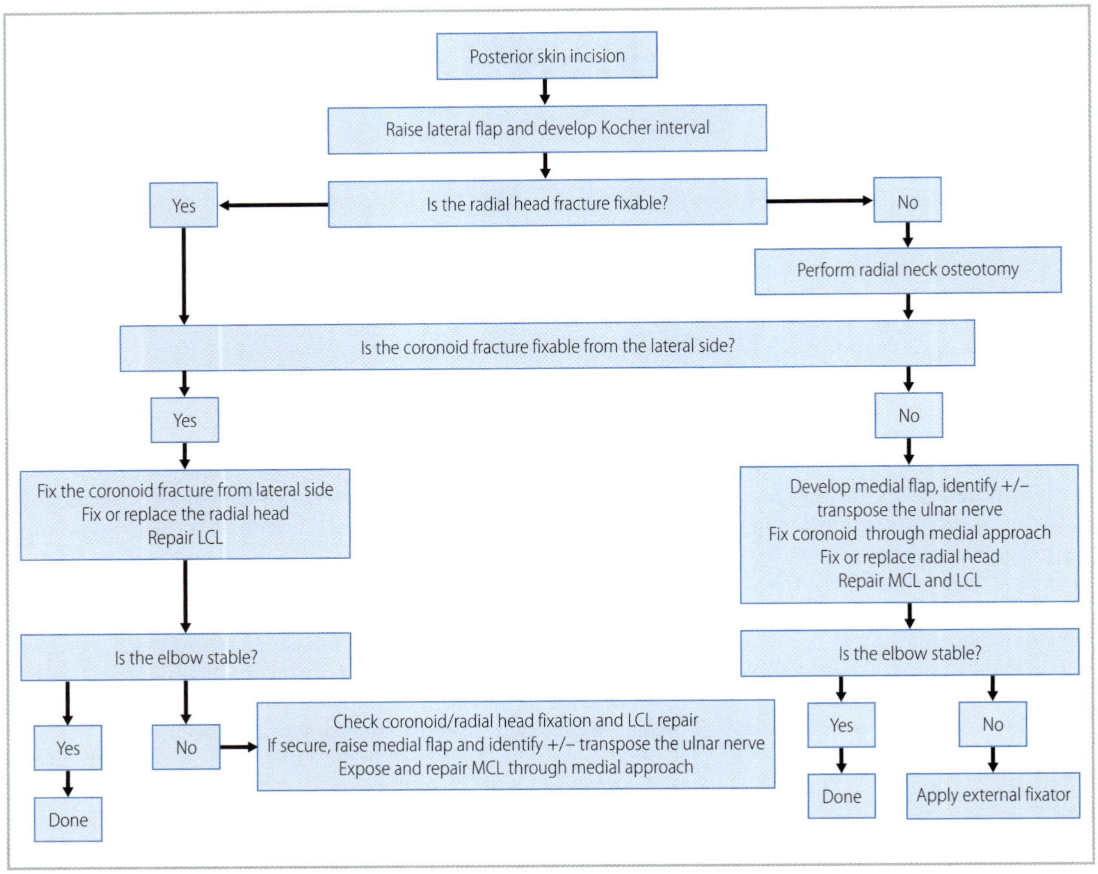

Figure 25.1 Algorithm for the surgical management of terrible triad injury of the elbow. ©2009 American Academy of Orthopaedic Surgeons. Reprinted from the Journal of the American Academy of Orthopaedic Surgeons, Volume 17(3), pp 137–151 with permission.

Coronoid fractures associated with terrible triad injuries are typically Regan and Morrey type I or II. Type I coronoid fractures usually do not require repair. Elbow joint stability is not significantly improved following repair of a small tip fracture (Beingessner et al. 2007). With larger coronoid fragments, fixation is usually achieved with screws or, rarely, a plate. With comminuted fractures, an alternative is to reattach the fragments and the anterior capsule to the coronoid process using transosseous suture fixation.

Fixation of the coronoid fracture fragment provides support against posterior forces, acts as a varus buttress, and prevents rotatory moments. Careful reduction of the ulnohumeral articular surface may reduce the risk of post-traumatic arthritis.

CONTRAINDICATIONS

Rarely, terrible triad injuries may be treated non-operatively. If it is unsafe for a patient to have anesthesia due to concomitant injuries or medical comorbidities, the injury is treated non-operatively. In a medically stable patient, a number of criteria need to be fulfilled to consider non-operative management. These include obtaining a concentric reduction of both the ulnohumeral and the radiocapitellar joints by closed means. The reduction should be stable through a functional range of motion and allow for active motion after two or three weeks. A fracture of the radial head, in itself, will not require surgery if there is minimal displacement with no block to elbow motion. For non-operative management the coronoid fracture should be a small tip fracture, typically a Regan and Morrey type I. Additionally, regular weekly radiographs are required for the first month to ensure that the reduction has been maintained.

TECHNIQUE

Surgery can be performed under regional or general anesthesia. The patient is positioned supine, and the affected limb is draped free. A sterile tourniquet is used. The arm is held across the chest, with an assistant on the opposite side of the table to assist in positioning and retraction. Preoperative imaging (including three-dimensional computerized tomography with the humerus subtracted) and fluoroscopy should be available for use intraoperatively.

Skin incision

Two types of skin incision may be used. Our preference an extensile posterior skin incision. We then raise a full-thickness fasciocutaneous flap, starting on the lateral side. The medial flap is raised only if medial exposure is required. The alternative is to use a direct lateral incision, with an additional medial incision if it is deemed necessary during the procedure.

The posterior skin incision has several advantages. It allows access for both medial and lateral approaches to the elbow. As there are fewer cutaneous nerves posteriorly, the risk of neuroma is reduced. Also, although longer in length, it is more cosmetic in its location. The possible disadvantages include seroma or hematoma formation and flap necrosis, but these are rare in our experience.

Lateral exposure

The injury is initially exposed from the lateral arthrotomy. The injured structures are identified and classified from superficial to deep.

Once identified, surgical repair and stabilization are carried out in reverse, that is, with the deeper structures addressed first, followed by the superficial structures (**Fig. 25.2**).

The lateral approach is done through the Kocher interval (between anconeous and extensor carpi ulnaris). If there is a defect in the common extensor origin, it is incorporated into the approach. Releasing a portion of the extensor origin from the lateral supracondylar ridge of the humerus can improve the exposure. Distally, the annular ligament is incised and later repaired.

Deep to the extensor origin, the LCL is assessed. Often a bare lateral epicondyle is encountered, consistent with a complete proximal avulsion of the LCL (**Fig. 25.2c**). The radial head is next assessed. A decision needs to be made whether stable fixation of the radial head fracture is possible. If there is concern about stability of the fixation due to the degree of fracture comminution and/or osteoporosis, a radial head implant is preferred. In the scenario of a fixable radial head fracture, attention is next turned to the fracture of the coronoid process. If the radial head fracture is not salvageable, an arthroplasty is recommended and a radial neck osteotomy is performed in preparation for prosthetic implantation. The radial neck osteotomy and removal of the remaining head fragments markedly improve coronoid exposure from the lateral side (**Fig. 25.2d**).

When the fracture of the radial head is amenable to fixation, visualization of the coronoid injury is more difficult. Several maneuvers can assist with exposure of the coronoid fracture from the lateral arthrotomy. The fragments of the radial head, if loose, can be temporarily removed to improve visualization. Alternatively, the fragments can be hinged distally on their intact soft-tissue attachments. Finally, the elbow joint can be subluxated posterolaterally to deliver the coronoid into the field of view (**Fig. 25.3**).

Coronoid fixation

Fixation of the coronoid fracture depends predominantly on its size and the degree of comminution (Ring 2006). Type I fractures generally do not require fixation, as biomechanical studies have demonstrated minimal improvements in elbow joint stability.

Type II fractures are generally fixed from the lateral side, using retrograde cannulated screws. A large reduction forceps is used to reduce the coronoid fragment through the lateral arthrotomy. A targeting device can then be used to pass cannulated screw guide wires from the subcutaneous border of the ulna into the reduced coronoid fracture fragment (**Fig. 25.4**).

If the fragments are too comminuted, suture fixation through transosseous tunnels may be performed. A non-absorbable suture is passed through the anterior joint capsule adjacent to the coronoid fracture fragments. The suture should provide a firm hold on the capsule, but not penetrate the brachialis muscle to the extent that the deeper neurovascular structures are put at risk. Transosseous tunnels are then created from the subcutaneous border of the ulna into the base of the coronoid fracture surface. A suture-passer device is used to retrieve the capsular sutures through the tunnels. These sutures are then tied over a bone bridge on the subcutaneous border of the ulna (**Fig. 25.2f**).

If we are unable to address the coronoid fracture from the lateral arthrotomy or plate fixation is required, a medial exposure of the coronoid process is performed.

FIXATION OF THE RADIAL HEAD

Open reduction and internal fixation of the fracture of the radial head is carried out using standard techniques and implants. Alternatively, newer fracture-specific implants, such as cannulated headless compression screws or anatomic plates, may be used (see Chapter 20).

Arthroplasty of the radial head

When the fracture of the radial head is deemed unreconstructable, due to the degree of comminution or poor bone quality, arthroplasty is recommended. Several metallic implant designs are commercially available and none has demonstrated clinical superiority. Ideally, the implant should be metallic or an equivalent solid to resist joint forces, and have modularity to assist with correct implant sizing. Insertion of a correctly sized radial head implant is important to prevent over-lengthening or 'over-stuffing' of the joint, which has been associated with accelerated capitellar wear, joint incongruency, loss of flexion, and pain. Ideally, the excised fragments of the native radial head should be pieced together to function as a template to ensure the chosen implant has the correct thickness and diameter.

Repair of the lateral collateral ligament

Typically in terrible triad injuries, the LCL complex and common extensor origin are avulsed from the lateral epicondyle. A variety of repair techniques have been described (Cohen 2008). These include using transosseous tunnels or suture anchors to repair the LCL and the common extensor origins as a single layer or as separate layers.

Our preference is to use transosseous tunnels to perform a double-layered repair. A running locking suture is passed through the LCL complex and the posterolateral joint capsule, leaving two proximal suture ends. Next, the isometric point on the lateral epicondyle is identified and a hole is created with a 2.5 mm drill. This is followed by two additional drill tunnels, starting on the posterior cortex of the lateral column directed toward the isometric point drill hole. These two drill tunnels are then connected with a curved needle, which also functions as a suture passer, shuttling one LCL suture through each tunnel (**Fig. 25.2g,h**). Once both suture limbs are transosseous through their individual tunnels, the elbow is reduced; the sutures are tensioned with the elbow in 90° of flexion and then tied over a bone bridge on the posterior aspect of the lateral column (deep layer of the repair). The second layer of the repair (superficial layer) is the side-to-side repair of the extensor origin.

Medial exposure

There are three reasons for a medial exposure: significant preoperative ulnar nerve dysfunction necessitating exploration; inability to fix the coronoid fracture from the lateral side; and persistent instability due to MCL insufficiency. We will outline our approach in the latter two scenarios.

Coronoid fixation from the medial side

To fix fractures of the coronoid process from the medial side, we use a flexor carpi ulnaris (FCU) splitting approach. This is accomplished by elevating a full-thickness medial fasciocutaneous flap, followed by identification and transposition of the ulnar nerve. The coronoid process is approached through the floor of the ulnar nerve by elevating the humeral head of the FCU and the flexor-pronator origin. The muscle is carefully elevated from distal to proximal, with care to identify the fracture fragments and the anterior bundle of the MCL. The fracture is carefully reduced to reconstruct the coronoid process and plate fixation is performed. Our preference is intraoperatively to

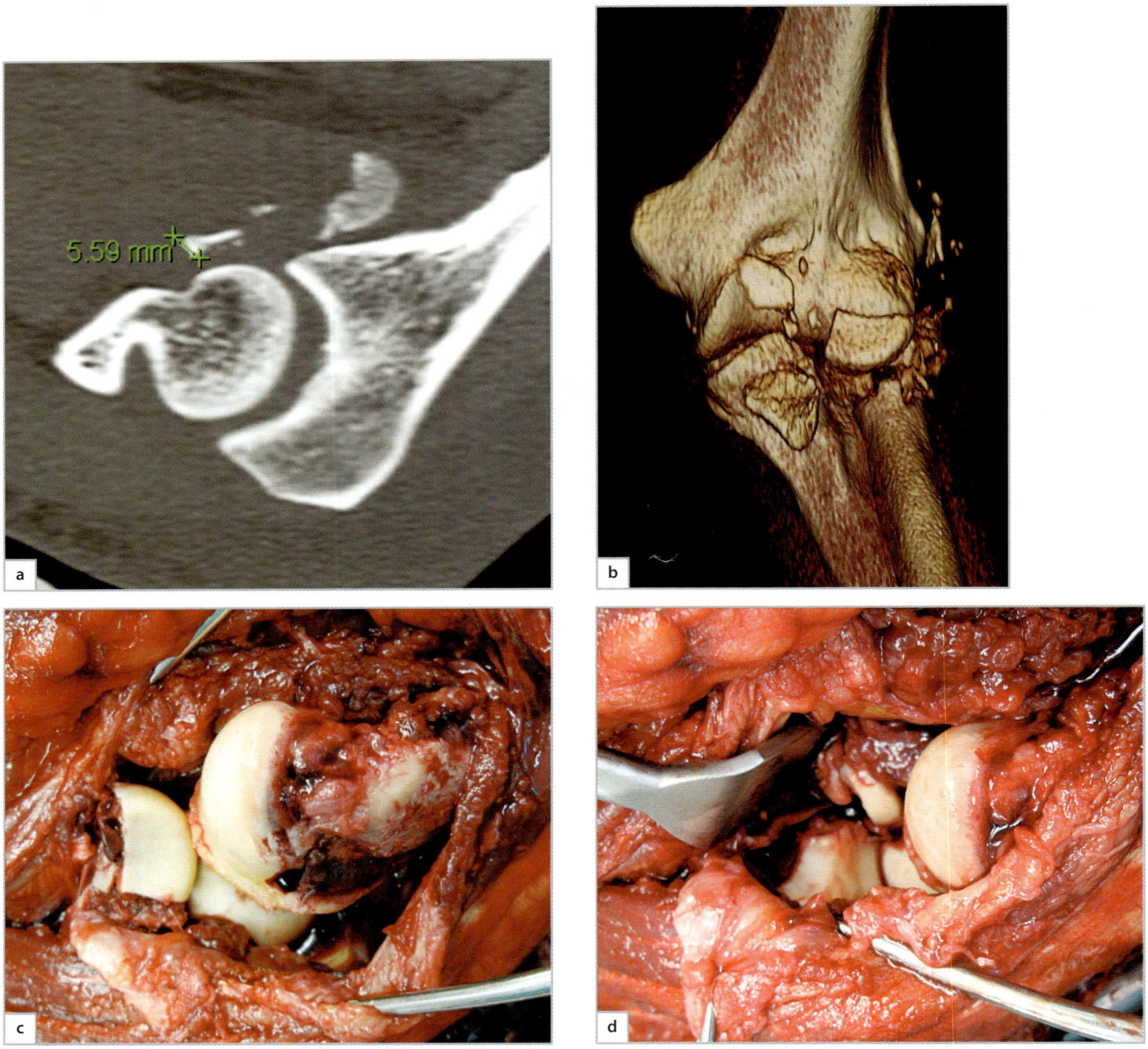

Figure 25.2 Terrible triad injury comprising a Regan and Morrey type II coronoid fracture in association with a comminuted radial head and neck fracture. ***(Contd)***

contour 2.0 mm or 2.4 mm mini-fragment plates. To fix smaller coronoid fracture fragments from the medial side, a limited flexor–pronator split may also be used.

Repair of the medial collateral ligament

The stability of the elbow joint is assessed following repair of the lateral structures and the coronoid process. The joint is placed through a range of motion, from flexion to extension, in supination, pronation, and neutral forearm rotation. If the elbow joint remains congruous from 30° to full flexion, in one or more positions of forearm rotation, MCL repair is not necessary. Infrequently, where the elbow joint remains unstable, we perform a transosseous repair of the MCL.

To repair the MCL, we recommend identification of the ulnar nerve and that consideration be given to anterior subcutaneous transposition. Typically, portions of the flexor–pronator origin will be ruptured off the medial epicondyle. Through these defects, the anterior bundle of the MCL and the flexor–pronator origin can be repaired to the medial epicondyle. In cases where the flexor–pronator origin is intact, we use a flexor–pronator-splitting approach that is in line with the sublime tubercle and medial epicondyle.

Use of external fixators (see Chapter 26)

Rarely, an elbow external fixator is required for persistent instability following repair of the osseous and ligamentous structures in a terrible triad injury. Both static and hinged external fixators can be used (McKee et al.1998). Hinged external fixators allow for early passive and

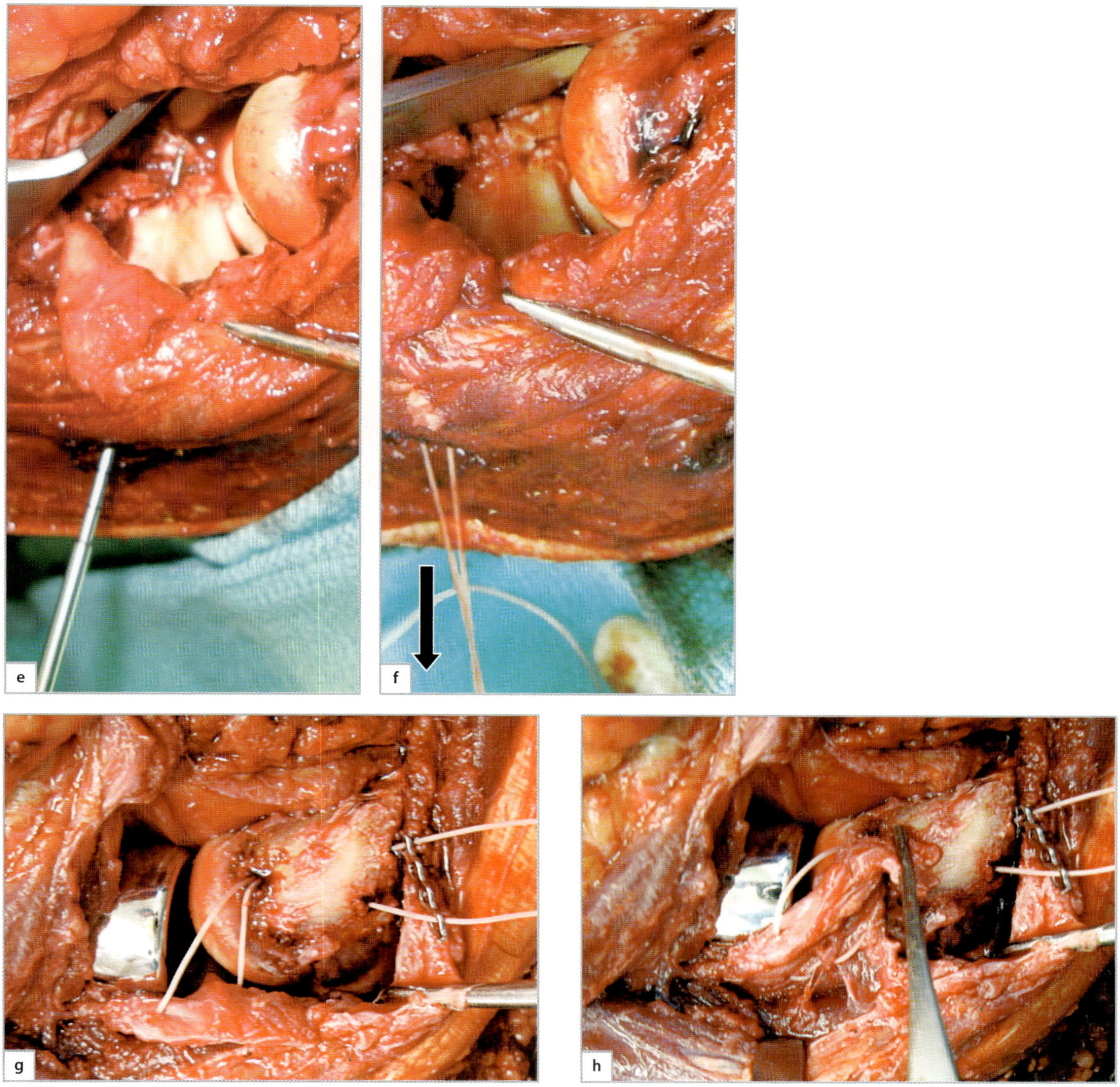

Figure 25.2 Terrible triad injury comprising a Regan and Morrey type II coronoid fracture in association with a comminuted radial head and neck fracture. ***(Contd)***

active motion. For large arms or after a lengthy surgical procedure, we recommend a static external fixation, due to relatively quick and easy application.

Pearls and pitfalls

It is critical to use a correctly sized implant for radial head arthroplasty (Athwal et al. 2010). The native radial head should be used as a template whenever possible. If the native radial head falls between sizes, the implant with the smaller diameter or length is selected. Similarly, where the resection or fracture line through the radial neck is oblique, the minimum height should be used.

If the native radial head is unavailable for templating, the following guidelines are helpful. The proximal portion of the radial head implant should be flush with the proximal aspect of the lesser sigmoid notch. Additionally, no clinical gapping should be observed at the lateral ulnohumeral joint with the elbow reduced.

REHABILITATION

The rehabilitation protocol is primarily dependent on the fluoroscopic examination of the elbow performed prior to leaving the operating room. Residual instability, position of immobilization, and safe arc of motion are determined.

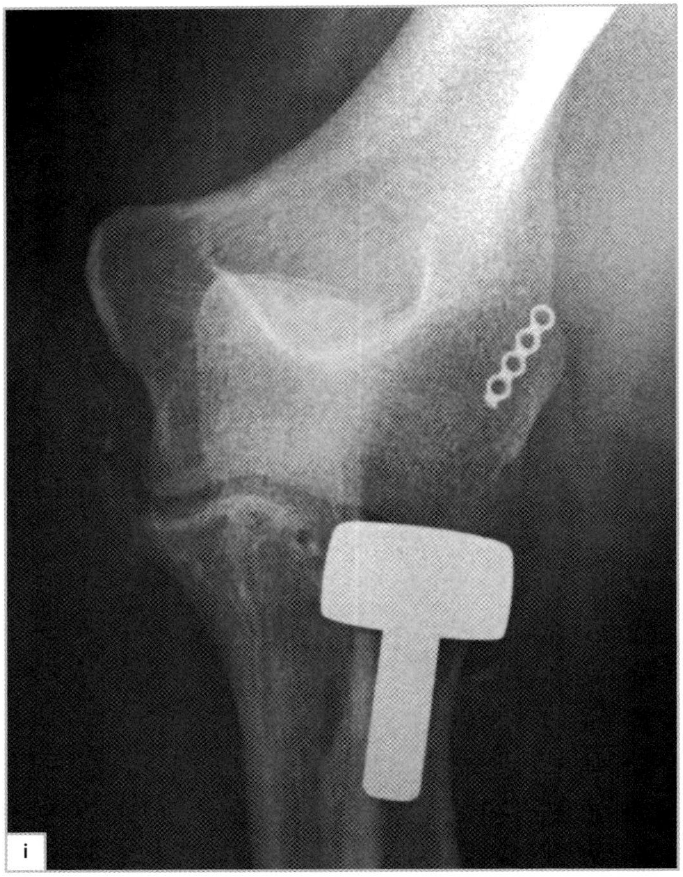

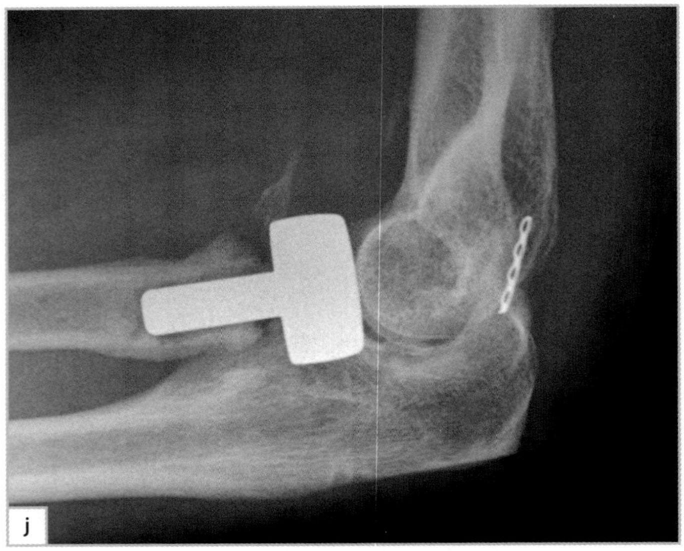

Figure 25.2 Terrible triad injury comprising a Regan and Morrey type II coronoid fracture in association with a comminuted radial head and neck fracture. (a)Sagittal computerized tomography scan and (b) a three-dimensional reconstruction. (c) Lateral approach to the elbow demonstrates complete avulsion of the lateral collateral ligament complex and capsule from the lateral epicondyle and posterior capitellum. As the fracture of the radial head was highly comminuted, a radial neck osteotomy was conducted in preparation for radial head arthroplasty. Additionally, removal of the fragments of the radial head allowed better visualization of the type II coronoid fracture (d). As the coronoid fracture was comminuted, suture fixation was done via two transosseous tunnels, starting on the subcutaneous border of the ulna and exiting into the coronoid fracture surface (e). The coronoid fracture was then reduced by tensioning and tying the sutures (black arrow) exiting the subcutaneous border of the ulna (f). After coronoid fixation, radial head arthroplasty was performed, followed by lateral collateral ligament repair (g). The lateral collateral ligament complex was repaired to the isometric point on the lateral epicondyle by a transosseous technique (h); an alternative technique is to use suture anchors. In this case, the sutures securing the lateral collateral ligament were tied over a bone bridge reinforced with a metal plate due to generalized osteopenia. Six-month follow-up anteroposterior (i) and lateral (j) radiographs demonstrate a reduced elbow joint with clinically insignificant heterotopic ossification.

Elbow range of motion is usually initiated two to five days after surgery. When the MCL is intact, the elbow is immobilized at 90° of flexion with the forearm in pronation to protect the repaired LCL. If the LCL is securely repaired and the MCL exhibits some laxity, the forearm is placed in supination. If both the MCL and the LCL have been repaired, neutral forearm rotation is used. When active elbow range of motion is initiated, full active flexion is permitted, with full pronation and supination in the flexed position. Active extension is done in the position of forearm rotation that maximizes stability. For example, with an MCL-deficient elbow, extension is permitted with forearm supination. With an MCL-intact elbow with residual LCL laxity, extension is done in forearm pronation to augment the lateral side. If residual instability is of concern, an overhead, gravity-assisted protocol can be used. This maneuver is performed with the patient supine and the arm overhead, as gravity adds to elbow joint compression and helps reduce patient apprehension. Isometric exercises of the elbow flexors and extensors are also important in maintaining joint reduction.

A resting splint with the elbow at 90° of flexion and the forearm in the appropriate position of rotation is used for the first four to six weeks. Night extension splinting may be initiated at six weeks to regain extension, if required. Strengthening is generally started at 8–12 weeks.

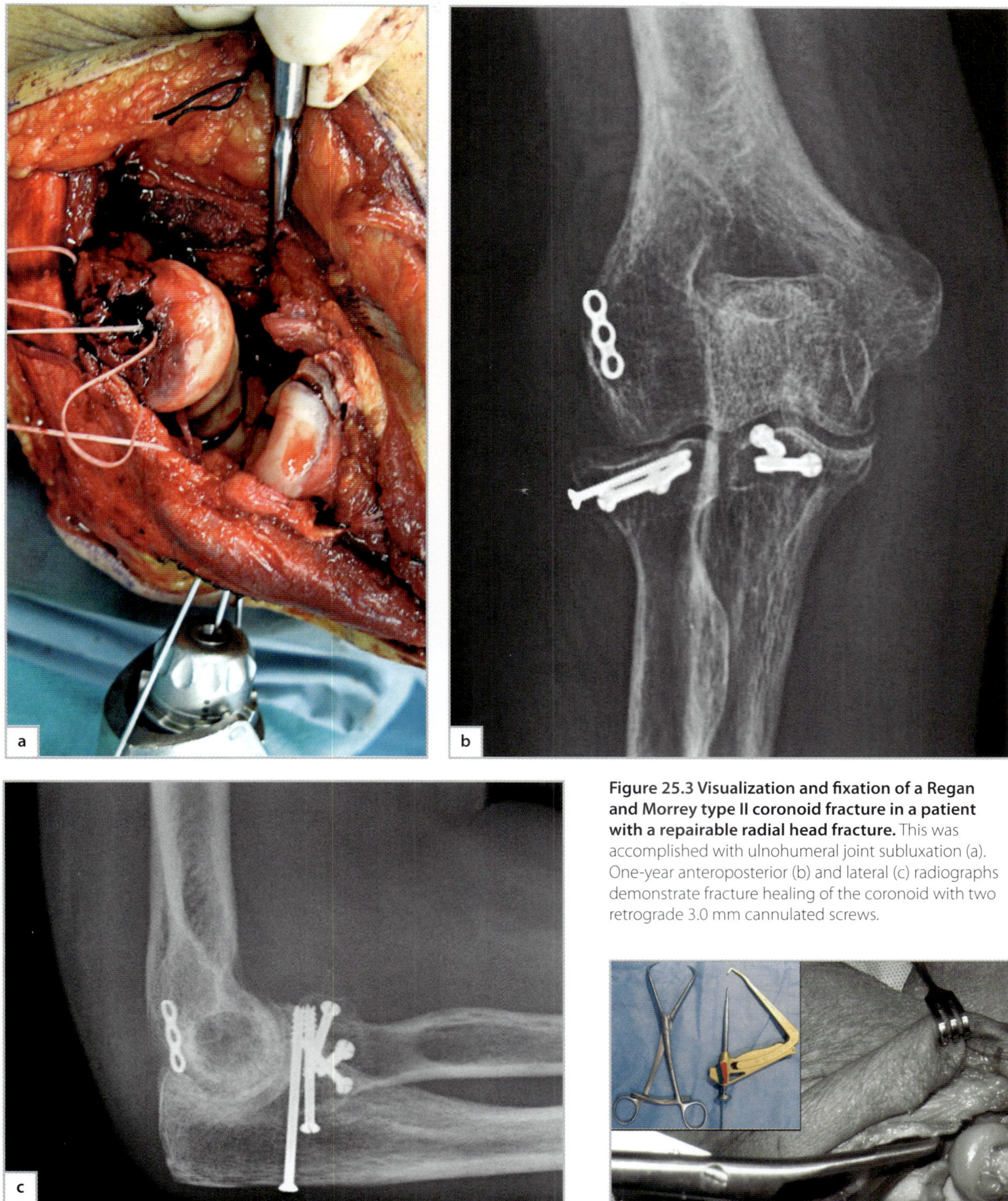

Figure 25.3 **Visualization and fixation of a Regan and Morrey type II coronoid fracture in a patient with a repairable radial head fracture.** This was accomplished with ulnohumeral joint subluxation (a). One-year anteroposterior (b) and lateral (c) radiographs demonstrate fracture healing of the coronoid with two retrograde 3.0 mm cannulated screws.

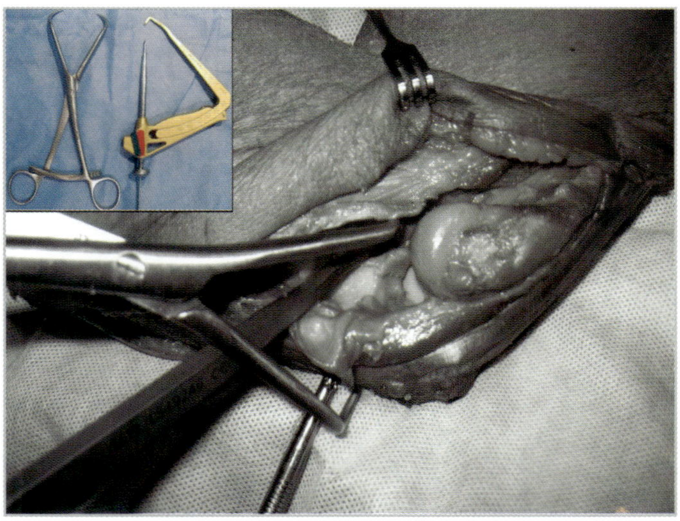

Figure 25.4 **Retrograde cannulated screw fixation of the coronoid.** This was accomplished with a large reduction forceps and a targeting device (inset). The targeting device allows insertion of a cannulated screw guide wire into the reduced coronoid fracture fragment.

REFERENCES

Athwal GS, Frank SG, Grewal R, et al. Determination of correct implant size in radial head arthroplasty to avoid overlengthening: surgical technique. J Bone Joint Surg Am 2010;92:250–257.

Beingessner DM, Dunning CE, Gordon KD, et al. The effect of radial head excision and arthroplasty on elbow kinematics and stability. J Bone Joint Surg Am 2004;86:1730–1739.

Beingessner DM, Stacpoole RA, Dunning CE, et al. The effect of suture fixation of type I coronoid fractures on the kinematics and stability of the elbow with and without medial collateral ligament repair. J Shoulder Elbow Surg 2007;16:213–217.

Broberg MA, Morrey BF. Results of treatment of fracture-dislocations of the elbow. Clin Orthop Relat Res 1987;216:109–119.

Cohen MS. Lateral collateral ligament instability of the elbow. Hand Clin 2008;24:69–77.

Hotchkiss RN. Fractures and dislocations of the elbow. In: Rockwood Jr CA, Green DP, Bucholz RW, Heckman JD, eds. Rockwood and Green's Fractures in Adults, vol. 1, 4th edn. Philadelphia, PA: Lippincott-Raven, 1996: 929–1024.

Mathew PK, Athwal GS, King GJW. Terrible triad injury of the elbow: current concepts. J Am Acad Orthop Surg 2009;17:137–151.

McKee MD, Bowden SH, King GJ. Management of recurrent, complex instability of the elbow with a hinged external fixator. J Bone Joint Surg Br 1998;80:1031–1036.

McKee MD, Schemitsch EH, Sala MJ, O'Driscoll SW. The pathoanatomy of lateral ligamentous disruption in complex elbow instability. J Shoulder Elbow Surg 2003;12:391–396.

O'Driscoll SW, Jupiter JB, Cohen MS, et al. Difficult elbow fractures: pearls and pitfalls. Instr Course Lect 2003;52:113–134.

Pugh DMW, Wild LM, Schemitsch EH, et al. Standard surgical protocol to treat elbow dislocations with radial head and coronoid fractures. J Bone Joint Surg Am 2004;86:1122–1130.

Regan W, Morrey B. Fractures of the coronoid process of the ulna. J Bone Joint Surg Am 1989;71:1348–1354.

Ring D. Fractures of the coronoid process of the ulna. J Hand Surg Am 2006;31:1679–1689.

Ring D, Quintero J, Jupiter JB. Open reduction and internal fixation of fractures of the radial head. J Bone Joint Surg Am 2002;84:1811–1815.

Chapter 26 External fixators for the management of elbow instability

Surbhi Panchal, Anand M. Murthi

INTRODUCTION

Elbow dislocations (either simple or with fracture) are a common injury and can be challenging and devastating because of the potential for resulting limited motion or increased elbow instability. Elbow instability can have several causes. It can be created acutely by a simple or complex elbow dislocation, or it can be created by inadequate fixation, chronic disruption of the ligamentous support structures, or repetitive tearing (Sotereanos et al. 2007). There are various treatment options for these injuries, based on the patient's initial presentation. These include immobilization and therapy, pin stabilization, static or hinged external fixation, and open reduction and internal fixation. Because both bony and ligamentous structures can be affected, unstable elbows often will require a combination of these treatment options. Either a static or a hinged elbow external fixator may be applied to render eventual elbow stability and range of motion. A hinged external fixator allows the bony and ligamentous structures to heal while maintaining/allowing motion. A hinged external fixator specifically allows elbow joint motion along the ulnohumeral joint axis, to prevent contracture. A static external fixation device keeps the joint in one position, whereas a hinged external fixation device allows the joint to go through a range of motion. A hinged external fixator can be locked so that it acts as a static fixator. Often the ligamentous and bony disruption of the elbow does not allow application of a hinged external fixator. In these cases, a static fixator may be applied. This does not always lead to a stiff elbow, and range of motion may be started after removal of the static fixator. Eventual secondary procedures such as capsular releases may be necessary to reach maximum range of motion.

A hinged external fixator is used to allow bony and ligamentous structures to heal while preserving motion in the elbow joint. Hinged external fixators allow for maintenance of a stable and congruent joint, while allowing acutely injured soft tissues to heal in proper length relative to the joint. The hinged external fixator also allows distraction of the joint while maintaining the axis of rotation. This principle is important in the elbow joint, to prevent contractures that limit the functional range of motion. The elbow is described as a modified hinge joint because it allows flexion/extension as well as pronation/supination. The elbow has a flexion/extension range of motion of 0–150°, with the functional range of motion from 30° to 130°. The elbow has a supination/pronation range of motion of about 90° to 90° (180° total arc of motion), with a functional range of motion of 100° total arc. The external fixator is designed to maintain this range of motion for functionality. Bony stability is primarily provided by the ulnohumeral articulation, specifically the coronoid process. Primary ligamentous stability is provided by the anterior bundle of the medial collateral ligament and the lateral ulnar collateral ligament. The radial head provides an important secondary restraint, especially with valgus loads. Secondary restraint is also provided by the common flexor and extensor origins. Therefore, a hinged external fixator is used to preserve these articulations while providing support to allow the stable structures to heal.

Both static and hinged external fixators neutralize forces across the injured segment until the joint has healed enough to accept those forces. Fixator placement is planned preoperatively, but the final placement can be decided in surgery, when stability after fixation can be assessed. The balance is between immobilization, which allows healing of the injured structures, versus motion, which allows healing of the joint surfaces and prevents elbow contractures. Specifically in the elbow, heterotopic ossification and reduction in motion can occur rapidly if a static external fixator is applied. Although an external fixation device can be used as an isolated treatment option, it is often an adjunct to internal fixation and/or ligamentous repair.

Static external fixation of unstable elbow dislocations provides definitive concentric management of alignment after reduction of the dislocation. It is important to maintain alignment of the joint during the decrease in swelling of the limb after an extensive injury. Maintenance of alignment is also recommended if definitive stabilization will be delayed for several weeks secondary to patient characteristics such as polytrauma, obesity, or neurovascular compromise requiring intervention. The benefits of a static external fixator include stability and congruence of the joint; the risks include decreased final range of motion, post-traumatic arthritis in the elbow, and increased heterotopic ossification. The bony architecture of a complex fracture dislocation may exclude any planned range of motion, and in these cases a static fixator is the optimal choice.

Hinged external fixators are classified as uniplanar or multiplanar. Uniplanar external fixators may be easier to apply and are lower profile, but they offer less stability than a multiplanar fixator. A multiplanar fixator is more stable relative to the fixed axis; however, this means it is often more technically challenging to apply. There are several systems available, with similar characteristics. These fixators stabilize the distal humerus and ulna so that the elbow moves in a hinge-like motion around the fixed axis. The joint can also be distracted with the fixators, which is important in keeping the joint congruent. The most important feature of all these fixators is the establishment of the ulnohumeral axis of rotation between the lateral epicondyle and inferior to the medial epicondyle. Once this axis of rotation is established, the system can be placed onto the patient.

Several studies have demonstrated that a hinged external fixator provides stability for healing of the elbow joint while also providing controlled motion to allow for continuous elbow range of motion. McKee et al. (1998) treated 16 patients with elbow instability with hinged external fixation and found that only one had recurrent instability. These patients either had an unstable acute presentation or an unstable presentation after an open reduction and internal fixation of the injury. The mean arc of motion was 105° of flexion (range 65–150°), 76° of pronation (range 20–90°), and 75° of supination (range 15–90°). Complications included reflex sympathetic dystrophy, pin-tract infection, wound infection, and transient ulnar nerve palsy. The investigators concluded that the use of a hinged external fixator was an important advance in the management of elbows with instability.

Ruch and Triepel (2001) found that the average flexion angle was 97° after hinged external fixation in eight patients. The first group of patients had a hinged external fixator as an adjunct to bony and ligamentous repair, and the second group had the fixator as the only treatment. When patients were stratified, those with acute instability who underwent internal fixation had an average postoperative arc of motion of 120° (range 105–130°), while those for whom the fixator was the only treatment had an average arc of motion of 84° (range 75–95°). This study, although with a small number of patients, revealed that patient presentation may determine the postoperative function achieved with a hinged external fixator.

Jupiter and Ring (2002) treated five patients with chronically unreduced elbow dislocations. After adequate debridement to allow for concentric reduction of the joint, a Compass external fixator was placed. At an average follow-up of 38 months, all five patients had stable, concentric joints. These patients were able to regain full pronation and supination but had a 15° flexion contracture.

Ring et al. (2004) expanded these indications and included seven patients with 'terrible triad' injury and six with a posterior Monteggia-type injury. They assessed whether hinged elbow external fixators allow for a functional improvement both subjectively (to the patient) and objectively (to the surgeon). In these 13 patients, followed for an average of six weeks, the average Mayo Elbow Performance Score (MEPS) was 84, the average Disabilities of the Arm, Shoulder and Hand (DASH) score was 15, and flexion arc was 99°.

INDICATIONS

Elbow dislocations are the second most common type of major joint dislocation and are often the result of a fall onto an outstretched hand. They are divided into simple (no fracture) and complex (associated fracture), with about equal incidence. Further classification is by the direction of the dislocation, with the majority being posterolateral. After clinical reduction, it is useful to determine whether these dislocations are stable or unstable by putting them through a controlled range of motion. If the elbow can extend past 30° without subluxation or dislocation, the elbow is considered stable. If there is subluxation or dislocation during a controlled range of motion, an external fixator can be used to stabilize it. It is important to tell these patients that they will regain their flexion motion but may lose terminal extension (Sotereanos et al. 2007).

The treatment of complex elbow dislocations can be broadly characterized as non-operative and operative options (Tashjian and Katarincic 2006). Non-operative treatment of these injuries is adequate if the elbow is deemed stable after reduction. For example, often the treatment for fractures of the radial head is splint and gentle range of motion. If the joint is concentric then, under close supervision, treatment in a splint with active motion is sufficient. Operative treatment of this injury can include repair of the radial head, resection, or resection with lateral collateral ligament repair. An external fixation device may need to be placed to ensure stability.

The 'terrible triad' is a posterior dislocation, radial head fracture, and coronoid process fracture (see Chapter 25). Terrible triad fracture dislocations must be followed closely because stability is often not clear in these patients. For this reason, the surgeon will frequently elect surgical intervention to repair the coronoid as well as to address the radial head and lateral collateral ligament complex. Often an external fixation device is used to supplement an internal fixation. The type I fracture is the most common fracture of the coronoid, which houses the attachment of the elbow anterior capsule. This fracture leads to instability due to decreased anterior constraint. Each component should be managed to regain stability, which means the radial head should be repaired or replaced, and the coronoid fractures should be reconstructed. The dislocation should be reduced and maintained, possibly using an external fixator to preserve concentricity. Other operative interventions include the application of an external fixator to stabilize the elbow joint, pin fixation, and open reduction and internal fixation.

There are three main types of elbow instability that lead to treatment beyond splinting and range of motion exercises: posterolateral rotatory instability, varus posteromedial rotational instability, and olecranon fracture dislocations. Posterolateral rotatory instability is the most common and often results from a fracture of the radial head and coronoid process with partial disruption of the medial collateral ligament. Varus posteromedial rotational instability is often a result of a fracture of the anteromedial facet of the coronoid process, injury to the lateral collateral ligament, and olecranon fracture. Anterior olecranon fracture dislocations are often due to a direct blow to a flexed elbow, unlike the other two types of fracture dislocation. Fracture dislocations of the elbow are considered complex because both bony and ligamentous structures are involved, and final treatment of the injury can vary. Elbow dislocations may involve fractures of the radial head, medial epicondyle, lateral epicondyle, or coronoid process, or a combination of these structures. Fractures of the distal humerus such as trochlea shear fractures and complex fractures of the olecranon are also common (O'Driscoll et al. 2003). An external fixator device can be used to help treat the fracture while allowing for mobilization (Tan et al. 2005).

Instability can also be categorized as acute (within six weeks of a specific traumatic event) or chronic, and the assessment may change the physician's treatment algorithm. Acute instability results from fracture dislocations, which are defined as either simple or complex. Chronic elbow instability includes a wider range of conditions, from occasional subluxation to locked dislocation (Tashjian and Katarincic 2006). Malunion and non-union of the elbow create chronic instability due to decreased constraints. The success of hinged external fixation in the setting of chronic instability is not as predictable as the results of other treatment options, such as internal fixation. This can be attributed to the variable healing of soft tissues and the bony constraints of the joint, and therefore there is not a robust healing response as in an acute injury. These findings can also be attributed to the limited fixator designs that were initially available.

Hinged or static external fixation is a good treatment option for patients with severely comminuted fractures, where internal fixation may not be adequate to treat all intra-articular comminution. These patients may have either bony defects or soft-tissue defects that prevent ligamentous reconstruction. This type of fixation is also important for those patients who have had an attempted bony and/or ligamentous repair that has failed or is inadequate intraoperatively. Furthermore, a compromised soft-tissue envelope from burns or other injuries may exclude a splint or brace, and therefore an external fixator may be used.

External fixation is a good primary or adjunct treatment option for elbow instability (**Table 26.1**).

Table 26.1 Indications for the use of an external fixator

Indication	Specific injury/purpose
Acute instability	Elbow dislocation
Chronic instability	Posterolateral rotatory instability Varus posteromedial instability
Fracture dislocations	Fracture of the olecranon Fracture of the radial head Fracture of the distal humerus Fracture dislocation of the transolecranon
Terrible triad	Posterior dislocation, with fractures of the radial head and coronoid process
Contracture	For ligamentous healing in an elongated manner

CONTRAINDICATIONS

The main justification for not using a hinged external fixator is that the elbow is stable after surgical stabilization. Another reason for not using an external fixator is potential non-compliance of the patient. If the patient is unable to follow the appropriate motion protocol, then the risks of fixator failure, loosening, or pin-tract infection may outweigh the benefits and the device should not be used. Patient characteristics that may be associated with non-compliance include traumatic brain injury, multi-trauma, and inability to comply with detailed instructions. Applying a hinged external fixator is demanding for the surgeon, and use is demanding for the patient. If the elbow joint is deemed stable, or if the patient is not able to adhere to the postoperative treatment course, then the hinged external fixator should not be placed (**Table 26.2**).

TECHNIQUE

Patients are usually positioned supine. Placement of patient, table, and anesthesia should allow easy access to fluoroscopic imaging of the elbow and upper extremity. A rolled towel or sandbag placed under the ipsilateral scapula may assist in patient positioning. The elbow axis of rotation is at the center of the capitellum and trochlear segments of the distal humerus, and is visible on both anatomical landmarks and on a radiograph. Studies have shown that the center of rotation is an area 2–3 mm in diameter in the center of the trochlea (Chen and Julka 2010). On the medial aspect of the elbow, this point is slightly anterior and inferior to the medial epicondyle. On the lateral aspect, the axis lies just distal to the lateral epicondyle, at the center of the projection of the curvature of the capitellum. After determining the correct starting point for the axis, the pin is slowly advanced parallel to the joint and the position is verified on the lateral and anteroposterior fluoroscopic images. On the lateral image ideally there is only a dot visible in the epicondyle, and on the anteroposterior view the pin line indicates that the pin is parallel to the joint line (**Fig. 26.1**). The pin is advanced up to the second cortex if it is a uniplanar system or through the second cortex for a multiplanar system.

Table 26.2 Contraindications for the use of an external fixator

Contraindication	Reason
Stability of the elbow joint	If joint is stable, it is advisable to avoid use of the fixator device to save surgeon time and patient inconvenience
Non-compliance of the patient	Fixator loosening, pin-tract infection, humerus/ulna fracture

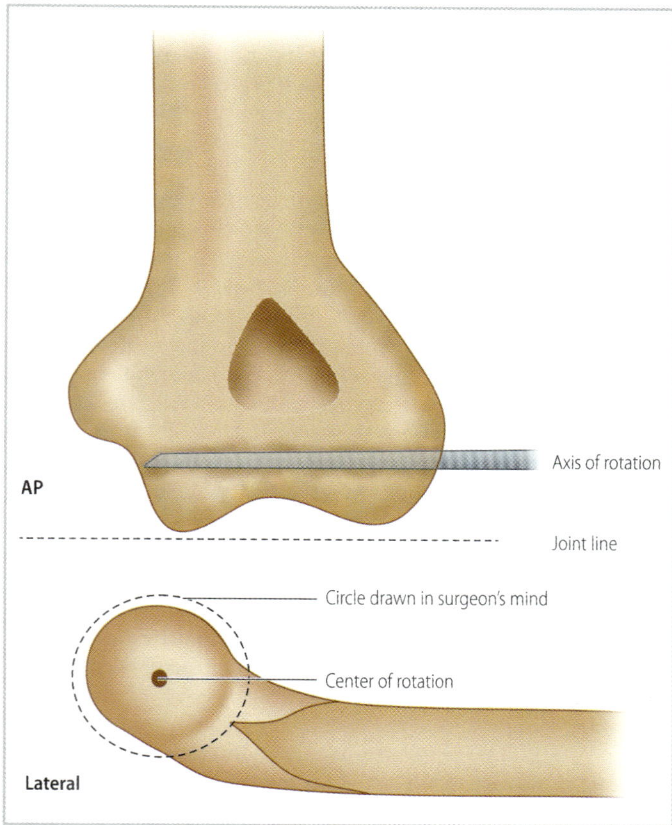

Figure 26.1 Illustration of elbow showing axis of rotation. The anteroposterior (AP) view demonstrates that the axis of rotation is parallel to the joint line. The lateral view demonstrates that the center of rotation lies just distal to the lateral epicondyle at the center of the projection.

It is also important that the axis of rotation be internally rotated 3–8° with respect to the epicondylar axis, and it must form an angle of 82–86° with the longitudinal axis of the humerus. Anatomic landmarks are the tuberosity of the lateral collateral ligament origin on the lateral epicondyle and the medial epicondyle (anterior and inferior as described above). Exact placement of this pin for the axis of rotation is important because 5 mm of translation or angulation can result in a fourfold increase in resistance to flexion (Chen and Julka 2010).

Once the axis-of-rotation pin is placed, then the order for applying external fixator pins is to some extent dependent on the manufacturer's instruction guide. The humeral and ulnar pins are placed in a typical fashion. Usually smaller pins are used in the lateral aspect of the ulna. Pins do not necessarily need to be parallel if some small angulation is necessary due to the anatomy of the elbow and fracture pattern. The humeral arm of the fixator is aligned with the anterior cortex of the humerus.

The hinged external fixator is provisionally put on for reduction, and then all hinges are tightened to the company's instructions. Some external fixator systems have several links, to allow movement of the device with respect to the axis-of-rotation pin. These additional links create different degrees of freedom so that valgus/varus or translation can be adjusted. These adjustments can be made after viewing an anteroposterior (AP) radiograph or fluoroscopic image to determine proper alignment. Once the devices are tightened, the surgeon can move the patient's elbow through a controlled range of motion under fluroroscopy to ensure that the device is centered. While putting the elbow through a range of motion, the surgeon notes whether the joint is concentric or eccentric and whether adjustments to the external fixator could be made. Caution should be used when placing pins to make sure neurovascular structures are protected. Also, to prevent iatrogenic fracture, pins should be placed centrally in the humerus and ulna, and not unicortically or through the thin cortical outer rim of bone (**Table 26.3**).

Various external fixator devices have been developed that can be used in the elbow. The Dynamic Joint Distractor II by Stryker Howmedica Osteonics (Mahwah, NJ) is a low-profile uniplanar hinged external fixator. This allows use of the Hoffman II Compact external fixation system, which is available in most hospitals. This system also allows for unilateral or bilateral application of the external fixation device. The Synthes Arm hinge also allows for combination with the large external fixator system that is readily available. This device is convenient to use and has a low profile.

Devices designed specifically for the elbow joint can also be used (Tan et al. 2005). The Orthofix by Intavent Orthofix Ltd (Berkshire, UK) is a unilateral uniplanar hinged external fixation system. This joint-specific system is less bulky and has fewer modular elements than general fixator devices. Because this system was designed for the elbow, a large degree of rotation and angulation is allowed for satisfactory pin placement. This system requires adequate knowledge of the device by the surgeon and manufacturer representative, to ensure appropriate placement.

Another system developed specifically for the elbow joint is the OptiROM, by Biomet EBI (Parsippany, NJ). This fixator can be placed radiographically along the fixation axis and therefore avoids additional pin placement along the axis of rotation. This is especially important when placing the hinged external fixator for additional stability after placement of internal fixation, such as suture anchors or screws.

The Compass hinge by Smith and Nephew (Memphis, TN) is a multiplanar external fixation system. This fixator is versatile, but it is technically demanding to apply. The manufacturer representative and surgeon should be well versed in placement of the device. Advantages of this device include a radiolucent frame, provision for valgus/varus alignment for stability, and a gear mechanism that allows for passive range of motion as well as the expected active range of motion. An important potential disadvantage is the bulk of the frame, which may lead to soft-tissue problems in the extremity or along the torso.

Table 26.3 External fixator technique

Issue to be addressed	Technique/factors to consider
Axis of rotation	Center of rotation lies at the center of the capitellum and trochlear spool Axis is parallel to joint and seen on radiographs
Placement of external fixation	Lateral humeral pins usually used, spread to bone to protect neurovascular structures, especially radial nerve When placing medial humeral pins, protect ulnar nerve when going medially Place pins bicortically to prevent iatrogenic fractures
Decision regarding uniplanar versus multiplanar	Uniplanar advantages: stabilityUniplanar disadvantages: potential for contracture Multiplanar advantages: joint motion Multiplanar disadvantages: ulnar nerve irritation

Illustrative case

A patient presented after a trauma that resulted in an elbow transolecranon fracture dislocation. Although not apparent in the films, this patient had both bony and ligamentous damage to the elbow (**Fig. 26.2**), and therefore an external fixator was placed to help with stability after placement of the internal fixation and to aid in holding of the elbow in a concentric position while the bone healed (**Figs 26.3, 26.4**). Placing the fixator up against the normal elbow to set at the proper length and position prior to affixing may be helpful in such cases (**Fig. 26.5**). The fixator offloads the stress on the internal fixation. Placement of the hinged external fixator also allowed healing of the ligamentous structures that were injured during the initial trauma and primarily repaired (medial and lateral collateral ligamentous complexes). Despite anatomic repair of the fractures and ligaments, the elbow remained unstable intraoperatively. The adjunctive use of the elbow fixator rendered a stable elbow at final follow-up, with a functional arc of motion of 20–140° extension to flexion (**Fig. 26.6**).

Placement of the external fixator can also be used in those patients who would not be stable in a sling due to a large midsection body habitus (**Figs 26.7, 26.8**). This patient was treated solely with a hinged external fixator for a complex terrible triad injury that had failed prior attempts

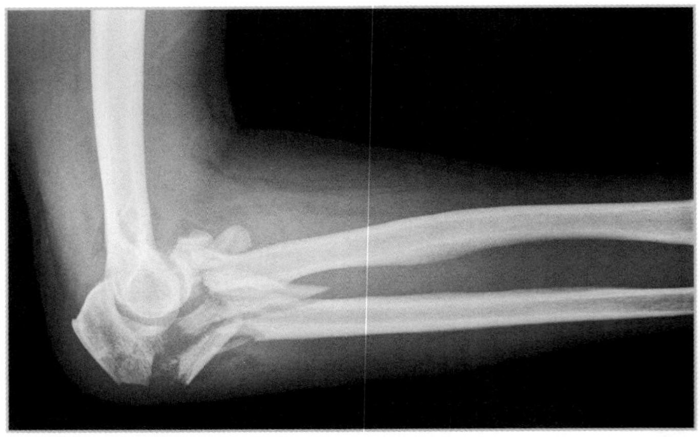

Figure 26.2 Lateral radiograph of the initial injury. Transolecranon fracture dislocation with comminuted proximal ulna, coronoid, and radial head.

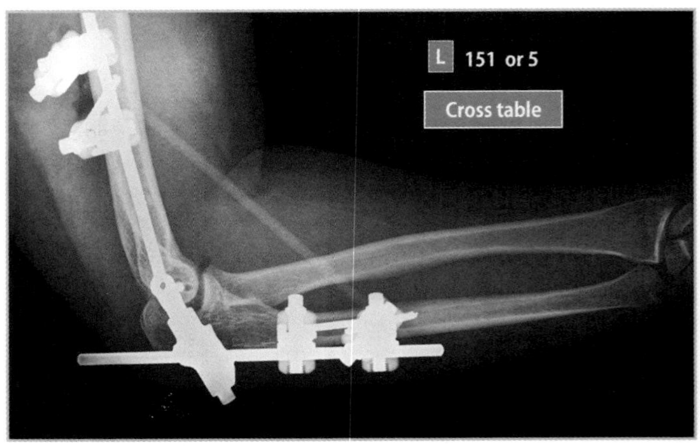

Figure 26.3 External fixator measured against contralateral elbow to set alignment for injured elbow.

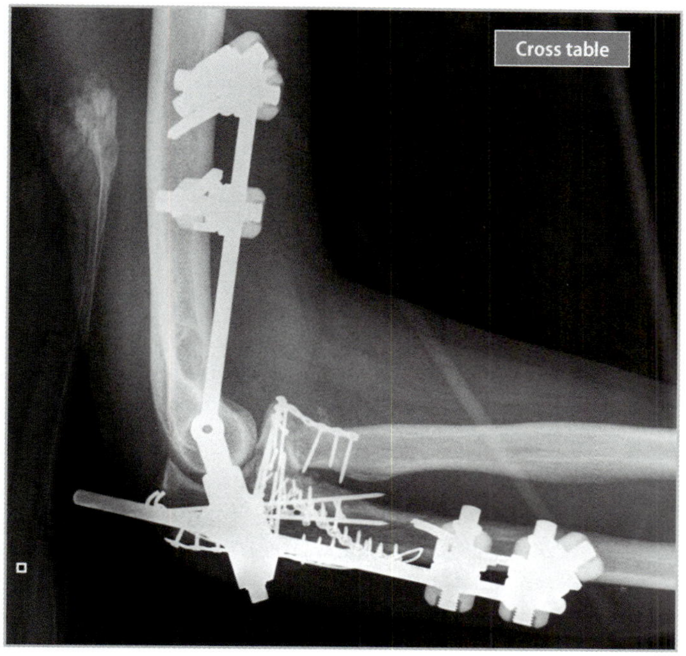

Figure 26.4 External fixator applied after open reduction and internal fixation of the radial head, coronoid, and proximal ulna.

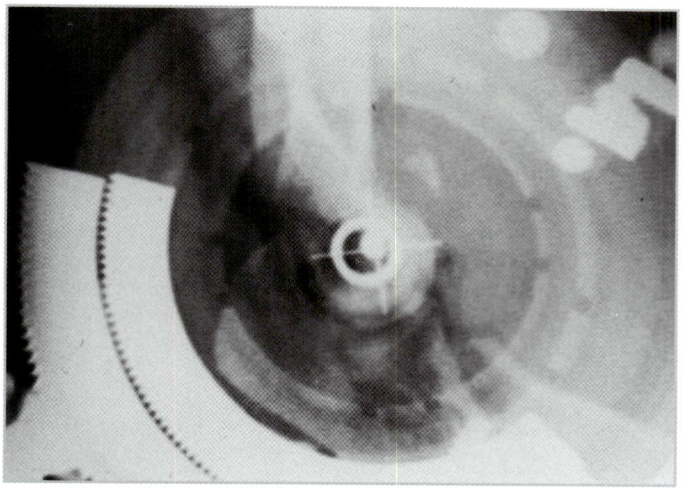

Figure 26.5 Intraoperative lateral fluoroscopy image of hinged external fixator placed over joint to help set alignment.

at surgical reconstruction. The arc of motion with the hinged external fixator allowed early range of motion and upon removal of the fixator at eight weeks provided a stable construct without further intervention.

Pearls and pitfalls

When placing fixator pins caution is needed to ensure that neurovascular structures are protected. Pins should be placed centrally in the humerus and ulna and not unicortically or through the thin cortical outer rim of bone, to prevent iatrogenic fracture. When using a hinged external fixator, a complete fluoroscopic evaluation must be performed to ensure a stable, concentric arc of motion with ulnohumeral joint line

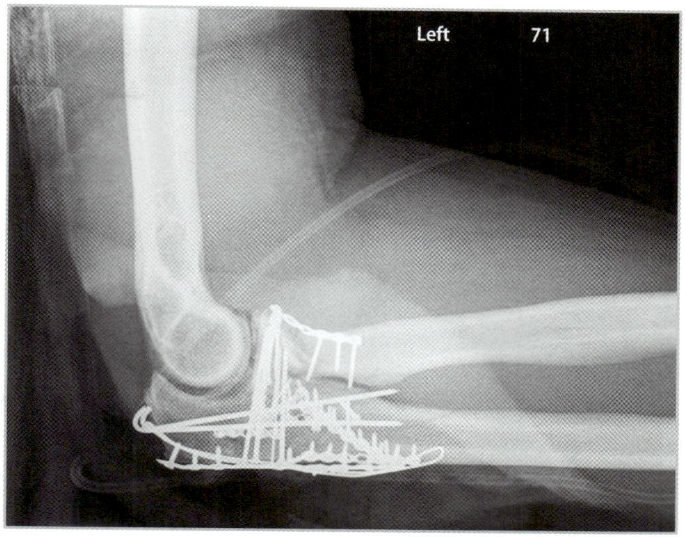

Figure 26.6 Lateral radiograph at one-year follow-up showing congruent elbow joint and healed fractures.

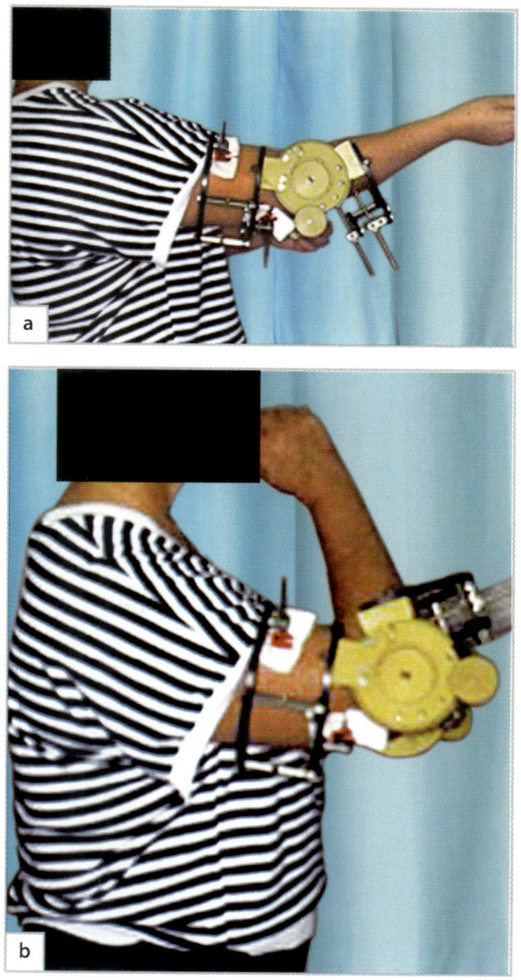

Figure 26.7 Postoperative clinical photographs. (a) Extension of elbow joint with hinged external fixator. (b) Flexion of elbow joint with hinged external fixator.

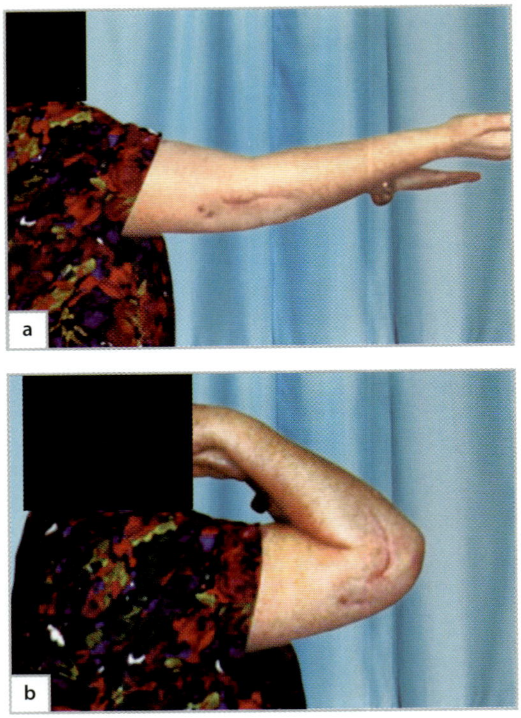

Figure 26.8 Follow-up clinical photographs. (a) Maintenance of elbow extension after removal of hinged external fixator. (b) Maintenance of elbow flexion after removal of hinged external fixator

congruence on both the lateral and anteroposterior views. If there is a question of instability or malalignment, then the fixator must be readjusted or placed in a static mode if this renders the joint concentric.

Axis of rotation

- On the medial aspect of the elbow, the axis is slightly anterior and inferior to the medial epicondyle.
- On the lateral aspect, the axis lies just distal to the lateral epicondyle.

- The pin is driven parallel to the joint line as seen on anteroposterior fluoroscopy view.
- Tissues should always be spread down to bone prior to placement of fixator pins, to protect neurovascular structures. Irrigation while drilling will prevent bone necrosis.

Uniplanar versus multiplanar system

- The decision whether to use a uniplanar or a multiplanar system has to weigh stability against joint motion.

Rehabilitation

- Pin-tract care is crucial.
- Motion (with a hinged fixator) should be started as soon as the patient is comfortable and able to perform active assisted stable motion exercises.

REHABILITATION

Rehabilitation of the elbow joint once the hinged external fixator device is placed is personalized for each patient. It is not possible to specify the details of a program because the indications for placing these devices are so varied. All patients should be assessed for neurovascular competence. Traditionally, acute elbow dislocations are moved sooner than elbows with chronic instability. Close follow-up of the patient's instability and concentricity of the joint is required as a controlled increase of the range of motion is allowed. Extension blocks are available to provide motion stops if there is concern about instability with too much motion. Physiotherapy can be used to increase active range of motion in a controlled manner, and the patient is encouraged to begin passive range of motion soon after surgery.

Movement of the elbow joint and removal of the external fixation device are dictated by the injury as well as the surgeon. Removal of the external fixator is done when there is adequate healing of the bony and ligamentous elements of the original injury. Healing can be determined by bony healing in serial radiographs, a decrease in pain, and the ability of the patient to use the elbow joint. Traditionally, the external fixator is removed approximately three weeks after a surgery for stiffness and six weeks after surgery for fracture.

FURTHER READING

Marsh JL, Phistkul P. Hinged external fixators in elbow reconstruction. In: Yamaguchi K, King GJW, McKee MD, O'Driscoll SWM (eds). Advanced Reconstruction Elbow. Rosemont, IL: AAOS, 2007: 393–402.

Morrey BF, Hotchkiss RN. External fixators of the elbow. In: Morrey BF (ed.). The Elbow and Its Disorders, 3rd edn. Philadelphia, PA: WB Saunders, 2000: 457–467.

Morrey BF, Hotchkiss RN. Articulated external fixators. In: Morrey BF (ed.). Master Techniques in Orthopaedic Surgery: The Elbow, 2nd edn. Philadelphia, PA: Lippincott, Williams & Wilkins, 2002: 139–160.

REFERENCES

Chen NC, Julka A. Hinged external fixation of the elbow. Hand Clin 2010;26:423–433.

Jupiter JB, Ring D. Treatment of unreduced elbow dislocations with hinged external fixation. J Bone Joint Surg Am 2002;84:1630–1635.

McKee MD, Bowden SH, King GJ, et al. Management of recurrent, complex instability of the elbow with a hinged external fixator. J Bone Joint Surg Br 1998;80:1031–1036.

O'Driscoll SW, Jupiter JB, Cohen MS, et al. Difficult elbow fractures: pearls and pitfalls. Instruct Course Lect 2003;52:113–134.

Ring D, Hannouche D, Jupiter JB. Surgical treatment of persistent dislocation or subluxation of the ulnohumeral joint after fracture-dislocation of the elbow. J Hand Surg Am 2004;29:470–480.

Ruch DS, Triepel CR. Hinged elbow fixation for recurrent instability following fracture dislocation. Injury 2001;32 Suppl 4:SD70–78.

Sotereanos DG, Darlis NA, Wright TW, et al. Unstable fracture-dislocations of the elbow. Instruct Course Lect 2007;56:369–376.

Tan V, Daluiski A, Capo J, Hotchkiss R. Hinged elbow external fixators: indications and uses. J Am Acad Orthop Surg 2005;13:503–514.

Tashjian RZ, Katarincic JA. Complex elbow instability. J Am Acad Orthop Surg 2006;14:278–286.

Chapter 27 Reconstruction of non-unions of the distal humerus

Marco Vennettilli, Graham J. W. King

INDICATIONS AND CONTRAINDICATIONS

The indications to proceed with reconstruction depend on the presence of bony fragments of sufficient size and quality to accept fixation. Synovial pseudarthrosis and peripheral sclerosis of the fracture fragments are not contraindications to open reduction and internal fixation. One of the most important factors when deciding to proceed with reconstruction is determining the patient's expectations for function.

Physiologic age also factors into the decision to proceed with reconstruction, insofar as it correlates with bone quality, functional demands, and the probability of a long-term satisfactory result with total elbow arthroplasty. However, physiologic age is used qualitatively, with no strict age criterion being used in the decision to proceed with open reduction and internal fixation or elbow arthroplasty.

Contraindications to attempted reconstruction are the lack of sufficient distal bone stock to accept fixation, significant joint arthrosis, osteoporosis, comminution, and active infection. Patients who are unable or unwilling to commit to a postoperative therapy program would also be a contraindication to undertaking reconstruction.

TECHNIQUE

The goals of reconstruction are anatomic restoration of the articular surface, compression at the supracondylar level, and fixation stable enough to allow for early motion. Capsular releases are often necessary to restore motion to the elbow joint and reduce excessive stresses on the internal fixation which occur with joint stiffness. Anterior subcutaneous ulnar nerve transposition is performed routinely with distal humeral reconstruction if not performed during the index procedure.

History

Non-union of the distal humerus typically presents with pain, stiffness, a sense of instability, and weakness. The clinician should seek to elicit a history of infection such as prolonged wound drainage, fevers, chills or malaise. It is also important to enquire about weakness, paresthesia or dysesthesia in the ulnar nerve distribution and to put these symptoms into context with the patient's functional limitations and expectations.

As with any revision surgery, the details of any previous procedure should be verified by obtaining the operative reports. Such reports are important to ensure the appropriate equipment is available for hardware removal, as screwdrivers, for example, often differ from system to system. The history should also document the functional disabilities in both vocations and avocations which are present as a result of the distal humeral non-union. Medical and surgical history (including medications and allergies), as well as social history, should also be obtained to evaluate the patient's suitability for revision surgery. The use of tobacco, alcohol or illicit drugs should also be elicited as they can influence the success of any reconstructive surgery. Excessive narcotic use should raise the suspicion of a chronic regional pain syndrome.

Physical examination

The physical examination should begin with an inspection for the number and location of surgical scars. The quality of skin and subcutaneous tissue should be noted, particularly over any bony or hardware prominence. Atrophy of the ulnar intrinsics of the affected limb should be noted. Fluctuance may be noted with a very mobile non-union; however, warmth or erythema would raise more concern about infection. The neurovascular examination should include testing for weakness of the ulnar intrinsic hand muscles, gross sensory changes, and two-point discrimination in the distributions of the radial, ulnar, and median nerves.

When assessing for range of motion it is important to note that significant mobility can occur at the site of non-union (**Fig. 27.1a–c**). An attempt should be made to determine the degree of mobility at the non-union site versus the elbow joint itself; however, this is often difficult without the assistance of fluoroscopy. Stiffness of the shoulder and hand should be evaluated, as it can affect positioning at surgery, as well as the functional outcome. Skin and vasomotor changes should be evaluated to identify evidence of a complex regional pain syndrome. A general physical examination should be completed to ensure the patient is medically suitable for surgical reconstruction.

Investigations

Imaging is essential when planning surgery. Orthogonal and oblique radiographs are helpful to assess the size of the distal fragments in an effort to determine whether or not reconstruction is possible. Radiographic interpretation of the size of the distal fragments can be affected by rotation (Jupiter 2008). This potential error should be considered when deciding between open reduction and internal fixation, or arthroplasty. Computerized tomography is routinely obtained preoperatively to evaluate the size and quality of the fragments, even in the presence of residual hardware. Minimum requirements for a successful reconstruction are the presence of both the medial and lateral aspects of the trochlea, or the presence of the medial trochlea and the capitellum (Sabo 2010). The medial and lateral epicondyles with their attached collateral ligaments are also necessary for a stable elbow.

Blood tests are obtained (including complete blood count, erythrocyte sedimentation rate, and C-reactive protein). Joint aspiration is not routinely performed unless there are concerns based on history, physical examination, radiographs, or blood tests. Intraoperative samples are routinely sent for culture. Frozen sections to identify white blood cells are also helpful to diagnose infection. Patients are given postoperative antibiotics covering Gram-positive organisms until the culture results are available.

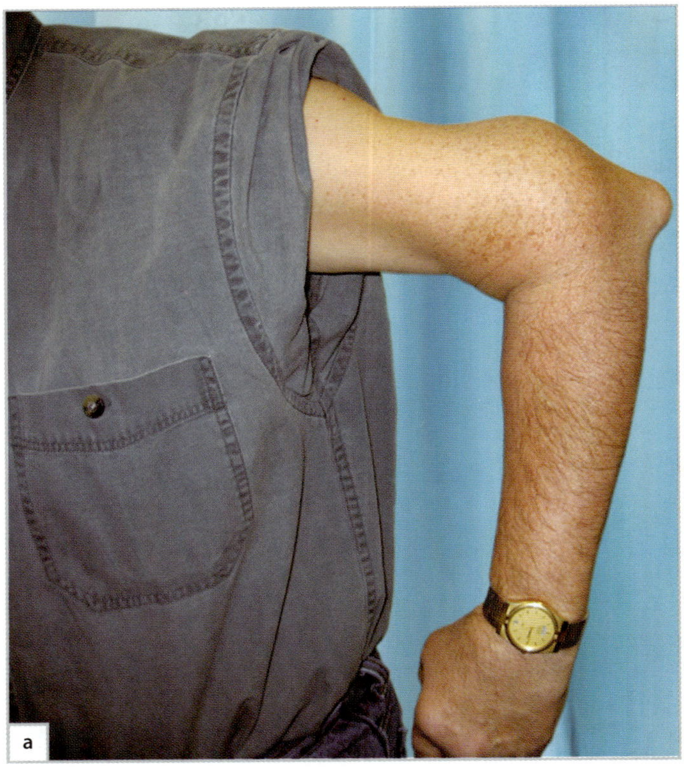

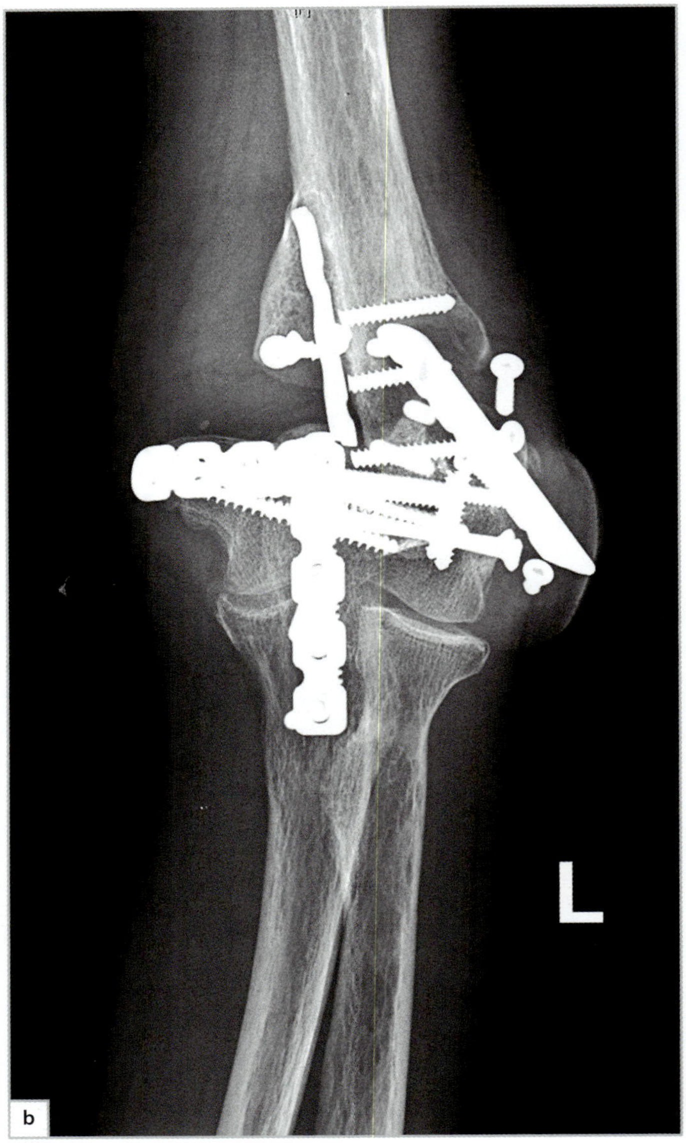

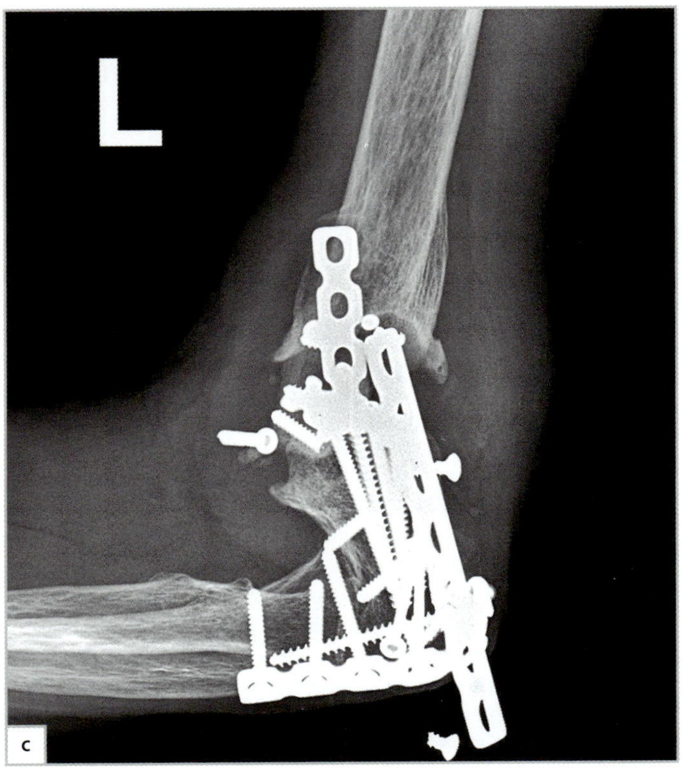

Figure 27.1 Chronic mobile non-union. *(Contd)*

Electrical studies are performed to document the function of peripheral nerves if the history or physical examination suggests neurologic deficits. Ultrasound can be used to document the location of the ulnar nerve and any compression, and magnetic resonance imaging can be useful to evaluate the ulnar nerve, bone vascularity, and possible infection in the absence of hardware.

Surgical reconstruction

The patient is positioned in the supine, prone or lateral decubitus position, under regional or general anesthesia. If the supine position is used, an assistant or robotic arm-holder is required to stabilize the arm during surgery. If the prone or lateral decubitus position is used,

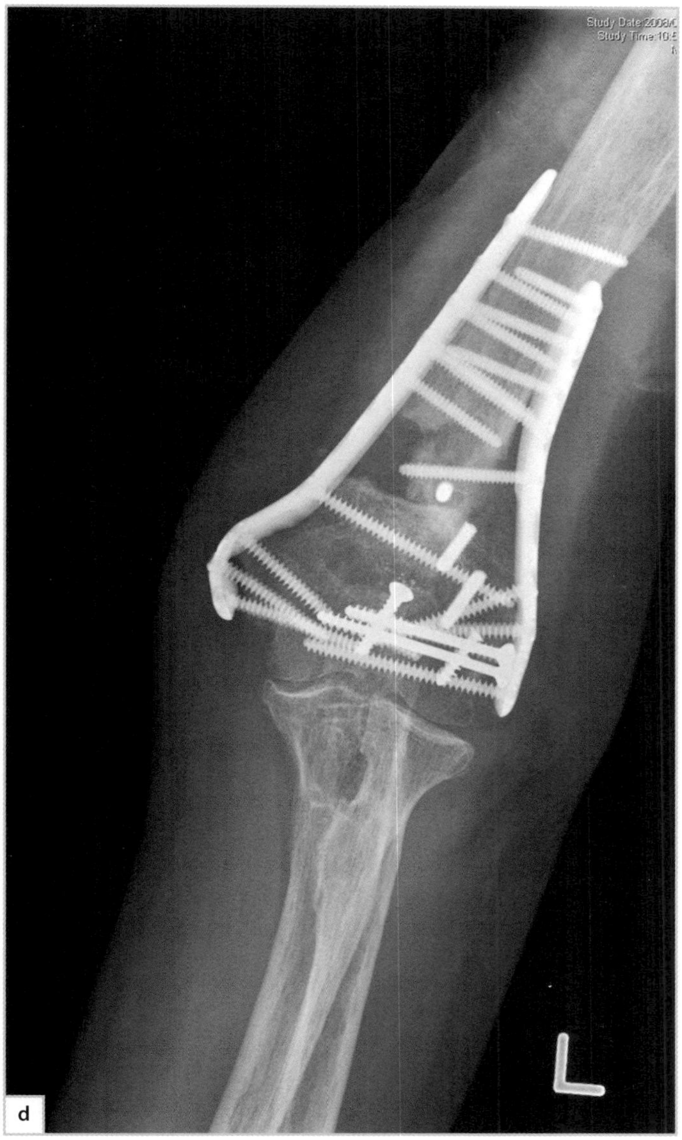

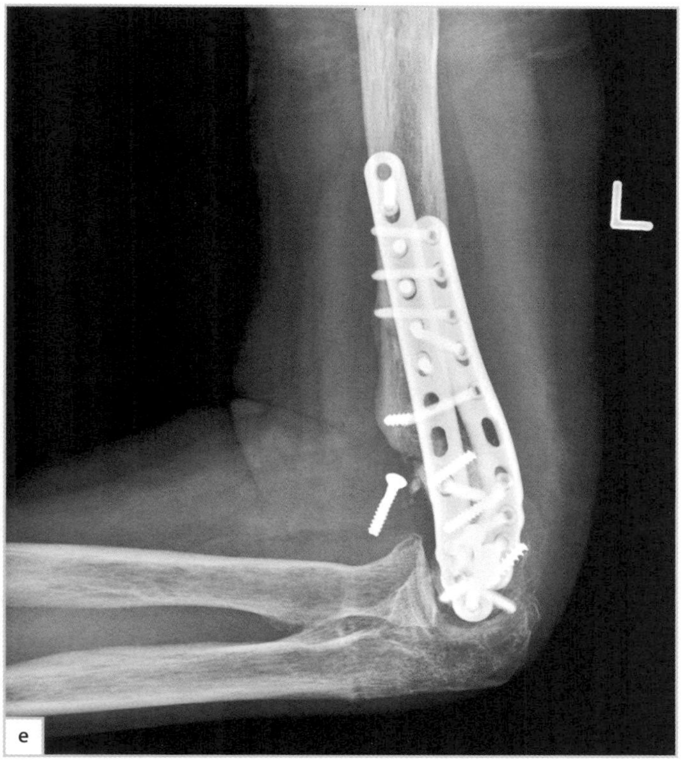

Figure 27.1 Chronic mobile non-union. ***(Contd)***

care should be taken to pad all bony prominences; the arm is then placed on a well padded support. These positions all give excellent access to the humerus, as well as to the ipsilateral or contralateral iliac crest for bone graft harvest. A sterile tourniquet is used in all cases, to maximize the humeral exposure.

Previous skin incisions are used where possible. A posterior midline incision just medial to the tip of the olecranon is preferred, as it affords adequate exposure of both the medial and the lateral columns. The incision is extensile and allows for identification of the ulnar nerve, for either transposition or neurolysis, depending on the nerve's location following previous surgery. Identification of the ulnar nerve can be challenging in the presence of scar tissue. The safest place to locate the ulnar nerve is outside the zone of previous surgery in the proximal portion of the incision, at the medial border of the triceps, posterior to the intermuscular septum. It is then exposed from proximal to distal under loupe magnification, and neurolysis and transposition are completed if the patient has ulnar nerve symptoms preoperatively. If the nerve was not transposed during the previous surgery, a subcutaneous transposition is performed at this time. If the nerve has been previously transposed it still must be identified and followed, to avoid injury during surgery.

Deep exposure of the non-union is accomplished using a triceps-on, Alonso-Llames approach (Alonso-Llames 1972) if the non-union is extra-articular. The fascia lateral to the triceps is incised to expose the lateral column and hardware. If lateral dissection is required more than 10 cm proximal to the lateral epicondyle, the radial nerve is identified as it leaves the spiral groove and is protected during the remainder of the procedure. This exposure can be extended distally into a Boyd exposure, giving access to the olecranon for osteotomy if required. An olecranon osteotomy is preferred for all intra-articular non-unions. This algorithm can be followed whether or not an olecranon osteotomy had been used in a previous procedure. An olecranon osteotomy should be avoided if an intraoperative conversion to an elbow arthroplasty is a possibility; the triceps should be left on or detached as a triceps-splitting or triceps-peel approach, as described by Bryan and Morrey (1982).

Debridement

Unlike with acute fractures, significant capsular contracture and intra-articular adhesions are to be expected. A posterior capsulectomy is performed as part of the approach to the non-union. Fibrous tissue

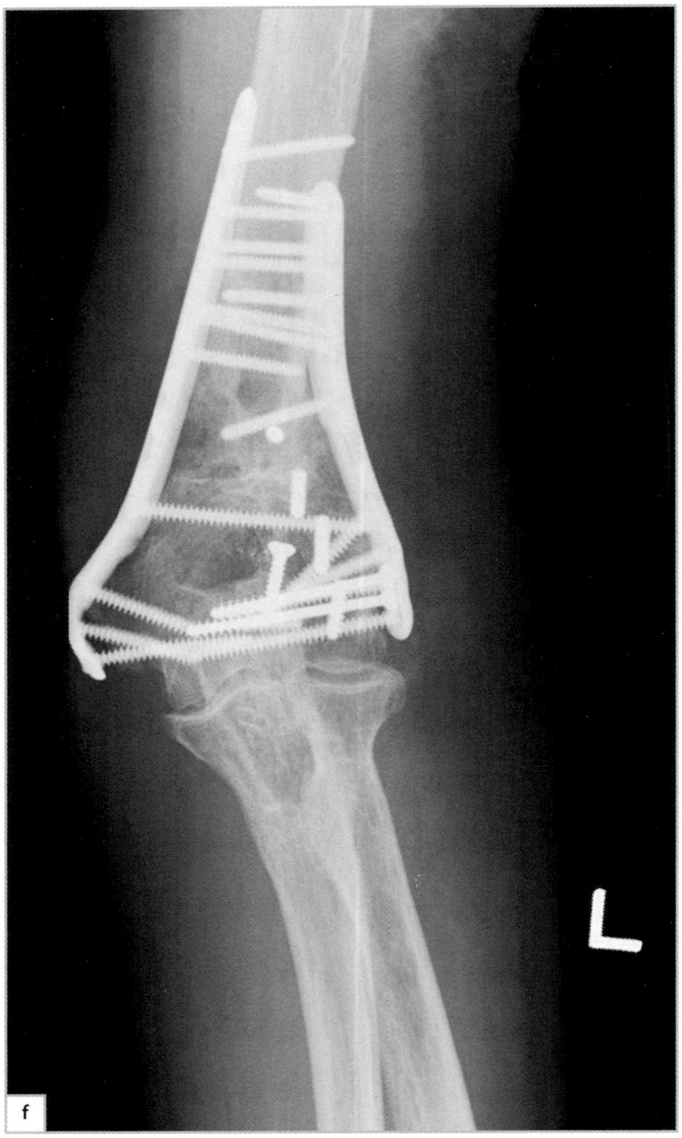

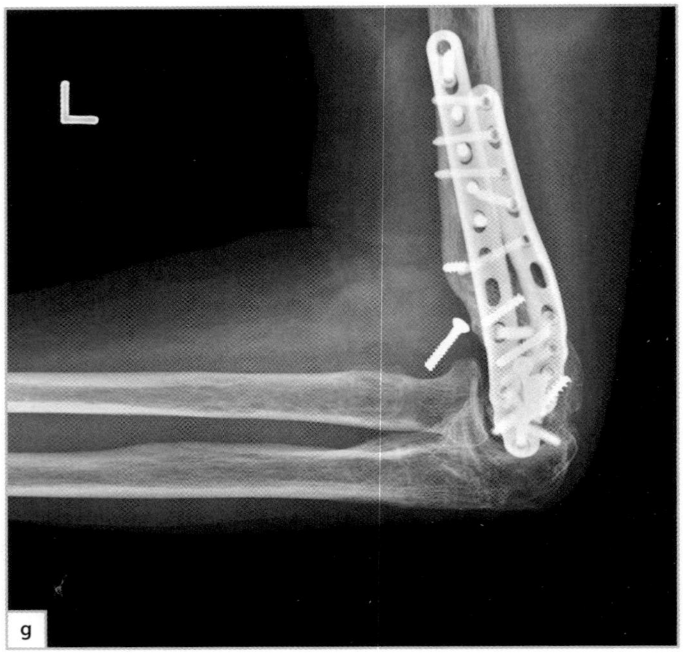

Figure 27.1 Chronic mobile non-union. (a) Clinical photograph of a large supracondylar deformity without accompanying erythema. Anteroposterior (b) and lateral (c) radiographs demonstrate failure and migration of the insufficient hardware, as well as cortical erosion. Postoperative anteroposterior (d) and lateral radiographs (e) demonstrate healing after revision to a parallel-plate construct with the use of corticocancellous autograft. Anteroposterior (f) and lateral (g) radiographs at one year demonstrate bony healing across the metaphyseal defect.

and any synovial pseudarthrosis are resected until viable bone is encountered at the non-union site. Rongeurs and curettes are preferred for debridement over motorized burrs. The tourniquet may be deflated to assess for bleeding bone surfaces as an indication of viability. If there is a partial ankylosis of the joint, care should be taken to carefully separate the articular surfaces to avoid shearing off the cartilage. The medullary canals of the fracture fragments are cannulated proximally with a 3.5 mm drill bit and distally with a 2 mm drill bit. Care should be taken to avoid detaching the collateral ligaments from the epicondyles during debridement.

Once the fracture fragments are mobilized, the anterior joint capsule can be released or excised by working anteriorly through the non-union site. The decision to perform a capsulectomy versus a release depends on the magnitude of the preoperative contracture and the amount of scar tissue present.

Fixation

Reconstitution of the articular surface should be performed first, using small wires for provisional fixation. A non-articulating corticocancellous autograft can be placed between the medial aspect of the trochlea and the capitellum to reconstitute the articular width of the distal humerus in the setting of intercondylar bone loss. It is important to maintain the integrity of the medial and lateral collateral ligaments and to provide secure fixation of the condyles, to maintain stability.

Once the articular surface has been reconstructed, it is important to achieve good bony contact and compression with the metaphysis using compression plating. Humeral shortening is achieved using an apex distal chevron osteotomy to improve cortical contact and mechanical stability (**Fig. 27.2e**). Humeral shortening is well tolerated up to 2 cm in the ambulatory population and carries the additional benefit of decreasing tension in the soft-tissue envelope. Biomechanical data have shown that significant loss of extension strength can begin with as little as 1 cm of shortening, which may be more significant for patients who require load-bearing through the arm for transfers (Hughes et al. 1997).

When lengthening of the humerus is required, this may be accomplished with structural or vascularized autograft. Non-vascularized corticocancellous autograft is the procedure of choice when the bone defect is 4 cm or less, in the absence of infection and with adequate

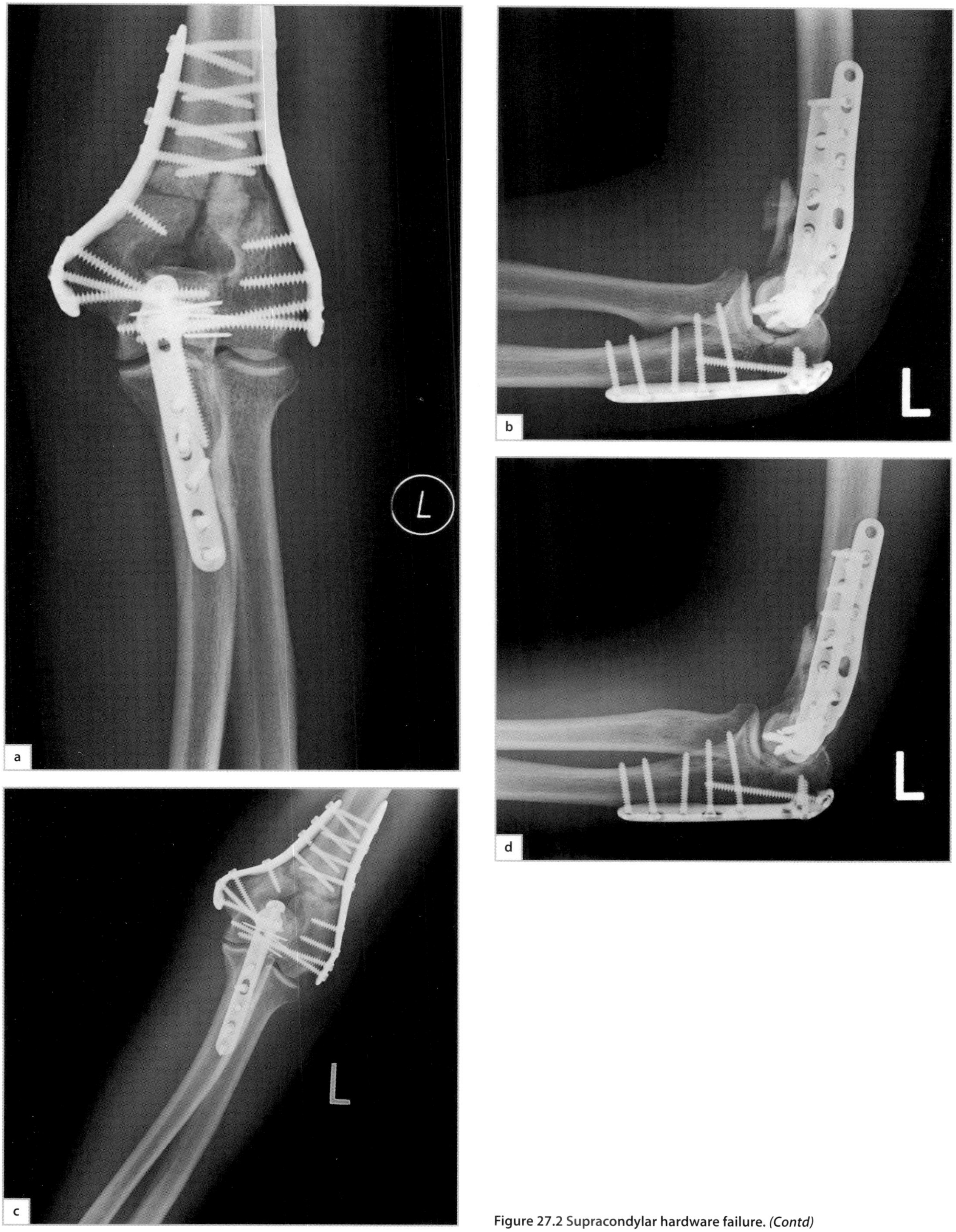

Figure 27.2 Supracondylar hardware failure. *(Contd)*

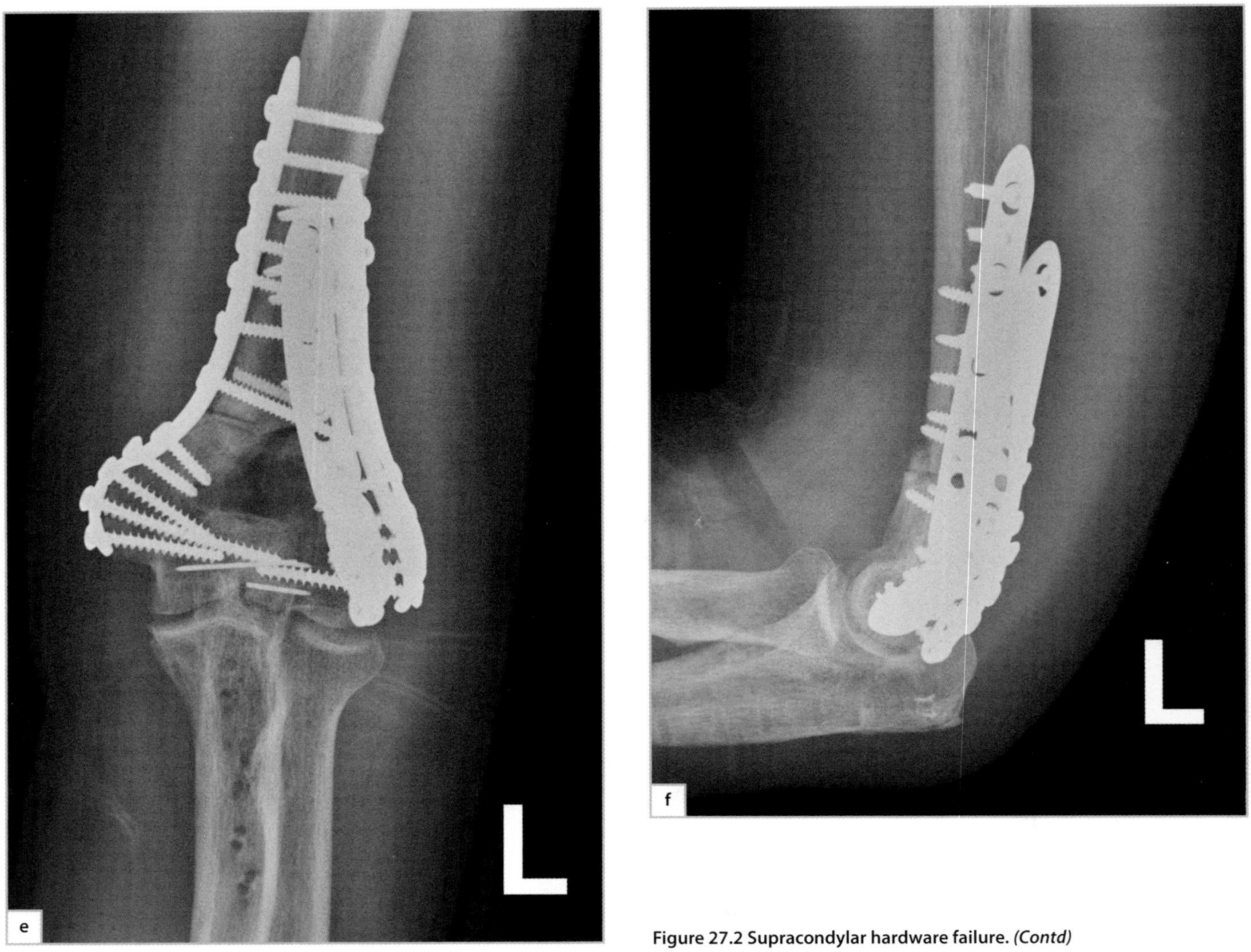

Figure 27.2 Supracondylar hardware failure. *(Contd)*

skin coverage (**Fig. 27.1d**). For recalcitrant non-unions, or when the previous conditions are not met, vascularized free tissue transfer is more appropriate (Beredjiklian et al. 2005). The fibula is the most common choice of graft to reconstruct either the medial or the lateral columns. Additional structural graft may be required from the iliac crest, depending on the nature of the metaphyseal defect.

Provisional fixation of the articular block to the humeral shaft is accomplished with stout smooth Kirschner wires (K-wires). It is critically important to ensure the articular block is correctly oriented in relation to the metaphysis. In addition to restoring the normal valgus carrying angle, fixation must occur in the correct rotational orientation and with the distal articular surface flexed approximately 30°, to allow for full elbow flexion and extension. Once the optimal position of the articular block on the metaphysis has been determined and provisional fixation achieved, the number and location of plates is assessed. While precontoured plates typically save time in the setting of acute fractures of the distal humerus, some contouring is often required when managing non-unions, because humeral shortening alters the normal shape of the bone. Strong, robust plates are required to reduce the incidence of hardware failure prior to fracture union. The plates are fixed to the articular block using cancellous screws as long as possible, to maximize purchase in the distal bone. Ideally, each screw should pass through a plate. Locking screws may be beneficial to augment fixation.

With the articular block reduced and internally fixed, attention can be turned to proximal fixation. The supracondylar interface will have been shaped to allow for coaptation of the articular block prior to application of the plates. If a structural bone graft is to be used it can be incorporated at this time. If a vascularized bone graft is to be used, space should be left for this so that microsurgical anastomosis can take place after internal fixation.

The steps to obtain compression and fixation at the supracondylar level are very similar. Fixation can begin either medially or laterally. When available, an oval plate hole is used for initial fixation, to give some stability while allowing further proximal translation to augment compression and stability. A large tenaculum is used to compress the non-union by placing one tine on the articular block and the opposing tine proximally on the metaphysis. In this orientation, the compression approaches a vector perpendicular to one side of the chevron interface. With compression applied, a screw can be placed proximally through the plate in dynamic compression mode. The tenaculum is removed and the process is repeated on the other column. The remainder of the proximal cortical screws can then be placed to complete the fixation. The goal is to achieve at least three screws proximal to the fracture site on both the medial and the lateral sides. The medial and lateral plates should end at different lengths, to lessen the effect of a stress riser. A third plate can also be applied, to improve fixation where necessary (**Fig. 27.2g,h**).

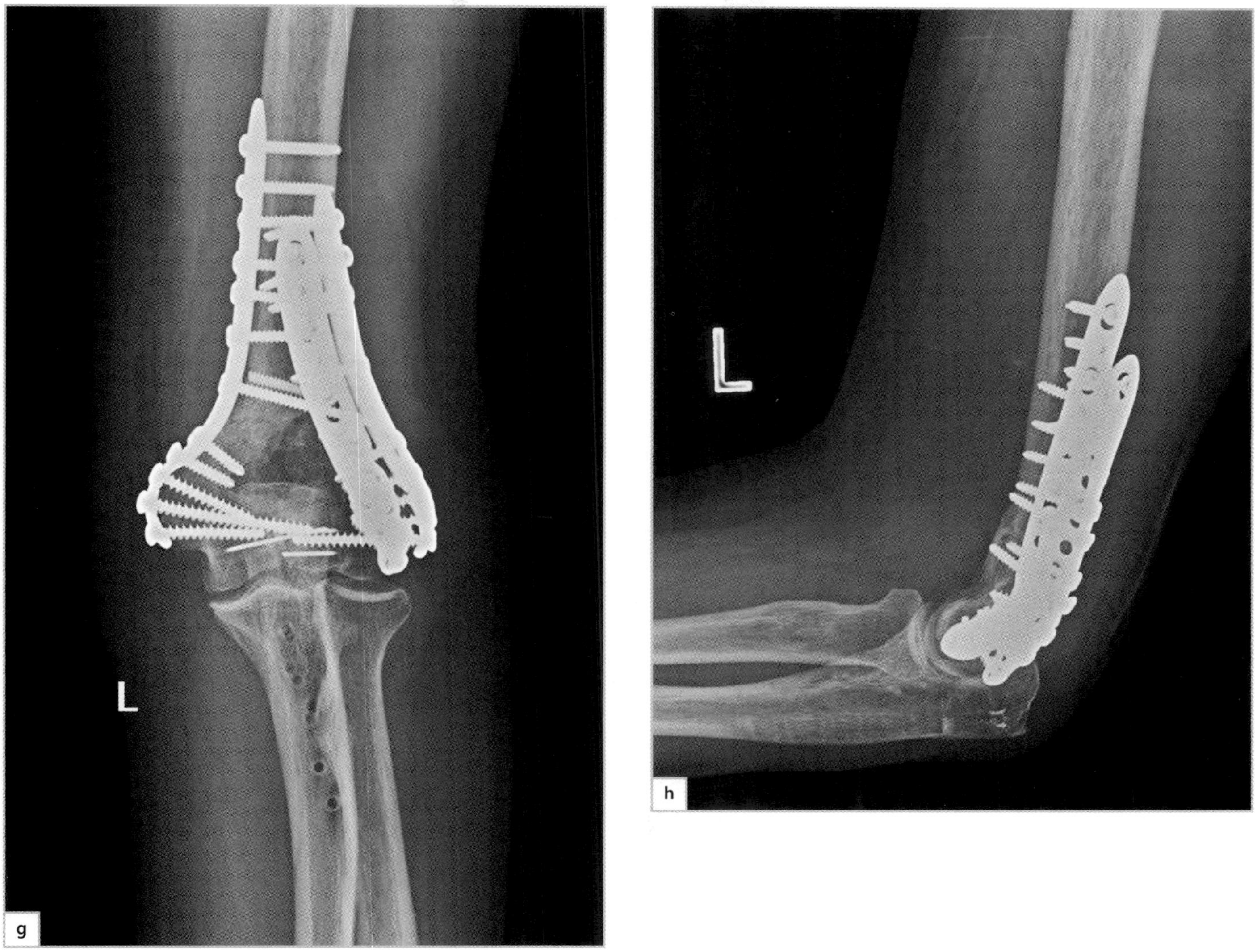

Figure 27.2 Supracondylar hardware failure. Anteroposterior (a) and lateral (b) radiographs of a parallel-plate construct used to reconstruct a comminuted intra-articular and extra-articular open fracture of the distal humerus. (c,d) Failure of the proximal screws is noted at four-month follow-up. Anteroposterior (e) and lateral (f) postoperative radiographs following a chevron osteotomy through the metaphysis to allow compression after removal of non-viable bone. The osteotomy site is visible on the anteroposterior radiograph. Due to an elevated erythrocyte sedimentation rate as well as inflammation noted at the time of debridement, the patient was placed on intravenous antibiotics for six weeks, in spite of negative cultures. Anteroposterior (g) and lateral (h) radiographs demonstrate healing at the osteotomy site one year postoperatively.

After removal of any temporary fixation the range of motion is tested. This allows for the assessment of crepitus as well as bony or hardware impingement. With shortening or reconstruction of the metaphysis, there is a loss of the normal contour of the coronoid and olecranon fossae. If bony impingement limits full range of motion, resection of the olecranon and coronoid tips can be helpful. The recreation of fossae will also improve motion and relieve impingement. This may be performed at the initial procedure or at a subsequent procedure once the graft has been incorporated.

Type of fixation

While the treatment of distal humeral non-unions using fine-wire circular external fixation has been reported (Ilizarov 1991), most surgeons prefer to use internal fixation. Plate fixation provides maximal stability and allows for early range of motion. Precontoured plates specific to the distal humerus are available, offering both compression and fixed-angle options. Unfortunately, some contouring of these plates is commonly required in the setting of non-unions, as humeral shortening and residual callus lead to a non-anatomic shape of the distal humerus. Fixed-angle screws can be used to improve fixation in osteoporotic bone. In the absence of precontoured elbow plates, surgeon-contoured 3.5 mm dynamic compression plates can provide adequate fixation. Contoured pelvic reconstruction plates have been used with success for the management of acute fractures of the distal humerus but more robust plates are preferred in the setting of non-unions. One third of tubular plates are weak and therefore not recommended for this application, as are compression screws or tension-band constructs in isolation.

The choice of parallel or orthogonal plate configurations is based on the geometry of the fracture. Both plate configurations have advantages and neither has been demonstrated to be clinically superior in a randomized trial. Parallel plating offers the advantage of bi-column purchase with each of the distal screws. When considered in isolation, an orthogonal plate configuration is biomechanically stronger than a parallel configuration. However, when fracture fragments and the plates are considered together as a fixation construct, the quality of the screw purchase has a significant effect on construct stability (Schuster et al. 2008, Windolf et al. 2010) (**Fig. 27.3e,f**). For this reason, parallel-plate constructs can provide equivalent or better stability (Zalavras 2011). When distal comminution is present, or when fractures in the coronal plane are being addressed, placing the lateral column plate posteriorly can be advantageous. If necessary, two lateral column plates, one posteriorly and one laterally, can be used to ensure stability and maximize the potential for healing (**Fig. 27.2g,h**). The issue of avascular necrosis with extensive lateral column dissection does not seem to be a significant concern in the adult patient; however, detachment of the lateral collateral ligament has been reported (Lu et al. 2010). Based on published series, the greater concern with non-union of the distal humerus appears to be a lack of stability (Mitsunaga 1982, Ackerman and Jupiter 1988, Helfet et al. 2003, Jupiter 2008). The most frequent site of non-union has consistently been reported to be the supracondylar level in cases of metaphyseal and articular involvement (**Fig. 27.2c**). This has been attributed to the combination of stresses placed on this region by motion of the elbow and inadequate stability of fixation constructs. With adequate stability there have been high rates of union reported with revision surgery at both the supracondylar and the intra-articular levels (Mitsunaga et al. 1982, Ring et al. 2006).

Pearls and pitfalls

Pearls

- Ensure there are bleeding bone surfaces after the debridement to improve the probability of union. Deflating the tourniquet will help in this very important assessment.
- Good bone contact and compression are needed. With adequate debridement, there will likely be a mismatch in shape between fracture fragments. Once articular congruity has been achieved, the apposition of cancellous surfaces should be optimized in order to maximize healing potential and allow for compression. A chevron osteotomy is a reliable way to maximize to bony contact and to allow for compression at the supracondylar level (**Fig. 27.2e,f**).
- Remove coronoid and olecranon tips. This improves elbow motion if the olecranon and coronoid fossae are compromised by hardware placement, fragment debridement, or humeral shortening. Excessive removal of the articular surface should be avoided, as this can result in elbow instability and can detach the brachialis and triceps insertions.
- Recreate the coronoid and olecranon fossae. In the setting of humeral shortening, deepening the fossae with a burr will often be necessary to allow for adequate motion.
- Autogenous bone graft is recommended. The use of cancellous autograft harvested from the iliac crest is standard in distal humeral non-union surgery. Consideration is given to corticocancellous or vacularized grafts where there has been significant loss of supracondylar bone.

Pitfalls

- Failure to consider the possibility of infection. Revision fixation and bone grafting in the setting of infection will likely result in recurrent failure. The appropriate preoperative investigations and intraoperative cultures are recommended. When in doubt, the reconstruction should be staged.
- Inadequate fixation. Parallel plating is preferred in the setting of low distal humeral non-unions, due to the improved fixation achieved in the distal fragments. There should be no hesitation to add a third posterior plate when necessary.
- Failure to identify and transpose the ulnar nerve. Anterior transposition is performed routinely for distal humeral non-unions. This is both to protect the nerve during surgery as well as to avoid compression from fracture callous and scar tissue that will occur in the vicinity of the hardware.
- Excessive distal soft-tissue stripping. Elbow instability as a consequence of detaching the humeral origins of the collateral ligaments precludes a good clinical result. Lateral plates should be placed on top of the lateral ligament origin on the lateral epicondyle (Lu et al. 2010). Dissection anteriorly on the medial epicondyle should be avoided while placing medial plates. Soft-tissue stripping may also predispose to the development of avascular necrosis of the articular segment.

ALTERNATIVES TO RECONSTRUCTION

It is not always possible to determine the feasibility of reconstruction prior to exposing the fracture. While it would be beyond the scope of this chapter to discuss all possible alternatives to reconstruction, they should be discussed briefly, for completeness. Prior to a reconstructive procedure, the surgeon should have a plan for dealing with infection, and have considered the alternatives of total elbow arthroplasty, distal humeral allograft, resection arthroplasty, and arthrodesis.

In the case of infection, whether discovered preoperatively or intraoperatively, a thorough irrigation and debridement are required, with intraoperative cultures obtained prior to antibiotic treatment. Immobilization is achieved with either an external splint or a static external fixator; a postoperative antibiotic regimen is instituted, adequate for the organisms cultured. Antibiotic-impregnated spacers can be helpful to fill dead space and elute a high local concentration of antibiotics. Thin-wire external fixation of infected or comminuted fractures has been described (Ring et al. 1999). This technique has the advantage of allowing for elbow joint motion while stabilizing the fracture. This is a viable alternative for those familiar with the application and perioperative care of these devices.

Conversion to a total elbow arthroplasty is the most frequent alternative to reconstruction of distal humeral non-unions in the elderly (see Chapter 28). For the purposes of this chapter, it is worth reiterating that an olecranon osteotomy should be avoided to expose the non-union if an elbow arthroplasty is being considered. While the presence of an olecranon osteotomy does not preclude a total elbow arthroplasty, it does complicate the procedure.

In the young patient with greater functional expectations than an arthroplasty would permit, a distal humeral allograft may be considered. This procedure is most commonly reserved for reconstruction after removal of a tumor; however, it has been described in the post-traumatic scenario (Breen et al. 1988, Dean et al. 1997). Humeral allografts are associated with a significant rate of complication, including infection, resorption, and non-union. In the largest reported series, 16 of 23 allografts remained viable after an average of eight years of follow-up (Breen et al. 1988).

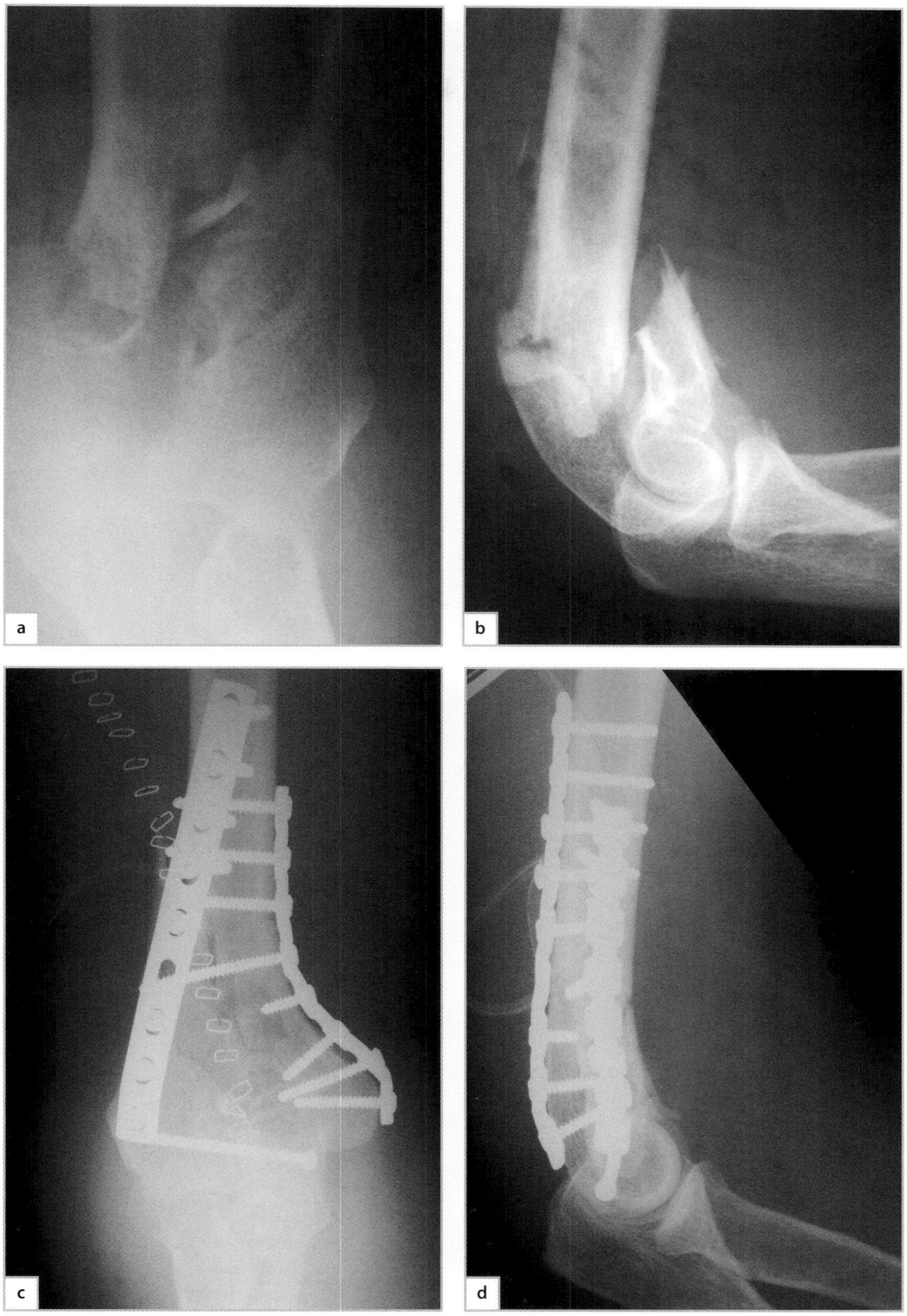

Figure 27.3 Failure of distal fixation. ***(Contd)***

The medically frail, low-demand patient may benefit from resection arthroplasty, particularly in the setting of a previous infection, which makes failure of a total elbow arthroplasty more likely. The goal of this procedure is a passively mobile joint with minimal pain and function of the hand with the arm at the side.

Arthrodesis is a rarely used option in the elbow joint. While it provides greater stability and the potential for loading through the elbow joint, the decreased range of motion of the upper arm is extremely limiting. When performed electively for bone loss, a trial of cast immobilization should be considered prior to a fusion. This option is not recommended without lengthy patient discussion. Preservation of the triceps mechanism is important, as it allows conversion to an elbow arthroplasty when the patient is older.

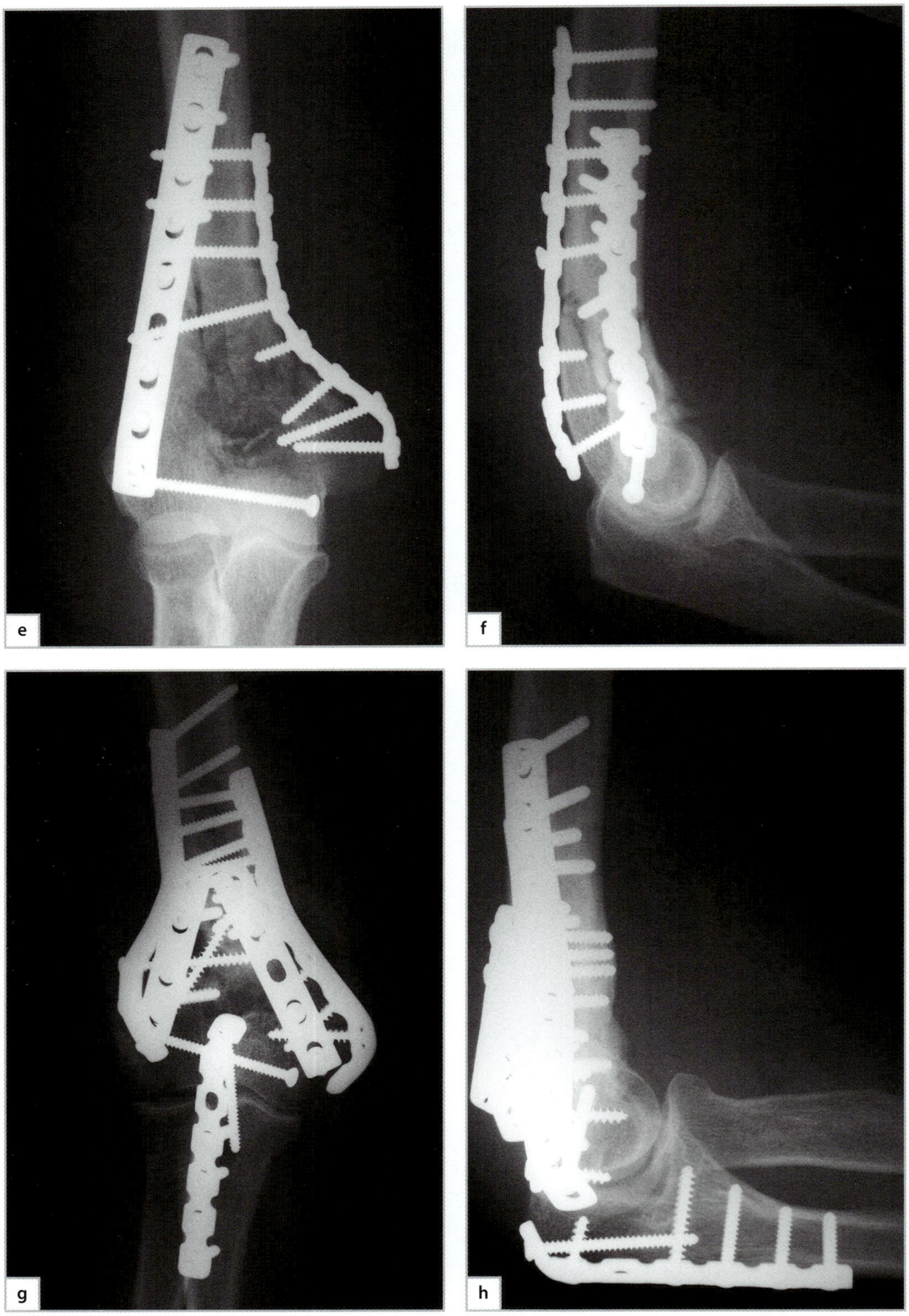

Figure 27.3 Failure of distal fixation. Anteroposterior (a) and lateral (b) radiographs of comminuted intra-articular open fracture. (c,d) Initial fixation with a posterolateral 3.5 mm low-contact dynamic compression plate and a medial reconstruction plate. (e,f) Distal fixation failure was first noted at five-week follow-up, prompting the first of two revision procedures (open reduction and internal fixation). Anteroposterior (g) and lateral (h) radiographs obtained after the second revision procedure. Distal fixation was obtained with a four-plate construct,resulting in fracture union without evidence of avascular necrosis.

REHABILITATION

Active motion is initiated when the soft tissues are suitable. In the elderly it may be wise to delay mobilization for 10 days to allow for early soft-tissue healing. In most patients active and active assisted range of motion is initiated within 24–48 hours. Patients are fitted with a sling (collar and cuff style), to be worn between exercises during waking hours, as well as a thermoplastic anteriorly based extension splint, to be worn at night.

The patient is asked to flex and extend the elbow repeatedly, to the point of mild discomfort, every alternate hour throughout the day for approximately 30 minutes. The range of motion is reassessed weekly by a therapist. With increasing range of motion it is necessary to refashion the extension splint for night-time use (Chinchalkar and Szekeres 2004).

After radiographic signs of early healing, the sling is discontinued and passive stretching and static progressive splinting are implemented to improve motion if required. Computerized tomography scans using metal-reduction protocols can be helpful to evaluate healing, which may be difficult using plain radiographs in the presence of substantial hardware. Strengthening exercises are initiated to allow optimal return of function.

COMPLICATIONS

The most common complication of revision open reduction and internal fixation is prominent hardware (Mitsunaga 1982, Ackerman and Jupiter 1988, Helfet et al. 2003, Jupiter 2008). Some 20–30% of patients will experience discomfort significant enough to merit hardware removal. Lateral column plates and olecranon osteotomy plates tend to be the most problematic in this regard.

Other complications are related to radial or ulnar nerve palsy. Radial nerve palsy is typically caused by retraction and tends to recover; however, lateral plates can be inadvertently applied on top of the radial nerve if proximal exposure is inadequate. With subcutaneous transposition and neurolysis of the anterior ulnar nerve, permanent and severe nerve symptoms can be minimized; however, transient symptoms are common.

The average postoperative arc of motion has been reported to vary between 76° and 90°. The range of motion is not as great as that seen after primary procedures. Stiffness severe enough for patients to request surgical contracture release has been reported to occur in approximately 8% of patients with distal humeral non-unions. Static progressive splinting is preferred over manipulation under anesthesia, due to the risk of disrupting the fixation or causing a fracture. When operative intervention is required for improved range of motion, an open contracture release is typically preferred, due to the presence of hardware, the variable position of the nerves, and extensive scarring, which increases the risk of an arthroscopic release. An open contracture release can be combined with hardware removal if healing is complete. Post-traumatic arthritis can be expected with intra-articular fractures and non-unions and is likely related to the initial injury severity and the duration of non-union.

The incidence of deep infection has been reported to be as low as 4% in the setting of open reduction and internal fixation for distal humeral non-union. This low rate is likely reflective of a prudent concern for this complication preoperatively. Preoperative testing for inflammatory markers, aspiration for culture where indicated, prophylactic antibiotics, meticulous debridement, rigid stability, and planning for adequate soft-tissue coverage are all of great importance in revision elbow surgery. Any concern regarding the quality of the soft-tissue envelope should be addressed with a preoperative plastic surgery consultation. Risk factors for infection include high-energy open injuries, a history of infection or wound breakdown, and multiple previous operations.

With careful patient selection, meticulous fixation technique, and early elbow motion, persistent non-union is uncommon. Successful union has been reported for over 90% of patients, and as many as 98% in specialist centers.

REFERENCES

Ackerman G, Jupiter JB. Non-union of fractures of the distal end of the humerus. J Bone Joint Surg Am 1988;70:75–83.

Alonso-Llames M. Bilaterotricipital approach to the elbow. Its application in the osteosynthesis of supracondylar fractures of the humerus in children. Acta Orthop Scand 1972;43:479–490.

Beredjiklian PK, Hotchkiss RN, Athanasian EA, et al. Recalcitrant non-union of the distal humerus: treatment with free vascularized bone grafting. Clin Orthop Relat Res 2005;(435):134–139.

Breen T, Gelberman RH, Leffert R, Botte M. Massive allograft replacement of hemiarticular traumatic defects of the elbow. J Hand Surg Am 1988;13:900–907.

Bryan RS, Morrey BF. Extensive posterior exposure of the elbow. A triceps-sparing approach. Clin Orthop Relat Res 1982;(166):188–192.

Chinchalkar SJ, Szekeres M. Rehabilitation of elbow trauma. Hand Clin 2004;20:363–374.

Dean GS, Holliger EH, Urbaniak JR. Elbow allograft for reconstruction of the elbow with massive bone loss. Long term results. Clin Orthop Relat Res 1997;(341):12–22.

Helfet DL, Kloen P, Anand N, Rosen HS. Open reduction and internal fixation of delayed unions and non-unions of fractures of the distal part of the humerus. J Bone Joint Surg Am 2003;85:33–40.

Hughes RE, Schneeberger AG, An KN, et al. Reduction of triceps muscle force after shortening of the distal humerus: a computational model. J Shoulder Elbow Surg 1997;6:444–448.

Ilizarov GA. Transosseous Osteosynthesis. Heidelberg: Springer-Verlag, 1991.

Jupiter JB. The management of non-union and malunion of the distal humerus – a 30-year experience. J Orthop Trauma 2008;22:742–750.

Lu HT, Guitton TG, Capo JT, Ring D. Elbow instability associated with bicolumnar fracture of the distal humerus: report of three cases. J Hand Surg 2010;35:1126–1129.

Mitsunaga MM, Bryan RS, Linscheid RL. Condylar n on-unions of the elbow. J Trauma 1982;22:787–791.

Ring D, Jupiter JB. Operative treatment of osteochondral non-union of the distal humerus. J Orthop Trauma 2006;20:56–59.

Ring D, Jupiter JB, Toh S. Salvage of contaminated fractures of the distal humerus with thin wire external fixation. Clin Orthop Relat Res 1999;(359):203–208.

Sabo MT. Effect of coronal shear fractures of the distal humerus on elbow kinematics and stability. J Shoulder Elbow Surg 2010;19:670–680.

Schuster I, Korner J, Arzdorf M, et al. Mechanical comparison in cadaver specimens of three different 90-degree double-plate osteosyntheses for simulated C2-type distal humerus fractures with varying bone densities. J Orthop Trauma 2008;22:113–120.

Windolf M, Maza E, Gueorguiev B, et al. Treatment of distal humeral fractures using conventional implants. Biomechanical evaluation of a new implant configuration. BMC Musculoskelet Disord 2010;11:172.

Zalavras CG. Biomechanical evaluation of parallel versus orthogonal plate fixation of intra-articular distal humerus fractures. J Shoulder Elbow Surg 2011;20:12–20.

Chapter 28 Reconstruction of malunions of the distal humerus

Reza Omid, Leesa M. Galatz

INDICATIONS

Malunions involving either the distal shaft or the distal articular surface of the humerus occur in both the adult and the pediatric populations. The complexity of treating the malunion varies greatly with fracture location and pattern. Treatment ranges from simple capsular release and osteophyte removal to complex arthroplasty reconstruction. Factors which influence treatment decision making include location of the fracture (specifically, intra- versus extra-articular), degree of functional disability, and condition of the articular surface. Malunions of the distal humerus occur in multiple planes – transverse, coronal, and sagittal – and typically involve deformity in at least two and sometimes all three planes. Varus and extension malunions are the most common.

Preoperative evaluation entails thorough radiographic evaluation and a clear understanding of normal anatomy. In addition to anteroposterior, lateral and oblique radiographs, a computerized tomography (CT) scan with accompanying three-dimensional reconstruction reveals the deformity and allows development of surgical strategy. Some patients with an apparent malunion may actually have a non-union on one side of the joint, which should be apparent on advanced imaging studies (McKee et al. 1994). A non-union may indicate infection, especially if previous surgery has been performed. Advanced imaging facilitates evaluation of the plane of deformity and articular congruity.

The normal adult elbow has a valgus carrying angle of 11–16° (6–8° of valgus at the distal humerus). On the lateral view, the articular surface has a 30° anterior angulation with respect to the long axis of the humeral shaft. There is, in addition, 5–7° of internal rotation seen at the distal articular surface with respect to the axial plane. Functional range of motion has been shown to be an arc of motion encompassing 100° of flexion and extension, and 30–130° was shown to allow most activities of daily living (Morrey et al. 1981). More recently these results were revisited using modern techniques and an increased need for flexion was noted. The functional range of motion needed to perform more modern tasks was found to be 27–149° (Sardelli et al. 2011).

Physical examination reveals several important factors. The levels of pain and disability primarily determine the indication for surgery. Certainly, some malunion deformity may be well tolerated. On the other hand, the native elbow is a very congruent joint and even minor variances may lead to pain and loss of motion that are not well tolerated. Some deformity involving the distal humeral shaft may be of cosmetic concern as well, and while this is not a primary indication for surgery, some deformity, such as cubitus varus, may lead to ligament attenuation and associated pathology as well.

O'Driscoll et al. (2001) provided an excellent biomechanical explanation for tardy posterolateral rotatory lateral instability (PLRI) secondary to cubitus varus; this was later confirmed in a biomechanical study (Beuerlein et al. 2004). In the elbow with varus deformity, the triceps vector is shifted from a lateral vector to a medial vector, imparting an internal rotation stress on the olecranon. This internal rotation stress overloads the lateral ulnar collateral ligament, leading to attenuation of the ligament and PLRI. Based on this work, elbows with less than 15° of varus angulation may be effectively treated with ligament reconstruction. However, angulation of over 15° should be addressed with an osteotomy (O'Driscoll et al. 2001).

Malunions can be divided into two general categories – intra-articular or extra-articular, although some may involve both. Intra-articular malunions lead to pain, loss of motion, and post-traumatic arthrosis, and often are treated with arthroplasty. Success has been reported (Cobb and Linscheid 1994, Marti and Doornberg 2009) with non-arthroplasty options, however, and should be considered in patient younger than 70 years. Treatment of extra-articular malunion is less complex in many circumstances. A clear appreciation of the planar deformity allows correction using a variety of surgical techniques. Deformities in the coronal plane are addressed using a closing or opening wedge osteotomy. For example, varus malunions are treated with a lateral closing-wedge osteotomy with or without reconstruction of the lateral collateral ligament (LCL). Extension malunions, on the other hand, may be treated with recontouring ostectomy of the distal humerus (Blaine et al. 2007). Procedures can be performed with or without capsular release to allow for improved range of motion, as needed.

Decision making in the treatment of intra-articular malunion is much more complex. The age of the patient and the degree of arthrosis are significant factors. In an elderly patient (over 70 years) with arthrosis, a total elbow arthroplasty may be the best option; however, in younger patients successful attempts at salvage with intra-articular osteotomies have been described. Alternatively, osteocapsular arthroplasty (capsular release with debridement of impinging osteophytes) or interposition arthroplasty can be considered in younger patients, given the poor longevity of elbow arthroplasty in the setting of post-traumatic arthrosis in young, active patients.

Arthrodesis of the elbow is very debilitating and should be considered only if no other reconstructive option is available. This is more of a historical option, as most patients will not be satisfied with an elbow arthrodesis.

CONTRAINDICATIONS

Contraindications include active infection, non-compliant patients, and patients with unreasonable expectations. Another contraindication for a non-arthroplasty reconstruction is significant intra-articular arthrosis. In this setting, interpositional arthroplasty, hemiarthroplasty, or total elbow arthroplasty with or without simultaneous osteotomy is considered. Arthroplasty for a malunited distal humerus may lead to early failure, due to eccentric loading of the implants; therefore, arthroplasty should be a last resort for these patients. Simultaneous correction of deformity is recommended to obviate the eccentric wear.

Both extension and varus deformities can result in symptoms of ulnar nerve entrapment. The ulnar nerve can also become symptomatic after restoration of flexion in an elbow with long-standing contracture.

In these situations, ulnar nerve transposition should be an important part of any procedure, open or arthroscopic, in order to prevent long-term consequences or injury to the nerve.

TECHNIQUES

Varus malunion

There are multiple types of osteotomies described for varus malunion, including lateral closing wedge, medial opening wedge, step-cut osteotomies, and dome osteotomies. We prefer the lateral closing wedge osteotomy for treatment of cubitus varus.

Preoperative planning

Proper planning of an osteotomy to treat a distal humerus malunion is essential. Preoperative anteroposterior radiographs of both elbows at known magnification are first obtained. The desired correction is then determined by calculating the ulnohumeral angle of the affected elbow and aiming for a correction of 10–15° of valgus.

Patient positioning

General anesthesia without peripheral nerve blocks is preferred for reconstructive elbow surgery, to allow for accurate postoperative neurologic assessment. The patient is positioned supine with an arm-holder keeping the elbow flexed across the chest for access to both sides of the joint. If intraoperative fluoroscopy is needed, the arm is abducted with the C-arm fluoroscope perpendicular to the bed.

Technique

A non-sterile tourniquet is used and a posterior midline incision is made, creating full-thickness skin flaps medially and laterally. The ulnar nerve is addressed first if transposition is planned. The nerve is decompressed 8–10 cm proximal to the medial epicondyle, with care to excise a portion of the medial intermuscular septum, and the decompression is carried 4 cm distal to the medial epicondyle, between the two heads of the flexor carpi ulnaris. The medial antebrachial cutaneous nerve is identified and protected during exposure of the ulnar nerve. A vessel loop is passed around the nerve and used to provide gentle retraction. The nerve is subcutaneously transposed anteriorly at the end of the operation with the use of a small sling of flexor–pronator fascia. The lateral and medial columns are exposed, followed by circumferential exposure of the humerus at the level of the proximal metaphysis, to allow for the osteotomy, leaving the triceps in continuity with the olecranon. The exposure of the lateral column is carried distally to Kocher's interval, between the extensor carpi ulnaris and anconeus.

Preoperative templating determines the amount of bone necessary to correct 10–15° of valgus at the ulnohumeral joint. Kirschner wires (K-wires) are used to guide the osteotomy intraoperatively. Hohmann retractors are placed anteriorly and posteriorly around the humerus to protect the soft tissues. The osteotomy is performed with an oscillating saw. The distal cut is made as distal as possible without violating the olecranon fossa. It is important to keep the osteotomy in the metaphyseal bone, to allow for better healing. Lag screw fixation is inadequate, and plates are used to provide stability and compression across the osteotomy site. Precontoured plates are available but may need some alteration to conform to the humeral anatomy. If the lateral step-off does not allow for use of a precontoured plate, a 3.5 mm reconstruction plate can be used instead. The osteotomy site should be fixed in compression, as with other fractures (**Figs 28.1, 28.2**).

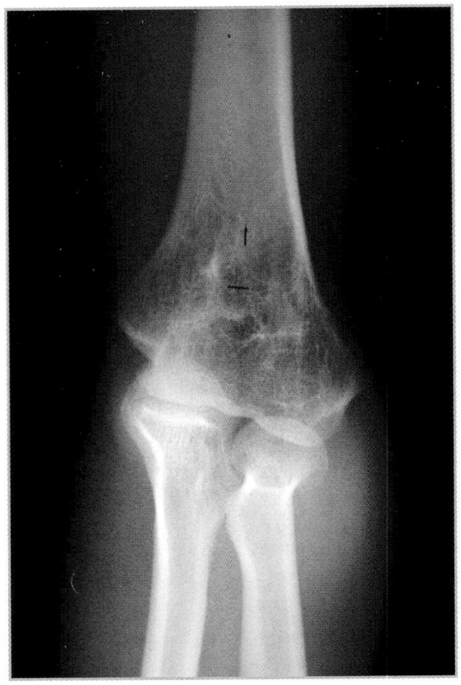

Figure 28.1 Varus malunion. Note the varus deformity at the joint level. Normally there is 6–8° valgus at the distal humerus in the coronal plane.

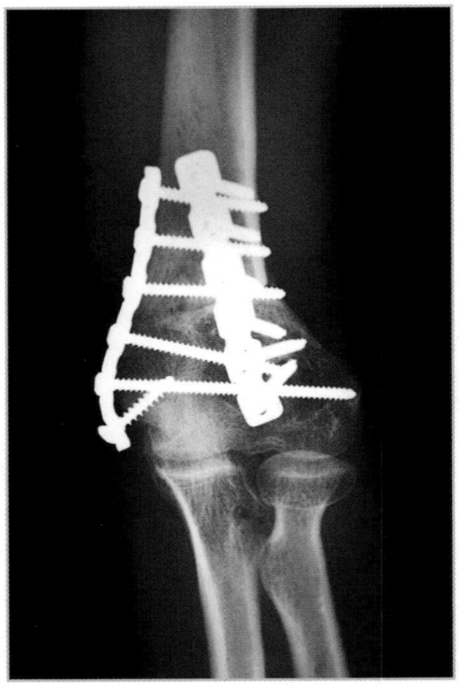

Figure 28.2 Lateral closing wedge osteotomy. Note the correction at the joint surface to neutral axis.

Once the mechanical axis of the elbow is restored, the LCL complex is assessed for competency. Commonly, severe varus deformity leads to attenuation of the lateral ligamentous complex and subtle PLRI. A ligamentous reconstruction is necessary to restore tissue and elbow stability.

The exposure is carried distally from the lateral column approach through Kocher's interval. A 3 mm burr is used to create two holes in the ulna for passage of the tendon graft. The first is at the crista supranatoris, located where the supinator crest blends with the radial notch, which is the anatomic insertion site of the LCL. The second is located 1.25 cm proximal and slightly posterior to the first, along the lateral joint line. The isometric point on the lateral side of the humerus is then determined and a 3 mm burr is used to create a third hole for entry of the graft.

Many techniques have been described for ligament reconstruction, but the authors generally prefer the docking technique (Rohrbough et al. 2002). The entry point of the graft on the humeral side may err slightly anterosuperior to the isometric point, so that tension on the graft occurs in extension, which is the unstable position for a laterally insufficient elbow. Two 2 mm drill holes are then made anterior and posterior to the supracondylar ridge, about 1.5 cm apart, proximal to the entry site, and used to tie sutures over a bone bridge. Several autologous graft sources can be used for reconstruction, including palmaris longus, plantaris, or gracilis. A graft length of 15 cm is usually sufficient for LCL reconstruction. Before the graft is secured, the elbow is held in 30° flexion, with the forearm in full pronation.

The medial triceps can often be involved in the pathology, causing translation or snapping over the medial epicondyle with flexion and extension of the elbow. If this is the case, the medial band of the triceps is detached and reattached to the lateral triceps.

Postoperative care

A Hemovac drain is placed for 24 hours and the arm is immobilized in 60–90° flexion for 7–10 days. If the LCL was also reconstructed, then a custom elbow brace is fabricated to immobilize the arm at 90° with the forearm in pronation. The range-of-motion protocol includes flexion and extension in pronation to 30° for three weeks. Thereafter, the elbow may be extended to full extension in pronation for an additional three weeks. Pronation and supination are performed with the elbow bent more than 90° during the immobilization period. Weight bearing is limited until six weeks postoperatively, by when bony union should have occurred.

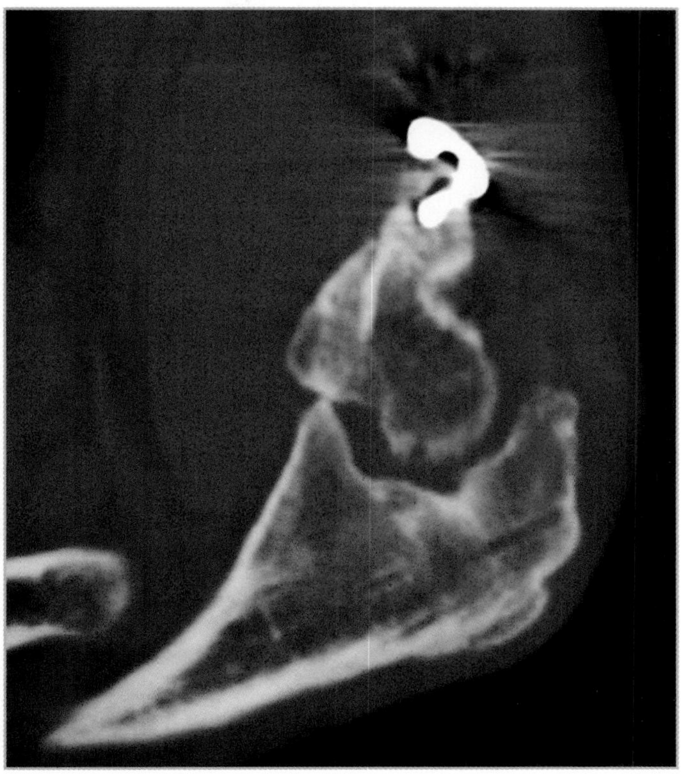

Figure 28.3 Extension malunion. The distal humerus is typically at 30° of anterior angulation in the sagittal plane. Here the patient demonstrates posterior angulation at the distal humerus as well as a large osteophyte impinging on the coronoid, limiting flexion.

Extension malunion

Extension malunions present a different mechanical problem. The bony deformity limits elbow flexion and extension, but can often be treated without an osteotomy (Blaine et al. 2007). The goal is to remove all bony sites of impingement and allow for a greater range of motion (**Fig. 28.3**). This can be achieved with debridement of the olecranon and especially the coronoid fossae. The patient's hand should be able to reach the mouth and body areas that require self-grooming; the goal is to attain approximately 145° flexion.

Preoperative planning

Preoperative range of motion is assessed with the use of a goniometer. Preoperative imaging with radiographs and a CT scan is essential to identify all sites of impingement, including osteophytes. The amount of overlap between the coronoid tip and coronoid fossa is determined, and estimations are made for the amount of bone resection needed.

Patient positioning

General anesthesia is provided and the patient is placed in the lateral decubitus position. We use a non-sterile tourniquet with the arm resting in a well padded arm-holder off the side of the bed.

Arthroscopic technique

A standard 4.0 mm, 30° arthroscope with a low-flow cannula is used in all elbow arthroscopy procedures. Pump pressures are low to avoid soft-tissue insufflation. Cannulae are generally not used, to allow for greater mobility of the instruments.

A proximal anteromedial portal is established initially. Depending on the amount of deformity and the location of osteophytes, portals can be adjusted to allow for a more successful entry into the joint. Osteophytes can cause divergence of portals, in which case adjustments are necessary. On the medial side, osteophytes can prevent proper entry into the joint, so a more distal anteromedial portal (at the joint line and 1–2 cm anterior to the medial epicondyle) can be used. Also laterally, a more distal portal allows for easier access to the anterior humerus with the instruments; however, this places the radial nerve at greater risk, so appropriate precautions have to be taken.

The appropriate amount of bone resection is estimated preoperatively, but care must be taken not to compromise the posterior cortical bone or the medial and lateral columns. The coronoid and radial fossae must be cleared to accept the coronoid and radial head, respectively. Care must be taken to avoid excessive bone resection, as this can cause formation of a stress riser, which can lead to a supracondylar distal humerus fracture. Any osteophytic bone at the coronoid tip is excised. If a flexion contracture exists, an anterior capsulectomy is performed, with a capsular biter from lateral to medial, under direct visualization. The muscle belly of the brachialis is visible once the anterior capsulectomy is complete.

Posterior capsulectomy and debridement of posterior osteophytes may not be necessary, as the loss of flexion is most often due to the loss of normal 30° anterior angulation (in the sagittal plane) of the joint line. Loss of flexion can sometimes be due to contracture of the posterior band of the medial collateral ligament and release of this band is necessary to obtain proper flexion angles. Experienced arthroscopists may consider arthroscopic release; however, this tissue forms the floor of the cubital tunnel, and so the intervention can place the ulnar nerve at risk. An open approach to posterior band release is entirely appropriate in most circumstances.

Open technique

A non-sterile tourniquet is used and a posterior midline incision is made, creating full-thickness skin flaps. The ulnar nerve is addressed first if transposition or release of the posterior band of the medial collateral ligament is planned. A lateral column approach generally allows excellent exposure to the distal humerus, but alternatively a medial 'over the top' approach can be used if more work is necessary on the medial side (Kasparyan and Hotchkiss 1997). If a lateral approach is used, the supracondylar ridge of the lateral column is exposed and dissection is developed both anteriorly (reflecting the brachialis anteriorly) and posteriorly (reflecting the triceps posteriorly). The dissection distally is between the pronator and flexor carpi ulnaris. Preoperative evaluation determines the location and amount of bone resection necessary and protective measures are taken to avoid compromising the structural integrity of the humerus by violating cortical bone, just as in arthroscopic surgery. The coronoid and radial fossae are contoured to accept the coronoid and radial head, respectively. Coronoid osteophytes are removed if present, and an anterior (and possibly posterior) capsulectomy is performed. If there is significant posterior osteophyte formation, a limited triceps split may be used to access them, but posterior impingement is usually not the cause of loss of motion in extension malunions. Manipulation is not recommended after a recontouring ostectomy.

Postoperative care

With open procedures, a Hemovac drain is placed for 24 hours. The arm is splinted and elevated for 24 hours, to reduce pain and swelling, but active assisted range-of-motion exercises are otherwise initiated soon thereafter. Night-time static splinting for four to six weeks is recommended.

Intra-articular malunions

Intra-articular malunions are the most difficult to treat. The articular incongruity presents a significant problem and cannot always be treated with non-arthroplasty options. In elderly patients (over 65 years old) with intra-articular malunions, elbow arthroplasty is the better option (**Figs 28.4, 28.5**). Rehabilitation is faster and easier, and the functional results are more predictable with elbow arthroplasty in this patient population. However, concerns over the longevity of an elbow prosthesis in the younger, more active patient with post-traumatic arthrosis make this a much less desirable option. Non-arthroplasty options include intra-articular osteotomies, arthroscopic osteocapsular arthroplasty, open ulnohumeral debridement, and interpositional/distraction arthroplasty.

Open ulnohumeral arthroplasty

Joint debridement, capsular release, and removal of osteophytes – a procedure termed ulnohumeral arthroplasty – is a modification of the original Outerbridge procedure, as popularized by Kashiwagi. The Outerbridge-Kashiwagi (OK) procedure was designed to remove loose bodies and hypertrophic osteophytes through a posterior approach and a fenestration of the olecranon fossa with a Cloward drill. This allows access to the anterior compartment and coronoid osteophytes.

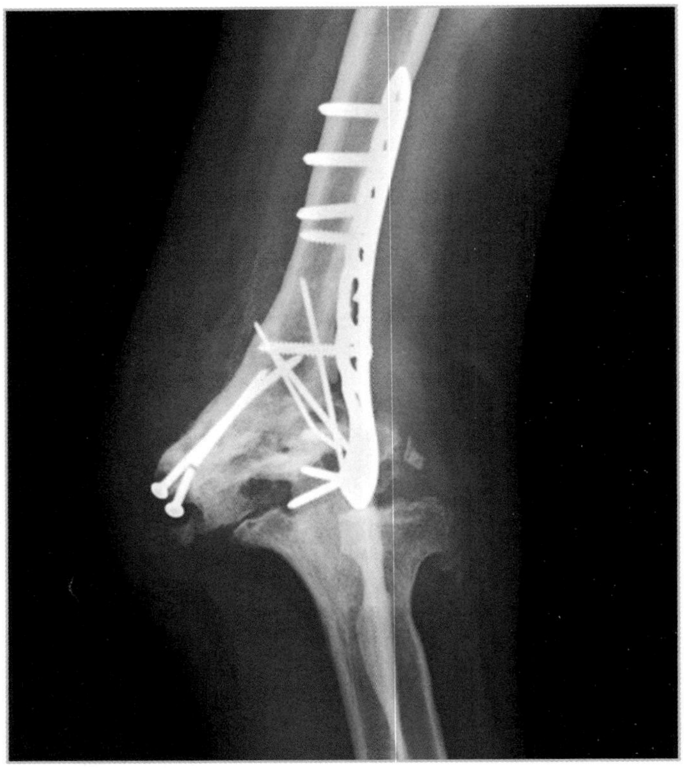

Figure 28.4 Intra-articular malunion. Note the severe destruction of the joint surface along with a valgus angulation of the distal humerus. Total elbow arthroplasty is the best option here, especially in elderly patients.

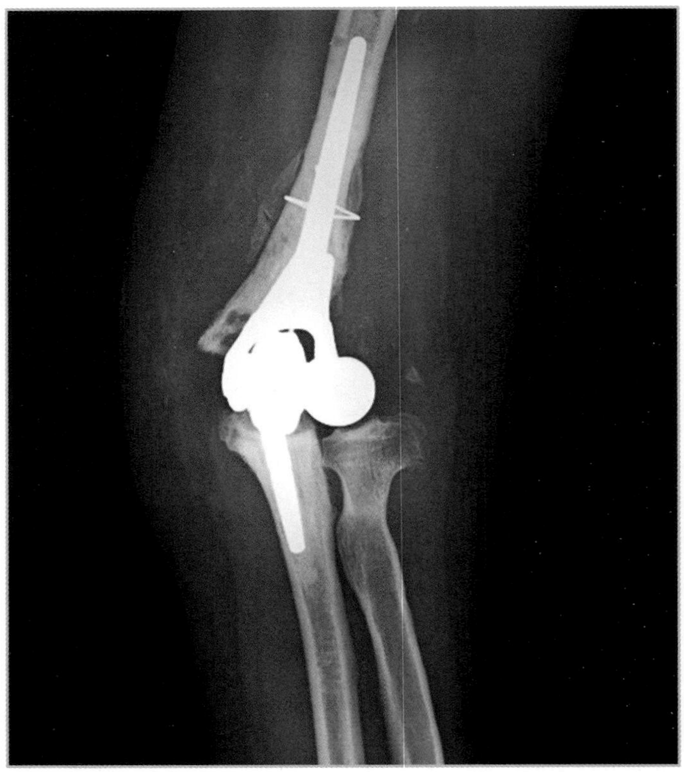

Figure 28.5 Total elbow arthroplasty. The mechanical axis has been slightly corrected and the arthrosis has been simultaneously addressed.

The use of a trephine to fenestrate the fossa (as opposed to a clower drill) eliminates the debris generated by a burr and provides a clean bone resection. Although a limited anterior capsular release can be accomplished through the trephinated fossa, open anterior capsulectomy and resection of osteophytes on the radiocapitellar joint are performed through a medial or lateral column approach.

Arthroscopic osteocapsular arthroplasty

O'Driscoll described a procedure for reshaping the bones (removal of osteophytes), and removing loose bodies, in combination with a complete anterior and posterior caspulectomy in order to restore motion to the arthritic elbow as an alternative to traditional open ulnohumeral arthroplasty (O'Driscoll 2007). This is a technically challenging procedure and requires considerable arthroscopic experience in the elbow.

Interpositional distraction arthroplasty

Use of interpositional distraction arthroplasty is limited to young, low-demand patients with loss of elbow function due to degenerative ulnohumeral arthritis. The procedure is typically indicated for patients too young for arthroplasty and should be thought of as a temporizing procedure. Several tissues have been used, including fascia, Achilles allograft, and dermis. Ligament reconstruction is necessary to provide stability. Once the tissue has been interposed, a distracting external fixator is placed to allow for motion of the elbow while simultaneously protecting the interposition graft as well as the ligament reconstruction. External fixation is used for approximately four to six weeks. The results are variable and highly surgeon dependent.

Distal humerus hemiarthroplasty/total elbow arthroplasty

Distal humerus hemiarthroplasty is a relatively new option and is not widely available. It may present a viable option in the future as product development and operative techniques evolve. Elbow arthroplasty should be considered as the last option in a younger, more active patient. Concerns over longevity and functional results in this population preclude its routine use. The results of arthroplasty in patients with a malunion of the distal humerus are generally inferior to results in patients without malunion. Patients with an altered mechanical axis may have eccentric wear of the polyethylene, leading to premature failure. Arthroplasty designs allowing implantation of an unlinked but stable prosthesis may hold promise in this difficult patient population.

Results

There is very little evidence to support any of these treatment options; however, three case series show improvement in function after reconstruction for malunion of the distal humerus. Cobb and Linscheid (1994) reported on three patients with intercondylar malunions treated with an intra-articular derotational wedge osteotomy and insertion of a tricortical iliac bone graft. Motion was improved in all patients (mean increase of 65°), and at 7.6 years' follow-up none required conversion to total elbow arthroplasty. One patient, however, did require conversion to an interpositional arthroplasty at 1.3 years. McKee et al. (1994) reported on 13 patients with intra-articular distal humeral malunion or non-union following trauma. After a mean follow-up of 25 months, the average arc of motion was 97° (an average gain of 54°), with no progressive radiographic degeneration. O'Driscoll et al. (2001) recommended that patients with varus malunion >15° should have an osteotomy for correction but patients with less deformity (<15°) may be simply treated with ligament reconstruction alone. They reported on 21 patients treated with either osteotomy alone (4 patients), osteotomy with ligament reconstruction (7 patients) or ligament reconstruction alone (10 patients) for longstanding cubitus varus. At an average of three-year follow-up, the Mayo Elbow Performance Score indicated good or excellent results for 19 of the 22 limbs and fair or poor results for three limbs.

Pearls and pitfalls

Complications of reconstructive elbow surgery include wound problems, heterotopic ossification (HO), infection, neurovascular injury, and intraoperative as well as postoperative fractures. Delicate soft-tissue handling is mandatory. Full-thickness skin flaps with sharp dissection should be used. Minimizing subcutaneous dissection is helpful in preventing seroma/hematoma formation. A drain should be used on all open procedures, to try to minimize hematoma formation.

Although there is no literature addressing HO prophylaxis with elbow reconstruction surgery, several general principles can be used. Prophylaxis with indomethacin given for six weeks postoperatively or 700 cGy radiation given preoperatively or postoperatively for HO prevention has been described. Indications for prophylaxis are controversial and there is no evidence-based consensus. If HO is seen preoperatively and resected as part of the procedure, then strong consideration should be given to prophylaxis. Classically, patients with head injury or burns should also be given consideration; however, this is more for the acute setting. Routine use of HO prophylaxis is not recommended.

Infection risk is high with elbow reconstruction surgery. Standard sterile technique is used as well as preoperative antibiotics. The use of an occlusive iodine-impregnated drape to seal off all areas of exposed skin is also recommended. Patients must be made aware of the increased risk with revision surgery as well.

Nerve injury is more likely in the post-traumatic and revision setting. A sound knowledge of the anatomy around the elbow is essential to safe surgery. The ulnar nerve is always exposed and possibly transposed, depending on the case, and particular care must be used when handling the nerve in patients with flexion contractures. If a patient lacks flexion for several years, the nerve can accommodate to a shorter length and scar to adjacent soft tissues. Restoration of flexion without addressing the ulnar nerve can cause a traction injury to it.

CONCLUSIONS

Treatment of malunions of the distal humeral is challenging. Many extra-articular malunions are relatively easily and successfully treated. However, intra-articular malunions leading to post-traumatic arthrosis remain particularly problematic. A thorough preoperative evaluation along with sound surgical judgment leads to appropriate surgical decision making. Future considerations include improvements in elbow arthroplasty to make it more applicable to younger and more active patients.

REFERENCES

Beuerlein MJ, Reid JT, Schemitsch EH, McKee MD. Effect of distal humeral varus deformity on strain in the lateral ulnar collateral ligament and ulnohumeral joint stability. J Bone Joint Surg Am 2004;86:2235–2242.

Blaine TA, O'Driscoll SW, Umansky SC, Kibler WB. Reconstruction of malunions of the distal humerus. In: K Yamaguchi, GJW King, MD McKee, SWM O'Driscoll, eds. Advanced Reconstruction: Elbow. Rosemont, IL: American Academy of Orthopaedic Surgeons, 2007: 363–373.

Cobb TK, Linscheid RL. Late correction of malunited intercondylar humeral fractures. J Bone Joint Surg Br 1994;76:622–666.

Kasparyan NG, Hotchkiss RN. Dynamic skeletal fixation in the upper extremity. Hand Clin 1997;13:643–663.

Marti RK, Doornberg J. Intra-articular osteotomy for distal humerus malunion. Case Report Med 2009; article ID 631306.

McKee M, Jupiter J, Toh CL, et al. Reconstruction after malunion and nonunion of intra-articular fractures of the distal humerus. J Bone Joint Surg Br 1994;76:614–621.

Morrey BF, Askew LJ, An KN, Chao EY. A biomechanical study of normal functional elbow motion. J Bone Joint Surg Am 1981;63:872–877.

O'Driscoll SW, Spinner RJ, McKee MD, et al. Tardy posterolateral rotatory instability of the elbow due to cubitus varus. J Bone Joint Surg Am 2001;83:1358–1369.

O'Driscoll. Arthroscopic osteocapsular arthroplasty. In: K Yamaguchi, GJW King, MD McKee, SWM O'Driscoll, eds. Advanced Reconstruction: Elbow. Rosemont, IL: American Academy of Orthopaedic Surgeons, 2007:59–68.

Rohrbough JT, Altchek DW, Hyman J, et al. Medial collateral ligament reconstruction of the elbow using the docking technique. Am J Sports Med 2002;30:541–548.

Sardelli M, Tashjian RZ, MacWilliams BA. Functional elbow range of motion for contemporary tasks. J Bone Joint Surg Am 2011;93:471–477.

Chapter 29 Total elbow replacement for elbow fractures

Bernard F. Morrey, Joaquin Sanchez-Sotelo

INTRODUCTION

Replacement for fractures of the elbow typically includes management of the acute fracture as well as post-traumatic arthrosis and non-union. This chapter focuses on elbow replacement for the acute fracture and for the established non-union.

ELBOW REPLACEMENT FOR ACUTE FRACTURE OF THE DISTAL HUMERUS

Indications

The indication for semiconstrained total joint replacement for acute fracture is becoming more clear and accepted (Srinivasan et al. 2005), largely based on data from controlled studies (Frankle et al. 2003, Prasad and Dent 2008, McKee et al. 2009). Of course, the treatment of choice for most displaced intra-articular fractures of the elbow joint remains open reduction and internal fixation (ORIF) (Mitsunaga et al. 1982, Helfet et al. 2003, Huang et al. 2005). But this is not the best treatment for all patients. In a review of nine studies of osteosynthesis of fractures of the distal humerus, fair to poor outcomes were reported in 25% of cases, and there was a high complication rate – in one series 70% of patients required secondary procedures (Mitsunaga et al. 1982).

In the older patient (>65 years), usually a female with osteoporosis and an extensively comminuted fracture, for whom osteosynthesis is unreliable, replacement is the treatment of choice (Kamineni and Morrey 2004, Srinivasan et al. 2005, Prasad and Dent 2008, McKee et al. 2009). This should not result in a high number of individuals needing a replacement, even in busy trauma centers. The fact that at the Mayo Clinic, a level-1 trauma center, only two or three acute fractures of the humerus per year are treated by total joint replacement emphasizes our strict selection criteria and emphasizes the role of ORIF in those amenable to this treatment. Virtually all of the literature reports the outcome of linked devices (Garcia et al. 2002, Helfet et al. 2003, Armstrong and Yamaguchi 2004, Lee et al. 2006, Charissoux et al. 2008, Jost et al. 2008), although one recent study documented acceptable outcomes with an unlinked implant (Kalogrianitis et al. 2008). If an already arthritic elbow (e.g. in a patient with rheumatoid arthritis) is fractured, it should be replaced if the joint was symptomatic prior to the fracture (Jost et al. 2008). It is a mistake to attempt ORIF in elderly patients who meet the proper indications for replacement, as failure of ORIF is associated with poorer outcomes with the subsequent arthroplasty, compared with an acute prosthetic replacement (Mighell et al. 2005, Prasad and Dent 2008).

Contraindications

Any fracture of the distal humerus that can be reliably fixed should be so treated (Helfet et al. 2003, Huang et al. 2005, Srinivasan et al. 2005). Open wounds must be rendered 'safe' by debridement prior to replacement.

Technique

With increasing experience, the operative technique for elbow replacement for acute fractures has evolved. There are several important aspects that should be emphasized. If encountered in the first 12 hours, a type I open wound may be treated in a single stage after careful and thorough debridement. A type II or III open fracture must first be irrigated and debrided to avoid deep sepsis. Total elbow replacement is performed at the second stage. Fractures requiring replacement usually involve fracture of the humeral articulation and some degree of column involvement. Hence, when the fracture fragments are removed, the triceps can be left attached to the olecranon in most instances (McKee et al. 2003).

Approach

A posterior midline skin incision is used and the hematoma is evacuated. From the medial aspect, the ulnar nerve is always identified and freed from the medial fragment. The flexor–pronator muscle group is completely released from the fractured medial epicondyle; the extensor mass is next dissected from the fractured lateral condyle. The triceps is elevated from the posterior medial, posterior lateral aspect of the humerus. Working from both sides of the triceps attachment, all remaining fracture fragments are excised (**Fig. 29.1**). A bone graft is prepared from the removed fragments and placed behind the flange of the humeral implant. Since the triceps attachment to the olecranon is left intact, rapid functional recovery is anticipated. The humerus is usually 'delivered' to the lateral margin of the triceps. Sometimes, the fracture is such that it is more convenient to expose the humerus at the medial margin of the triceps. The fracture and circumstances dictate this exposure. Reconstruction of the condyles is not necessary, and should be avoided, as it is time consuming and may be a source of pain (**Fig. 29.2**). Since up to 8 cm of distal humerus can be resected and still managed with an off-the-shelf long flanged Coonrad/Morrey device, there is no need to fix any of the fracture elements (**Fig. 29.3**).

In cases of acute fracture, we prefer the 15 cm (6 inch) humeral stem. The extended flange is used for fractures in which more than 5 cm of distal humerus is involved. A trial reduction is carried out and the proper depth of humeral insertion is defined, but in general replicates the normal axis position when dealing with the acute injury.

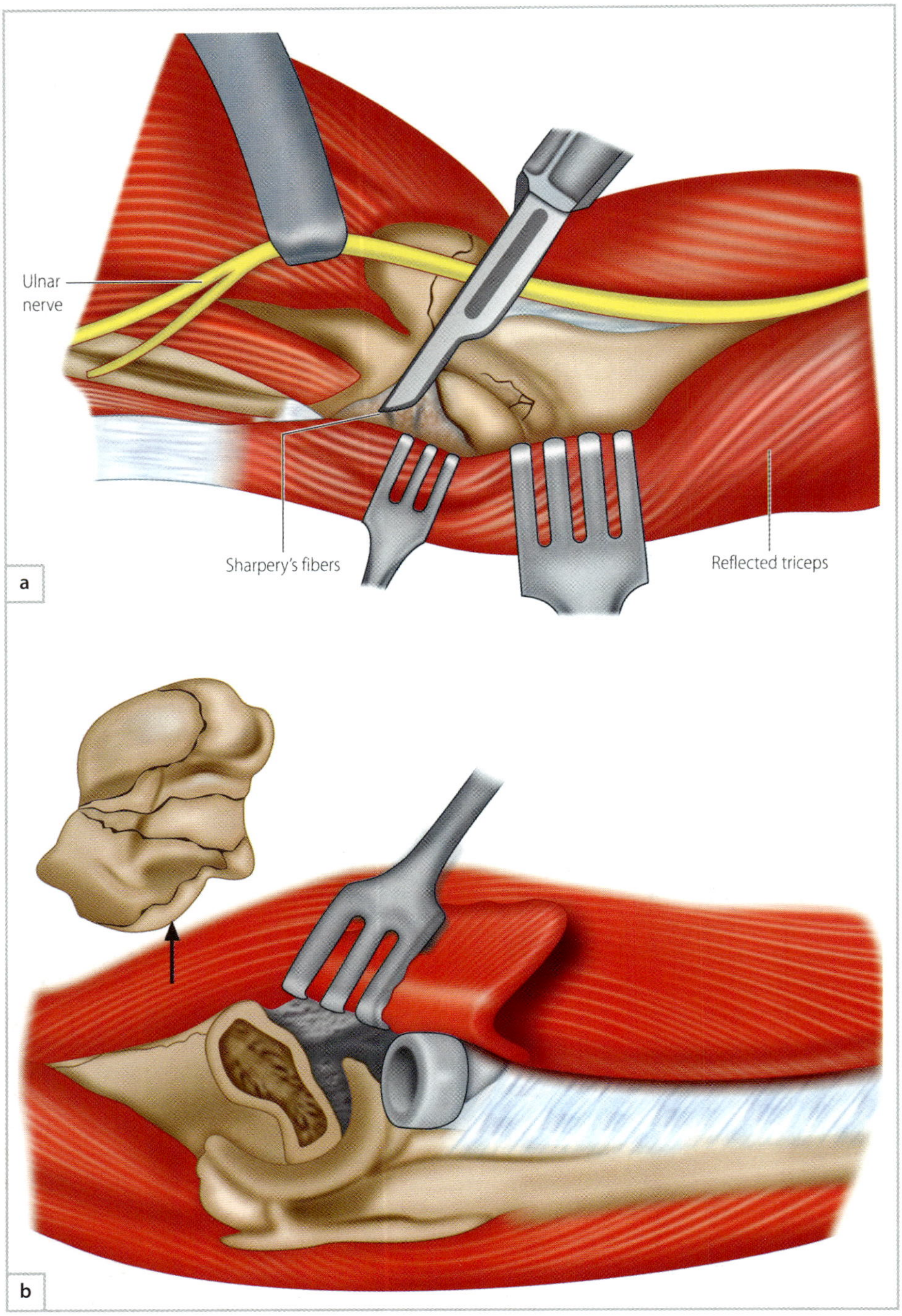

Figure 29.1 For acute fractures and non-union of the distal humerus, the fracture fragments are completely excised, releasing all tissue. This is done both medially (a) and laterally (b), allowing implantation without removal of the triceps.
By permission of Mayo Foundation for Medical Education and Research. All rights reserved.

Preparation of the humerus

The humerus is easily prepared with minimal rasping, since the bone is typically osteoporotic and there is loss of distal humeral bone (given the fracture). If remnants of intact humerus prevent correct implant positioning, a trial implant is used to direct any additional preparation of the distal humerus. If the fracture obliterates the roof of the olecranon, the depth of insertion is estimated by the soft-tissue tension after the ulna has been prepared (**Fig. 29.4**). Note that failure to properly account for soft-tissue tension puts shear stress on the ulnar implant and can lead to loosening (Cheung and O'Driscoll 2007). Landmarks for rotational alignment include the medial intermuscular septum and the triangular shape of the anterior distal humerus.

Preparation of the ulna

For the ulna preparation, approximately 25–30% of the triceps attachment is released from the medial attachment of the olecranon. The forearm is internally rotated, and the canal is exposed from the medial aspect of the greater sigmoid notch. The tip of the olecranon process is removed to allow access down the canal (**Fig. 29.5**). This is the most difficult step, especially if the triceps attachment has been maintained. Palpating the subcutaneous border of the proximal ulna and the proximal shaft serves as reliable landmarks to enter the canal safely. The ulna is first entered with a high-speed burr at the base of the coronoid. In older patients the ulna is usually atrophic and the canal can be prepared with little difficulty. Care must be taken,

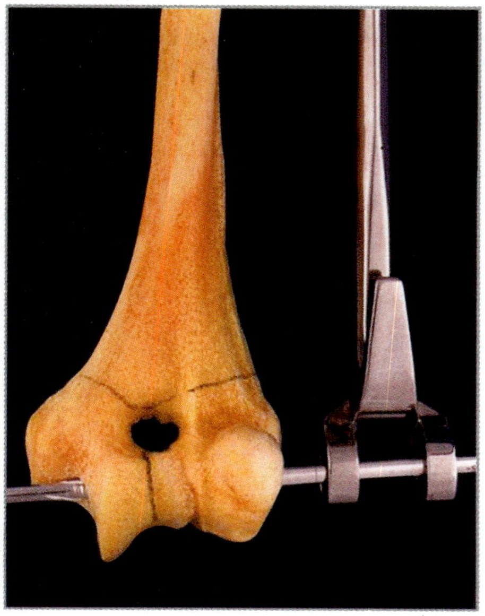

Figure 29.2 With bone loss at the level of the roof of the olecranon fossa, the axis of rotation remains at the anatomic level.

however, to ensure the rasp is down the canal, is not 'flexed', and is properly rotated. As noted above, this is the most challenging part of the procedure. Special care must be taken to ensure proper depth of insertion and that the ulnar plane of flexion is perpendicular to the 'flat' surface of the ulna.

Trial reduction

A trial reduction is important to ensure proper depth of insertion and to ensure the humeral component can articulate with the ulnar component. If this is not the case, ulnar bone must be trimmed to allow easy articulation of the two components. As noted above, the proper depth of humeral insertion is determined by the roof of the olecranon. When this landmark is not present, axial traction applied to the forearm when flexed 90° provides a reasonable estimate of proper humeral position. The position of the humeral component is thus noted and is marked on the implant. The key here is to assure the ulnar component: is properly seated; is properly rotated; and articulates freely with the humeral component, without impingement.

Cementation and insertion

Both canals are thoroughly cleaned with pulsatile lavage and dried. Depending on the surgeon's experience, both implants may be inserted simultaneously. If the surgeon is unsure or inexperienced, it is best to cement the ulna first. To every 40 g of cement, 1 g of vancomycin is added. We usually use 60–80 g of cement, since an injector system is also used. Absence of the distal humerus facilitates coupling of the implant. However, this can be difficult, hence the value of performing a trial reduction. Note that by flexing and extending the articulate joint, a final setting of the implant is realized and elimination of any contracture is assured.

Closure

At the end of the procedure, since the triceps has been minimally disturbed, no formal repair is necessary. The flexor and extensor origins are sewn to the margin of the triceps and the ulnar nerve is transected anteriorly. If the triceps has been reflected, it is reattached to the olecranon with two no. 5 non-absorbable sutures placed through the olecranon in the manner described previously. Both techniques of triceps management allow immediate use of the joint. A compression dressing and elevation of the extremity are recommended for about two days, followed by gentle active range of motion, as tolerated. Formal physiotherapy is not necessary and the patient is usually discharged from hospital on day 2.

Pearls and pitfalls

Pearls

- Do the replacement as soon as possible.
- Resect all fracture segments. Fix nothing.
- If the patient had pre-existing arthritis, release the anterior capsule.
- Find and free the ulnar nerve as the first step to the deep exposure.
- Leave the triceps attachment on the olecranon.
- Reflection of a portion of the medial triceps attachment is the most significant, non- intuitive step. By retracting the released portion, rotation of the ulna is facilitated and the exposure is enhanced.
- Palpate the proximal ulna during preparation, to avoid violating the cortex.
- Take note of the easiest manner to articulate the device with the trial reduction.
- If an aggressive soft tissue of the elbow has also been required, it will recontract. This is addressed during recovery with a night splint and patient counseling.

Pitfalls

- Malposition of the humerus, rotation, and depth of insertion.
- Inadequate exposure of the ulna.
- Violation of the ulnar canal.
- Not removing a sufficient amount of the olecranon process to properly prepare the ulnar canal.
- Malposition of the ulna, especially rotation.
- Osseous impingement preventing articulation.
- Failure to reapproximate flexor and extensor origins to the margin of the triceps.

Results

Since the original description by Cobb and Morrey (1997), an increasing number of reports have confirmed the initial findings (Gambirasio et al. 2001, Garcia et al. 2002, Charissoux et al. 2008). In short, the procedure is about 90% successful in the first two to five years after surgery (**Table 29.1, Fig. 29.6**). The complication rate is about 10% (Cobb and Morrey 1997, Kamineni and Morrey 2004, McKee et al. 2009). There is, though, little long-term information on this patient population.

Of particular importance are two prospective, randomized studies comparing ORIF and replacement. Both studies found replacement the superior choice, especially where the fracture is so comminuted that ORIF is unreliable (Frankle et al. 2003, McKee et al. 2009). Further, the complication rate, range of motion, and operative time all favored replacement in both these studies.

Complications/reoperations

There are fewer complications associated with replacement than with ORIF (Frankle et al. 2003, Kamineni and Morrey 2004, McKee et al. 2009). The complications that do occur are, for the most part, those associated with the elbow and with fractures in general. These include wound problems, ulnar nerve symptoms, sepsis, and residual pain. Complications associated with the mechanical failure of the device are uncommon, especially if the pre-coat surface finish was not used on the ulnar component.

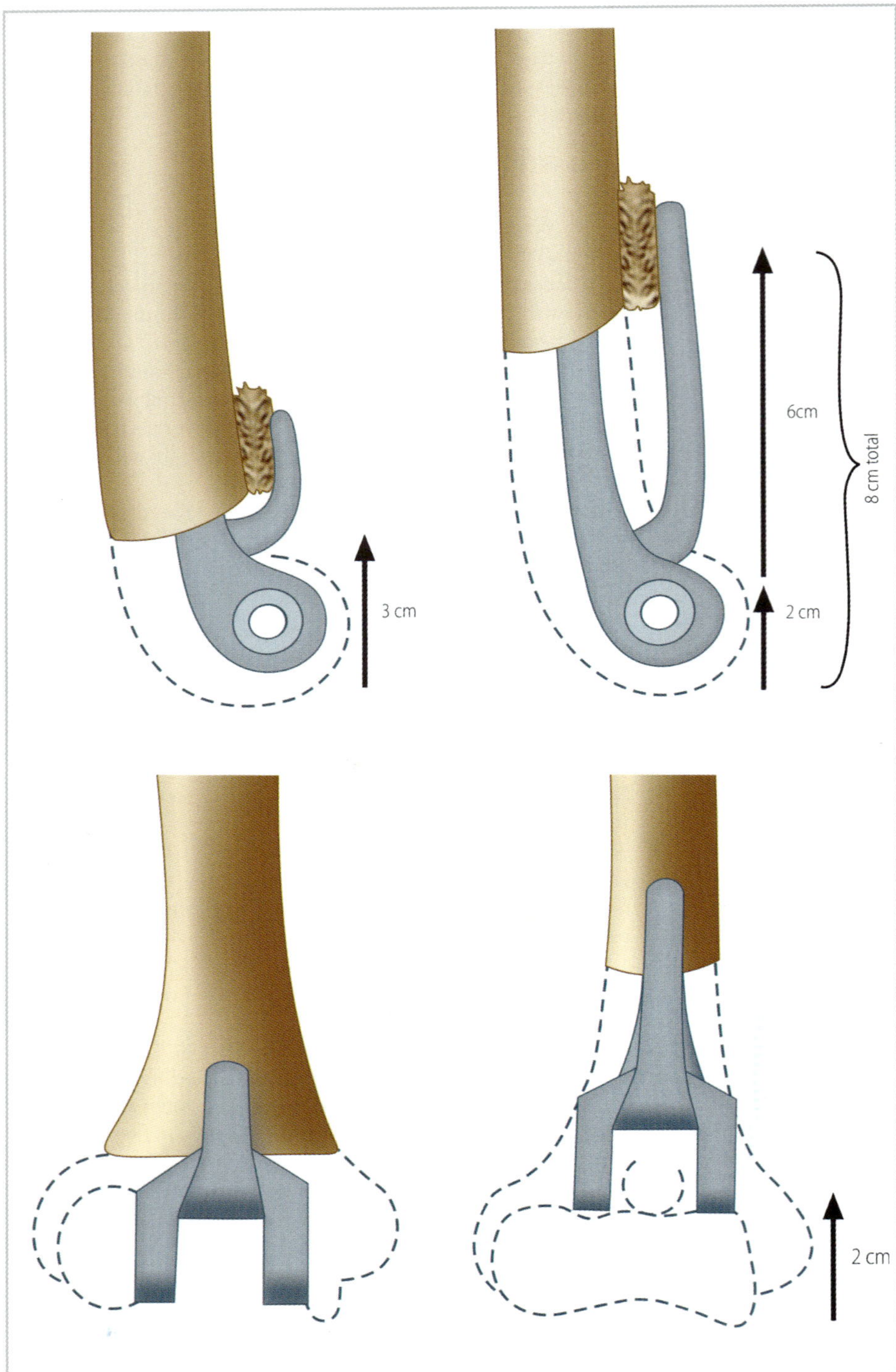

Figure 29.3 Using an extended flange and allowing 2 cm of shortening, up to 8 cm of distal humeral bone loss can be addressed by this system. By permission of Mayo Foundation for Medical Education and Research. All rights reserved.

Rehabilitation

Unlike the shoulder, the rehabilitation program in our practice is simple. Use of the elbow and arm as tolerated is recommended (with the recognition of the permanent weight-lifting restriction of 2.5 kg). Swelling in the postoperative period after acute fracture must be monitored but formal physiotherapy is not used and is not considered to be advisable. In this context, if concern exists regarding the wound, motion is deferred and the elbow is immobilized in extension and assessed every three or four days. The only other issue is avoiding a flexion contracture. If this is a problem or potential problem we use a Mayo elbow brace (Don Joy), adjusted to a position in extension that causes discomfort but not excessive pain, at night.

Conclusion

Semi-constrained Coonrad/Morrey total elbow replacement for acute fractures of the distal aspect of the humerus can be a very reliable treatment in a specific group of elderly patients but is not an alternative to osteosynthesis in younger patients

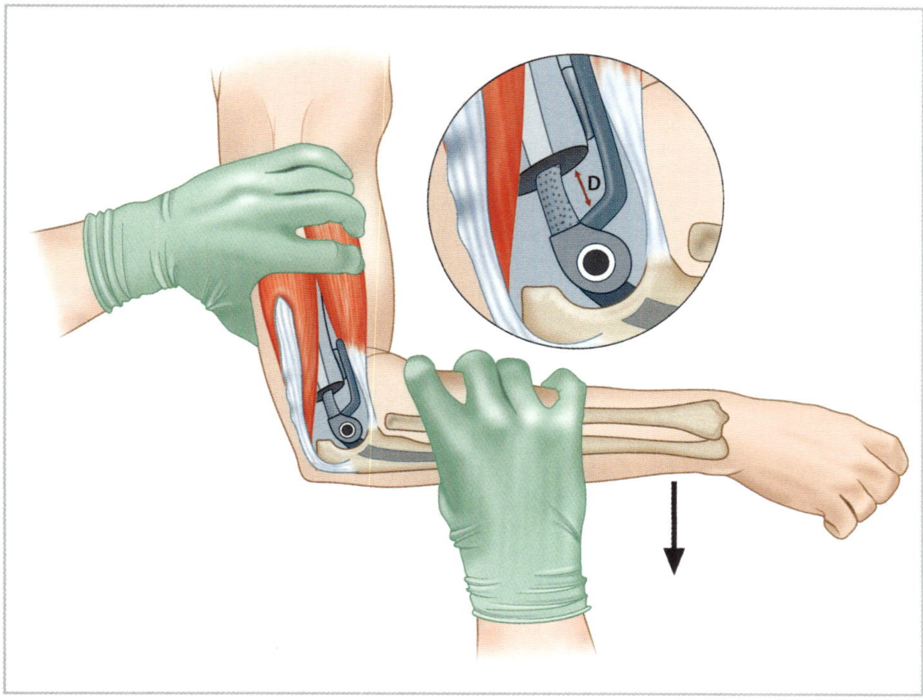

Figure 29.4 With severe distal humerus bone loss, the depth of insertion is determined by placing the forearm at 90° flexion and applying traction to the forearm. The position of the humerus defines the proper depth of insertion. By permission of Mayo Foundation for Medical Education and Research. All rights reserved.

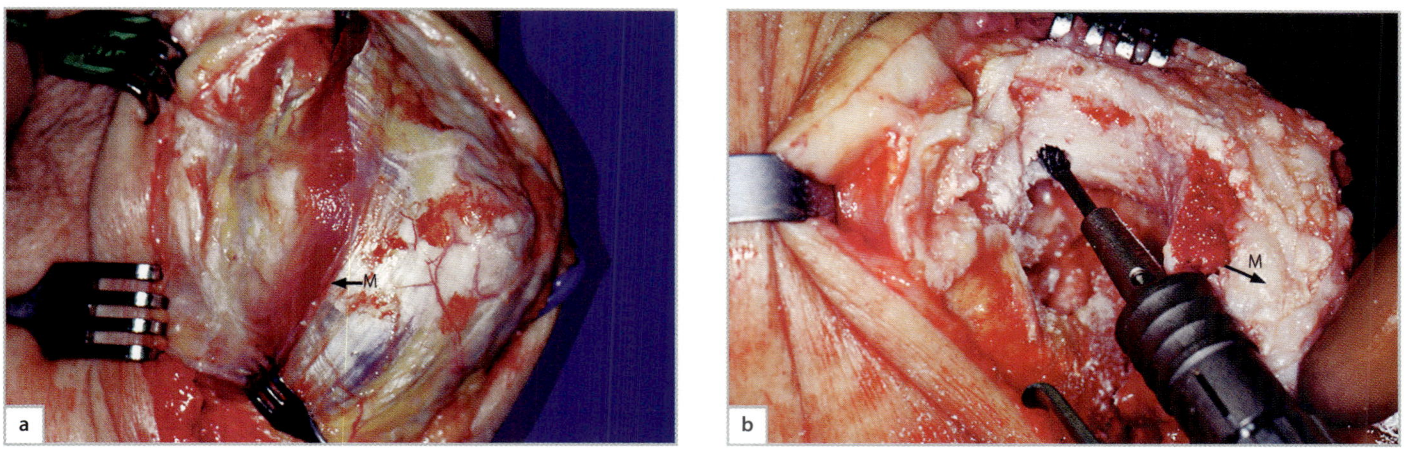

Figure 29.5 Preparation of the ulna. (a) The ulna is best prepared by releasing the medial aspect of the triceps attachment, M. (b) rotating the ulna and approaching the canal from the medial aspect of the ulna are simplified by releasing the medial portion of the triceps attachment, M.

Table 29.1 Summary of reported results

Study	Number of patients	Length of follow-up (years)	Percentage of sample with satisfactory outcome
Cobb and Morrey (1997)	21	5	92
Frankle	12	2	92
Ray	7	3	100
Gambirasio et al. (2001)	7	3	100
Garcia et al. (2002)	16	3	94
Kamineni and Morrey (2004)	42	6.5	93
Overall	84	4.5	94

ELBOW REPLACEMENT FOR NON-UNION OF THE DISTAL HUMERUS

Indications

The management of non-union of the distal humerus is strongly based on, and should be stratified according to, the activity and age of the patient (Morrey and Adams 1995). For young, active individuals we continue to perform osteosynthesis. The two essential pathologic requirements of osteosynthesis are: an intact or near normal articulation; and adequate distal bone to establish rigid fixation and a balanced reduction. The two technical requirements are: the need to expose, protect, and translocate the ulnar nerve; and the need to aggressively

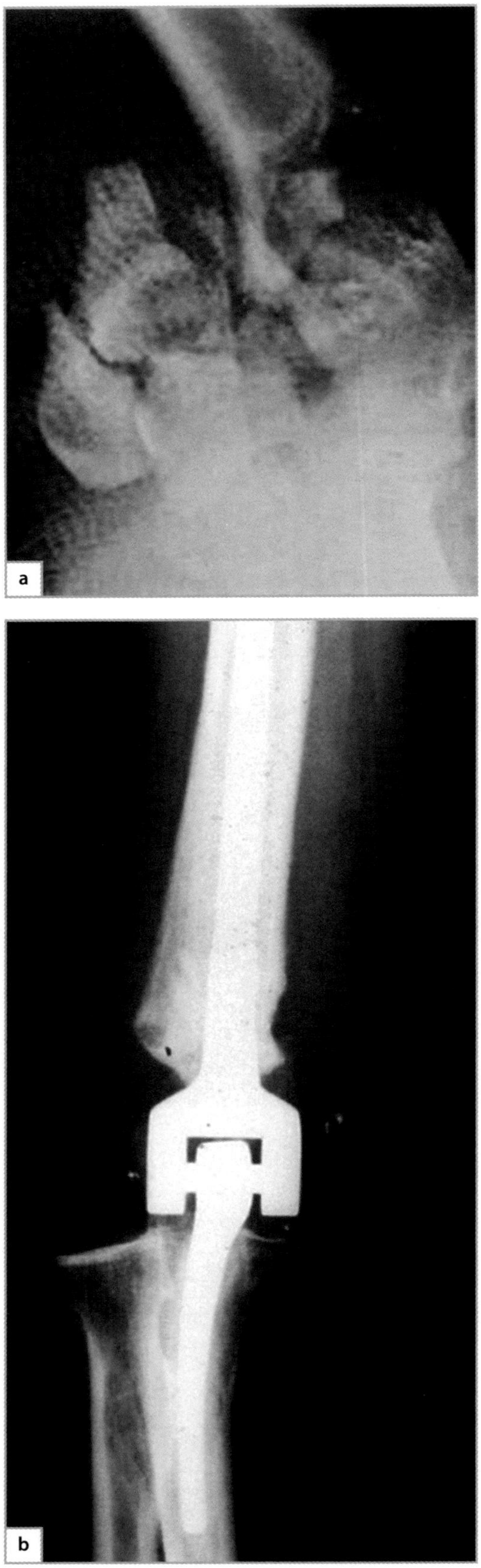

Figure 29.6 A 71-year-old woman with a comminuted fracture of the distal humerus. (a) Preoperative radiograph. Patient is asymptomatic with essentially normal function after joint replacement at five years (b).

free the contracted capsular tissue (Ackerman and Jupiter 1988, Ring et al. 2003). The same essential considerations are necessary when performing a replacement procedure.

Other reconstructive techniques that might be considered are a hemi-replacement or interposition arthroplasty, although the deformity and instability that are usually present are a relative contradiction for both (Morrey and Adams 1995, Ramsey et al. 1999). Further, absence of intact collateral origins at the humerus further precludes this as a reliable option, unless the non-union is after a shear fracture, or unless it is a very distal transarticular non-union. We have performed osteosynthesis and then proceeded to reconstruct the arthritic joint with an interposition arthroplasty. However, this is an unpredictable strategy and is viable only in the young patient without deformity at the site of the non-union.

Contraindications

Replacement is avoided in the face of recent sepsis, lack of motor control, or in those with unrealistic expectations. We try to avoid prosthetic replacement in the younger, active patient.

Technique (Morrey and Adams 1995)

Exposure

The elbow is exposed through a posterior midline skin incision, and the ulnar nerve is identified and treated according to the location of the nerve and preoperative symptoms. Regardless, it is always identified and protected. Importantly, the extensor mechanism is left undisturbed and the procedure is performed working on both sides of the triceps unless an associated olecranon non-union or triceps detachment provides the opportunity for exposure (**Fig. 29.7**).

Preparation

Retained hardware is removed and the non-united distal humerus is resected subperiosteally and saved for bone grafting behind the flange of the humeral component. At this point a careful assessment of the soft-tissue envelope contracture is carried out and extensive release is performed, as necessary. The goal is to obtain varus/valgus balance as well as to restore flexion and extension motion. Tissue samples are sent for pathology and microbiology testing to rule out infection. The working space created by resection of the distal humerus is sufficient to instrument the canals and implant the components. Preparation of the humerus is straightforward. Exposure of the ulnar canal may be improved by partial detachment of the triceps from the olecranon on the medial side, as highlighted above.

Implantation

The surgical technique for implantation of a linked elbow arthroplasty is described above. Use of a 15 cm (6 inch) humeral component provides secure fixation. In the presence of severe humeral bone loss, an implant with a longer flange may be cemented 'proud' to compensate for part of the lost humeral length, as noted above for the management of an acute fracture. If severe contracture of the triceps mechanism has occurred, the preference is to place the humeral component 2–3 cm more proximal, to relax this contracture. As above, antibiotic-impregnated cement is used and injected down the canals with an

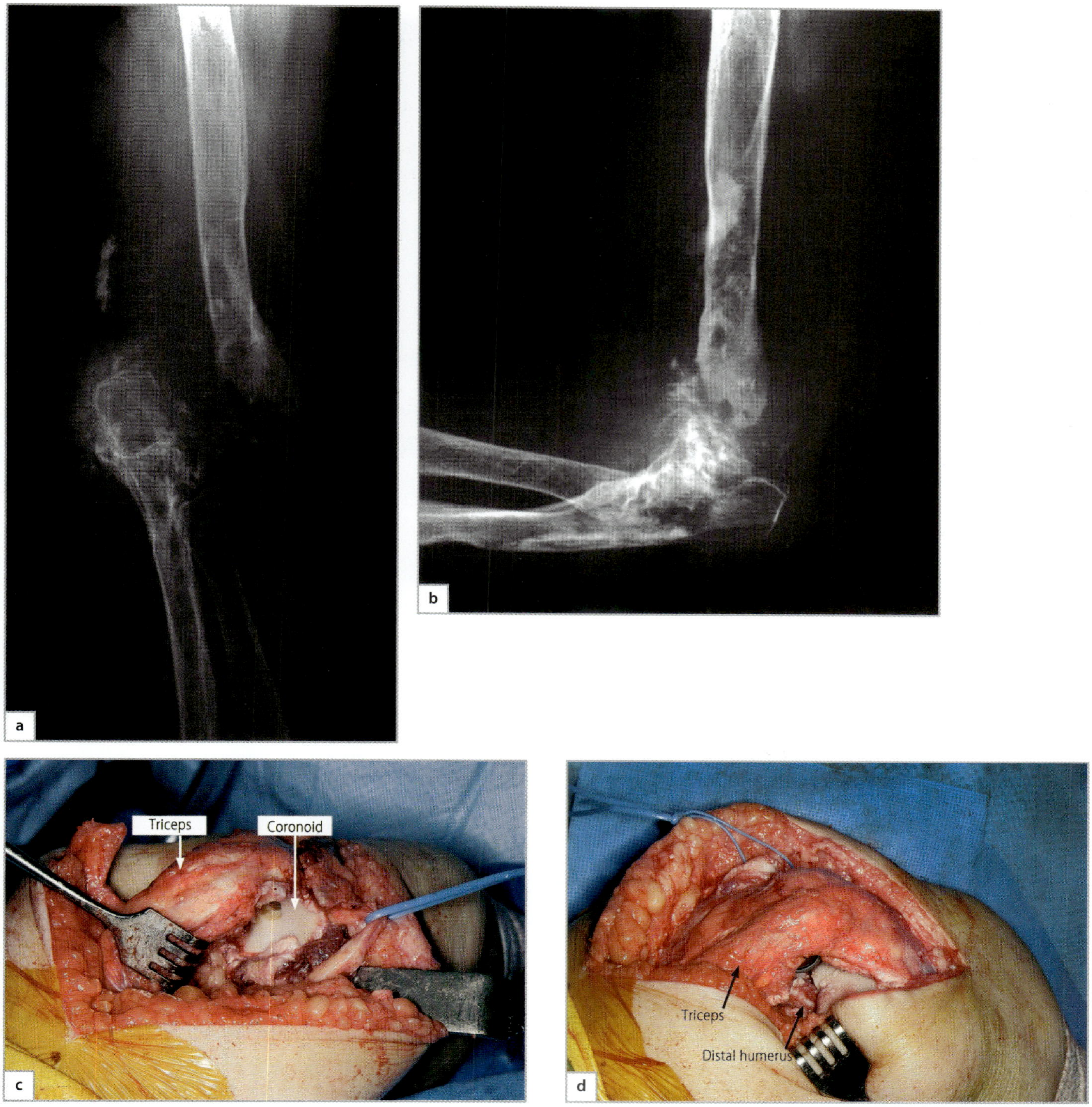

Figure 29.7 Linked elbow arthroplasty may be performed working on both sides of the triceps in patients with non-union of the distal humerus. ***(Contd)***

injector system. The implants may be fully seated prior to interlocking, as the articular windows at the medial and lateral side of the elbow after removal of the united distal humerus bone allow interlocking.

Closure

Since the dissection is often extensive, we release the tourniquet prior to closure or prior to cementation. In the latter instance it is reinflated for the cementation process. At the end of the procedure, the common extensor and common flexor muscle groups are sutured to the lateral and medial triceps fascia to seal the joint space and maintain the strength of the forearm muscles. Drains are occasionally used if the bleeding seems excessive after efforts at hemostasis.

Postoperative management

After surgery, the elbow is placed in full extension in a bulky dressing with an anterior plaster splint and kept elevated to minimize swelling. Active assisted range of motion may be initiated on

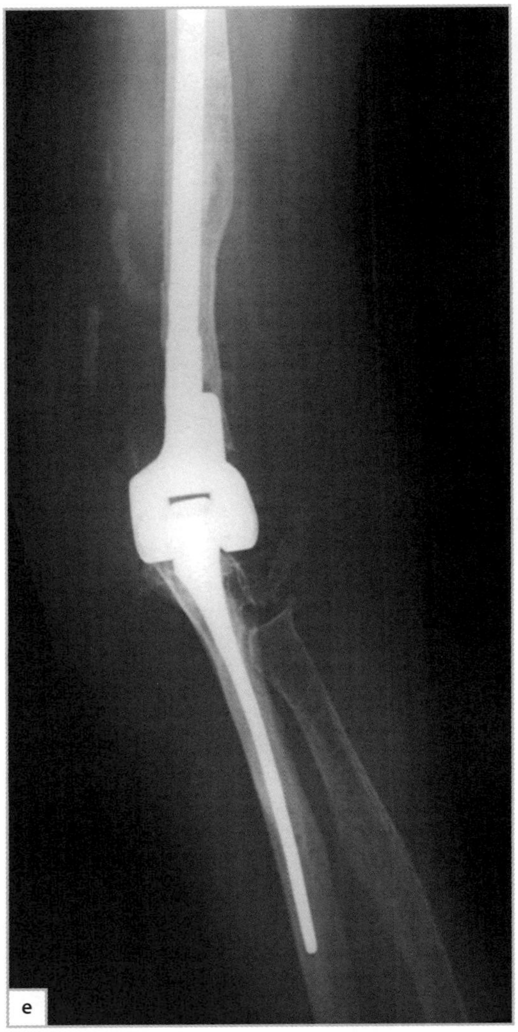

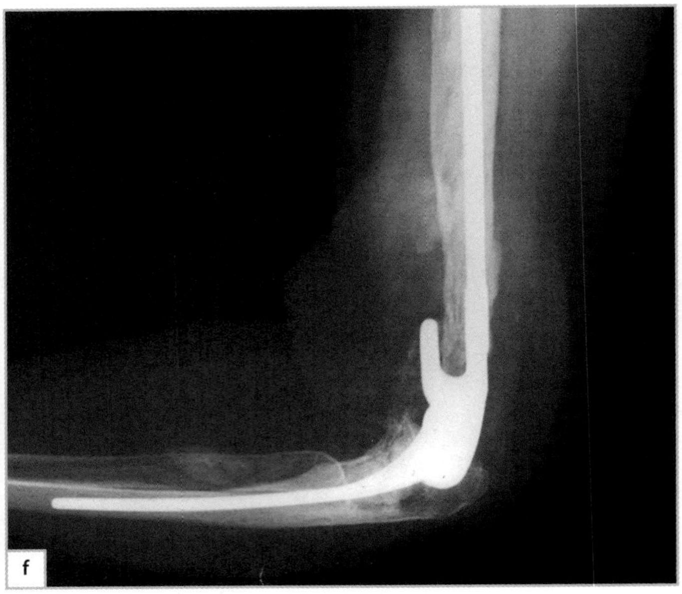

Figure 29.7 Linked elbow arthroplasty may be performed working on both sides of the triceps in patients with non-union of the distal humerus. (a) Fragment resection from the medial side. (b) Humeral rasping leaving the triceps attached. (c) Preparation of the ulna, with the triceps on. (d) Components implanted. (e,f) Postoperative radiographs showing adequate component positioning and resected medial and lateral condyles.

postoperative day 1 or 2. Once the surgical wound is healed, no additional protection is needed, as the implants are fixed with cement and the extensor mechanism is left completely undisturbed. Usually, patients regain functional elbow motion within the first three months after surgery. Improvement is seen up to one year after surgery.

Outcomes

Total elbow arthroplasty has been shown in several studies to provide satisfactory results in a large proportion of well selected patients. Morrey and Adams (1995) reported on 36 consecutive patients with an average age of 68 years who underwent total elbow arthroplasty for a distal humeral non-union. At an average follow-up of four years, results were satisfactory in 86% of the patients. There was no or mild pain in 91% and motion was improved in most patients. Complications included deep infection in two cases, polyethylene wear or particulate synovitis requiring surgery in three cases, and transient ulnar neuropathy in two cases.

The Mayo Clinic experience with total elbow arthroplasty for distal humerus non-unions has been updated recently (Cil et al. 2008). Ninety-two consecutive total elbow arthroplasties performed for the treatment of a distal humeral non-union were reviewed at an average follow-up of 6.5 years (range 0.5–20.3 years). There were 22 men and 69 women with an average age of 65 years at the time of elbow replacement. Seventy-six elbows (83%) had undergone prior surgery, with an average of two previous operations (range 1–10). Five elbows had had at least one prior operation due to infection. Before surgery, 86% of the patients complained of moderate or severe pain. At most recent follow-up, 79% of the patients had no pain or mild pain. Mean extension was improved from 37° to 22° and average flexion from 106° to 135°. Joint stability was restored in all patients, including nine with a grossly flailing elbow (**Fig. 29.8**). Complications included aseptic loosening in 16 (four with periprosthetic fractures), component fracture in five, deep infection in five (three with previous infection), and bushing wear in one. At most recent follow-up, 85% of the patients were satisfied with their outcome. Survivorship was 95.7% at two years, 82.1% at five years, and 65.3% at 10 and 15 years (**Fig. 29.9**). The risk of implant failure was increased in patients less than 65 years old, with two or more prior surgeries, and a history of previous infection.

Some concerns have been raised about the effect of humeral condyle resection on elbow and forearm strength. However, McKee et al. (2003) reported on 32 patients who had undergone total elbow arthroplasty with preservation (16 cases) or resection (16 cases) of the humeral condyles. There were no statistically significant differences

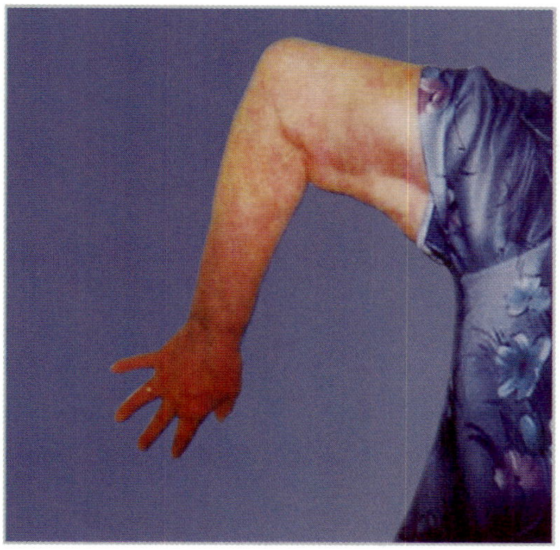

Figure 29.8 Patients with dysfunctional instability are unable to control the position of the arm.

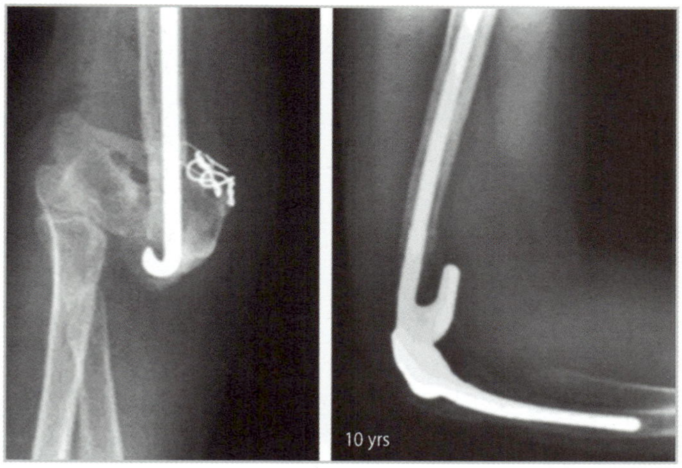

Figure 29.9 Treatment of a patient with non-union of the distal humerus and dysfunctional instability. (a) Postoperative result. (b) Linked elbow arthroplasty provided a successful clinical outcome for 16 years.

in elbow flexion and extension, forearm pronation and supination, or grip strength. Both groups also had similar overall results according to the Mayo Elbow Performance Score.

Our preference is to resect the non-united fragments in order to preserve the extensor mechanism intact and replace the elbow joint with a linked implant. Condylar resection does not seem to affect pain, strength, or function with the design used by the authors. However, when arthroplasty is indicated in this condition, the potential for complications and implant failure in the long term should be recognized.

REFERENCES

Ackerman G, Jupiter JB. Non-union of fractures of the distal end of the humerus. J Bone Joint Surg Am 1988;70:75–83.

Armstrong AD, Yamaguchi K. Total elbow arthroplasty and distal humerus elbow fractures. Hand Clin 2004;20:475–483.

Charissoux J-L, Mabit C, Fourastier J, et al. Comminuted intraarticular fractures of the distal humerus in elderly patients. [In French.] Rev Chir Orthop Reparatrice Appar Mot 2008;94 (4 Suppl):S36–62.

Cheung EV, O'Driscoll SW. Total elbow prosthesis loosening caused by ulnar component pistoning. J Bone Joint Surg Am 2007;89:1269–1274.

Cil A, Veillette C, Sanchez-Sotelo J, Morrey BF. Linked elbow replacement: a salvage procedure for distal humeral nonunion. J Bone Joint Surg Am 2008;90:1939–1950.

Cobb TK, Morrey BF. Total elbow arthroplasty as primary treatment for distal humeral fractures in elderly patients. J Bone Joint Surg Am 1997;79:826–832.

Frankle MA, Herscovici D Jr, Di Pasquale TG, et al. A comparison of open reduction and internal fixation and primary total elbow arthroplasty in the treatment of intraarticular distal humerus fractures in women older than age 65. J Orthop Trauma 2003;17:473–480.

Gambirasio R, Riand N, Stern R, Hoffmeyer P. Total elbow replacement for complex fractures of the distal humerus. An option for the elderly patient. J Bone Joint Surg Br 2001;83:974–978.

Garcia JA, Mykula R, Stanley D. Complex fractures of the distal humerus in the elderly. The role of total elbow replacement as primary treatment. J Bone Joint Surg Br 2002;84:812–816.

Helfet DL, Kloen P, Anand N, Rosen HS. Open reduction and internal fixation of delayed unions and nonunions of fractures of the distal part of the humerus. J Bone Joint Surg Am 2003;85:33–40.

Huang TL, Chiu FY, Chuang TY, Chen TH. The results of open reduction and internal fixation in elderly patients with severe fractures of the distal humerus: a critical analysis of the results. J Trauma 2005;58:62–69.

Jost B, Adams RA, Morrey BF. Management of acute distal humeral fractures in patients with rheumatoid arthritis. A case series. J Bone Joint Surg Am 2008;90:2197–2205.

Kalogrianitis S, Sinopidis C, El Meligy M, et al. Unlinked elbow arthroplasty as primary treatment for fractures of the distal humerus. J Shoulder Elbow Surg 2008;17:287–292.

Kamineni S, Morrey BF. Distal humerus fractures treated with noncustom total elbow replacement. J Bone Joint Surg Am 2004; 86:940–947.

Kamineni S, Morrey BF. Distal humeral fractures treated with noncustom total elbow replacement. Surgical technique. J Bone Joint Surg Am 2005;87:41–50.

Lee KT, Lai CH, Singh S. Results of total elbow arthroplasty in the treatment of distal humerus fractures in elderly Asian patients. J Trauma 2006;61:889–892.

McKee MD, Pugh DM, Richards RR, et al. Effect of humeral condylar resection on strength and functional outcome after semiconstrained total elbow arthroplasty. J Bone Joint Surg Am 2003;85:802–807.

McKee MD, Veillette CJH, Hall JA, et al. A multicenter, prospective, randomized, controlled trial of open reduction – internal fixation versus total elbow arthroplasty for displaced intra-articular distal humeral fractures in elderly patients. J Shoulder Elbow Surg 2009;18:3–12.

Mighell MA, Dunham RC, Rommel EA, Frankle MA. Primary semi-constrained arthroplasty for chronic fracture-dislocations of the elbow. J Bone Joint Surg Br 2005;87:191–195.

Mitsunaga MM, Bryan RS, Linscheid RL. Condylar nonunions of the elbow. J Trauma 1982;22:787–791.

Morrey BF, Adams RA. Semiconstrained elbow replacement for distal humeral nonunion. J Bone Joint Surg Br 1995;77: 67–72.

Prasad N, Dent C. Outcome of total elbow replacement for distal humeral fractures in the elderly: a comparison of primary surgery and surgery after failed internal fixation or conservative treatment. J Bone Joint Surg Br 2008;90:343–348.

Ramsey ML, Adams RA, Morrey BF. Instability of the elbow treated with semiconstrained total elbow arthroplasty. J Bone Joint Surg Am 1999;81:38–47.

Ring D, Gulotta L, Jupiter JB. Unstable nonunions of the distal part of the humerus. J Bone Joint Surg Am 2003;85:1040–1046.

Srinivasan K, Agarwal M, Matthews SJ, Giannoudis PV. Fractures of the distal humerus in the elderly: is internal fixation the treatment of choice? Clin Orthop 2005;434:222–230.

Index

Note: Page numbers with suffix *f* and *t* refer to figures and tables respectively.